2003

Race, Ethnicity, and Health

Race, Ethnicity, and Health

A Public Health Reader

Thomas A. LaVeist, Editor

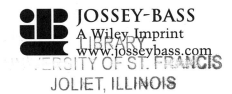

JOSSEY-BASS
A Wiley Imprint
www.josseybass.com

Published by Jossey-Bass
A Wiley Imprint
989 Market Street, San Francisco, CA 94103-1741 www.josseybass.com

Jossey-Bass books and products are available through most bookstores. To contact Jossey-Bass directly call our Customer Care Department within the U.S. at 800-956-7739, outside the U.S. at 317-572-3986, or by fax at 317-572-4002.

Jossey-Bass also publishes its books in a variety of electronic formats. Some content that appears in print may not be available in electronic books.

Library of Congress Cataloging-in-Publication Data
Race, ethnicity, and health : a public health reader / Thomas A. LaVeist, editor. — 1st ed.
    p. ; cm.
   Includes bibliographical references and index.
   ISBN 0-7879-6451-4 (alk. paper)
   1. Minorities—Health and hygiene—United States. 2. Discrimination in medical care—United States. 3. Health services accessibility—United States.
   [DNLM: 1. Health Services Accessibility—United States. 2. Blacks—United States. 3. Ethnic Groups—United States. 4. Health Status—United States. 5. Hispanic Americans—United States. 6. Socioeconomic Factors—United States. WA 300 R1183 2002] I. LaVeist, Thomas Alexis.

RA563 .M56 R325 2002
  362.1'089'00973—dc21
                                     2002013059

Printed in the United States of America
FIRST EDITION
PB Printing   10 9 8 7 6 5 4 3 2 1

CONTENTS

SOURCES

Chapter 2: Nancy Krieger, "Shades of Difference: Theoretical Underpinnings of the Medical Controversy on Black/White Differences in the United States, 1830–1870," *International Journal of Health Services,* 17(2):259–78, 1987.

Chapter 3: Vanessa Northington Gamble, "Under the Shadow of Tuskegee: African Americans and Health Care," *American Journal of Public Health,* 87(11):1773, 1997.

Chapter 4: William A. Vega and Hortensia Amaro, "Latino Outlook: Good Health, Uncertain Prognosis," *Annual Review of Public Health,* 15:39–67, 1994 Annual Reviews.

Chapter 5: Thomas A. LaVeist, "Segregation, Poverty, and Empowerment: Health Consequences for African Americans," *Milbank Quarterly,* 71(1):41–64, 1993.

Chapter 6: Richard Cooper, "A Note on the Biologic Concept of Race and Its Application in Epidemiologic Research," *American Heart Journal,* 108(3 Part 2):715–22, 1984.

Chapter 7: Thomas A. LaVeist, "Beyond Dummy Variables and Sample Selection: What Health Services Researchers Ought to Know About Race as a Variable," *Health Services Research,* 29(1):1–16, 1994.

Chapter 8: Carles Muntaner, F. Javier Nieto, and Patricia O'Campo, "The Bell Curve: On Race, Social Class, and Epidemiologic Research," *American Journal of Epidemiology,* 144(6):531–535, 1996.

Chapter 9: David E. Hayes-Bautista and Jorge Chapa, "Latino Terminology: Conceptual Bases for Standardized Terminology," *American Journal of Public Health,* 77(1):61–68, 1987.

Chapter 10: Robert M. Mayberry, Fatima Mili, and Elibabeth Ofili, "Racial and Ethnic Differences in Access to Medical Care." *Medical Care Research and Review,* 57(Supplement):108–45, 2000.

Chapter 11: Kevin Fiscella, Peter Franks, Mark P. Doescher, and Barry G. Saver, "Disparities in Health Care by Race, Ethnicity and Language Among the Insured: Findings from a National Sample," *Medical Care,* 40(1):52–59, 2002.

Chapter 12: Arline T. Geronimus, "Black/White Differences in the Relationship of Maternal Age to Birthweight: A Population-Based Test of the Weathering Hypothesis," *Social Science and Medicine,* Feb; 42(4):589–97, 1996.

Chapter 13: W. Parker Frisbie, Youngtae Cho, and Robert A. Hummer, "Immigration and the Health of Asian and Pacific Islander Adults in the United States," *American Journal of Epidemiology,* 153(4):372–80, 2001.

Chapter 14: Richard J. David and James W. Collins, "Differing Birth Weight Among Infants of U.S.-Born Blacks, African-Born Blacks, and U.S.-Born Whites," *New England Journal of Medicine,* 337(17):1209–1214, 1997.

Chapter 15: Gopal K. Singh and Stella M. Yu, "Adverse Pregnancy Outcomes: Differences Between US- and Foreign-born Women in Major US Racial and Ethnic Groups," *American Journal of Public Health,* 86(6):837–43, 1996.

Chapter 16: Luisa Franzini, John C. Ribble, and Arlene M. Keddie, "Understanding the Hispanic Paradox," *Ethnicity and Disease,* Autumn; 11(3):496–518, 2001.

Chapter 17: Camara Phyllis Jones, "Levels of Racism: A Theoretic Framework and a Gardener's Tale," *American Journal of Public Health,* 90(8):1212–5, 2000.

Chapter 18: Rodney Clark, Norman B. Anderson, Vernessa R. Clark, and David R. Williams, "Racism as a Stressor for African Americans. A Biopsychosocial Model," *American Psychologist,* 54(10):805–16, 1999.

Chapter 19: Elizabeth A. Klonoff and Hope Landrine, "Is Skin Color a Marker for Racial Discrimination? Explaining the Skin Color-Hypertension Relationship," *Journal of Behavioral Medicine,* 23(4):329–38, 2000.

Chapter 20: Sherman A. James, "John Henryism and the Health of African Americans," *Culture Medicine and Psychiatry,* 18(2):163–182, 1994.

Chapter 21: David R. Williams and Chiquita Collins, "Racial Residential Segregation: A Fundamental Cause of Racial Disparities in Health," *Public Health Reports,* Sept.–Oct., Vol. 16, 2001.

Chapter 22: David R. Williams and Chiquita Collins, "US Socioeconomic and Racial Differences in Health: Patterns and Explanations," *Annual Review of Sociology,* 21:349–386, 1995 Annual Reviews.

Chapter 23: Michelle Pearl, Paula Braverman, and Barbara Abrams, "The Relationship of Neighborhood Socioeconomic Characteristics to Birthweight Among 5 Ethnic Groups in California," *American Journal of Public Health,* 91(11):1808–1814, 2001.

Chapter 24: Kimberley Morland, Steve Wing, Ana Diez Roux, and Charles Poole, "Neighborhood Characteristics Associated with the Location of Food Stores and Food Service Places," *American Journal of Preventive Medicine,* 22(1):23–9, 2001.

Chapter 25: R. Sean Morrison, Sylvan Wallenstein, Dana K. Natale, Richard S. Senzel, and Lo-Li Huang, "'We Don't Carry That'—Failure of Pharmacies in Predominantly Non-white Neighborhoods to Stock Opioid Analgesics," *New England Journal of Medicine,* 342:1023–1026, 2000.

Chapter 26: Robert D. Bullard, "Solid Waste Sites and the Black Houston Community," *Sociological Inquiry,* 53(2/3):273–288, 1983.

Chapter 27: Thomas A. LaVeist, John M. Wallace Jr, "Health Risk and Inequitable Distribution of Liquor Stores in African American Neighborhoods," *Social Science and Medicine,* Aug; 51(4):613–7, 2000.

Chapter 28: Marsha Lillie-Blanton, James C. Anthony, and Charles R. Schuster, "Probing the Meaning of Racial/Ethnic Group Comparisons in Crack Cocaine Smoking," *Journal of the American Medical Association,* Feb 24; 269(8):993–7, 1993.

Chapter 29: Knox H. Todd, Christi Deaton, Anne P. D'Adamo, and Leon Goe, "Ethnicity and Analgesic Practice," *Annals of Emergency Medicine,* Jan; 35(1):11–6, 2000.

Chapter 30: Kevin A. Schulman, Jesse A. Berlin, William Harless, Jon F. Kerner, Shyrl Sistrunk, Bernard J. Gersh, Ross Dube, Christopher K. Taleghani, Jennifer E. Burke, Sankey Williams, John M. Eisenberg, and Jose J. Escarce, "The Effect of Race and Sex on Physicians' Recommendations for Cardiac Catheterization," *New England Journal of Medicine,* Feb 25; 340(8):618–26, 1999.

Chapter 31: Betsy Sleath, Bonnie Svarstad, and Debra Roter, "Patient Race and Psychotropic Prescribing During Medical Encounters," *Social Science and Medicine,* 34:227–238, 1998.

Chapter 32: Michelle van Ryn and Jane Burke, "The Effect of Patient Race and Socio-economic Status on Physicians' Perception of Patients," *Social Science and Medicine,* 50:813–828, 2000.

Chapter 33: Jeff Whittle, Joseph Conigliaro, C. B. Good, and Monica Joswiak, "Do Patient Preferences Contribute to Racial Differences in Cardiovascular Procedure Use?" *Journal of Internal Medicine,* May; 12(5):267–73, 1997.

Chapter 34: Chamberlain Diala, Carles Muntaner, Christine Walrath, Kim Nickerson, Thomas LaVeist, and Philip Leaf, "Racial Differences in Attitudes Toward Professional Mental Health Care and in the Use of Services," *American Journal of Orthopsychiatry,* Vol. 70, no. 4 (October), pp. 455–464, 2000.

Chapter 35: Lisa Cooper-Patrick, Joseph J. Gallo, Junius J. Gonzales, Hong Thi Vu, Neil R. Powe, Christine Nelson, and Daniel E. Ford, "Race, Gender, and Partnership in the Patient–Physician Relationship," *Journal of the American Medical Association,* Aug 11; 282(6):583–9, 1999.

Chapter 36: Somnath Saha, Miriam Komaromy, Thomas D. Koepsell, and Andrew B. Bindman, "Patient-Physician Racial Concordance and the Perceived Quality and Use of Health Care," *Archives of Internal Medicine,* 159(9):997–1004, 1999.

Chapter 37: Jersey Chen, Saif S. Rathore, Martha J. Radford, Yun Wang, and Harlan M. Krumholz, "Racial Differences in the Use of Cardiac Catheterization After Acute Myocardial Infarction," *New England Journal of Medicine,* 344(19), 1443–1449, 2001.

THE AUTHORS

Barbara Abrams, D.P.H., School of Public Health, University of California, Berkeley

Anne P. D. Adamo, M.D., Department of Emergency Medicine, Emory University, Atlanta

Hortensia Amaro, Ph.D., School of Health Professions, Bouve College of Health Sciences, Northeastern University, Boston

Norman B. Anderson, Ph.D., Chief Executive Officer, American Psychological Association, Washington, D.C.

James C. Anthony, Ph.D., Department of Mental Hygiene, Bloomberg School of Public Health, Johns Hopkins University, Baltimore

David E. Hayes Bautista, Ph.D., Center for the Study of Latino Health and Culture and the School of Medicine, University of California, Los Angeles

Jesse A. Berlin, Sc.D., Center for Clinical Epidemiology and Biostatistics and Department of Biostatistics and Epidemiology, University of Pennsylvania School of Medicine, Philadelphia

Andrew B. Bindman, M.D., Primary Care Research Center, Division of General Internal Medicine, San Francisco General Hospital; Department of Medicine, University of California, San Francisco

Paula Braveman, M.D., M.P.H., School of Medicine, University of California, San Francisco

Jane Burke, Department of Health Policy, Management, and Behavior, University at Albany School of Public Health, Rensselaer

Jennifer E. Burke, M.A., M.S., RAND Health Program, Santa Monica

Jorge Chapa, Ph.D., Latino Studies Program, Indiana University, Bloomington

Jersey Chen, M.D., M.P.H., Section of Cardiovascular Medicine, Department of Medicine, Yale University School of Medicine, New Haven

Youngtae Cho, Ph.D., Population Research Center, Department of Sociology, University of Texas, Austin

Rodney Clark, Department of Psychology, Wayne State University, Detriot

Vernessa R. Clark, Ph.D., Department of Psychology, Morehouse College, Atlanta

Chiquita Collins, Ph.D., Department of Sociology, University of Texas, Austin

James W. Collins Jr., M.D., M.P.H., The Feinberg School of Medicine, Northwestern University, Chicago

Joseph Conigliaro, M.D., M.P.H., School of Medicine, University of Pittsburgh, Pittsburgh

Richard Cooper, M.D., Division of Cardiology, Department of Medicine, Cook County Hospital, Chicago

Lisa Cooper-Patrick, M.D., M.P.H., Department of Medicine and Department of Health Policy and Management, Johns Hopkins University School of Medicine, Baltimore

Richard J. David, M.D., Division of Neonatology, Cook County Children's Hospital, Chicago, and the Department of Pediatrics, School of Medicine, University of Illinois, Chicago

Christi Deaton, R.N., Ph.D., Nell Hodgson Woodruff School of Nursing, Emory University, Atlanta

Chamberlain Diala, Ph.D., M.P.H., Department of Health Policy and Management, Johns Hopkins University, Baltimore

Ana Diez Roux, M.D., Ph.D., Division of General Medicine and Department of Epidemiology, Columbia University, New York

Mark P. Doescher, M.D., M.S.P.H., Department of Family Medicine, University of Washington School of Medicine, Seattle

Ross Dubé, Interactive Drama Inc., Bethesda

John M. Eisenberg, M.D., Agency for Healthcare Research and Quality, Department of Health and Human Services, Washington, D.C.

José J. Escarce, M.D., Ph.D., RAND Health Program, Santa Monica

Kevin Fiscella, M.D., M.P.H., Department of Family Medicine, Department of Community and Preventive Medicine, University of Rochester School of Medicine, Rochester

Daniel E. Ford, M.D., M.P.H., Department of Medicine and Department of Health Policy and Management, Johns Hopkins University School of Medicine, Baltimore

Peter Franks, M.D., Department of Family and Community Medicine, University of California, Davis

Luisa Franzini, Ph.D., Center for Society and Population Health, University of Texas Health Science Center, School of Public Health, Houston

W. Parker Frisbie, Population Research Center, Department of Sociology, University of Texas, Austin

Joseph J. Gallo, M.D., M.P.H., School of Medicine, University of Pennsylvania, Philadelphia

Vanessa Northington Gamble, M.D., Ph.D., independent researcher

Bernard J. Gersh, M.B., Ch.B., D.Phil., Mayo Medical School, Rochester, Minnesota

Leon Goe, M.H.S., Department of Emergency Medicine, Emory University, Atlanta

C. B. Good, M.D., M.P.H., Section of General Internal Medicine, Pittsburgh Veterans Affairs Medical Center, and Division of General Internal Medicine, University of Pittsburgh Medical Center, Pittsburgh

Junius J. Gonzales, M.D., Services Research and Clinical Epidemiology, Branch Division of Services and Intervention Research, National Institute of Mental Health, Bethesda

William Harless, Ph.D., Interactive Drama Inc., Bethesda

Lo-Li Huang, B.A., Hertzberg Palliative Care Institute, Department of Geriatrics and Adult Development, Mount Sinai School of Medicine, New York

Robert A. Hummer, Population Research Center, Department of Sociology, University of Texas, Austin

Camara Phyllis Jones, M.D., M.P.H., Ph.D., Centers for Disease Control and Prevention, Atlanta

Monica Joswiak, M.P.H., Section of General Internal Medicine, Pittsburgh Veterans Affairs Medical Center, Pittsburgh

Arlene M. Keddie, M.S.P.H., Center for Society and Population Health, University of Texas Health Science Center, School of Public Health, Houston

Jon F. Kerner, Ph.D., National Cancer Institute, National Institutes of Health, Bethesda

Elizabeth A. Klonoff, Department of Psychology, San Diego State University, San Diego

Thomas D. Koepsell, M.D., M.P.H., Department of Epidemiology, University of Washington, Seattle

Miriam Komaromy, M.D., Adult Genetics Clinic, University of California, San Francisco

Nancy Krieger, Department of Health and Social Behavior, Harvard School of Public Health, Boston

Harlan M. Krumholz, M.D., Section of Cardiovascular Medicine, Department of Medicine, and the Section of Chronic Disease Epidemiology, Department of Epidemiology and Public Health, Yale University School of Medicine, and the Yale-New Haven Hospital Center for Outcomes Research and Evaluation, New Haven

Hope Landrine, Rebecca and John Moores UCSD Cancer Center, University of California, San Diego

Philip J. Leaf, Ph.D., Department of Mental Hygiene, Bloomberg School of Public Health, Johns Hopkins University, Baltimore

Marsha Lillie-Blanton, Dr.P.H., Henry J. Kaiser Family Foundation, Washington, D.C.

Robert M. Mayberry, M.S., M.P.H., Ph.D., Morehouse School of Medicine, Atlanta

Fatima Mili, M.D., Ph.D., Centers for Disease Control and Prevention, Atlanta

Kimberly Morland, Ph.D., Department of Epidemiology, School of Public Health, University of North Carolina, Chapel Hill

R. Sean Morrison, M.D., Hertzberg Palliative Care Institute, Department of Geriatrics and Adult Development, Mount Sinai School of Medicine, New York

Carles Muntaner, M.D., Ph.D., Department of Behavioral and Community Health, University of Maryland School of Nursing, Baltimore

Dana K. Natale, M.A., Hertzberg Palliative Care Institute, Department of Geriatrics and Adult Development, Mount Sinai School of Medicine, New York

Christine Nelson, R.N., NYLCare Health Plans of the Mid-Atlantic, Greenbelt

Kim J. Nickerson, Ph.D., Minority Fellowship Program, American Psychological Association, Washington, D.C.

F. Javier Nieto, Department of Health Services, University of Wisconsin Medical School, Madison

Patricia O'Campo, Ph.D., Department of Population and Family Health Sciences, Bloomberg School of Public Health, Johns Hopkins University, Baltimore

Elizabeth Ofili, M.D., M.P.H., F.A.C.C., Morehouse School of Medicine, Atlanta

Michelle Pearl, Ph.D., Sequoia Foundation, California Department of Health Services, San Francisco

Charles Poole, Sc.D., Department of Epidemiology, University of North Carolina, Chapel Hill

Neil R. Powe, M.D., M.P.H., M.B.A., Department of Medicine and Department of Health Policy and Management, Johns Hopkins University School of Medicine, Baltimore

Martha J. Radford, M.D., Section of Cardiovascular Medicine, Department of Medicine, Yale University School of Medicine, and the Yale-New Haven Hospital Center for Outcomes Research and Evaluation, New Haven

Saif S. Rathore, M.P.H., Section of Cardiovascular Medicine, Department of Medicine, Yale University School of Medicine, New Haven

John C. Ribble, M.D., Center for Society and Population Health, University of Texas Health Science Center, School of Public Health, Houston

Debra Roter, Dr.P.H., Bloomberg School of Public Health, Johns Hopkins University, Baltimore

Somnath Saha, M.D., M.P.H., Health Services Research and Development, Department of Veterans Affairs, Puget Sound Health Care System, Seattle

Barry G. Saver, M.D., M.P.H., Department of Family Medicine, University of Washington School of Medicine, Seattle

Kevin A. Schulman, M.D., Fuqua School of Business, Duke University School of Medicine, Durham

Charles R. Schuster, Ph.D., Substance Abuse Research Division and the Addiction Research Institute, Wayne State University, Detroit

Richard S. Senzel, M.R.P., Hertzberg Palliative Care Institute, Department of Geriatrics and Adult Development, Mount Sinai School of Medicine, New York

Gopal K. Singh, Ph.D., National Cancer Institute, National Institutes of Health, Bethesda

Shyrl Sistrunk, M.D., Division of General Internal Medicine, Georgetown University Medical Center, Washington, D.C.

Betsy Sleath, Ph.D., School of Pharmacy and Cecil G. Sheps Center for Health Services Research, University of North Carolina, Chapel Hill

Bonnie Svarstad, Ph.D., School of Pharmacy and Department of Sociology, University of Wisconsin, Madison

Christopher K. Taleghani, M.D., Clinical Economics Research Unit, Georgetown University Medical Center, Washington, D.C.

Knox H. Todd, M.D., M.P.H., Department of Emergency Medicine, Emory University, Atlanta

Michelle van Ryn, Ph.D., M.P.H., Center for Chronic Disease Outcomes Research, Minneapolis Veterans Medical Center, and the Department of Epidemiology, University of Minnesota School of Public Health, Minneapolis

William A. Vega, Ph.D., professor of psychiatry, Robert Wood Johnson Medical School, New Jersey

Hong Thi Vu, M.H.S., Department of Medicine, Johns Hopkins University School of Medicine, Baltimore

John M. Wallace Jr., Ph.D., Institute for Social Research and School of Social Work, University of Michigan, Ann Arbor

Sylvan Wallenstein, Ph.D., Department of Biomathematical Sciences, Mount Sinai School of Medicine, New York

Christine Walrath, Ph.D., Department of Mental Hygiene, Bloomberg School of Public Health, Johns Hopkins University, Baltimore

Yun Wang, M.S., Yale University School of Medicine, and the Yale-New Haven Hospital Center for Outcomes Research and Evaluation, New Haven

Jeff Whittle, M.D., M.P.H., Section of General Internal Medicine, Pittsburgh Veterans Affairs Medical Center, and Division of General Internal Medicine, University of Pittsburgh Medical Center, Pittsburgh

David R. Williams, Ph.D., M.P.H., Department of Sociology and Survey Research Center, Institute for Social Research, University of Michigan, Ann Arbor

Sankey Williams, M.D., Division of General Internal Medicine, University of Pennsylvania School of Medicine, Philadelphia

Steve Wing, Ph.D., Department of Epidemiology, University of North Carolina, Chapel Hill

Stella M. Yu, Sc.D., M.P.H., Bureau of Maternal and Child Health, Health Resources and Services Administration, Rockville

THE EDITOR

Thomas A. LaVeist is director of the Center for Health Disparities Studies and associate professor at the Johns Hopkins University, Bloomberg School of Public Health, where he teaches courses in minority health and public health policy. He is a frequent visiting lecturer on minority health issues at other universities and at professional conferences and workshops. He often consults to federal agencies on minority health issues and racial disparities in health. He has conducted several important studies of minority health. His research on minority health has been funded by the National Institutes of Health, the Centers for Disease Control, the Commonwealth Fund, the Russell Sage Foundation, and the Kaiser Family Foundation.

LaVeist received his B.A. degree from the University of Maryland, Eastern Shore, and his Ph.D. degree in medical sociology from the University of Michigan. His dissertation was awarded the Roberta G. Simmons Outstanding Dissertation Award, for the best doctoral dissertation in medical sociology, by the American Sociological Association in 1989. He held a postdoctoral fellowship in public health at the University of Michigan School of Public Health. He joined the Johns Hopkins faculty in 1990 and was appointed a fellow of the Brookdale Foundation in 1992. He has published numerous articles in scientific journals. He is also the author of *The DayStar Guide to Colleges for African American Students* (2000) and coauthor of the forthcoming *Getting Paid, Financial Aid: 7 Easy Steps to Help Black Families Cover the College Bill.*

ACKNOWLEDGMENTS

I will be eternally grateful to the members of the Editorial Board and the Advisory Committee who patiently waded through numerous drafts and revisions of this book. They provided me with encouragement and criticism, both of which were precisely what I needed at various points in the process. While these advisors were kind enough to provide me with valuable feedback during the selection process, the final article selections were my own. Any omissions, therefore, should be attributed to my misjudgment, not theirs.

EDITORIAL BOARD

Harold W. Neighbors, Ph.D., School of Public Health, University of Michigan

H. Jack Geiger, M.D., M.P.H., City University of New York Medical School

Eleanor A. Walker, Ph.D., R.N.C., Department of Nursing, Bowie State University

Carol Itatani, Ph.D., Department of Biological Sciences, California State University, Long Beach

Kirk A. Johnson, Ph.D., Bowdoin College

Marjorie Kagawa-Singer, R.N., Ph.D., School of Public Health, University of California, Los Angeles

Joseph Telfair, Dr.P.H., M.S.W., M.P.H., School of Public Health, Univeristy of Alabama, Birmingham

Jeffrey J. Guidry, Ph.D., Texas A&M University

Ronald L. Braithwaite, Ph.D., Rollins School of Public Health, Emory University

Robert M. Mayberry, M.S., M.P.H., Ph.D., Morehouse School of Medicine

Cliff Broman, Michigan State University

Carles Muntaner, Ph.D., School of Nursing, University of Maryland

Hortensia Amaro, Ph.D., Bouve College of Health Sciences, Northeastern University

David T. Takeuchi, University of Washington

Joyce Rasin, Ph.D., R.N., School of Nursing, University of North Carolina

Camera Jones, M.D., Ph.D., Centers for Disease Control and Prevention

David R. Williams, Ph.D., M.P.H., Institute for Social Research, University of Michigan

Keith Witfield, Ph.D., Pennsylvania State University

ADVISORY COMMITTEE

Cathy J. Tashiro, Ph.D., R.N., Jay S. Kaufman, Ph.D., Chiquita A. Collins, Ph.D., Barbara Joyce-Nagata, Ph.D., R.N., Marian McDonald, Don Barr, Carl M. Toney, P. A., Hilda R. Heady, Daniel E. Korin, M.D., F.A.A.P., Fernando Elijovich, M.D., Randy Reiter, Ph.D., M.P.H., Arlene S. Bierman, M.D., M.S., Elmer R. Freeman, M.S.W., Bella Mody, Shelia Bunch, Ph.D., Oivia Carter-Pokras, Ph.D., Chandra

Ford, M.P.H., M.L.I.S., Doris A. Fields, Elmer R. Freeman, Douglas Taylor, David Allen, Judy Kaplan, Richard David, M.D., Gavin Kearney, Dabney Evans, M.P.H., C.H.E.S., Lillian Stokes, Ph.D., R.N., William D. Corser, Ph.D., R.N., Dee Judd, Stephanie Ann Farquhar, Ph.D., Clarissa Agee Shavers, Ava E. Lewis, Ph.D., R.N., Alice Furumoto-Dawson, Chaya Gordon, M.P.H., Carla King, Ph.D., R.N., Clarence Spigner, M.P.H., Dr.P.H., Denice Curtis, D.D.S., M.P.H., Gilbert C. Gee, Doris Lassiter, George T. Rowan, Ph.D., Jessica M. Robbins, Jon M. Hussey, Ph.D., M.P.H., Kausar S. Khan, Patricia A. Keener, M.D., Lucie Ferguson, R.N., M.P.H., Ph.D., Lukowa Kidima, Ph.D., M.P.H., Memoona Hasnain, M.D., M.H.P.E., Ph.D., Neena Murgai, Ph.D., M.P.H., Elsie R. Pamuk, Stan Wanat, Ph.D., Beth Stanger, Vickie D. Ybarra, R.N., M.P.H., Barbara Gottlieb, M.D., M.P.H., Isabel C. Scarinci, Ph.D., M.P.H., Joan M. Prince, Ph.D., June Morrison-Jones, Kimberly R. Barber, Linda Holmes, Luisa N. Borrell, D.D.S., Ph.D., Mary Canales, R.N., Ph.D., Michael Root, Creshelle R. Nash, M.D., M.P.H., Preety Gadhoke, Gopal Sanrakan, M.D., Dr.P.H., Stephanie Y. Crawford, Ph.D.

TABLES AND FIGURES

Tables

Figures

Race, Ethnicity, and Health

CHAPTER ONE

Introduction

Why We Should Study Race, Ethnicity, and Health

Thomas A. LaVeist

During the twentieth century there was a literal and figurative change in the "face of America." At the beginning of the century racial issues were essentially concerns with relations between black and white Americans. However, by the end of the century the relative sizes of American racial and ethnic groups had changed, and Latinos and Asian Americans made up a sizable proportion of the U.S. population. According to projections from the U.S. Census Bureau (summarized in Figure 1.1), this pattern is part of a long-term trend. During the twenty-first century U.S. racial and ethnic minorities are expected to constitute a steadily larger minority and eventually a majority of the U.S. population.

Another important trend that has unfolded during the twentieth century is the steadily improving health profile of Americans. As Figure 1.2 shows, early in the century the average white American lived fewer than fifty years. Life expectancy for African Americans was around thirty-five years. By the end of the century, life expectancy for all Americans exceeded sixty-five years, yet the disparities among racial and ethnic groups remained generally constant. As racial and ethnic minorities come to make up a larger percentage of the total population, the overall health statistics in the United States will increasingly reflect the health status of those minorities. Consequently, it is becoming increasingly important to monitor the health status of racial and ethnic minorities, and finding ways to improve minority health has taken on heightened urgency.

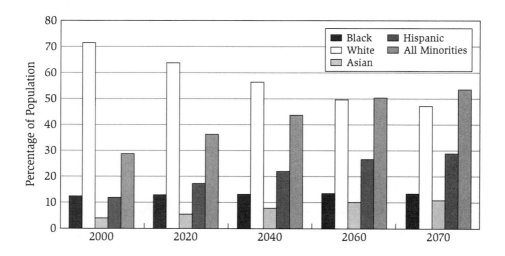

Figure 1.1 Projected Racial Diversity in the United States in the Twenty-First Century.

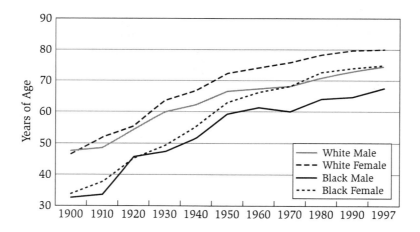

Figure 1.2 U.S. Life Expectancy by Race, 1900–1997.

There are substantial differences among the health profiles of U.S. racial and ethnic groups.[1] Researchers have demonstrated this fact for centuries.[2-4] Figure 1.3 shows mortality rates for U.S. racial and ethnic groups for the year 2000. African Americans have the worst health profile, and Asian Americans have the fewest health problems. Such disparities in health status are well documented

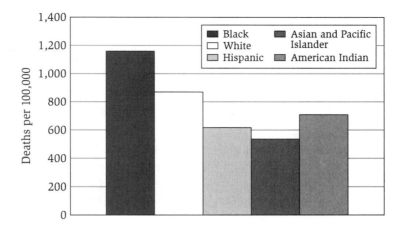

Figure 1.3 U.S. Age-Adjusted Death Rates by Race and Hispanic Origin, 1996–1998.

Source: Eberhardt, M. S., Ingram, D. D., Makuc, D. M., et al. (2001). Urban and rural health chartbook. In *Health, United States, 2001.* Hyattsville, MD: National Center for Health Statistics, p. 164, table 29.

and widely known. However, research on race, ethnicity, and health is controversial, probably owing in part to the thorny role that race has played in U.S. history and contemporary culture.[5] Because of this history, race engenders emotion, and emotion is often the antidote to rational thought. Some have called for an end to research on race and health.[6–9] Medical journal editors now discourage the use of the term *race* in submitted manuscripts. In fact, physical anthropologists no longer recognize race as a valid concept.[10,11] Other disciplines have also begun to debate the viability of the concept of race.[12,13]

The argument against continuing to conduct research on race and health goes like this:

Proposition 1. Race is not a valid biological concept, therefore

Proposition 2. Race is not a valid scientific concept, therefore

Proposition 3. Continuing to document racial differences in health bolsters pseudoscientific and even racist arguments about the existence of biological differences between what we call races and thus about the genetic inferiority of certain groups.

Although it is easy to be sympathetic to propositions one and three, it is at the second proposition that the reasoning goes astray. The problem is in using biology as the arbiter of what is scientific. As knowledge of human genomic makeup has unfolded, it has become increasingly clear that the widely held belief that there are biological differences between racial groups is incorrect. However, even though race may be a biological fiction, it is nevertheless—as the articles in this reader demonstrate—a profoundly important determinant of health status and health care quality.

THE PURPOSE OF THIS BOOK

So what is race, and why do racial disparities exist? These are the central questions this book is designed to address by bringing together a set of articles and chapters previously published in scientific journals and books. Together, these materials provide an overview of our current state of knowledge as we attempt to answer these questions.

The chapters in this book address race, ethnicity, and health only in the United States. I set this limitation because different cultures and countries respond differently to race and ethnicity. This being the case, I felt it best to address the broader international context in a separate volume. Moreover, this compilation is not intended to be merely a listing of the "best" articles in minority health. My goal has been to compile a set of articles with range and depth that will provide an overview and a strong foundation for those interested in learning about health disparities that reflect race and ethnicity.

An advisory committee and an editorial board, made up of experts in minority health, were kind enough to provide me with valuable feedback during the selection process. However, the final selections were my own, and any omissions should be attributed to my judgment (or misjudgment) alone.

ORGANIZATION OF THIS BOOK

Race, Ethnicity, and Health is divided into seven parts. The chapters in Part One provide a historical and political context for the study of research on race, ethnicity, and health. Nancy Krieger addresses the history of the ways in which race has been used as a political tool in health and public policy. Vanessa Gamble's classic article on the Tuskegee Syphilis Study details the long-term consequences of mistrust resulting from that experience. William Vega and Hortensia Amaro offer a profile of the health of the Latino population, noting once-ignored differences from other minority populations. Thomas LaVeist addresses political aspects of minority status and health, demonstrating the interrelationships among political power, racial segregation, poverty, and health.

In Part Two we move to discussions of the theoretical and conceptual underpinnings of race and ethnicity. These chapters address the questions, what is race, and how should it be used in health research? Richard Cooper looks at the social forces that give rise to racial differences; Thomas LaVeist describes the caution and skepticism required of researchers who employ race as a variable; Carles Mutaner, F. Javier Nieto, and Patricia O'Campo address the methodological, empirical, and ethical weaknesses of arguments for a biological basis for certain racial differences; and David Hayes-Bautista and Jorge Chapa offer a conceptual analysis of the terminology used in the United States for persons of Latin American origin.

The two chapters in Part Three, by Robert Mayberry, Fatima Mili, and Elizabeth Ofili and by Kevin Fiscella and colleagues, summarize findings on disparities in health care access, utilization, and quality. The chapters in Part Four then seek to explain why racial and ethnic variations in health status exist. These chapters address a variety of hypotheses, including Arline Geronimus's weathering hypothesis and Sherman James's John Henryism theory. Chapters by W. Parker Frisbie, Youngtae Cho, and Robert Hummer; Richard David and James Collins; Gopal Singh and Stella Yu; and Luisa Franzini, John Ribble, and Arlene Keddie examine the interrelationships among immigration, assimilation, and acculturation. A well-known paradox in the health literature is that although Latinos (especially Mexican Americans) have a generally worse health profile than white Americans, Mexican immigrants have better health than white and Mexican Americans. However, as their time in the United States extends, their health status begins to approximate that of Mexican Americans. As Singh and Yu demonstrate, similar findings exist for African and Asian immigrants.

Another possible explanation for health disparities is exposure to racism. The chapters by Camara Jones and by Rodney Clark et al. describe the theoretical basis for this hypothesis, and David Williams and Chiquita Collins and also Elizabeth Klonoff and Hope Landrine discuss empirical tests. The final chapters in Part Four explore the idea that disparities among the racial and ethnic groups are caused by differential exposure to health risks. Michelle Pearl, Paula Braveman, and Barbara Abrams and also Williams and Collins examine socioeconomic status. Kimberly Morland et al. demonstrate that food stores are less available in minority communities, and R. Sean Morrison et al. demonstrate that pharmacies in those communities are less likely to carry pain medication. Limited availability of products that sustain good health is typically accompanied by overavailability of products injurious to health, as discussed by Robert Bullard (solid waste sites), Thomas LaVeist and John Wallace (liquor stores), and Marsha Lillie-Blanton, James Anthony, and Charles Schuster (crack cocaine).

In Part Five we turn to the health care system and examine the role of health care providers in producing health disparities. Knox Todd and colleagues demonstrate that African American patients were less likely than white patients to receive pain medication when they came to a hospital emergency room.

Schulman and colleagues show that African American women were less likely than white men to be referred for heart surgery. Betsy Sleath, Bonnie Svarstad, and Debra Roter discuss the racial differences they found in the prescribing of psychotropic medications. And Michelle van Ryn and Jane Burke explore physicians' attitudes toward African American and white patients.

Part Six of this reader presents two views of patient factors in health care disparities. Numerous studies have found (as, for example, Schulman et al. did) that there are racial differences in the receipt of heart surgery. Most of these studies have speculated that the difference is caused by patient preferences, that is, African American patients prefer not to have the procedure. Jeff Whittle et al. provide a good test of the patient preference hypothesis. Then Chamberlain Diala and colleagues study racial differences in patients' attitudes toward use of mental health services.

Finally, Part Seven presents three important discussions about provider-patient interaction. Lisa Cooper-Patrick et al. and Somnath Saha et al. test whether matching patients and doctors by race has a benefit in terms of patients' perception of their health care experience. And Jersey Chen and colleagues test whether matching patients and doctors by race has an effect on the racial disparity in the receipt of heart surgery.

Notes

1. National Center for Health Statistics. (2001). *Health, United States, 2001, with Urban and Rural Health Chartbook*. Hyattsville, MD: Author.

2. Savitt, T. (1982). The use of blacks for medical experimentation and demonstration in the old South. *J South Hist, 48*(3), 331–348.

3. Byrd, W. M., & Clayton, L. A. (1992). An American health dilemma: A history of blacks in the health system. *J Natl Med Assoc, 84*(2), 189–200.

4. Jones, C. P., LaVeist T. A., & Lillie-Blanton, M. (1991). "Race" in the epidemiologic literature: An examination of the *American Journal of Epidemiology, 1921–1990. Am J Epidemiol, 134*(10), 1079–1084.

5. Krieger, N. (1987). Shades of difference: Theoretical underpinnings of the medical controversy on black/white differences in the United States, 1830–1870. *Int J Health Serv, 17*(2), 259–278.

6. Stolley, P. D. (1999). Race in epidemiology. *Int J Health Serv, 29*(4), 905–909.

7. Fullilove, M. T. (1998). Comment: Abandoning "race" as a variable in public health research—an idea whose time has come. *Am J Public Health, 88*(9), 1297–1298.

8. Osborne, N. G., & Feit, M. D. (1992). Using race in medical research. *JAMA, 267*(2), 275–279.

9. Leslie, C. (1990). Scientific racism: Reflections on peer review, science and ideology. *Soc Sci Med, 31*(8), 891–905.

10. Brace, C. L. (1964). On the race concept. *Curr Anthropol, 5,* 313–320.

11. Livingston, F. B. (1962). On the non-existence of human races. *Curr Anthropol, 3,* 279–281.

12. Scarr, A. (1988). Race and gender as psychological variables. *Am Psychol, 43*(1), 56–59.

13. Betancourt, H., & Lopez, S. R. (1993). The study of culture, ethnicity and race in American psychology. *Am Psychol, 48,* 229–237.

PART ONE

BACKGROUND: HISTORICAL AND POLITICAL CONSIDERATIONS

CHAPTER TWO

Shades of Difference

Theoretical Underpinnings
of the Medical Controversy
on Black-White Differences
in the United States, 1830–1870

Nancy Krieger

The Negro races stand at the lowest point in the scale of human beings. . . . It
is clear they are incapable of self-government and that any attempt to improve
their condition is warring against an immutable force of nature.
—Dr. Josiah C. Nott, 1851 (p. 370)[1]

From Nat Turner's revolt in 1831 to the defeat of the Confederacy in 1865, doctors in the United States made it their business to be involved in the great debate about slavery. For these physicians, the fate of the nation hinged on one key question which medical science alone could answer: are blacks innately inferior to whites and therefore fit only to be slaves? That one set of doctors proclaimed "yes" while another declared "no" is not surprising: the question of slavery polarized every sector of society and literally split the nation in two. What is striking, however, is that physicians of all political persuasions, ranging from reactionary to abolitionist, invoked the exact same authority—science—to justify their contradictory conclusions.

The controversy raises a critical question: how could opposing doctors use the same scientific principles to vindicate their profoundly different views? What I will argue is that in fact they did *not* use the same science, that their sciences differed in *essence*, not just in application. Intrinsic to the debate were issues of fact and necessity, permanence and change, cause and effect, and above all else, the role of biology in human affairs. The majority of doctors asserted, on the

I would like to thank the following people for helping me sharpen my questions and ideas: Mary Bassett, Ros Baxandall, Linda Burnham, Ruth Hubbard, Mark Nelson, Melinda Paras, Robert Proctor, and Margo Sercaz. I would also like to thank Mary Bassett for helping me locate many of the medical articles dating from the 1800s.

basis of what would now be called reductionist, biological determinist, and ahistorical assumptions, that innate racial differences—as reflected by racial disparities in health—required blacks to be slaves and whites to be masters. In contrast, antislavery physicians (and especially the first generation of black doctors) utilized what would now be termed a historical and antireductionist approach to contend that social factors rooted in the need for cheap black labor determined both the diseases and stature of blacks enslaved in the South and impoverished in the North. The controversy, then, was much more than a question of obvious political manipulation of an allegedly neutral science: clashing worldviews entered into the very assumptions upon which the competing scientific theories were based.

Politics, moreover, set the terms, tempo, and tenor of the medical debate. Which paradigm attained scientific prominence and political significance depended primarily not on academic merit, but on the prevailing forms of the social relations of capitalist exploitation and racial oppression. As long as Northern industrialists and Southern planters mutually supported slavery, the doctrine of innate racial differences held sway. Their eventual schism, however, not only provoked the Civil War but also created new conditions that enabled many physicians to perceive the underlying role of social class in producing the vast majority of black-white health differences. Yet this insight—occasioned by changes in social relations, not by technological breakthroughs—was short-lived, the new science soon muted by the deliberate destruction of Reconstruction.

Comprehending the course of the past century's polemic on racial differences, then, can do more than clarify how the content and development of scientific theory is historically bound to both the technical level and social relations of the society in which it is conceived. By starkly revealing the resonance between scientific theory and politics, especially in a field in which people are both the subject and object of inquiry, analysis of this debate can also help expose the premises of contemporary racist science, and suggest steps for the development of a progressive alternative.

PRELUDE TO THE DEBATE: ON THE ORIGINS OF SLAVERY AND SCIENTIFIC RACISM

The discovery of gold and silver in America, the extirpation, enslavement and entombment in the mines of the aboriginal population, the beginning of the conquest and looting of the East Indies, the turning of Africa into a warren for the commercial hunting of black-skins, signalised the rosy dawn of the era of capitalist production. . . . [T]he veiled slavery of the wage-workers in Europe needed, for its pedestal, slavery pure and simple in the new world.
—Karl Marx, 1867[2]

Ever since the beginning of the African slave trade in the fifteenth century, Europeans engaged in the hunting and selling of human beings sought a higher justification than simply profit. They found it in the Bible. God permitted Christians to enslave infidels, Africans were infidels, and therefore enslaved Africans served as an ideal source of the labor that Europeans urgently needed to make the colonies of the New World prosper for the greater glory of God and King. Unfortunately, infidels could convert. To circumvent the contradiction of Christian slavery, Europeans again consulted the Bible and found a foolproof rationale: marked by their color, Africans were descendants of Ham, cursed son of Noah, consigned by God to a fate of perpetual servitude (pp. 90–91).[3]

North American colonists, like other enterprising Europeans, quickly grasped the value of a color-coded system of labor. From the outset, the problem of land and labor loomed large: too few people and too much land meant that the wealth of the new territories could be secured only by importing labor. White indentured servants and convicts comprised the initial colonial workforce. They were, however, too few in number and notoriously difficult to distinguish from free yeomen if they escaped. After colonial attempts to enslave Native Americans failed, the settlers turned to African labor, ever thankful that, by making Europeans white and Africans black, God had provided an easy way to identify runaway slaves.

The first shipment of slaves arrived in North America in 1619, by way of Jamestown, Virginia. By the end of the century, a color-coded system of slavery was firmly entrenched. This socially determined division of labor not only proved profitable but also forged a new social relation—that of black oppression–white supremacy—which soon became both the law and belief of the land (pp. 193–194).[3]

Slavery fueled the primitive capital accumulation process that financed the Industrial Revolution in both colonial America and imperial England.[4] The nefarious triangle trade of slaves, rum, and sugar spurred on not just the economy of the South but the industry of the North. By the mid-1700s, the Puritan states were the greatest slave carriers of the New World (p. 245).[3] Rising prosperity led to increased economic and political tension with the motherland. The conflict ultimately exploded into war. As revolutionaries waged the American War of Independence, they proclaimed the natural rights of man as justification; shortly thereafter, their stance served as inspiration to the democratic revolutions carried out by the nascent French bourgeoisie and working class in 1789 and the Haitian slaves in 1791.

The liberation of Haiti intensified the ongoing debate about slavery within the newly emergent United States. If all men innately possessed the natural right to liberty (women were a different matter), how could slavery be justified? To bolster their arguments, proponents and opponents alike turned to the rising authority of the age: science.

Impelled by the ferment of their times, leading scientists—scions of the merchant class—eagerly took up the question of slavery. Enthralled by taxonomy, they queried if blacks and whites differed enough to be labeled distinct species, created separately but not equally by God; if so, then blacks were neither entitled to the natural rights of whites, nor protected by God's ban on enslaving one's brethren. While the politically cautious eschewed the heretical belief that all humans had not descended from Adam and Eve, their opponents declared that, in this rational era, facts not faith must buttress argument. During the following decades, the debate waxed and waned, its content as concerned with religious implications as with scientific evidence. By the 1820s, a fragile truce emerged favoring the faithful theory of unity of species (pp. 10–18).[5] Though numerous differences remained, one tenet was clear: whatever the origin of blacks might be, they clearly were inferior to whites *now;* any scientist who voiced an opinion to the contrary was the exception, not the rule.

THE 1830s–1840s: SLAVERY, STATISTICS, AND BLACK DISEASES

Domestic slavery, instead of being a political evil,
is the cornerstone of our republican edifice.
—George McDuffie, Governor of South Carolina, 1835 (p. 369)[1]

Physicians in the 1830s and 1840s lived in raucous times. Rapid territorial and industrial expansion, under the reign of King Cotton, simultaneously spawned a vigorous new defense of slavery by Southern planters, Northern textile manufacturers, and the innumerable merchants who profited from and connected the two, as well as an increasingly militant and national abolitionist movement (pp. 203–204),[1] (p. 392).[3] This heightened controversy also spurred a new round of medical debate about black-white differences, one which not only reopened old questions but posed new ones as well.

Though the physicians who entered the fray perceived and depicted themselves as scientists whose quest for truth transcended petty politics, they were not a disinterested lot—economically, politically, or ideologically. Many Southern doctors received a guaranteed annual income by hiring their services to plantations, and often supplemented their earnings at the auction block, where, for a fee, they inspected slaves to see if they were fit to be sold.[6] Likewise, physicians in the North had little incentive to raise an antiracist ruckus: free blacks offered no lucrative patronage, and wealthy Northerners avoided abolitionist zealots. Moreover, as aspiring white professionals, doctors were eager to halt the growth of rapidly proliferating populist health movements in the 1830s. To secure the franchise on medical practice, physicians nationwide actively lobbied state legislatures to pass allopath-only licensing laws.[7] Under such circumstances, most doctors had more to lose than gain if they challenged the authority of government by questioning either the legal or moral basis of slavery.

Political considerations affected not only physician participation in but the social significance of the medical debate on racial differences. Its rise to a matter of state in the mid-1830s occurred not because of any new scientific discoveries but because slavery proponents faced two new challenges. One was to justify why slavery, rather than wage labor, should be extended to territories newly wrested from both Native Americans and Mexicans; the other was to crush the increasingly influential abolitionist movement. Pro-slavery politicians therefore began trumpeting scientific proof of black inferiority not because they suddenly thought science should rule society but because science alone could lend a legitimacy and authority capable of offsetting the abolitionists' moral and religious clout.

Turning to the medical literature, these politicians found that numerous physicians had already scientifically confirmed what slaveholders had always intuitively known: blacks, by virtue of their biology, were destined to be slaves. Moreover, the legions of studies supporting this view were neither "fringe" science nor the result of crass data manipulation. Instead, their prevalence and legitimacy was a product of the unspoken beliefs of the age.

In this period, the eternal now of God's creation pervaded all theory. Despite scientists' growing ability to make wondrous new combinations of *preexisting* materials and to measure progress with increasingly sophisticated statistical methodologies,[8] most still believed that the essential properties of fixed types remained unchanged; truly there was nothing new under the sun. Further dominating their beliefs were five additional assumptions, all of which hinged on unstated philosophical principles:

1. The Baconian belief that neutral and objective science should not sully itself with politics.
2. The Cartesian belief that the character of any system can be completely defined solely through detailed examination of its ontologically prior constituent parts.
3. The view that dissimilarity is equivalent to inequality.
4. The equation of measurement and neutrality with objectivity.
5. The conflation of the empirically real with the historically necessary.

While none of these assumptions was explicitly racist, they nonetheless provided the theoretical and ideological backbone for a racist science.

Within this framework, Occam's razor provided a presumably objective parsimonious hypothesis that was in fact highly partisan: racial disparities stemmed primarily from fixed biological traits, rather than from the black and white populations' historical and social relationship to each other. Logic therefore demanded that if empirical evidence could demonstrate the existence of racial differences, then the diverse races differed fundamentally, were not equal, and therefore could never experience similar health profiles nor occupy equal positions in society. These beliefs, combined with the axiom that the authority of science hinged upon the verifiability of data, consequently ensured that the rising volume of medical debate in the 1830s and 1840s would center on three themes: the accuracy, validity, and interpretation of the alleged findings.

To appreciate the controversy's context, it is first necessary to examine the standard science of the day, and an unexceptional review of black diseases written by Dr. E. M. Pendleton of Sparta, Georgia, in 1849 provides a typical illustration of how the era's ideology thoroughly penetrated the medical discourse.[9] Wedded to the notion that innate differences underlay black-white disparities in disease, Pendleton attributed utmost importance to the least racial divergence in rates or intensity and discovered evidence of black inferiority everywhere he looked. For example, although he conceded that "different modes of living" might affect health (whites, after all, suffered more from maladies linked to the "evils of civilization"), Pendleton's explanation of why twice as many blacks as whites with tuberculosis died of the disease (28 percent versus 14 percent) was the common belief[10-12] that blacks were not "suited for the cold even of our temperate climate"—not that black slaves were forced to live in crowded, poorly heated, leaky cabins without adequate clothing or blankets and were overworked to boot. Similarly, to account for why diseases of the brain and nervous system killed a minutely greater proportion of afflicted whites than blacks (5.4 percent versus 4.4 percent), Pendleton averred that the mental apparatus of whites was "brought into much greater activity" and made of "more delicate fiber" than that of blacks.[9]

Turning to the endemic fevers that plagued the South, Pendleton generally affirmed the majority view that blacks were *less* susceptible than whites to ailments such as malaria[13,14] and yellow fever.[15,16] Yet, after observing that "the fresh imported African can sustain the deathly climate of our rice fields far better than whites," Pendleton also noted that "people in miasmatic districts" often "undergo a kind of acclimation . . . and afterwards become less subject" to these fevers,[9] a phenomenon also reported by a few other physicians.*[17,18] Despite the conflicting data, Pendleton and the rest of the medical community clearly favored the evidence for innate as opposed to acquired immunity, as well as for

---

*In retrospect, both sets of observations probably were "true": some racial differences in susceptibility may genuinely have existed (because the sickling trait does confer partial immunity to certain strains of malaria and is more prevalent among people from regions where malaria is endemic, such as Africa and the Mediterranean), and many slaves may have acquired immunity to both diseases either in Africa or on the plantations (pp. 25–26, 241).[19]

the miasmatic rather than contagionist theory of disease transmission. That they did so illustrates how, in periods when the technical limitations of science prevent definitive tests of the contending hypotheses (none could have identified the virus which caused yellow fever or the malaria protozoa, let alone the sickling trait), social beliefs readily fill scientific vacuums.[20]

Only one set of diseases initially left Pendleton grasping for an explanation: those pertaining to women. Having thought that "the delicate white female would have much oftener demand for the physician than the coarse muscular negress," Pendleton was amazed to discover that black women had higher rates than white women for both "diseases peculiar to women" (12.4 versus 6.4 per hundred) and miscarriages (3.9 versus 0.8 per hundred). Interpreting these puzzling results as best he could, Pendleton stated:

> This table [of disease data] either teaches that slave labor is inimical to the procreation of the Species from exposure, violent exercise, etc., or as the planters believe, the blacks are possessed of a secret by which they destroy the foetus at an early stage of gestation. . . . In philosophizing upon this immense difference we are led to the conclusion from the facts within our knowledge, that it originates from the unnatural tendency of the African female to destroy her offspring [p. 649].[9]

Given the choice, Pendleton—like most of his peers—studiously avoided the dangerous notion that the South's "peculiar institution" could make slaves sick, and instead attributed racial disparities in health to the "peculiar constitution" of the blacks themselves.

The routine emphasis on racial differences expressed in such reviews inevitably provoked doctors to wonder, once again, whether blacks and whites were even the same species. To answer this question, a new generation of investigators created a novel science. Called "ethnology," the discipline's pioneering work appeared in 1840, when Dr. Samuel G. Morton published *Crania America*. Morton's central thesis was that the various human races had remained unchanged in their physical and mental constitution since the time of their separate creations.[5] As proof, Morton initially presented measurements of the cranial capacity of current and ancient human skulls, and then later argued in his internationally acclaimed *Crania Aegyptiaca* (published in 1844) that the existence of black slavery in ancient Egypt clearly proved that black inferiority was a divinely inspired fact of nature which politics could never change. Aware of the timeliness of his findings, Morton personally sent a copy of *Crania Aegyptiaca* to none other than Senator John C. Calhoun, the South's most illustrious defender of slavery (pp. 40, 62).[5]

The first physician to employ Morton's thesis in the medical controversy on racial differences was Dr. Josiah C. Nott, a wealthy and highly educated proslavery Southerner (pp. 65–69).[5] In 1843, Nott published a widely read and extremely controversial article in the highly respected *Boston Medical and Surgical Journal.* Entitled "The Mulatto a Hybrid—Probable Extermination of the Two Races if the Whites and Blacks Are Allowed to Intermarry,"[21] it articulated what was to become the ruling hypothesis of his times. Nott's piece contested two prevalent beliefs: that hybrids resulting from the mating of distinct species were invariably sterile, and that blacks "benefited" from the infusion of "white blood." Instead, Nott conjectured that in certain cases hybrids might simply be less fertile and more feeble than their parents. Applying this hypothesis to humans, Nott suggested that mulattoes should be viewed as a sickly, bastard breed whose very existence proved blacks and whites were separate species.

To prove his case, Nott cited a smattering of Morton's cranial measurements and a handful of vital statistics and insanity rates derived from the 1840 Census.[21] Claiming that these data clearly showed mulattoes to be of "intermediate intelligence," "less capable of endurance and shorter lived," and "less prolific" than either blacks or whites, Nott also reiterated the Census's apparent finding that freedom drove blacks mad.† Appealing to the common sense of his times, Nott therefore concluded (emphasis in original):

> The Caucasian, Ethiopian, Mongol, Malay and American may have been distinct creations, or may be mere varieties of the same species produced by external causes acting through many thousand years; but this I do believe, *that at the present day the Anglo-Saxon and the Negro races are, according to the common acceptation of the terms distinct species, and that the offspring of the two is a hybrid.* Look first upon the Caucasian female with her rose and lily skin, silky hair, Venus form, and well-chiseled features—and then upon the African wench, with her black and odorous skin, woolly head and animal features—next compare their whole anatomical structure, and say whether they do not differ as much as the swan and the goose, the horse and the ass, or the apple and the pear tree [p. 30].[21]

Nott's provocative conjecture immediately gained many supporters, but prompted a few rebuttals as well. The most powerful was written by Dr. Samuel Forry, editor of the *New York Journal of Medicine.*[23] In his critique, Forry systematically showed that Nott's conclusion rested not only on fabricated data, but also on dubious assumptions that had nothing to do with nature and everything to do with politics. Reminding his readers to "bear in mind that *figures* are not *facts,* and hence the necessity of ascertaining the correctness of data represented by numerals," Forry first sharply enquired how Nott obtained data on mulattoes from the 1840 Census since the *only* racial categories employed by

---

†The data showed that the farther north blacks lived, the higher their insanity rates—a fact that Calhoun triumphantly declared to Congress and the world as "proof" that "the African is incapable of self-care and sinks into lunacy under the burden of freedom."[22]

the Census were "white" and "black," *not* "mulatto." Second, Forry also urged caution regarding interpretation of the black insanity rates, noting that a French study had recently shown that better ascertainment of insanity in urban regions artificially inflated rural-urban differences in rates. One year later, Forry was to join with other prominent scientists in demonstrating the thoroughly fraudulent nature of the Census insanity data.‡[24]

Apart from questions of accuracy, Forry critiqued Nott's tendency to "absolutize" difference and to equate difference with inferiority. Using Nott's own data, Forry showed that—contrary to what Nott alleged—black and white cranial capacity overlapped considerably. Attacking the validity of Nott's interest in skull sizes in the first place, Forry exclaimed "how absurd is the idea of taking the whole mass of the brain as a standard of moral and intellectual power!"[23] Forry also derided Nott's construction of "race" as an absolute and static category. Pointing to variations in skin color, hair texture, and physique *within* as well as between different African tribes, Arabic nations, and European communities, Forry adduced that "the Negro and the European are two extremes which, as in every other particular in which the various tribes of human kind differ, press into each other by insensible gradations."[23] Exposing the link between Nott's distorted reasoning and reactionary politics, Forry concluded:

> In the laudable desire no doubt to advance science, [Nott] has unfortunately made a retrograde movement in human knowledge. . . . And it has ever been thus, by denying an equality in the original endowments of certain families of the human race, that writers have attempted to justify the institution of perpetual servitude [p. 167].[23]

The dominance of pro-slavery politics, however, ensured that Nott's unsubstantiated hypothesis rapidly gained almost axiomatic status. By the end of the 1840s, the medical debate seemed almost over, with victory (measured by volume, if nothing else) going to the proponents of innate racial differences. Yet, just as voices such as Forry's were apparently to be drowned out forever, they received unexpected encouragement—not from scientific colleagues or abolitionist crusaders, but from a break in the national consensus of those who wielded power as to whether slavery best utilized the resources of the fast-growing nation.

---

‡The history of the exposure of the fallacious 1840 Census data is well recounted by Deutsch.[22] In 1844, Dr. Edmund Jarvis, a specialist in mental disorders and one of the founders of the American Statistical Association in 1839, demonstrated that Northern black insanity rates had been greatly inflated by virtue of the Census listing more "insane blacks" than the total number of blacks recorded as living in the region.[25] When coupled with the Southern tendency to treat black insanity as insubordination and to exclude black patients from insane asylums, this gross inaccuracy therefore meant that the alleged correlation between latitude and insanity, between freedom and madness, was completely spurious.

THE 1850s: THE POLITICS OF NO POLITICS AND THE FIRST GENERATION OF BLACK DOCTORS

The abolitionist theory that the Negro is only a lampblacked white man is the cause of all those political agitations threatening to dissolve our union.
—Dr. Samuel A. Cartwright, 1851 (p. 194)[26]

Battles about black disease and inferiority broke out yearly in the pages of medical journals in the 1850s, replacing the somewhat more sporadic spats of the 1830s and 1840s. As violence and bloodshed increasingly accompanied the rapidly proliferating political crises of the 1850s—themselves a consequence of the struggle between industrial capitalists of the North and landholding slave-owners of the South for control of the nation's economy, government, and ever expanding territories (p. 3)[27]—the debate on slavery grew ever more encompassing and divisive. In a decade commencing with the passage of the draconian Fugitive Slave Act and the subsequent rise of traffic on the Underground Railroad (p. 482),[1] punctuated by the appearance of Harriet Beecher Stowe's extraordinarily influential *Uncle Tom's Cabin* (pp. 112–115),[27] and culminating with the Republican Party's rise to power on the platform of "free labor, free land, and free markets" (pp. 206–207),[27] the medical controversy not surprisingly underwent a substantial change in both form and intensity.

From lecterns in the halls of science and government to podiums at mass rallies, doctors in both camps proclaimed their contradictory truths: blacks were—or were not—the equals of whites. Their escalated attacks marked a shift in content as well as style, for during the 1850s, two new groups with opposite agendas plunged into the medical fray: "apolitical" doctors and the first generation of black physicians.

The timing of their participation once again had more to do with politics than science. Self-declared apolitical physicians, alarmed at their pro-slavery colleagues' increasing tendency to mix fancy with fact and heresy with hypothesis, joined the debate to rescue the scientific integrity of their profession; throughout the decade they argued that medicine must be purged of politics in order to retain its objectivity. In marked contrast, the majority of black doctors asserted that the key question was not *whether* but *which* politics would inform medical thought. Moreover, they entered the debate in the early 1850s not because they were suddenly troubled or inspired, but because prior to this time they were not allowed to exist: until 1848, not one medical school in the United States permitted blacks to be students. Indeed, before this bitterly fought-for change in admissions policies, the number of university-trained black doctors practicing medicine in the United States could be counted on one finger: Dr. James McCune Smith, who had received his medical degree abroad in 1837, at the University of Glasgow (pp. 229, 268).[1]

Apart from Nott, one of the chief targets of both factions was Dr. Samuel A. Cartwright, a prominent Southern physician, diehard defender of slavery, and author of innumerable articles on the inferior status and diseases of blacks. In 1850, at the request of the Louisiana legislature, Cartwright and several other physicians embarked on a study of the health of the state's black population. The final report, authored by Cartwright and entitled "Diseases and Physical Peculiarities of the Negro Race,"[28] appeared in the prestigious *New Orleans Medical and Surgical Journal.* A typical example of Cartwright's work, its publication "excited a good deal of discussion," according to the editors of the journal, "both in and out of the Profession"—a remarkable feat in an era when reading medical journals was hardly a common practice among physicians, let alone the lay public. What explained its appeal was not only the report's governmental imprimatur but Cartwright's unusually explicit and imaginative defense of his essential thesis: that "the negro is a slave by nature."

After exhaustively detailing every racial difference imaginable—ranging from hair texture and brain size to bone density and hue of internal organs— Cartwright announced that he had discovered the ultimate physiological basis of black inferiority: their inability to consume as much oxygen as whites, a consequence of certain "peculiarities" of the black nervous system.[28] Not only did the allegedly larger nerves of blacks lead to "sensuality at the expense of intellect," but the "excessive nervous development" of their stomach, liver, and genitals caused blacks to have a "lymphatic temperament, in which the lymph, phlegm, mucus and other humors predominate over the red blood." Cartwright noted that

> It is the red vital blood, sent to the brain, that liberates their minds under the white man's control; and it is the want of a sufficiency of red, vital blood that chains their mind to ignorance and barbarism when in freedom [p. 694].[28]

He therefore inferred that oxygen deficiency explained black lethargy. Observing that blacks often compounded their dangerous condition by sleeping with blankets wrapped around their heads, Cartwright concluded that only slavery, the institution of forced labor, could provide the necessary antidote to blacks' natural torpor.

As additional proof, Cartwright proudly described and named two never before identified black diseases: "drapetomania, or the disease causing slaves to run away," and "dysesthesia Ethiopia, or hebetude of mind and obtuse sensibility of body" (but known by overseers as "rascality," for its symptoms included sleeping during the day and a tendency to "break, waste and destroy everything they handle").[28] Cartwright's discovery arose from his determinist logic: blacks naturally were slaves, behavior opposing one's nature is unnatural or sick, and hence, if black slaves attempted to escape or avoid work, they must be ill. Excessive kindness, not just cruelty, could therefore induce drapetomania for, according to Cartwright, treating blacks as the equal of whites contradicted their innate servility and drove them mad. As for dysesthesia, sloth-induced oxygen deprivation clearly was the cause; forcing the stricken slaves to do "invigorating labor" was therefore the only cure. With black diseases and black slavery neatly linked to one fundamental physiological cause, Cartwright declared that the verdict brought in by science was clear: "liberty, republican or free institutions, are not only unsuitable to the negro race, but actually poisonous to its happiness."[28]

Cartwright's article sparked a little war in defense of scientific integrity and apolitical medicine. Of the numerous rebuttals received by the *New Orleans Medical and Surgical Journal,* the editors decided to print only one, written by Dr. James T. Smith, a Louisiana surgeon;[29] two other critiques appeared in the *Charleston Medical Journal.*[30,31] All three charged Cartwright with supplying "imaginary facts" to prove his case. But while one suggested that Cartwright had used political clout to suppress dissenting views within his commission,[30] the other two accused Cartwright of substituting politically motivated speculation for scientific investigation. As Smith pointed out, even the most rudimentary analysis would have shown that blacks slept with blankets around their heads "not to obtain impure atmosphere, as it is said here, but in cold weather for the purpose of warming themselves . . . [and] in warm weather, to ward off the attacks of insects."[29] Likewise, one of the other critics declared that Cartwright had violated the apolitical essence of the "Baconian system" of science, and warned that (emphasis in original):

> The mind which is biased by political prejudices cannot do justice to a medical subject. . . . To mingle medicine and politics is an unholy contamination of the former, which no wily argument can justify, no apology atone for. Make our medical journals *politico-medical* organs, and farewell to science! farewell to truth! farewell to virtuous ambition! [p. 92].[31]

None of the three critiques, however, attacked either Cartwright's support for slavery or his fundamental belief in innate racial differences. Instead, by appealing to neutrality in the name of "objectivity," they implicitly endorsed the view that only those who explicitly *state* their politics *have* politics—and thus gave free rein to the period's prevailing racism and other unspoken prevalent beliefs. Consequently, their allegedly "apolitical" position not only was *highly* political but was tantamount to saying that because consensus exists, truth is known.

The limitations of these apolitical critiques accordingly allowed Cartwright the freedom to say that indisputable facts would eventually prove him right. In addition to writing numerous review articles explicating the biological basis of black inferiority—such as "Alcohol and the Ethiopian"[32] and "The Ethnology of the Negro or Prognathous Race"[33]—Cartwright also conducted an experiment in 1855 on 300 black slaves stricken with cholera to test his hypothesis that racial differences required racially distinct remedies even for the same disease. Conjecturing that cholera in blacks was more an affliction of the mind than the body, Cartwright marched the sick slaves at twilight to a clearing in the forest. There, the slaves were

> stripped, and greased with fat bacon. . . . [T]he grease was well slapped in with broad leather straps, marking time with the *tam tam,* a wild African dance that was going on in the center of the camp among all those who had the physical strength to participate in it. This procedure drove the cholera out of the heads of all who had been conjured into the belief that they were to die with the disease [p. 149].[34]

The only critical response the journal received was from a Dr. H. S. Wooten, who simply stated that while blacks and whites obviously differed in their physical and moral constitutions, too little was known to justify Cartwright's radical therapeutic approach; on the topic of Cartwright's barbaric treatment of the slaves, Wooten remained mute.[35] Similarly, Cartwright's disingenuous if not despicable call for Southern medical schools to promote the study of the "peculiarities" of black physiology[26]—uttered at a time when black slaves already comprised the overwhelming majority of "living subjects upon which professors could demonstrate operative techniques and the course and treatment of disease, as well as corpses for anatomy and dissection" (p. 282)[19]— received little censure and much support from his peers.[36]

While Cartwright delved ever deeper into medicine for the ultimate proof of black inferiority, Nott solicited evidence from every discipline imaginable. In 1853, Nott coedited *Types of Mankind,* a huge 800-page defense of Morton's theory of polygenesis and white supremacy. Containing essays by numerous eminent scientists, such as Harvard's internationally renowned biologist Louis Agassiz, the volume rapidly sold out and went through nine editions by the end of the century (pp. 162–163).[5] Its heretical stance, however, militated against universal acceptance: not only did several physicians revive the biblical tale of Ham as a more orthodox explanation of racial differences,[36-38] but one even cautioned that Nott's challenge to church teachings threatened "if not speedily checked, to revolutionize our social organization, and assimilate us, as a people, to infidel France,"[37] which had just experienced its 1848 revolution.

Relishing the controversy, in 1857 Nott coedited the equally determinist and blasphemous *Indigenous Races of the Earth.*[39] Published just one year after he translated Gobineau's *Essais sur l'inégalité des races* (the founding work of eugenics, which Nott tellingly dedicated to "the statesmen of America" (p. 174),[5] this new volume appeared the same year as the Supreme Court's notorious Dred Scott decision and provided ideological support for Chief Justice Tanney's declaration that blacks "had no rights which the white man was bound to respect" (pp. 217–219).[27] With topics ranging from paleontology to philology, Nott's tome[39] once again proffered proof of the eternal nature of white supremacy. While editors of both the *New Orleans Medical and Surgical Journal*[40] and the *Charleston Medical Journal*[41] praised the book as an "important work upon Anthropology," they avoided heresy by saying that Nott's essay on polygenesis did not offer conclusive proof of the theory of "Diversity of Origins." Apparently, only doctors who cared as little for religion as they did for politics in their science felt free to discredit Nott's work. Editors of the *American Journal of Medical Sciences,* for example, wrote a snide and stinging review in which they equated Nott's thesis with religious dogma and then declared that their journal lacked the space to give Nott's article the criticism it so richly deserved.[42]

The first generation of black doctors, however, could not simply dismiss findings that favored notions of "black inferiority," because others could charge that abolitionist views polluted their own science. Their critique therefore had to be at once powerful and subtle—powerful, because racist science justified the enslavement of millions; subtle, because both racist and antiracist science incorporated explicit, albeit contradictory, worldviews, and any errors in their exposure of the *inherent* role of politics *within* medicine could easily jeopardize their own claims to scientific truth.

Among the new extremely energetic and committed black physicians to develop this critique was Dr. John S. Rock. In the mid-1850s, Rock lectured throughout New England and the western states on topics such as "The Unity of the Human Races" and "Race and Slavery." Challenging the common belief that the allegedly greater resistance of blacks to malaria "proved" that blacks were "designed" for slavery, Rock scoffed at the idea that a country could be "good for slavery and not good for freedom!"[43] and countered that even if racial differences in susceptibility existed, why should such a finding mean blacks must be slaves? Moreover, beyond exposing the logical flaws that riddled racist science, Rock also showed that the main problem stemmed not from what such science looked at, but from what it ignored. As long as doctors refused to examine how slavery and poverty caused disease, they would have only biological rationales to explain racial differences in behavior and health.

Rock elaborated this novel analysis in a speech he presented at the first Crispus Attucks celebration, held on March 5, 1858, to protest the Dred Scott decision (pp. 225–226).§[27] Featured alongside such abolitionist luminaries as Wendell Phillips and William Lloyd Garrison, Rock attacked both the premises and the conclusions of racist science. At a time when Cartwright was popularizing the view that "it is no physical force which keeps [blacks] in submission,

---

§Crispus Attucks was the first citizen and first black to die in the American Revolution; he was killed during the Boston Massacre of March 5, 1770.

but the spiritual force of the white man's will,"[33] Rock averred that black slavery had nothing to do with innate black cowardliness but everything to do with white military superiority.[44] Then, in a tongue-in-check manner, Rock deliberately turned topsy-turvy the typical racist arguments of the day and showed just how much was in the eye of the beholder.

> I will not deny that I admire the talents and noble character of many white men. But I cannot say that I am particularly pleased with their physical appearance. If old mother nature had held out as well as she had commenced, we should, probably, have had fewer varieties in the races. When I contrast the fine, tough, muscular system, the beautiful, rich color, the full broad features and the gracefully frizzled hair of the Negro with the delicate physical organization, wan color, sharp features and lank hair of the Caucasian, I am inclined to believe that when the white man was created, nature was pretty well exhausted. But, determined to keep up appearances, she pinched up the features and did the best she could under the circumstances [p. 340].[43]

Ending with a denunciation of all who used biology to explain or sanction black slavery and degradation, Rock clearly stated the true cause of both: the white man's desire for cheap black labor.

One year later, Dr. James McCune Smith further advanced this nascent antiracist science by publishing a widely circulated and highly influential pamphlet entitled *On the Fourteenth Query of Thomas Jefferson's Notes on Virginia.*[45] Jefferson's famous query had been whether blacks and whites could ever live together as equals, given their physical differences; Smith's response was to expose the logical and biological flaws of Jefferson's argument. After reviewing the known anatomical evidence, Smith not only concluded that blacks and whites were more alike than different, but he also contested the definition of "race" as a natural category, stating:

> The fallacy in the argument has consisted in this: the variations in the black race have been arranged together and have been called this type of the race, and as such have been compared with, not the varieties, but the general type of the whites, and from this comparison, the illogical conclusion has been adduced that there is a permanent difference between these two races. This argument is about as conclusive as if we were to select all the white men in this city who have grey eyes, and to argue that because the color of their eyes differs from that of the remainder, therefore the two classes belong to different races [p. 227].[45]

Consequently, if "race" had any meaning, it was a *social* category, one whose political essence Smith revealed by explaining that "the term white is an arbitrary one, when used in contradistinction to black, the latter meaning the colored mixed race now enslaved in this Republic."[45] But if the designation of "race" was unscientific and the apparent racial differences trivial, then why did black and white populations exhibit such different patterns of disease?

To answer this question, Smith argued—perhaps for the first time ever in this debate—that apparently intrinsic traits could be the consequence not of innate factors, but of inherited, socially created environments.[45] To prove his point, Smith compared rates of bone deformities due to rickets (a condition he attributed to poor diet) in the *families* of blacks and poor whites. Finding the rates to be nearly equal, Smith concluded that blacks had rickets not because they were biologically "black," but because they were poor, and they were poor because they were blacks living in a racist society that either condemned blacks to slavery in the South or to a marginal existence as the most poorly paid workers (if employed at all) in the North. With the biological determinist argument now turned on its head—racial disparities in disease were an *effect* of racism, rather than *caused* by "race"—Smith began to advance the view that the health of individuals was not primarily a consequence of their innate constitution, but instead was a reflection of their intrinsic membership in groups created by the social relations of the society in which they lived.

As part of his efforts to place scientific investigations on a new footing, Smith also attacked the racist belief that "difference" equaled "inequality." Variation in skin color did not imply to Smith, as it did to Jefferson, that whites and blacks could not one day live together as peers. On the contrary, to Smith, differences were a source not of inequality and discord, but of diversity and strength. This was an uncommon view in 1859, but then 1859 was an uncommon year: the raid of John Brown and his abolitionist followers on Harper's Ferry to secure arms to wage war against slavery, and the publication of Darwin's *On the Origin of Species* signaled critical turning points in the political and medical controversy over slavery, one soon to reach its climax.

THE 1860s: CIVIL WAR, RECONSTRUCTION, AND THE RISE AND FALL OF AN ANTIRACIST SCIENCE

The present struggle between the South and North is, therefore, nothing but a struggle between two social systems, between the system of slavery and the system of free labor. The struggle was broken out because the two systems can no longer live peacefully side by side on the North American continent. It can only be ended with the victory of one system or another.
—Karl Marx, 1861 (p. 81)[46]

In the brief interval between the onset of the Civil War and the destruction of Reconstruction, a new candor emerged from the dregs of the medical debate, prompted not by any new scientific discovery, but by the inarguable transformation of black slaves from property to people. Four years of bloody warfare followed by emancipation destroyed the claim that blacks were slaves by nature. In the medical literature, scientific verities gave way to frank admissions of ignorance as the new stature of millions of freed blacks forced many physicians to acknowledge that much information about black physiology and disease was false. Meanwhile, upholders of black inferiority continued to defend their doctrine, certain that the eternal laws of nature would prevail over the transient laws of humankind. At the heart of the medical controversy in the 1860s was whether blacks and whites, in equal circumstances, might be equal—and at the heart of the political debate was whether such conditions would be permitted to exist.

Throughout the war, turmoil surrounded the question of what to do with the slaves. Vacillating between protecting the property of slave owners and granting liberty to the slaves (p. 396),[27] the Union moved to free the slaves only after it became clear that winning the war required emancipation (p. 324).[27] On January 1, 1863, the Emancipation Proclamation went into effect, and in February 1865, Lincoln outlawed slavery forever by signing the Thirteenth Amendment into law. One month later, Congress created the Freedman's Bureau to adjudicate the transition of previously enslaved blacks to freedom. The question of land and labor, however, once again loomed large. To preserve property relations, the bureau ensured that freed blacks would become sharecroppers rather than landowners by decreeing that each freedman and "loyal white" could receive at most only four acres of abandoned or confiscated plantations, and only by leasing the land at 6 percent of its value for three years and then paying the rest of the purchase price (p. 469).[27] Angrily responding to this regressive policy, Dr. John S. Rock exclaimed:

> Why talk about compensating masters? . . . What does society owe them? . . . It is the slave who ought to be compensated. The property of the South is by right the property of the slave [p. 192].[47]

Instead, the inheritance of the ex-slaves was to be yet more emiseration and exploitation.

During the war years, however, many physicians began to analyze past convictions in a new light. One 1865 paper described dissimilarities in the structure of the larynx of blacks and whites, but now its author mused that perhaps such differences did not necessarily imply "degradation."[48] Even more notably, an astonished Union army surgeon stationed in Tennessee in 1863 reported that blacks were as susceptible as whites to sunstroke and fevers and concluded that blacks "suffer from the same maladies and ought to be treated by the same remedies" as whites.[49] A similar freshness also characterized a comprehensive article on the health of 7,949 sick and wounded freed slaves and whites stationed in the District of Columbia, which was published in 1866 by yet another Union army physician, Dr. Robert Reyburn.[50] Noting that malaria ranked second only to typhoid among the black refugees, Reyburn observed:

> This significant fact is, we believe, a sufficient answer to, and refutation of, the
> statement so often reiterated in our textbooks, that the negro race are not
> subject to and do not suffer from malarious disease [p. 366].[50]

For other diseases, such as pneumonia, Reyburn concurred that reports of the higher prevalence in blacks than in whites apparently seemed correct. No new techniques of observation enabled Reyburn to discern the deficiency or accuracy of previously collected data. Instead, what had changed was the expectation that blacks and whites must differ for every disease in order to uphold the doctrine of innate racial differences.

The Civil War also prompted direct examination of the hypothesis that black health was primarily a function of the conditions under which blacks lived. For example, an 1865 article documented that the mortality rate of the poor was twice that of the rich in both Europe and the United States, while that of black slaves was seven times that of free blacks serving in English troops; the article thereby inferred that the poor health of black slaves stemmed from conditions of slavery, not from "race" per se.[51] Also rejecting the crude conflation of fact and necessity that had marked earlier works on racial differences in disease, Reyburn further observed in his 1866 study that

> the same causes which produce scrofula among the colored people, may be seen
> (to a limited extent) in operation among the poorer class of white people in
> many of the larger cities of the Union, and produce among them precisely
> the same result; in other words we believe that scrofula is nothing more than the
> effect produced upon the human system by unfavorable hygienic influences,
> and any races of man will suffer from it in the exact proportion as they are
> subjugated to these deleterious conditions [p. 367].[50]

As a result of comparing the health of blacks to poor whites, this new cohort of investigators began to develop not only an antiracist science but a class-conscious approach to the role of social conditions in the production of disease.

Others, however, clung to old hypotheses, but conceded that they needed new data to support their views. Most significant among this sector was the federal government itself, which continued to adhere to Nott's hybridity hypothesis (still unproven, twenty years later). In 1863, the Union appointed a commission, headed by Dr. S. G. Howe, to investigate the health of the newly freed "Colored Population."[52] This commission, in a unique admission of ignorance, sent a list of thirteen questions on the vital statistics of blacks and mulattoes to all major medical journals. Requesting that the editors both print the queries and strongly encourage their readers to reply, the letter complained that

> it is not known, from any wide circle of observation, whether the Mulattoes are
> as fertile as blacks and whites; whether they are also long lived: nor even

whether their breed can exist permanently; that is, whether its hybridity will
prevent its persistence [p. 478].[52]

As Howe's letter so succinctly stated, despite all that had been published for the
past thirty years, the "data do not exist."

In addition to implicitly supporting the view that blacks and whites were different species, the federal government also contributed to the ruin of Reconstruction as it helped reforge the national economy (pp. 199–202).[47] Its actions,
along with the rise of the Ku Klux Klan, not only ensured the continued impov-
erishment and ill health of blacks but also reinstated a climate in which upholders of scientific racism could publish freely.

In 1866, Nott reemerged to write a two-part article entitled "Instincts of the
Races."[53] Invoking his classic argument of "permanency of type," Nott argued
that Emancipation was bound to fail because of blacks' "instinctive dislike of
agricultural labor"; only under the compulsion of slavery would blacks work.
Aware, however, that Darwin's new theory of evolution threatened his beliefs,
Nott devised a clever defense. Conceding Darwin's brilliance in admitting history to the realm of biology, Nott countered that such notions had little bearing
on the thesis of black extinction as a consequence of emancipation (emphasis
in original):

> Forms that have been permanent for several thousand years must remain so at
> least during the life of a nation. It is true, there is a school of Naturalists among
> whom are numbered the great names of Lamarck, Geoffrey St. Hilaire, Darwin
> and others, which advocates the *development* theory, and contends not only that
> one type may be transformed into another, but that man himself is nothing more
> than a developed worm; but this school requires *millions of years* to carry out
> the changes by infinitesimal steps of progression. With such theories, or refine-
> ments of science, our present investigation has no connection, and the
> Freedmen's Bureau will not have the vitality enough to see the negro experiment
> through many hundred generations, and to direct the imperfect plans of
> Providence [p. 4].[53]

It remained for a new generation of physicians, spawned by post-
Reconstructionist America, to discover how the social Darwinist concept of "survival of the fittest" could be used to demonstrate that blacks were "slowly
succumbing to the rigors of competition." Reflecting the racism of their times,
these new doctors eagerly and successfully accepted the challenge; in the words
of one historian:

> The belief in the Negro's extinction became one of the most pervasive ideas in
> American medicine and anthropological thought during the late nineteenth
> century . . . a fitting culmination to the concept of racial inferiority in American
> life [p. 155].[54]

CONCLUSION

The new antiracist science never fully flourished, its progressive impulse squelched by the political realities of the times. No new technological break-throughs occasioned either its genesis or arrest, only changes in and transformations of the antagonistic social relationship of white supremacy and black oppression—a phenomenon rooted in, shaped by, and even influencing the development of capitalist relations in the United States. Yet, as the medical debate so clearly demonstrated, it was not simply a matter of politics—whether reactionary or progressive—influencing the application of a neutral science: it was a case of politics, of assumptions about how the world is or can be, that entered into the very practice, content, and even theory of the science itself.

A review of the past century's debate therefore clearly suggests that to combat the scientific racism of our own generation, we must rebut the notion of a "neutral science." Not only should we use political analysis to advance scientific theory, but we must also expose the intrinsic tension between the objective and the partisan that exists within any science—be it racist, radical, or more commonly and hence insidiously, liberal. While current racial biases may seem tame compared to their more virulent and florid forms of 100 years ago, they are equally pernicious. For example, despite general scientific agreement that the biological definition of "race" is an anachronism,[55] modern-day medical journals remain replete with racialized studies that compare the health of blacks and whites without ever addressing the role of social class in producing disease in either blacks *or* whites. Similarly, at the heart of the recent victim-blaming and policymaking *Report of the Secretary's Task Force on Black and Minority Health*[56] lies the all too familiar belief that the poorer health of minority communities is the result of numerous individuals making ill-informed "lifestyle choices," rather than a consequence of racial oppression and the disproportionate concentration of minorities in the lower strata of the working class.

Finally, as we continue the task of developing an explicitly antiracist, class-conscious science, we must also heed the main lesson of the past century's debate: social change, not science, resolved the question of whether blacks were innately inferior to whites and therefore fit only to be slaves. In his speech protesting the Dred Scott decision, Rock surmised that racist ideology would fade only "when the avenues of wealth are opened" to all, after which "the roughest looking colored man that you ever saw, or ever will see, will be pleasanter than the harmonies of Orpheus, and black will be a very pretty color."[44] The challenge is clear: if we are to defeat scientific racism, we must, in the tradition of Rock and so many others, participate in the political struggle to end racism itself.

Notes

1. Foner, P. S. (1983). *History of black Americans: From the emergence of the Cotton Kingdom to the eve of the Compromise of 1850* (Vol. 2). Westport, CT: Greenwood Press.

2. Marx, K. (1974). *Capital* (Vol. 1). New York: International, pp. 751, 759–760.

3. Foner, P. S. (1975). *History of black Americans: From Africa to the emergence of the Cotton Kingdom* (Vol. 1). Westport, CT: Greenwood Press.

4. Williams, E. (1944). *Capitalism and slavery.* New York: Capricorn Books, pp. 98–102.

5. Stanton, W. (1960). *The leopard's spots: Scientific attitudes toward race in America, 1815–1859.* Chicago: University of Chicago Press.

6. Fisher, W. (1968). Physicians and slavery in the antebellum Southern Medical Journal. *J Hist Med Allied Sci, 23*(1), 36–49.

7. Starr, P. (1982). *The transformation of American medicine.* New York: Basic Books.

8. Grob, G. (1976). Edward Jarvis and the federal census. *Bull Hist Med, 50,* 4–27.

9. Pendleton, E. M. (1849). Statistics of diseases of Hancock County. *South Med Surg J,* n.s. *5,* 647–654.

10. Emerson, G. (1831). Medical statistics: Consisting of estimates relating to the population of Philadelphia. *Am J Med Sci, 9,* 3–46.

11. Coates, B. (1844). On the effect of secluded and gloomy imprisonment on individuals of the African variety of mankind. *NY J Med, 4,* 91–95.

12. Caucasian and Negro races. (1844). *Boston Med Surg J, 30,* 244–245.

13. Caldwell, C. (1831). An essay on the nature and sources of the malaria or noxious miasma. *Am J Med Sci, 16,* 249–340.

14. Simmons, T. Y. (1831). Remarks on the climate of the lower country of South Carolina. *Am J Med Sci, 9,* 256–257.

15. Monnet, J. W. (1831). Epidemic yellow fever of Washington, Miss. *Am J Med Sci, 9,* 243–245.

16. Rossignol, H. (1848). Statistics of the mortality in Augusta, Georgia from 1839 to 1840. *South Med Surg J,* n.s. *4,* 658–663.

17. Drake, D. (1845). Diseases of the Negro populations. *South Med Surg J, 1,* 341–342.

18. Swados, F. (1941). Negro health on the antebellum plantations. *Bull Hist Med, 10*(3), 460–472.

19. Savitt, T. L. (1978). *Medicine and slavery: The diseases and health care of blacks in antebellum Virginia.* Urbana: University of Illinois Free Press.

20. Ackerknecht, E. H. (1948). Anticontagionism between 1821 and 1867. *Bull Hist Med, 22*(5), 562–593.

21. Nott, J. C. (1843). The mulatto a hybrid—Probable extermination of the two races if the whites and blacks are allowed to intermarry. *Boston Med Surg J, 26*(2), 29–32.

22. Deutsch, A. (1944). The first U.S. Census of the insane (1840) and its use as pro-slavery propaganda. *Bull Hist Med, 15,* 469–482.

23. Forry, S. (1843). Vital statistics by the Sixth Census of the United States, bearing upon the question of the unity of the human race. *NY J Med, 1,* 151–167.

24. Forry, S. (1844). On the relative proportion of centenarians, of deaf and dumb, of blind, and of insane, in the races of European and African origin, as shown by the Census of the United States. *NY J Med, 2,* 310–320.

25. Jarvis, E. (1844). Insanity among the coloured population of the free states. *Am J Med Sci, 7*(14), 71–83.

26. Cartwright, S. A. (1851). The diseases and physical peculiarities of the Negro race. *New Orleans Med Surg J, 8,* 187–194.

27. Foner, P. S. (1983). *History of black Americans: From the Compromise of 1850 to the end of the Civil War* (Vol. 3). Westport, CT: Greenwood Press.

28. Cartwright, S. A. (1850). Report on the diseases and physical peculiarities of the Negro race. *New Orleans Med Surg J, 7,* 691–715.

29. Smith, J. T. (1851). Review of Dr. Cartwright's report on the diseases and physical peculiarities of the Negro race. *New Orleans Med Surg J, 8,* 228–237.

30. *Charleston Med J,* (1851), *6,* 829–843.

31. *Charleston Med J,* (1852), *7,* 89–98.

32. Cartwright, S. A. (1853). Alcohol and the Ethiopian; Or, the moral and physical effects of ardent spirits on the Negro race, and some accounts of the peculiarities of that people. *New Orleans Med Surg J, 10,* 150–165.

33. Cartwright, S. A. (1858). Ethnology of the Negro or prognathous race: A lecture delivered November 30, 1857, before the New Orleans Academy of Science. *New Orleans Med Surg J, 15,* 149–163.

34. Cartwright, S. A. (1855). Remarks on dysentery among Negroes. *New Orleans Med Surg J, 11,* 145–163.

35. Wooten, H. S. (1855). Dysentery among Negroes. *New Orleans Med Surg J, 11,* 448–456.

36. Grier, S. L. (1853). The Negro and his diseases. *New Orleans Med Surg J, 9,* 752–763.

37. King, J. W. (1853). Review of J. C. Nott's "Geographical distribution of animals and the races of men." *South J Med Physical Sci, 1,* 366–370.

38. Ramsey, H. A. (1853). Letter to Dr. James Bryon on the Southern Negro. *South J Med Physical Sci, 1,* 301–302.

39. Nott, J. C. (1857). Acclimation; or, the comparative influence of climate, endemic and epidemic diseases, on the races of men. In J. C. Nott & G. Gliddon (Eds.), *Indigenous races of the earth; or new chapters of ethnological enquiry* (pp. 353–401). Philadelphia: Lippincott.

40. Editors. (1857). Indigenous races of the earth. *New Orleans Med Surg J, 14,* 138–142.

41. Editors. (1857). Indigenous races of the earth. *Charleston Med J, 12,* 650–653.

42. H. H. (Editors). (1857). Indigenous races of the earth. *Am J Med Sci, 34*(68), 468–470.

43. Levesque, G. A. (1980). Boston's black Brahmin: Dr. John S. Rock. *Civil War Hist, 54*(4), 326–346.

44. Link, E. P. (1967). The civil rights activities of three great Negro physicians (1840–1940). *J Negro Hist, 52*(3), 169–184.

45. Smith, J. M. (1859). On the fourteenth query of Thomas Jefferson's notes on Virginia. *The Anglo-African Magazine, 1*(8), 225–238.

46. Marx, K. Die Presse (Nov. 7, 1861/1971). In K. Marx & F. Engels, *The Civil War in the United States.* New York: International.

47. Zinn, H. (1980). *A people's history of the United States.* New York: Harper Colophon Books.

48. Gibb, G. (1865). The larynx of the Negro. *Chicago Med Examiner, 6,* 183–185.

49. Bryon, J. (1863). Negro regiments—Department of Tennessee. *Boston Med Surg J, 69*(1), 43–44.

50. Reyburn, R. (1866). Remarks concerning some of the diseases prevailing among the freedpeople in the District of Columbia (Bureau of Refugees, Freedmen and Abandoned Lands). *Am J Med Sci,* n.s. *51*(102), 364–369.

51. Half-yearly abstract. (1865). *Am J Med Sci,* n.s. *50,* 560.

52. Howe, S. G. (1863). The colored population: Mulattoes, etc. *Chicago Med J, 20,* 478–479.

53. Nott, J. C. (1866). Instincts of the races. *New Orleans Med Surg J, 19,* 1–16, 148–156.

54. Haller, J. S. (1970). The physician versus the Negro: Medical and anthropological concepts of race in the late nineteenth century. *Bull Hist Med, 44*(2), 154–167.

55. Kuper, L. (1975). Introduction. In L. Kuper (Ed.), *Race, science and society* (pp. 14–28). Paris: UNESCO Press.

56. U.S. Department of Health and Human Services. (1985). *Report of the Secretary's Task Force on Black and Minority Health: Vol. 1. Executive summary.* Washington, DC: U.S. Government Printing Office.

CHAPTER THREE

Under the Shadow of Tuskegee

African Americans
and Health Care

Vanessa Northington Gamble

O n May 16, 1997, in a White House ceremony, President Bill Clinton apologized for the Tuskegee Syphilis Study, the forty-year government study (1932 to 1972) in which 399 black men from Macon County, Alabama, were deliberately denied effective treatment for syphilis in order to document the natural history of the disease.[1] "The legacy of the study at Tuskegee," the president remarked, "has reached far and deep, in ways that hurt our progress and divide our nation. We cannot be one America when a whole segment of our nation has no trust in America."[2] The president's comments underscore that in the twenty-five years since its public disclosure, the study has moved from being a singular historical event to a powerful metaphor. It has come to symbolize racism in medicine, misconduct in human research, the arrogance of physicians, and government abuse of black people.

The continuing shadow cast by the Tuskegee Syphilis Study on efforts to improve the health status of black Americans provided an impetus for the campaign for a presidential apology.[3] Numerous articles, in both the professional and popular press, have pointed out that the study predisposed many African Americans to distrust medical and public health authorities and has led to critically low black participation in clinical trials and organ donation.[4-16]

The specter of Tuskegee has also been raised with respect to HIV/AIDS prevention and treatment programs. Health education researchers Dr. Stephen B. Thomas and Dr. Sandra Crouse Quinn have written extensively on the impact of the Tuskegee Syphilis Study on these programs.[17-19] They argue that "the legacy of this experiment, with its failure to educate the study participants and treat them adequately, laid the foundation for today's pervasive sense of black distrust of public health authorities" (p. 83).[19] The syphilis study has also been used to explain why many African Americans oppose needle exchange programs. Needle exchange programs provoke the image of the syphilis study and black fears about genocide. These programs are not viewed as mechanisms to stop the spread of HIV/AIDS but rather as fodder for the drug epidemic that has devastated so many black neighborhoods.[18,20] Fears that they will be used as guinea pigs like the men in the syphilis study have also led some African Americans with AIDS to refuse treatment with protease inhibitors.[21]

The Tuskegee Syphilis Study is frequently described as the singular reason behind African American distrust of the institutions of medicine and public health. Such an interpretation neglects a critical historical point: the mistrust predated public revelations about the Tuskegee study. Furthermore, the narrowness of such a representation places emphasis on a single historical event to explain deeply entrenched and complex attitudes within the black community. An examination of the syphilis study within a broader historical and social context makes plain that several factors have influenced, and continue to influence, African Americans' attitudes toward the biomedical community.

Black Americans' fears about exploitation by the medical profession date back to the antebellum period and the use of slaves and free black people as subjects for dissection and medical experimentation.[22,23] Although physicians also used poor whites as subjects, they used black people far more often. During an 1835 trip to the United States, French visitor Harriet Martineau found that black people lacked the power even to protect the graves of their dead. "In Baltimore the bodies of coloured people exclusively are taken for dissection," she remarked, "because the Whites do not like it, and the coloured people cannot resist."[24] Four years later, abolitionist Theodore Dwight Weld echoed Martineau's sentiment. "Public opinion," he wrote, "would tolerate surgical experiments, operations, processes, performed upon them [slaves], which it would execrate if performed upon their master or other whites."[25] Slaves found themselves as subjects of medical experiments because physicians needed bodies and because the state considered them property and denied them the legal right to refuse to participate.

Two antebellum experiments, one carried out in Georgia and the other in Alabama, illustrate the abuse that some slaves encountered at the hands of physicians. In the first, Georgia physician Thomas Hamilton conducted a series of brutal experiments on a slave to test remedies for heatstroke. The subject of these investigations, Fed, had been loaned to Hamilton as repayment for a debt owed by his owner. Hamilton forced Fed to sit naked on a stool placed on a platform in a pit that had been heated to a high temperature. Only the man's head was above ground. Over a period of two to three weeks, Hamilton placed Fed in the pit five or six times and gave him various medications to determine which enabled him best to withstand the heat. Each ordeal ended when Fed fainted and had to be revived. But note that Fed was not the only victim in this experiment; its whole purpose was to make it possible for masters to force slaves to work still longer hours on the hottest of days.[26]

In the second experiment, Dr. J. Marion Sims, the so-called father of modern gynecology, used three Alabama slave women to develop an operation to repair vesicovaginal fistulas. Between 1845 and 1849, the three slave women on whom Sims operated each underwent up to thirty painful operations. The physician himself described the agony associated with some of the experiments: "The first patient I operated on was Lucy. . . . That was before the days of anaesthetics, and the poor girl, on her knees, bore the operation with great heroism and bravery." This operation was not successful, and Sims later attempted to repair the defect by placing a sponge in the bladder. This experiment, too, ended in failure. He noted:

> The whole urethra and the neck of the bladder were in a high state of inflammation, which came from the foreign substance. It had to come away, and there was nothing to do but to pull it away by main force. Lucy's agony was extreme. She was much prostrated, and I thought that she was going to die; but by irrigating the parts of the bladder she recovered with great rapidity [pp. 236–237].[27]

Sims finally did perfect his technique and ultimately repaired the fistulas. Only after his experimentation with the slave women proved successful did the physician attempt the procedure, with anesthesia, on white women volunteers.

EXPLOITATION AFTER THE CIVIL WAR

It is not known to what extent African Americans continued to be used as unwilling subjects for experimentation and dissection in the years after emancipation. However, an examination of African American folklore at the turn of the century makes it clear that black people believed that such practices persisted. Folktales are replete with references to night doctors, also called student doctors and Ku Klux doctors. In her book, *Night Riders in Black Folk History,* anthropologist Gladys-Marie Fry writes, "The term 'night doctor' (derived from the fact that victims were sought only at night) applies both to students of medicine, who supposedly stole cadavers from which to learn about body processes, and [to] professional thieves, who sold stolen bodies—living and dead—to physicians for medical research" (p. 171).[28] According to folk belief, these sinister characters would kidnap black people, usually at night and in urban areas, and take them to hospitals to be killed and used in experiments. An 1889 *Boston*

Herald article vividly captured the fears that African Americans in South Carolina had of night doctors. The report read, in part:

> The negroes of Clarendon, Williamsburg, and Sumter counties have for several weeks past been in a state of fear and trembling. They claim that there is a white man, a doctor, who at will can make himself invisible, and who then approaches some unsuspecting darkey, and having rendered him or her insensible with chloroform, proceeds to fill up a bucket with the victim's blood, for the purpose of making medicine. After having drained the last drop of blood from the victim, the body is dumped into some secret place where it is impossible for any person to find it. The colored women are so worked up over this phantom that they will not venture out at night, or in the daytime in any sequestered place [p. 285].[29]

Fry did not find any documented evidence of the existence of night riders. However, she demonstrated through extensive interviews that many African Americans expressed genuine fears that they would be kidnapped by night doctors and used for medical experimentation. Fry concludes that two factors explain this paradox. She argues that whites, especially those in the rural South, deliberately spread rumors about night doctors in order to maintain psychological control over blacks and to discourage their migration to the North so as to maintain a source of cheap labor. In addition, Fry asserts that the experiences of many African Americans as victims of medical experiments during slavery fostered their belief in the existence of night doctors (p. 210).[29] It should also be added that, given the nation's racial and political climate, black people recognized their inability to refuse to participate in medical experiments.

Reports about the medical exploitation of black people in the name of medicine after the end of the Civil War were not restricted to the realm of folklore. Until it was exposed in 1882, a grave robbing ring operated in Philadelphia and provided bodies for the city's medical schools by plundering the graves at a black cemetery. According to historian David C. Humphrey, southern grave robbers regularly sent bodies of southern blacks to northern medical schools for use as anatomy cadavers (pp. 822–823).[23]

During the early twentieth century, African American medical leaders protested the abuse of black people by the white-dominated medical profession and used their concerns about experimentation to press for the establishment of black-controlled hospitals.* Dr. Daniel Hale Williams, the founder of Chicago's Provident Hospital (1891), the nation's first black-controlled hospital, contended that white physicians, especially in the South, frequently used black

---

*A detailed examination of the campaign to establish black hospitals can be found in Gamble, V. N. (1995). *Making a place for ourselves: The black hospital movement, 1920–1945.* New York: Oxford University Press.

patients as guinea pigs (p. 177).[30] Dr. Nathan Francis Mossell, who graduated, with honors, from Penn in 1882 and was the founder of Philadelphia's Frederick Douglass Memorial Hospital (1895), described the "fears and prejudices" of black people, especially those from the South, as "almost proverbial." He attributed such attitudes to southern medical practices in which black people, "when forced to accept hospital attention, got only the poorest care, being placed in inferior wards set apart for them, suffering the brunt of all that is experimental in treatment, and all this is the sequence of their race variety and abject helplessness" (p. 17).[31] The founders of black hospitals claimed that only black physicians possessed the skills required to treat black patients optimally and that black hospitals provided these patients with the best possible care (pp. 4–5).[32]

Fears about the exploitation of African Americans by white physicians played a role in the establishment of a black veterans hospital in Tuskegee, Alabama. In 1923, nine years before the initiation of the Tuskegee Syphilis Study, racial tensions had erupted in the town over control of the hospital. The federal government had pledged that the facility, an institution designed exclusively for black patients, would be run by a black professional staff. But many whites in the area, including members of the Ku Klux Klan, did not want a black-operated federal facility in the heart of Dixie, even though it would serve only black people.[†]

Black Americans sought control of the veterans hospital, in part because they believed that the ex-soldiers would receive the best possible care from black physicians and nurses, who would be more caring and sympathetic to the veterans' needs. Some black newspapers even warned that white southerners wanted command of the hospital as part of a racist plot to kill and sterilize African American men and to establish an "experiment station" for mediocre white physicians.[33] Black physicians did eventually gain the right to operate the hospital, yet this did not stop the hospital from becoming an experiment station for black men. The veterans hospital was one of the facilities used by the U.S. Public Health Service in the syphilis study.

During the 1920s and 1930s, black physicians pushed for additional measures that would battle medical racism and advance their professional needs. Dr. Charles Garvin, a prominent Cleveland physician and a member of the editorial board of the black medical publication *The Journal of the National Medical*

[†]For in-depth discussions of the history of the Tuskegee Veterans Hospital, see Gamble, *Making a place for ourselves*, pp. 70–104; Daniel, P. (1970). Black power in the 1920s: The case of Tuskegee Veterans Hospital. *J Southern Hist, 36,* 368–388; and Wolters, R. (1975). *The new Negro on campus: Black college rebellions of the 1920s.* Princeton, NJ: Princeton University Press, pp. 137–191.

Association, urged his colleagues to engage in research in order to protect black patients. He called for more research on diseases such as tuberculosis and pellagra that allegedly affected African Americans disproportionately or idiosyncratically. Garvin insisted that black physicians investigate these racial diseases because "heretofore in literature, as in medicine, the Negro has been written about, exploited and experimented upon sometimes not to his physical betterment or to the advancement of science, but the advancement of the Nordic investigator." Moreover, he charged that "in the past, men of other races have for the large part interpreted our diseases, often tinctured with inborn prejudices."[34]

FEARS OF GENOCIDE

These historical examples clearly demonstrate that African Americans' distrust of the medical profession has a longer history than the public revelations of the Tuskegee Syphilis Study. There is a collective memory among African Americans about their exploitation by the medical establishment. The Tuskegee Syphilis Study has emerged as the most prominent example of medical racism because it confirms, if not authenticates, long-held and deeply entrenched beliefs within the black community. To be sure, the Tuskegee Syphilis Study does cast a long shadow. After the study had been exposed, charges surfaced that the experiment was part of a governmental plot to exterminate black people.[35,36] Many black people agreed with the charge that the study represented "nothing less than an official, premeditated policy of genocide" (p. 12).[1] Furthermore, this was not the first or last time that allegations of genocide have been launched against the government and the medical profession. The sickle cell anemia screening programs of the 1970s and birth control programs have also provoked such allegations.[37–39]

In recent years, links have been made between Tuskegee, AIDS, and genocide. In September 1990, the article "AIDS: Is It Genocide?" appeared in *Essence,* a black woman's magazine. The author noted: "As an increasing number of African-Americans continue to sicken and die and as no cure for AIDS has been found some of us are beginning to think the unthinkable: Could AIDS be a virus that was manufactured to erase large numbers of us? Are they trying to kill us with this disease?" (p. 76).[40] In other words, some members of the black community see AIDS as part of a conspiracy to exterminate African Americans.

Beliefs about the connection between AIDS and the purposeful destruction of African Americans should not be cavalierly dismissed as bizarre and paranoid. They are held by a significant number of black people. For example, a 1990 survey conducted by the Southern Christian Leadership Conference found that 35 percent of the 1,056 black church members who responded believed that

AIDS was a form of genocide (p. 1499).[17] A *New York Times*–WCBS TV News poll conducted the same year found that 10 percent of black Americans thought that the AIDS virus had been created in a laboratory in order to infect black people. Another 20 percent believed that it could be true (p. A22).[41]

African Americans frequently point to the Tuskegee Syphilis Study as evidence to support their views about genocide, perhaps, in part, because many believe that the men in the study were actually injected with syphilis. Harlon Dalton, a Yale Law School professor and a former member of the National Commission on AIDS, wrote, in a 1989 article titled "AIDS in Black Face," that "the government [had] purposefully exposed Black men to syphilis" (pp. 220–221).[42] Six years later, Dr. Eleanor Walker, a Detroit radiation oncologist, offered an explanation as to why few African Americans become bone marrow donors. "The biggest fear," she claimed, "is that they will become victims of some misfeasance, like the Tuskegee incident where Black men were infected with syphilis and left untreated to die from the disease."[43] The January 25, 1996, episode of *New York Undercover,* a Fox Network police drama that is one of the top shows in black households, also reinforced the rumor that the U.S. Public Health Service physicians injected the men with syphilis.‡ The myth about deliberate infection is not limited to the black community. On April 8, 1997, news anchor Tom Brokaw, on *NBC Nightly News,* announced that the men had been infected by the government.[44]

Folklorist Patricia A. Turner, in her book *I Heard It Through the Grapevine: Rumor in African-American Culture,* underscores why it is important not to ridicule but to pay attention to these strongly held theories about genocide.[45] She argues that these rumors reveal much about what African Americans believe to be the state of their lives in this country. She contends that such views reflect black beliefs that white Americans have historically been, and continue to be, ambivalent and perhaps hostile to the existence of black people. Consequently, African American attitudes toward biomedical research are not influenced solely by the Tuskegee Syphilis Study. African Americans' opinions about the value white society has attached to their lives should not be discounted. As Reverend Floyd Tompkins of Stanford University Memorial Church has said, "There is a sense in our community, and I think it shall be proved out, that if you are poor or you're a person of color, you were the guinea pig, and you continue to be the guinea pigs, and there is the fundamental belief that Black life is not valued like White life or like any other life in America."[46]

---

‡From September 1995 to December 1995, *New York Undercover* was the top-ranked show in black households. It ranked 122nd in white households. Zurawik, D. (1996, May 14). Poll: TV's race gap growing. *Madison (Wisconsin) Capital Times,* p. 5D.

NOT JUST PARANOIA

Lorene Cary, in a cogent essay in *Newsweek,* expands on Reverend Tompkins's point. In an essay titled "Why It's Not Just Paranoia," she writes:

> We Americans continue to value the lives and humanity of some groups more than the lives and humanity of others. That is not paranoia. It is our historical legacy and a present fact; it influences domestic and foreign policy and the daily interaction of millions of Americans. It influences the way we spend our public money and explains how we can read the staggering statistics on black Americans' infant mortality, youth mortality, mortality in middle and old age, and not be moved to action [p. 23].[47]

African Americans' beliefs that their lives are devalued by white society also influence their relationships with the medical profession. They perceive, at times correctly, that they are treated differently in the health care system solely because of their race, and such perceptions fuel mistrust of the medical profession. For example, a national telephone survey conducted in 1986 revealed that African Americans were more likely than whites to report that their physicians did not inquire sufficiently about their pain, did not tell them how long it would take for prescribed medicine to work, did not explain the seriousness of their illness or injury, and did not discuss test and examination findings.[48] A 1994 study published in the *American Journal of Public Health* found that physicians were less likely to give pregnant black women information about the hazards of smoking and drinking during pregnancy.[49]

The powerful legacy of the Tuskegee Syphilis Study endures, in part, because the racism and disrespect for black lives that it entailed mirror black people's contemporary experiences with the medical profession. The anger and frustration that many African Americans feel when they encounter the health care system can be heard in the words of Alicia Georges, a professor of nursing at Lehman College and a former president of the National Black Nurses Association, as she recalled an emergency room experience. "Back a few years ago, I was having excruciating abdominal pain, and I wound up at a hospital in my area," she recalled. "The first thing that they began to ask me was how many sexual partners I'd had. I was married and owned my own house. But immediately, in looking at me, they said, 'Oh, she just has pelvic inflammatory disease'" (p. 52).[50] Perhaps because of her nursing background, Georges recognized the implications of the questioning. She had come face to face with the stereotype of black women as sexually promiscuous. Similarly, the following story from the *Los Angeles Times* shows how racism can affect the practice of medicine:

> When Althea Alexander broke her arm, the attending resident at Los Angeles County-USC Medical Center told her to "hold your arm like you usually hold

your can of beer on Saturday night." Alexander who is black, exploded. "What are you talking about? Do you think I'm a welfare mother?" The white resident shrugged: "Well aren't you?" Turned out she was an administrator at USC medical school.[51]

This example graphically illustrates that health care providers are not immune to the beliefs and misconceptions of the wider community. They carry with them stereotypes about various groups of people.

BEYOND TUSKEGEE

There is also a growing body of medical research that vividly illustrates why discussions of the relationship of African Americans and the medical profession must go beyond the Tuskegee Syphilis Study. These studies demonstrate racial inequities in access to particular technologies and raise critical questions about the role of racism in medical decision making. For example, in 1989, *The Journal of the American Medical Association* published a report that demonstrated racial inequities in the treatment of heart disease. In this study, white and black patients had similar rates of hospitalization for chest pain, but the white patients were one-third more likely to undergo coronary angiography and more than twice as likely to be treated with bypass surgery or angioplasty. The racial disparities persisted even after adjustments were made for differences in income.[52] Three years later, another study appearing in that journal reinforced these findings. It revealed that older black patients on Medicare received coronary artery bypass grafts only about a fourth as often as comparable white patients. Disparities were greatest in the rural South, where white patients had the surgery seven times as often as black patients. Medical factors did not fully explain the differences. This study suggests that an already existing national health insurance program does not solve the access problems of African Americans.[53] Additional studies have confirmed the persistence of such inequities.[54-58]

Why the racial disparities? Possible explanations include health problems that precluded the use of procedures, patient unwillingness to accept medical advice or to undergo surgery, and differences in severity of illness. However, the role of racial bias cannot be discounted, as the American Medical Association's Council on Ethical and Judicial Affairs has recognized. In a 1990 report on black–white disparities in health care, the council asserted:

> Because racial disparities may be occurring despite the lack of any intent or purposeful efforts to treat patients differently on the basis of race, physicians should examine their own practices to ensure that inappropriate considerations do not affect their clinical judgment. In addition, the profession should help increase the awareness of its members of racial disparities in medical treatment decisions by engaging in open and broad discussions about the issue. Such

discussions should take place as part of the medical school curriculum, in medical journals, at professional conferences, and as part of professional peer review activities [p. 2346].[59]

The council's recommendation is a strong acknowledgment that racism can influence the practice of medicine.

After the public disclosures of the Tuskegee Syphilis Study, Congress passed the National Research Act of 1974. This act, established to protect subjects in human experimentation, mandates institutional review board approval of all federally funded research with human subjects. However, recent revelations about a measles vaccine study financed by the Centers for Disease Control and Prevention (CDC) demonstrate the inadequacies of these safeguards and illustrate why African Americans' historically based fears of medical research persist. In 1989, in the midst of a measles epidemic in Los Angeles, the CDC, in collaboration with Kaiser Permanente and the Los Angeles County Health Department, began a study to test whether the experimental Edmonston–Zagreb vaccine could be used to immunize children too young for the standard Moraten vaccine. By 1991, approximately 900 infants, mostly black and Latino, had received the vaccine without difficulties. (Apparently, 1 infant died for reasons not related to the inoculations.) But the infants' parents had not been informed that the vaccine was not licensed in the United States or that it had been associated with an increase in death rates in Africa. The 1996 disclosure of the study prompted charges of medical racism and of the continued exploitation of minority communities by medical professionals.[60,61]

The Tuskegee Syphilis Study continues to cast its shadow over the lives of African Americans. For many black people, it has come to represent the racism that pervades American institutions and the disdain in which black lives are often held. But despite its significance, it cannot be the only prism we use to examine the relationship of African Americans with the medical and public health communities. The problem we must face is not just the shadow of Tuskegee but the shadow of racism that so profoundly affects the lives and beliefs of all people in this country.

Notes

1. The most comprehensive history of the study is Jones, J. H. (1993). *Bad blood* (expanded ed.). New York: Free Press.

2. Remarks by the president in apology for study done in Tuskegee (Press release). (1997, May 16). The White House, Office of the Press Secretary.

3. *Final report of the Tuskegee Syphilis Study Legacy Committee.* (1996, May 20). Vanessa Northington Gamble, chair, and John C. Fletcher, cochair.

4. Gamble, V. N. (1993). A legacy of distrust: African Americans and medical research. *Am J Prev Med, 9,* 35–38.

5. Roan, S. (1994, November, 1). A medical imbalance. *Los Angeles Times*.

6. Stevens, C. (1995, December 10). Research: Distrust runs deep; Medical community seeks solution. *Detroit News*.

7. Kadaba, L. S. (1993, September 13). Minorities in research. *Chicago Tribune*.

8. Steinbrook, R. (1989, September 25). AIDS trials shortchange minorities and drug users. *Los Angeles Times*.

9. Smith, M. D. (1991). Zidovudine: Does it work for everyone? *JAMA, 266,* 2750–2751.

10. Lyles, C. (1994, August 15). Blacks hesitant to donate; Cultural beliefs, misinformation, mistrust make it a difficult decision. *Virginian-Pilot*.

11. Wong, J. (1993, February 17). Mistrust leaves some blacks reluctant to donate organs. *Sacramento Bee*.

12. ABC News. (1994, April 6). *Nightline*.

13. Gaines, P. (1994, April 10). Armed with the truth in a fight for lives. *Washington Post*.

14. Henry, F. (1994, April 23). Encouraging organ donation from blacks. *Cleveland Plain Dealer*.

15. Swanson, G. M., & Ward, A. J. (1995). Recruiting minorities into clinical trials: Toward a participant-friendly system. *J Natl Cancer Inst, 87,* 1747–1759.

16. Wickham, D. (1997, May 21). Why blacks are wary of white MDs. *The Tennessean*, p. 13A.

17. Thomas, S. B., & Quinn, S. C. (1991). The Tuskegee Syphilis Study, 1932 to 1972: Implications for HIV education and AIDS risk education programs in the black community. *Am J Public Health, 81,* 1498–1505.

18. Thomas, S. B., & Quinn, S. C. (1993). Understanding the attitudes of black Americans. In J. Stryker & M. D. Smith (Eds.), *Dimensions of HIV prevention. Needle exchange* (pp. 99–128). Menlo Park, CA: Henry J. Kaiser Family Foundation.

19. Thomas, S. B., & Quinn, S. C. (1994). The AIDS epidemic and the African-American community: Toward an ethical framework for service delivery. In A. Dula & S. Goering (Eds.), *"It just ain't fair": The ethics of health care for African Americans* (pp. 75–88). Westport, CT: Praeger.

20. David L., Kirp, D. L., & Bayer, R. (1993, July). Needles and races. *Atlantic*, pp. 38–42.

21. Richardson, L. (1997, April 21). An old experiment's legacy: Distrust of AIDS treatment. *New York Times*, pp. A1, A7.

22. Savitt, T. L. (1982). The use of blacks for medical experimentation and demonstration in the old South. *J South Hist, 48,* 331–348.

23. Humphrey, D. C. (1973). Dissection and discrimination: The social origins of cadavers in America, 1760–1915. *Bull N Y Acad Med, 49,* 819–827.

24. Martineau, H. (1838). *Retrospect of western travel* (Vol. 1). London: Saunders & Ottley; New York: Harpers and Brothers, p. 140, quoted in Humphrey (n. 23), p. 819.

25. Weld, T. D. (1839). *American slavery as it is: Testimony of a thousand witnesses.* New York: American Anti-Slavery Society, p. 170, quoted in Savitt (n. 22), p. 341.

26. Boney, F. N. (1967). Doctor Thomas Hamilton: Two views of a gentleman of the old South. *Phylon, 28,* 288–292.

27. Sims, J. M. (1889). *The story of my life.* New York: Appleton.

28. Fry, G.-M. (1984). *Night riders in black folk history.* Knoxville: University of Tennessee Press.

29. Concerning Negro sorcery in the United States. (1890). *J Am Folk-Lore, 3.*

30. Link, E. P. (1969, July). The civil rights activities of three great Negro physicians (1840–1940). *J Negro Hist, 52.*

31. *Seventh annual report of the Frederick Douglass Memorial Hospital and Training School.* (1902). Philadelphia.

32. Green, H. M. (n.d., c. 1930). *A more or less critical review of the hospital situation among Negroes in the United States.*

33. Klan halts march on Tuskegee. (1923, August 4). *Chicago Defender.*

34. Garvin, C. H. (n.d.). The "New Negro" physician. Unpublished manuscript, box 1, Charles H. Garvin Papers, Western Reserve Historical Society Library, Cleveland, Ohio.

35. Taylor, R. A. (1991, December 10). Conspiracy theories widely accepted in U.S. black circles. *Washington Times,* p. A1.

36. Welsing, F. C. (1991). *The Isis papers: The keys to the colors.* Chicago: Third World Press, pp. 298–299. Although she is not very well known outside of the African American community, Welsing, a physician, is a popular figure within it. *The Isis Papers* headed for several weeks the best-seller list maintained by black bookstores.

37. Weisbord, R. G. (1973). Birth control and the black American: A matter of genocide? *Demography, 10,* 571–590.

38. Jones, A. S. (1990, December 23). Editorial linking blacks, contraceptives stirs debate at Philadelphia paper. *Arizona Daily Star,* p. F4.

39. Wilkinson, D. Y. (1974). For whose benefit? Politics and sickle cell. *The Black Scholar, 5,* 26–31.

40. Bates, K. G. (1990, September). AIDS: Is it genocide? *Essence, 76.*

41. The AIDS "plot" against blacks. (1992, May 12). *New York Times.*

42. Dalton, H. L. (1989, Summer). AIDS in blackface. *Daedalus, 118.*

43. Bates-Rudd, R. (1995, December 7). State campaign encourages African Americans to offer others gift of bone marrow. *Detroit News.*

44. *NBC Nightly News* (Transcript). (1997, April 8).

45. Turner, P. A. (1993). *I heard it through the grapevine: Rumor in African-American culture.* Berkeley: University of California Press.

46. National Public Radio. (1994, March 13). Fear creates lack of donor organs among blacks. *Weekend Edition.*

47. Cary, L. (1992, April 6). Why it's not just paranoia: An American history of "plans" for blacks. *Newsweek.*

48. Blendon, R. J. (1989). Access to medical care for black and white Americans: A matter of continuing concern. *JAMA, 261,* 278–281.

49. Rogan, M. D., et al. (1994). Racial disparities in reported prenatal care advice from health care providers. *Am J Public Health, 84,* 82–88.

50. Johnson, J., et al. (1991, September 16). Why do blacks die young? *Time.*

51. Nazario, S. (1990, December 20). Treating doctors for prejudice: Medical schools are trying to sensitize students to "bedside bias." *Los Angeles Times.*

52. Wenneker, M. B., & Epstein, A. M. (1989). Racial inequities in the use of procedures for patients with ischemic heart disease in Massachusetts. *JAMA, 261,* 253–257.

53. Goldberg, K. C., et al. (1992). Racial and community factors influencing coronary artery bypass graft surgery rates for all 1986 Medicare patients. *JAMA, 267,* 1473–1477.

54. Ayanian, J. D. (1993). Heart disease in black and white. *N Engl J Med, 329,* 656–658

55. Whittle, J., et al. (1993). Racial differences in the use of invasive cardiovascular procedures in the Department of Veterans Affairs medical system. *N Engl J Med, 329,* 621–627.

56. Peterson, E. D., et al. (1994). Racial variation in cardiac procedure use and survival following acute myocardial infarction in the Department of Veterans Affairs. *JAMA, 271,* 1175–1180.

57. Horner, R. D., et al. (1995). Theories explaining racial differences in the utilization of diagnostic and therapeutic procedures for cerebrovascular disease. *Milbank Q, 73,* 443–462.

58. Moore, R. D., et al. (1994). Racial differences in the use of drug therapy for HIV disease in an urban community. *N Engl J Med, 350,* 763–768.

59. Council on Ethical and Judicial Affairs. (1990). Black-white disparities in health care. *JAMA, 263,* 2346.

60. Cimons, M. (1996, June 17). CDC says it erred in measles study. *Los Angeles Times,* p. A11.

61. Glenn, B. (1996, July 21). Bad blood once again. *St. Petersburg Times,* p. 5D.

CHAPTER FOUR

Latino Outlook

Good Health, Uncertain Prognosis

William A. Vega
Hortensia Amaro

This article presents a profile of the health status of Hispanic (Latino) populations in the United States. The review is issue oriented and identifies those factors that have a continuing influence on Hispanic health. Heterogeneity is perhaps the most salient characteristic that defines Hispanic populations of the United States. Hispanic populations include native born, migrant, and immigrant peoples with distinctive national origins and regional settlement patterns.[85] This multigenerational migratory and social adjustment process has produced important cultural variations within and among the respective Hispanic ethnic groups. Moreover, the demographic structure of Hispanic populations is also varied and complex.[7] These historical, demographic, and sociocultural features shape the health and disease experience of Hispanics. Logically, respective Hispanic ethnic groups can be expected to vary in health status and to have differing needs for health services.

This review provides a demographic comparison of Hispanic ethnic groups in the United States, an assessment of health status for the largest Hispanic groups, a brief summary of services utilization issues, and a discussion of health promotion and disease prevention. Framing the overall presentation is a controversial issue that deserves careful consideration. Historically, the absence of comprehensive epidemiologic information on Hispanic morbidity and mortality resulted in lumping Hispanics into a larger social category of "minorities." Presumably, since Hispanics were exposed to similar underclass social conditions as other minorities, especially African Americans, generalizations derived from minority health profiles could be extended to cover Hispanics as well. However, the advent of dedicated studies on Hispanic health has demonstrated that some Hispanic groups diverge very significantly from the classic minority morbidity or mortality profiles. The reasons for these differences are not well understood. However, a number of researchers and Hispanic health advocates have concluded that Hispanics have a more favorable health profile than would be expected from their socioeconomic and minority status, and attribute this to sociocultural characteristics of Hispanics that operate as protective factors, or to selective immigration patterns.[47] Are Hispanics a super-healthy population with differing health promotion and services needs? One goal of this review is to provide a critical summary of information pertinent to this complex question.

DEMOGRAPHIC COMPOSITION OF HISPANIC ETHNIC GROUPS

There are approximately 21 million Hispanics in the United States according to the 1990 Census,[110] with an additional 3.5 million in Puerto Rico. Between 1980 and 1990, the Hispanic population increased by 53 percent, a rate of growth eight times higher than that of the white non-Hispanic population.[112] It has been estimated that by the year 2020 Hispanics will constitute the largest minority group in the United States. The rapid rate of increase is attributable to two facts: a continuing large influx of documented and undocumented immigrants and high cumulative fertility among the largest Hispanic ethnic group—Mexican Americans.

The age-sex profile of the U.S. Hispanic population based on the 1990 Census[111] demonstrates two outstanding features. First, a larger proportion of Hispanics than white non-Hispanics is under thirty years of age. Second, the large number of twenty- to twenty-nine-year-old males produces an asymmetry in gender by age with young adult males actually outnumbering females until age forty. This reflects, in part, the increased immigration from Mexico and Central America during the 1980s, and the results of the Immigration Reform and Control Act of 1986, which granted legal residence to approximately 2.5 million formerly undocumented individuals. About 71 percent of Hispanics in the United States are native born, with 29 percent being immigrants, and about two of three Hispanics speak Spanish at home.[90]

Sociodemographic differences between Hispanic ethnic groups are apparent in the 1990 Census data. Mexican-origin Hispanics constitute the largest subgroup, 64 percent, and are the youngest, with a median age of 24.1 years, and have the lowest education and income levels (median income = $12,527 for males and $8,874 for females). Only 44.1 percent of Mexican Americans have completed high school, and 69.6 percent of all Hispanics earning below the poverty level are of Mexican origin. The most striking contrast is with

Cuban-origin Hispanics. With a median age of 39.1, they are significantly older than either the Hispanic or non-Hispanic populations. Fully 14 percent of Cuban-origin Hispanics are sixty-five years of age or older, as contrasted with only 4.9 percent of the total Hispanic population. Cubans are also twice as likely to be college educated as the total Hispanic population, 20.2 percent compared to 9.2 percent, and Cubans are much less likely to have incomes (median = $19,336 for males and $12,880 for females) below the poverty level (15.2 percent). Puerto Ricans are a comparison group of considerable interest because they are U.S. citizens and have never been immigrants. Nevertheless, their demographic characteristics most closely resemble Mexican Americans although they are more likely to have completed high school (55.5 percent) and to have a higher income (median = $18,222 for males and $12,812 for females). However, a larger proportion of Puerto Ricans (33 percent) than Mexican Americans (28.4 percent) is living below the poverty line. The aggregated Central and South American origin group is older (median age = 28 years), better educated (58.5 percent high school graduates), and slightly less likely to live below the poverty level (18.5 percent) than the total Hispanic population. As a source of comparison, the following demographic profile of white non-Hispanics is provided: median age = 33.5 years; 79.6 percent are high school graduates; median income = $22,081 (males) and $11,885 (females); 11.6 percent live below the poverty level.

The variation in female-headed households among Hispanic ethic groups is profound, with 38.9 percent of Puerto Rican households contrasting with 19.6 percent of Mexican and 18.9 percent of Cuban-origin households being female-headed. Hispanic families are larger than non-Hispanic families, with Mexican-origin families being the largest and Cuban-origin families being the smallest.

Unemployment among Hispanics is generally 40 to 60 percent higher than among white non-Hispanics and somewhat lower overall than among African Americans. Cubans have the lowest unemployment rate, 6.4 percent, whereas Puerto Rican and Mexican American levels are almost twice as high, 10.3 percent and 10.7 percent, respectively. Hispanic employment is concentrated in lower status occupations such as service workers/laborers, and least likely to be found among professionals and managers. About 73.5 percent of Hispanic men and 40.2 percent of Hispanic women, as compared with 51.4 percent of non-Hispanic men and 24.6 percent of non-Hispanic women, were employed in service, production, and laborer occupations according to the 1990 Census.

Although Hispanics are in the process of becoming a national population, their regional distribution reflects historical migration and immigration patterns. Southwestern Hispanics are predominantly of Mexican origin; in the Northeast, Puerto Ricans are more numerous; and in South Florida, Cubans are the largest subgroup. However, immigration from the Caribbean Basin area, especially the

Dominican Republic, Colombia, Guatemala, El Salvador, Honduras, and Nicaragua, has sharply increased the numbers of people immigrating from this region in the past decade into Miami, New York, Chicago, Washington D.C., Los Angeles, Houston, and other major urban centers of the United States. About nine of ten Hispanics live in urban areas, but there are proportionately and numerically more Mexican Americans than other Hispanics in rural areas, in part because of the farm-labor component of the Mexican-origin subgroup.

Gleaning the implications of this demographic profile of Hispanics is difficult because it is not a static population. Immigration from Latin America continues, and the numbers of individuals from different sending nations, as well as their ultimate destinations, cannot be predicted with precision. It is very obvious that the past decade has decreased the educational level of foreign-born Hispanics, and by extension, their earning potential as well. Previous research has shown a consistent inverse relationship between socioeconomic status and morbidity or mortality in societies throughout the world.[102] Therefore, the potential impact of low economic mobility on health among Hispanics is a serious concern. Continuing problems with communicable diseases among immigrant populations are to be expected. The disproportionate number of young males in the Hispanic population portends public health problems such as accidental death, alcohol and drug abuse, serious psychiatric disorders, sexually transmitted diseases, and increasing suicide rates. The high cumulative fertility of certain Hispanic ethnic groups has implications for reproductive health and nutrition, and the increasing size of the Hispanic population over sixty-five suggests that health issues associated with later life will receive increasing attention.

From a public health perspective, the most vexing issue is the marginal socioeconomic and educational position of the U.S. Hispanic population. There are disturbing signs of increasing intergenerational poverty, reinforced by structural problems such as poor labor market conditions and a debilitated educational infrastructure. The critical question is whether, at this historical juncture, sufficient opportunity for social and economic mobility will be available to offset Hispanic population growth, and whether Hispanic cultural strengths can operate to mitigate the negative impact of structural factors on health and on the environments where Hispanics must live.

Mortality and Morbidity Indicators of Hispanic Populations

To reiterate, the health status of Hispanics arguably presents a paradox in public health[53,77,95,123] because they have a health profile that is as good or better than that of white non-Hispanics.[26,47] The evidence to support this position is ambiguous, and so are the potential implications. Generally, the data suggest that Puerto Ricans in the continental United States have a more jeopardized health status than Mexican Americans. In turn, Mexican Americans have a more jeopardized health status than Cuban Americans. Further, variations in health status among Hispanics necessitate that health data be disaggregated by Hispanic group. Therefore, data on Hispanics as an aggregate group do not represent an accurate picture of the health status of all Hispanic ethnic groups and loose generalizations can lead to erroneous conclusions and faulty public health strategies.

Limitations of Existing Data

Before discussing the issues identified above, it is important to note some severe limitations of available data. The 1985 Secretary's Task Force on Black and Minority Health report[115] was filled with apologies regarding the lack of Hispanic health data. Almost ten years later, the *Healthy People 2000* report was not able to propose Hispanic-specific initiatives for the majority of measurable objectives due to the continued lack of baseline data. The failure of U.S. health data systems to provide information on mortality and morbidity trends for Hispanic populations was noted in a 1992 report by the General Accounting Office.[38] *Health, United States, 1991,* which provides systematic analysis of health data by race, provides extremely limited health data by Hispanic ethnicity. The most useful data on Hispanics have come from a one time cross-sectional study, the Hispanic Health and Nutrition Examination Survey, which is now ten years old. Improvement in the nation's health data systems has been slow and limited.

Most national health data systems do not provide adequate data on the health of Hispanics because (a) they do not collect appropriate and accurate data on Hispanic ethnicity; (b) they do not sample sufficiently large numbers of Hispanics; or (c) they fail to tabulate and report data separately for Hispanics. Moreover, the Council of Scientific Affairs of the American Medical Association concluded, "Accurate estimates of Hispanic death rates are impossible to determine because, until 1988, the national model death certificates did not contain Hispanic identifiers. Although some states incorporated Hispanic origin on their death certificates, such reporting was not uniform and lacks precision."[25]

The most recent mortality statistics[73] present two additional limitations. First, 1990 mortality data that are based on Hispanic-origin population from forty-six states and the District of Columbia exclude Hispanics from New York City because more than 10 percent of death certificates had inadequate data for ethnicity.[73] Although the exclusion of New York City does not seriously affect the data's coverage of the Mexican American population (99 percent covered), the Cuban American population (92 percent covered) or the Other Hispanic population (81 percent covered), the Puerto Rican population (58 percent covered) is grossly underrepresented. Further, since about half of the deaths attributed to Puerto Ricans are accounted for by New York City, the mortality rates for Hispanics overall and for Puerto Ricans in particular are underestimated.[73] This is likely to introduce an underestimation of specific causes of death that are disproportionately found in the New York City Puerto Rican population (for example, infant mortality, HIV/AIDS, tuberculosis). A second limitation of currently available death statistics is that, for Hispanics, they provide only absolute numbers of deaths and the ranking of the causes of death. Due to inadequate denominator data from the Census,[74] detailed cause-specific death rates for Hispanic subgroups have not been calculated for Hispanics since 1979–1981. Death rates for 1987–1989 have been calculated for selected causes of death and overall death rates for Hispanics.[72]

In the following sections we present data on mortality and morbidity among Hispanics. When available, data are presented for the major Hispanic groups (that is, Mexican Americans, Puerto Ricans, and Cubans). It has become increasingly important to also understand the health status and health care needs of other Hispanic populations (for example, Central and South Americans) who represent a growing sector of the Hispanic population in the United States. These data are provided when available, but these groups are often not considered in the presentation of health data.

MORTALITY

Three commonly used mortality indicators are overall death rates, disease-specific death rates, and leading causes of death. For each of these, data are first presented for Hispanics overall; whenever data are available on specific Hispanic groups, such data are presented.

Death Rates for Hispanics

The most recently available overall death rates for Hispanics reflect 1988 deaths from twenty-six states and the District of Columbia.[72] These data have been published only for Hispanics as a whole and do not provide Hispanic group breakdowns. Although these data provide relatively good coverage for the overall Hispanic population (82 percent), they provide poor coverage of the Cuban population (32 percent).[72,74] Among fifteen- to twenty-four-year-olds,[34,72] the death rate for Hispanics (113 per 100,000) is greater than that for white non-Hispanics (95 per 100,000), but lower than for non-Hispanic blacks (145 per 100,000). Similarly, among twenty-five- to forty-four-year-olds, the death rate for Hispanics (185 per 100,000), is greater than that for non-Hispanics (149 per 100,000) and lower than for non-Hispanic blacks (367 per 100,000). In the youngest age group (one to fourteen years), Hispanics have rates similar to white non-Hispanics (30 per 100,000). However, in the older age groups (forty-five to sixty-five and sixty-five years and older), Hispanics (609 per 100,000 and 3,482 per 100,000, respectively) have much lower death rates than white non-Hispanics (790 per 100,000 and 5,106 per 100,000, respectively).

Death Rates for Specific Hispanic Groups

Mortality statistics that group all Hispanics together mask important differences in health conditions that affect specific groups. The most recent available data on overall death rates by Hispanic group come from fifteen reporting states, between 1979 and 1981, which included 45 percent of the Hispanic population.[61] However, the accuracy of these data might also differ among the various Hispanic groups. The average annual age-adjusted death rates for Hispanic groups reflect significant within-group variability. They are highest among Puerto Ricans (512.4 per 100,000) compared to other Hispanic groups (Mexican = 489.4; Cuban = 345.2; Other Hispanic = 341.3). Even among Puerto Ricans, however, the rate is lower than that for white non-Hispanics (529.5) and much lower than the rate for non-Hispanic blacks (795.6).

Disease-Specific Mortality Rates

Data on specific causes of death for Hispanics as a group indicate that of thirty-eight major categories representing seventy-two selected causes of death in 1979–1980, Hispanics have higher rates for twenty major categories: tuberculosis, meningococcal infection, septicemia, viral hepatitis, syphilis, all other infectious and parasitic diseases, diabetes mellitus, nutritional deficiencies, meningitis, pneumonia and influenza, chronic liver disease and cirrhosis, cholelithiasis and other disorders of the gallbladder, nephritis, nephrotic syndrome and nephrosis, complications of pregnancy-childbirth and the puerperium, certain conditions originating in the perinatal period, all other diseases, accidents and adverse effects, homicide and legal intervention, and all other external causes.[61] More recent data from 1987–1989,[72] which provide information on Hispanic death rates for four major causes of death, show continued increasing rates among Hispanics that surpass the rate for white non-Hispanics for deaths due to accidents and adverse effects (especially among fifteen- to forty-four-year-olds) and for homicide and suicide after age fourteen. Diseases of the heart and malignant neoplasms, the two leading causes of death by far, among Hispanics between 1987 and 1989 continue to be much lower than for white non-Hispanics.[72]

When disease-specific death rates are separated out by Hispanic group, it becomes clear that the above causes of death vary in importance across Hispanic groups (see Table 4.1). The average annual age-adjusted death rates for 1979–1981 indicate that Puerto Ricans have the highest overall age-adjusted death rates among Hispanic groups, and Cubans and Other Hispanics have the lowest rates.

Data on infant mortality also demonstrate the pattern of higher death rates among Puerto Ricans (10.2) who have a higher infant mortality rate than Mexican Americans (7.7), Cubans (7.6), and white non-Hispanics (7.4).[73] Data

Table 4.1. Average Annual Age-Adjusted Death Rates

Cause of Death	Mexican	Hispanic Puerto Rican	Cuban	Other Hispanic	Non-Hispanic White
All causes	489.4	512.4	345.2	341.3	795.6
Shigellosis and amebiasis	0.1	—	—	—	0.0
Certain other intestinal infections	0.1	0.0	—	0.1	0.2
Tuberculosis	1.5	1.1	0.4	0.5	0.4
Whooping cough	—	—	—	0.0	
Streptococcal sore throat, scarlatina, and erysipelas	0.0	—	—	—	0.0
Meningococcal infection	0.1	0.3	—	0.2	0.1
Septicemia	4.1	1.8	1.1	1.7	2.1
Acute poliomyelitis	—	—	—	—	0.0
Measles	—	—	—	—	0.0
Viral hepatitis	0.3	0.5	1.0	0.3	0.3
Syphilis	0.1	—	—	—	0.0
All other infectious and parasitic diseases	1.9	1.0	0.0	0.9	1.1
Malignant neoplasms	84.4	86.4	81.6	65.8	123.6
Benign neoplasms, carcinoma in situ, and neoplasms of uncertain behavior and of unspecified nature	1.3	1.9	0.9	1.0	1.7
Diabetes mellitus	18.6	16.8	6.1	7.7	8.8
Nutritional deficiencies	0.6	0.1	—	0.3	0.4
Anemias	0.6	0.6	—	0.7	0.7
Meningitis	0.5	0.5	0.0	0.4	0.4
Major cardiovascular diseases	186.9	202.6	141.1	130.8	240.6
Acute bronchitis and bronchiolitis	0.1	0.1	—	0.0	0.1
Pneumonia and influenza	11.4	18.1	7.5	9.0	11.3
Chronic obstructive pulmonary diseases and allied conditions	6.6	11.9	5.5	6.4	15.7
Ulcer of stomach and duodenum	1.1	1.6	1.0	1.3	1.6
Appendicitis	0.1	0.0	—	0.0	0.2

Table 4.1. (Continued)

Cause of Death	Mexican	Hispanic			Non-Hispanic
		Puerto Rican	Cuban	Other Hispanic	White
Hernia of abdominal cavity and intestinal obstruction without mention of hernia	1.4	0.5	0.6	0.7	1.2
Chronic liver disease and cirrhosis	14.7	34.2	9.2	12.8	9.4
Cholelithiasis and other disorders of gallbladder	1.6	0.7	0.2	0.8	0.7
Nephritis, nephrotic syndrome, and nephrosis	0.1	0.0	—	0.0	0.2
Infections of kidney	0.6	0.5	—	0.5	0.6
Hyperplasia of prostate	0.1	0.2	—	0.1	0.2
Complications of pregnancy, childbirth, and the puerperium	0.2	0.3	0.0	0.0	0.1
Congenital anomalies	5.0	5.0	1.6	5.0	5.4
Certain conditions originating in the perinatal period					
All other diseases-residual	32.7	31.6	14.2	22.2	28.9
Accidents and adverse effects	46.9	25.5	19.5	27.9	36.8
Suicide	8.2	9.2	12.4	6.9	11.3
Homicide and legal intervention	24.7	35.3	20.9	18.8	5.2
All other external causes	1.1	6.4	3.0	2.9	1.6

from 1983–1985, which did not exclude Puerto Ricans in New York City, showed a higher infant mortality rate among Puerto Ricans (12.3), which represents a 41 percent excess neonatal mortality and a 29 percent excess postneonatal mortality compared to the rates for children of white non-Hispanic mothers.[72] The reliability of these estimates for Mexican Americans has also been questioned due to underreporting in the U.S.-Mexico border region.

Leading Causes of Death

There are also important differences between Hispanics and white non-Hispanics in the leading causes of death. The ten leading causes of death among Hispanics are diseases of the heart, malignant neoplasms, accidents and adverse effects, cerebrovascular diseases, homicide and legal intervention, diabetes mellitus, pneumonia and influenza, HIV infection, chronic liver disease and cirrhosis, and certain conditions generating in the perinatal period. Data from deaths in 1989 indicate that whereas among Hispanics homicide and legal intervention, HIV infection, and certain conditions in the perinatal period rank in the ten leading causes of death, among white non-Hispanics, these three categories are not found among the ten leading causes of death.[71] Conversely, white non-Hispanics have three leading causes of death not found among the ten leading causes for Hispanics: chronic obstructive pulmonary disease and allied conditions, suicide, and atherosclerosis. Some of these differences are attributable to age differences between these groups. However, the following leading causes of death consistently rank higher among Hispanics than white non-Hispanics across the same age categories: homicide and legal intervention (fifteen to sixty-four years of age), and HIV infection (one to sixty-four years of age).[71] Among Hispanics aged forty-five years and over, chronic liver disease also ranks higher than it does among white non-Hispanics. The 1990 data indicate that HIV changed from the sixth to the eighth leading cause of death, although this is surely an artifact of the exclusion of deaths from New York City.

Morbidity Among Hispanics

Indicators of health status, such as the incidence of chronic conditions and infectious diseases, other measures of illness such as bed-disability days, and health behaviors, also vary across Hispanic groups.

Table 4.2 presents a summary of research studies documenting excess morbidity related to certain chronic conditions among Hispanics. Studies summarized in Table 4.2 show that much of the data on morbidity among Hispanics has been obtained in community-specific studies, many of which focus on Mexican Americans in San Antonio, Texas, or in California and on Puerto Ricans in New York City or Connecticut. The Hispanic Health and Nutrition Examination Survey conducted between 1982 and 1984 is the only study that systematically provides data on all of the major Hispanic groups (Mexican Americans, Puerto Ricans, and Cuban Americans). In some cases, studies have compared data for Puerto Ricans living on the island. However, as shown in Table 4.2, there are few studies that provide such comparisons.

Table 4.2 shows diseases and conditions for Hispanic groups relative to non-Hispanic whites. For example, while the rates of diabetes among Cubans are similar to those for white non-Hispanics, Mexican Americans and Puerto Ricans have rates two to three times higher.[35] Diabetes in Mexican Americans is also associated with a rate of complications, especially end-stage renal disease and retinopathy, that is six times higher than among white non-Hispanics.[99] Higher

Table 4.2. Summary of Reported Evidence of Excess Morbidity Among Hispanic Populations as Compared to Non-Hispanic Whites (NHWs)

Disease	Evidence	Geographic Area/Year of Data/Hispanic Group	Reference
Cancer			
Overall rates	Lower overall incidence rates for Hispanics (RR = .88)	Dade County, FL, 1982–83 Hispanic (67% Cuban)	105
	Standardized incidence rates (SIR) for all invasive cancers higher for men (SIR = 1.16) and lower for women (SIR = .77) compared to NHW and higher than for Hispanics in Puerto Rico (males: SIR = 1.99; females: SIR = 1.39)	Connecticut, 1980–86 Puerto Rican born CT, residents and residents of Puerto Rico	83
	Incidence lower (320/100,000) than for NHW (392) and higher than for those in Puerto Rico (245) for men and women	New York City, 1982–85 Hispanic (60% PR)	124
Lung	Lower risk (RR = .88)	Dade County, FL, 1982–83 Hispanic (67% Cuban)	105
	SIR significantly reduced for females (SIR = .57) but not for males (SIR = .94)	Connecticut, 1980–86 (see above)	83
	Incidence rates for males and females lower than (51.5 vs. 73.2) and higher for NHW than for residents of Puerto Rico (22.9)	New York City, 1982–85 Hispanic (60% PR)	124
Stomach	Increased incidence (SIR = 2.65, females; SIR = 2.91, males)	Connecticut, 1980–86 (see above)	83
	Increased incidence (RR = 2.1, females; RR = 2.2, males)	California, 1991 Mexican American	66
	Highest incidence rates per 100,000 in Puerto Rico (11.3/24.4), followed by Hispanics in NYC (10.3/18.7) and NHW (7/13.4) (female/male)	New York City, 1982–85 Hispanic (60% PR)	124
	Lower risk (RR = .61)	Dade County, FL, 1982–83 Hispanic (67% Cuban)	105
Reproductive system	Cervical cancer: higher incidence (SIR = 1.81; RR = 2.3) or rates (2.5 times) found in four regions	Studies in Florida, Connecticut, New York City, California, 1980s M-A, PR, C-A	66, 83, 105, 124
	Anglos get pap smears and mammograms more often	U.S., 1987–88 California, 1989 Hispanic (majority Puerto Rican)	15, 30
	Lower rate incidence in other reproductive organs: breast cancer	New York City, 1982–85; Connecticut 1980–86 Hispanic (PR)	83, 124

(Continued)

Table 4.2. Summary of Reported Evidence of Excess Morbidity Among Hispanic Populations as Compared to Non-Hispanic Whites (NHWs). (Continued)

Disease	Evidence	Geographic Area/Year of Data/Hispanic Group	Reference
	corpus uteri and ovary	New York City, 1982–85; Connecticut 1980–86 Hispanic (PR)	83, 124
	testicular (RR = .17)	Florida, 1982–83 Hispanic (67% Cuban)	105
Gall bladder	Increased incidence for females (RR = 4.9)	California, 1991 Mexican American	66
	Increased incidence among men and women (RR = 5.45)	Dade County, FL, 1982–83 Hispanic (67% Cuban)	105
Buccal cavity and pharynx	Higher rates than for NHW among males (23 vs 14.3)	New York City, 1982–85 Hispanic (60% PR)	124
Oral cavity, larynx, thyroid, and esophagus	Higher rates in larynx (RR = 1.58) and thyroid (RR = 3.12)	Dade County, FL, 1982–83 Hispanic (67% Cuban)	105
	Higher SIR of esophageal cancer for males (RR = 2.76) and females, and of oral cavity for males (RR = 2.29)	Connecticut, 1980–86 Puerto Rican born CT residents	83
	Lower rate of esophageal cancer	Dade County, FL, 1982–83 Hispanic (67% Cuban)	105
Liver	Twice as prevalent for males	New York City, 1982–85 Hispanic (60% PR)	124
Other sites	Higher rates of leukemia among males	Connecticut, 1980–86 (see above)	83
	Lower rates or relative risk in following sites: skin (melanoma), rectum, kidney, pancreas, colon, Kaposi's sarcoma	Studies in California, New York City, Florida, Connecticut, 1980–86 M-A, PR, C-A	66, 83, 105, 124
Cardiovascular Disease (including coronary artery disease)	Mortality declining more slowly among Hispanics than overall decline	Meta-analysis M-A, PR, C-A[†]	16
	Slightly lower age-adjusted prevalence rates of Rose angina for Mexican American women	Samples from 3 areas of U.S.A., 1982–84 M-A, PR, C-A	53a
	Lower cardiovascular mortality for Mexican American men; no ethnic difference for women	San Antonio, 1979–88 Mexican American	64
Risk factors Cholesterol	Women had lower HDL cholesterol and higher triglycerides than NHW; no difference for total cholesterol or LDL; similar pattern for men but not significant	Florida Cuban	52a
Hypertension	More prevalent, and higher rates of untreated or unrecognized cases	Meta-analysis M-A, PR, C-A	16

Table 4.2. (Continued)

Disease	Evidence	Geographic Area/Year of Data/Hispanic Group	Reference
	Acculturation and age are stronger predictors of hypertension than poverty among older Mexican Americans	Samples from 3 areas of U.S.A., 1982–84 M-A, PR, C-A	32
Children's Illnesses Asthma	Similar prevalence compared to NHW children; possibly higher morbidity related to poverty and limited insurance and health coverage	San Antonio, 1988–89 Mexican American	126
Birth outcomes	Similar low birthweight (LBW) prevalence as compared to NHW (6.2%/5.6%) with greater risk for Puerto Ricans (9.3%)	U.S. sample and samples from 3 areas of U.S.A.; 1987 and 1982–84 M-A, PR, C-A	63
	Higher prevalence LBW babies among U.S.-born Puerto Rican, Mexican and Cuban women than among foreign or island-born women in all age groups	U.S. sample and samples from 3 areas of U.S.A.; 1987 and 1982–84 M-A, PR, C-A	63
	Premature births more common among 3 Hispanic groups than among NHW women: highest for Puerto Ricans	U.S. sample and samples from 3 areas of U.S.A.; 1987 and 1982–84 M-A, PR, C-A	63
Chronic medical conditions (CMC)	Puerto Rican children at greater risk for CMC than Mexican or Cuban American or NHW children	U.S. sample and samples from 3 areas of U.S.A.; 1987 and 1982–84 M-A, PR, C-A	63
Diabetes	Rates of NIDDM* 3 times higher	San Antonio, 1979–82 Mexican American	45
	Mexican American diabetics have higher levels of glycemia and clinical proteinuria (OR = 2.82)	San Antonio, 1979–82 Mexican American	45
	Prevalence 2 to 3 times greater for Puerto Ricans and Mexican Americans	Sample from 3 areas of U.S.A., 1982–84 M-A, PR, C-A†	35, 46
	Prevalence increases initially among migrant populations as they "modernize"; may then decline again for men and maybe women	San Antonio, 1989 Mexican American	100
	Higher acculturation and, among women, higher SES associated with linear decline in obesity and diabetes	San Antonio, 1979–82 Mexican American	49
Related factors end-stage renal disease (ESRD)	Relative disparity for ESRD: 17% of diabetics and 22% of those seeking care for ESRD	Colorado, 1982–89 Hispanics in CO	21

(Continued)

Table 4.2. Summary of Reported Evidence of Excess Morbidity Among Hispanic Populations as Compared to Non-Hispanic Whites (NHWs). (Continued)

Disease	Evidence	Geographic Area/Year of Data/Hispanic Group	Reference
Obesity/ overweight	Increase in age-adjusted incidence rate (1982–89) (Hispanics 770%, Blacks 440%, NHW 190%)	Colorado, 1982–89 Hispanics in CO	21
	Higher prevalence among Hispanics; highest for Mexican Americans; higher among women and low SES	Texas and U.S. sample, 1982–84 Mexican American and other Hispanics	78
	Prevalence of obesity 31–34% for men and 38–42% for women among Hispanics	Sample from 3 areas of U.S.A., 1982–84 M-A, PR, C-A[†]	81
	Body mass index (BMI) decreased for women as SES increased; high acculturation related to decrease in BMI	Texas, 1979–82 Mexican American	49, 100
Glucose intolerance	Higher prevalence particularly among Mexican Americans and Puerto Ricans	Sample from 3 areas of U.S.A., 1982–84 M-A, PR, C-A	35
	Higher prevalence of hyperinsulinemia among nondiabetic Mexican Americans relative to nondiabetic NHWs	San Antonio, 1982–84 Mexican American	100

*NIDDM = non-insulin-dependent diabetes mellitus.

[†]M-A = Mexican American; PR = Puerto Rican; C-A = Cuban American.

prevalences of factors related to diabetes, such as obesity, proteinuria, and glucose intolerance, have also been documented among Mexican Americans and Puerto Ricans.[35,45,78,81,100]

Rates of cardiovascular disease and related factors, such as cholesterol levels, among Hispanics have been reported to be similar or lower than among white non-Hispanics, while other factors such as diabetes and obesity show higher rates in Hispanics.[27] Some studies have reported that high blood pressure is more prevalent among Mexican Americans and Cubans than among white non-Hispanics.[16,31] However, other research indicates that Hispanics have similar or lower levels of high blood pressure compared to white non-Hispanics.[65,98] Most studies have consistently shown, however, that Hispanics have higher rates of untreated or unrecognized cases of high blood pressure.[16,27,31,65,98]

Data from state cancer registries generally indicate lower overall rates of cancer among Hispanics, although for some cancers some Hispanic groups have higher rates. For example, studies of Hispanics in Connecticut and New York City (primarily Puerto Ricans)[83,124] and California (the majority Mexican Americans)[66] have documented increased incidence of stomach cancer in these groups, whereas data from Hispanics in Dade County, Florida (primarily Cubans), show lower rates than among white non-Hispanics.[105] Disproportionately high cervical cancer rates (a two times higher relative risk) have been found among Hispanic women in Connecticut, New York, and California compared to white non-Hispanics.[66,83,124] There is also evidence of increased rates of gallbladder cancer among Hispanics in California[66] and male and female Hispanics in Dade County, Florida;[105] cancer of the buccal cavity and pharynx among Hispanic men in New York City;[124] cancer of the larynx and thyroid among Hispanic men and women in Dade County, Florida;[105] cancer of the esophagus for Hispanic men and women, and cancer of the oral cavity among Hispanic men in Connecticut.[83] There are higher rates of cancer of the liver and leukemia among Hispanic men than among white non-Hispanics men in New York City and Connecticut.[83,124]

Infectious diseases disproportionately affect Hispanics.[101] Increased rates of immunizable diseases, such as measles, rubella, congenital rubella, tetanus, and pertussis, have been documented among Hispanics living in the Southwestern United States and in the Northeast.[101] Higher rates of bacterial gastrointestinal diseases, parasites, and other tropic-endemic diseases have been found among Hispanics living primarily in the Southwest and among Hispanic farmworkers in other geographic regions compared to white non-Hispanics.[101]

The incidence of tuberculosis is two times higher among Hispanics (18.3 per 100,000) as it is among white non-Hispanics (9.1 per 100,000).[114] The higher rates of tuberculosis have been documented among Hispanics living in New York City and in the Southwest.[101] The rates of primary and secondary syphilis are five times greater among Hispanic women (10.7 per 100,000) and men (22.8) compared to rates among white non-Hispanics (1.8 and 2.9, respectively).[28] Other sexually transmitted diseases such as congenital syphilis, chancroid, chlamydia, and gonococcus have been demonstrated to affect Hispanics disproportionately and to be on the increase in this population. The increase in syphilis (24 percent) in Hispanics has been especially striking compared to that in Hispanic men (7 percent) and the minimal increase observed in white non-Hispanics.[101]

The cumulative incidence rate for adults diagnosed with AIDS is 3.3 times higher among Hispanics; Puerto Ricans largely account for AIDS cases among Hispanics. They are seven times more likely than non-Hispanic whites to be diagnosed with AIDS.[93,94] Rates of AIDS cases among Hispanics in the Southwest are at levels similar to those in the white non-Hispanic population; rates for Hispanics in Florida fall between the two.[18,101] AIDS cases have especially disproportionately increased among Hispanic children (23 percent of pediatric AIDS cases) and women (20 percent of cases in women). Rates of HIV infection are also higher among Hispanics, especially in the Northeast, as demonstrated by higher rates of HIV antibody among U.S. military service applicants, active duty military personnel, women attending family planning clinics, adolescents entering the Job Corps program, and blood donors.[19,20]

Rates of depression symptomatology and lifetime history of depression have been reported to be higher among Puerto Ricans when compared to rates obtained for the general population and for other Hispanic groups.[67] Data on bed-disability days and activity limitation suggest that Puerto Rican children under seventeen years of age have over two times the number of bed-disability days[43] and 50 percent more Puerto Rican children have some type of activity limitation due to an illness (6.2) than do non-Hispanics whites (5.1; 4.0) or black children (4.7; 3.7).[113]

Risk Behaviors

Certain behaviors or risk factors associated with negative health outcomes and impaired psychosocial development are also more prevalent among Hispanics compared to non-Hispanics. For example, pregnancy among girls age seventeen and younger is more prevalent among Hispanics (158 per 1,000) than white non-Hispanics (71.1 per 1,000) and close to that of blacks (186 per 1,000).[121] Relatively little is known about family planning among Hispanic women. It remains inconclusive whether Hispanic women initiate intercourse at an older age and engage in sexual intercourse less often than other women. Paradoxically, relatively low rates of sexual intercourse among Mexican American teenage girls coincide with high fertility rates as a result of relatively low rates of use of contraceptives and low rates of abortion. Factors related to contraception decisions are not well understood, but Hispanic women may simply have more desire to have children than women in other ethnic groups. Similarly, little is known about sexual behavior among Hispanic women. In all of these areas considerably more comparative research is needed. Hispanic women (Mexican American = 39 percent; Puerto Rican = 37 percent; Cuban = 34 percent) are also more likely to be overweight than white non-Hispanic women (27 percent).[25,78,81]

Use of marijuana and cocaine varies greatly by Hispanic group and is more common among Puerto Ricans of both genders compared to women and men in other Hispanic groups.[1] Puerto Rican women (30.3 percent) also have higher age-adjusted smoking rates than Mexican American (23.8 percent) and Cuban (24.4 percent) women.[48]

In summary, the health status of Hispanics, as reflected in morbidity and mortality patterns, differs greatly among Hispanic subgroups. While patterns vary for specific diseases, Puerto Ricans in the continental United States demonstrate a more unfavorable health profile than Mexican Americans. Although more sparse, the mortality and morbidity data on Cubans indicate that they are generally in better health than other Hispanics. The relatively low death rate among Mexican Americans, who share many of the economic disadvantages of

Puerto Ricans and blacks, has presented a public health paradox. This pattern runs counter to the well-documented gradient effect of socioeconomic status on health.[53,77,95,123]

Health Status and Acculturation

There is evidence that the health habits and health status of Hispanic immigrants deteriorate with length of stay in the United States, as well as in succeeding generations, due to increased acculturation. The process of acculturation and the type of cultural contact experienced in migration among Hispanics is stressful because of the disruption of attachments to supportive networks, and the concomitant tasks of adapting to the economic and social systems in the host culture.[86,118] The work of Vega and colleagues[120] has provided evidence that the social support provided by networks of family and friends among immigrant Mexican women plays a critical role in adaptation to life in this country. The Hispanic migrant is also likely to experience discrimination, prejudice, and exclusion that frustrates expectations of improved social and economic status with increased adoption of the dominant culture's values. At the same time, the immigrant/migrant is faced with incorporating into his or her identity a newly acquired "minority status." Berry[10] describes responses to these conditions and notes the vulnerability of the individual who, in the process of adaptation, abandons all or major parts of her or his cultural values and identification and assimilates into the dominant society. This assimilation may include the abandonment of culturally tied health beliefs and the loss of culturally tied resources and social support networks, which may place her or him at risk.[52]

Other evidence indicates that some forms of cultural "adaptation" or acculturation are harmful to the health of Hispanics. The following health indicators worsen with increased acculturation: rates of infant mortality,[8] low birthweight,[8,44,63] overall cancer rates,[30,83,124] high blood pressure,[32] and adolescent pregnancy.[121]

Certain behaviors also increase with acculturation. These include decreased fiber consumption,[30] decreased breast feeding,[25] increased use of cigarettes,[48] increased alcohol consumption—especially in younger women[14,39,58,60,76] and driving under the influence of alcohol,[22] and increased use of illicit drugs.[1,75,80,82,86,92] Some studies have also documented that depressive symptomatology increases with acculturation,[13,42,52,67,79,96] although the relationship between depression and acculturation remains controversial.[86]

The relationship between acculturation and risky behaviors or jeopardized health is often striking. For example, the rate of adolescent pregnancy is twice as high among Hispanics born in the United States as among those born outside the continental United States.[121] Furthermore, the rate of low birthweight infants born to second-generation Mexican American women is almost two times higher than that among comparable first-generation women.[44] Use of illicit drugs increases with acculturation.[1,75,80,82,92,117] Data from the Hispanic HANES indicate that marijuana use is eight times higher among Mexican Americans and five times greater among Puerto Ricans who are highly acculturated than it is among those who are not acculturated, even after sociodemographic factors are controlled.[1] Also, use of cocaine is associated with acculturation among Mexican Americans and Puerto Ricans.[1] Moreover, drug use and acculturation conflicts are related to increased suicide attempts among Hispanic adolescents.[116] Use of cigarettes among Mexican American women is significantly lower among those with low levels of acculturation (19 percent) compared to those with high levels of acculturation (28 percent).[48]

There are, however, some exceptions to the trend toward worsening health and health habits with acculturation. Dietary habits (intake of total calories and fat), for example, improve with acculturation.[30,99] Body mass index,[27] diabetes, and obesity[49,100] also decrease with increased socioeconomic status and acculturation.

The acculturation process involves adaptation not only at the individual level but also at the level of family and community. Szapocznik and colleagues[80,92,103] have described the effects of acculturation and its differential impact on generations within the family. Their work has demonstrated that gender and age mediate the experience of adaptation to a new culture. The effects of acculturation on the social character and group dynamics within communities and accompanying negative effects on health have been documented in other immigrant populations, such as the studies of the Roseto community.[29] The Roseto effect points to the need to understand the impact that community structure and organization have on the acculturative process and the health of Hispanics.

Research is needed to address a series of profound questions. First, we must understand the selective factors that operate in the migration process and how these shape immigrants' health status and risk behaviors. We also need to understand the nature of social networks, social support systems, and the organization and cohesion of the varied communities where Hispanics live and work.[84,86,120] Finally, research is needed to better understand Hispanic immigrants' experience of discrimination and its impact on social, environmental, and behavioral health risks.

HEALTH SERVICES UTILIZATION ISSUES

Key questions remain about Hispanic health services utilization patterns: Do Hispanics underutilize health services? If they do, which Hispanics are underutilizing, and why? A cursory review of the literature on services utilization clearly suggests that Hispanics, as a composite population, use almost all forms of health care at a rate below that of white non-Hispanics. However, these differences are clearly attributable to the utilization behavior of Mexican Americans,[11,51,55,107] who have lower mortality rates for the leading chronic diseases.

Factors held responsible for Hispanic health use behaviors include selective migration;[12,13] personal,[47] cultural,[23,24,37,48,51,56,88,89,97,104,108,109,122] and social characteristics;[54] and structural barriers.[9,43,91,106] Although cultural beliefs affect the use of health services, very little empirical evidence supports the assertion that indigenous beliefs, cultural practices, or uses of healers are offsetting use of orthodox medical providers in any significant way.[3,17] Similarly, no consistent relationship has been discerned between various indicators of acculturation and physician utilization.[59]

Structural barriers to access include financial constraints and features of medical providers that deter or discourage potential or actual clients. Hispanics are less likely than other ethnic groups to have a regular medical provider or physician[9] or to have health insurance.[106] The Mexican American population, with its large numbers of undocumented and seasonal workers, is much less likely to have public health insurance coverage and more likely to work for employers who do not provide private health insurance.[106] In the absence of financial barriers, as among Hispanics who are eligible for Medicaid, rates of use of health services are higher than for other populations.[108] However, even when financial barriers are removed, provider characteristics (for example, location, language, and cultural competence) mediate access to health services among Hispanics.[3,11,40,57]

Only a few (that is, two to five[33]) well-conceived theoretical models have been tested empirically with Hispanics to evaluate the relative contribution of explanatory factors to the use of health services. Analytical models of Hispanic services utilization need to be elaborated that supersede, and hopefully improve, traditional behavioral models,[2,41,62,125] by including additional indicators that reflect the Hispanic cultural and social experiences.[6] Another set of factors to be considered is contextual, occasioned by differences in provider characteristics that facilitate or act as barriers to care.

The advent of publicly assisted universal health coverage for large numbers of currently uninsured Hispanics will permit a direct test of whether intrinsic ethnic group factors (for example, the notion that Mexican Americans are "super healthy") or structural factors (for example, the low availability of public health insurance) are responsible for low utilization among Mexican Americans, and among other Hispanic ethnic groups as well. Furthermore, it will be possible to assess the impact of unanticipated high-level Hispanic enrollment on public and private health care providers, and how these providers change procedures and clinical practices to accommodate the needs of Spanish-speaking clients. Indeed, bilingualism and multicultural competency may become much more highly valued and rewarded abilities among medical professionals as a result.

PREVENTION, HEALTH PROMOTION, AND PUBLIC HEALTH POLICY FOR HISPANICS

The fact that many Hispanics have no primary care provider of choice implies irregularity of preventive screening that in turn reduces prophylactic immunization or early detection and effective management of disease. To correct this situation, the National Institutes of Health are funding intramural and extramural projects to increase awareness of health issues, using various communication models. These initiatives emphasize the need for regular health screening for major diseases such as cancer, AIDS, and heart disease. There is increasing emphasis on health promotion and disease prevention projects to reduce smoking, alcohol consumption, risky sexual behaviors, and illicit drug use. More recently, these NIH initiatives have included the provision of technical assistance to design and implement community-based interventions, interaction with and use of social networks, design of media messages and campaigns, and the development of informational materials appropriate for interventions in multilingual or multicultural environments. Much remains to be learned in this area, but this earnest effort is a solid beginning. Continuing experimentation and dissemination of technical information is needed so that practitioners and researchers can keep abreast of the growing complexity of the U.S. Hispanic population and the rapid pace of knowledge development.

The economic and educational gap between Hispanics and white non-Hispanics has direct consequences for Hispanic public health status by increasing community disintegration and risky behaviors. In Hispanic communities, lack of opportunity fosters conflicts among Hispanic youth that are directly related to acculturation. Unhealthy lifestyles and gang membership among urban adolescents and young adults proliferate in this environment. Regardless of improvements in access to care, medical care providers are unlikely to reduce the incidence of street violence, rising teen suicide, and sexual or physical abuse in families. Furthermore, the prevention of diseases such as AIDS depends on the primacy Hispanics assign to behavioral changes in the context of the harsh and debilitating inner-city environment. Is it possible to prevent disease in communities where the basic requirements of physical survival are so burdensome, where public safety is questionable, and educational systems are in total disarray? Not in the long run, and certainly not in the short run.

The most fundamental and effective method to lower the incidence of morbidity and mortality among Hispanics may be through health promotion and prevention, but only if these activities can be linked to employment and improved economic opportunities. Prevention activities are frequently limited by their narrow scope, which restricts the number of individuals who can be reached, or are too costly to sustain. To overcome this limitation, health must become the business of the Hispanic community in direct and tangible ways.

Increased training and employment opportunities as allied health professionals and as community health outreach workers are needed in Hispanic communities. Health media messages must be disseminated to communicate accurate information competently in homes, schools, community locations, and work sites. These activities could counteract among low-income Hispanics the influences of alcohol and tobacco industry advertising and their high-visibility financial support of Hispanic community cultural events. All intervention strategies, regardless of type, carry the burden of demonstrating that they are imparting something of local and personal value to community members. And these tactics must be implemented creatively, drawing on the aesthetic and spiritual qualities of Hispanic families and communities.[47]

Despite a low prevalence of many health problems among some Hispanic groups, population growth will increase the magnitude of many common public health problems. For example, a recent epidemiologic study of perinatal substance use, which used anonymous urine screening in California hospitals, found that Hispanic women, who constitute about one-quarter of all women in the state, had a 6.8 percent prevalence of alcohol-exposed infants.[119] The prevalence for African American women was 11.6 percent, almost twice as high as for Hispanic women. Nevertheless, because Hispanic women constitute a disproportionately large fraction of the birthing population, they were responsible for almost one-half, as compared to one-tenth for African Americans, of alcohol-exposed infants born in California in 1992. The implication of this finding is that health promotion and intervention are important public health activities within Hispanic communities, low prevalence rates notwithstanding. Current activities in this field are highly encouraging and, with persistence, may bring about fundamental changes in the way health is perceived and maintained among Hispanics in the United States. As Muñoz has forcefully argued, there is nothing intrinsic to Hispanic culture to suggest a lesser concern with health issues or an innate resistance to interventions.[68,69]

Notes

1. Amaro, H., Whitaker, R., Coffman, J., & Heeren T. (1990). Acculturation and marijuana and cocaine use: Finding from the HHANES 1982–84. *Am J Public Health, 80*(Suppl.), 54–60.

2. Andersen, R., & Newman, J. F. (1973). Societal and individual determinants of medical care utilization in the United States. *Milbank Mem Fund Q, 51,* 95–124.

3. Andersen, R. M. (1968). *A behavioral model of families' use of health services.* Chicago: University of Chicago Press.

4. Andersen, R. M., Giachello, A. L., & Aday, L. A. (1986). Access of Hispanics to health care and cuts in services: A state-of-the-art overview. *Public Health Rep, 101,* 238–252.

5. Andersen, R. M., Zelman, L. S, Giachello, A. L., Aday. L. A., & Chiu, G. (1981). Access to medical care among the Hispanic population of the Southwestern United States. *J Health Soc Behav, 22,* 78–89.

6. Angel, R., & Cleary, P. D. (1984). The effects of social structure and culture on reported health. *Soc Sci Q, 65,* 814–288.

7. Bean, F. D., & Tienda, M. (1987). *The Hispanic population of the United States.* New York: Russell Sage Foundation.

8. Becerra, J., Hogue, C., Atrash, H., & Perez, N. (1991). Infant mortality among Hispanics. *JAMA, 265,* 217–221.

9. Berkanovic, E., & Telesky, C. (1985). Mexican-American, black-American and white-American differences in reporting illnesses, disability and physician visits for illness. *Soc Sci Med, 20,* 567–577.

10. Berry, J. W. (1980). Acculturation as varieties of adaptation. In A. M. Padilla (Ed.), *Acculturation: Theory, models and some new findings* (pp. 9–25). Boulder, CO: Westview Press.

11. Brown, J. P. (1992). Oral health of Hispanics: Epidemiology and risk factors. In A. Furino (Ed.), *Health policy and the Hispanic* (pp. 132–143). Boulder, CO: Westview Press.

12. Burnam, M. A., Hough, R. L., Escobar, J. I., Karno, M., Timbers, D. M., et al. (1987). Six-months prevalence of specific psychiatric disorders among Mexican Americans and non-Hispanic whites in Los Angeles. *Arch Gen Psychiatry, 44,* 687–694.

13. Burnam, M., Hough, R., Karno, M., Escobar, J., & Telles, C. (1987). Acculturation and lifetime prevalence of psychiatric disorders among Mexican Americans in Los Angeles. *J Health Soc Behav, 28,* 89–102.

14. Caetanno, R. (1987). Acculturation and drinking patterns among U.S. Hispanics. *Br J Addict, 82,* 789–799.

15. Caplan, L. S., Wells, B. L., & Haynes, S. (1992). Breast cancer screening among older racial/ethnic minorities and whites: Barriers to early detection. *J Gerontol, 47,* 101–110.

16. Caralis, P. V. (1990). Hypertension in the Hispanic-American population. *Am J Med, 88*(Suppl. 3B), 3B–9S.

17. Casas, M. M., & Keefe, S. M. (Eds.). (1978). *Family and mental health in the Mexican American community.* Los Angeles: Spanish Speaking Mental Health Resource Center.

18. Castro, K. G., Valdiserri, R. O., & Curran, J. W. (1992). Perspectives on HIV/AIDS epidemiology and prevention from the 8th International Conference on AIDS. *Am J Public Health, 82,* 1465–1470.

19. Centers for Disease Control. (1987). Trends in immunodeficiency virus infection among civilian applicants for military service—United States: Oct. 1985–Dec. 1986. *Morbid Mortal Wkly Rep, 36,* 273–276.

20. Centers for Disease Control. (1988). Prevalence of human immunodeficiency virus antibody in U.S. active-duty military personnel, April 1988. *Morbid Mortal Wkly Rep, 37,* 461–463.

21. Centers for Disease Control. (1992). Incidence of treatment of end-stage renal disease attributable to diabetes mellitus, by race/ethnicity—Colorado: 1982–1989. *Morbid Mortal Wkly Rep, 41,* 845–848.

22. Cherpitel, C. J. (1992). Acculturation, alcohol consumption, and casualties among United States Hispanics in the emergency room. *Int J Addict, 27,* 1067–1077.

23. Chesney, A. P., Chavira, J. A., Hall, R. P., & Gary, H. E. (1982). Barriers to medical care of Mexican-Americans: The role of social class, acculturation and social isolation. *Med Care, 20,* 883–891.

24. Clark, M. (1959). *Health in the Mexican-American culture.* Berkeley: University of California Press.

25. Council of Scientific Affairs of the American Medical Association. (1991). Hispanic health in the United States. *JAMA, 265,* 248–252.

26. Delgado, M. (1990). Hispanic adolescents and substance abuse: Implications for research, treatment and prevention. In A. R. Stiffman & L. E. Davis (Eds.), *Ethnic issues in adolescent mental health* (pp. 303–320). Newbury Park, CA: Sage.

27. Derenowski, J. (1990). Coronary artery disease in Hispanics. *J Cardiovasc Nurs, 4,* 13–21.

28. Division of STD/HIV Prevention. (1991). *Sexually transmitted disease surveillance, 1990.* Atlanta: Centers for Disease Control.

29. Egolf, B., Lasker, J., Wolf, S., & Potvin, L. (1992). The Roseto effect: A 50-year comparison of mortality rates. *Am J Public Health, 82,* 1089–1092.

30. Elder, J. P., Castro, F. G., deMoor, C., Mayer, J., Candelaria, J., et al. (1991). Differences in cancer risk-related behaviors in Latino and Anglo adults. *Medicine, 20,* 751–763.

31. Espino, D. V., Burge, S. K., & Moreno, C. A. (1991). The prevalence of selected chronic diseases among the Mexican American elderly: Data from the 1982–1984 Hispanic Health and Nutrition Examination Survey. *J Am Board Fam Pract, 4,* 217–222.

32. Espino, D. V., & Maldonado, D. (1990). Hypertension and acculturation in elderly Mexican Americans: Results from 1982–84 Hispanic HANES. *J Gerontol, 45,* M209–213.

33. Estrada, A. L., Trevino, F. M., & Ray, L. A. (1990). Health care utilization barriers among Mexican Americans: Evidence from HHANES 1982–84. *Am J Public Health, 80*(Suppl.), 27–31.

34. Fingerhut, L. A., & Makuc, D. M. (1992). Mortality among minority populations in the United States. *Am J Public Health, 82,* 1168–1170.

35. Flegal, M. K., Ezzatti, T. M., Harris, M. I., Haynes, S. G., Juarez, R. Z., et al. (1991). Prevalence of diabetes in Mexican Americans, Cubans, and Puerto Ricans

from the Hispanic Health and Nutrition Examination Survey, 1982–1984. *Diabetes Care, 14*(Suppl. 3), 628–638.

36. Fox, S. A., & Stein, J. A. (1991). The effect of physician-patient communication on mammography utilization by different ethnic groups. *Med Care, 29,* 1065–1083.

37. Garrison, V. (1975). Espiritismo: Implications for provisions of mental health services to Puerto Rican populations. In H. Hodges & C. Hudson (Ed.), *Folktherapy.* Miami: University of Miami Press.

38. General Accounting Office. (1992). *Hispanic access to health care: Significant gaps exist.* Washington, DC: U.S. Government Printing Office.

39. Gilbert, M. (1989). Alcohol consumption pattern in immigrant and later generation Mexican American women. *Hisp J Behav Sci, 9,* 299–313.

40. Ginzberg, E. (1991). Access to health care for Hispanics. *JAMA, 265,* 238–241.

41. Goldsmith, H .F., Jackson, D. J., & Hough, R. L. (1988). Process model of seeking mental health services: Proposed framework for organizing the research literature on help-seeking. In *Needs assessment: Its future* (pp. 49–64) (Mental Health Service System Report Series BN No. 8). Rockville, MD: National Institute of Mental Health.

42. Griffith, J. (1983). Relationship between acculturation and psychological impairment in adult Mexican Americans. *Hisp J Behav Sci, 5,* 431–459.

43. Guendelman, S., & Schwalbe, J. (1986). Medical care utilization by Hispanic children: How does it differ from black and white peers? *Med Care, 24*(10), 925–937.

44. Guendelman, S. S., Gould, J., Hudes, M., & Eskenazi, B. (1990). Generational difference in perinatal health among the Mexican American population: Findings from HHANES, 1982–1984. *Am J Public Health, 80,* 61–65.

45. Haffner, S. M., Mitchell, B. D., Pugh, J. A., Stern, M. P., Kozlowski, M. K., Hazuda, H. P., et al. (1989). Proteinuria in Mexican Americans and non-Hispanic whites with non-insulin-dependent diabetes mellitus. *JAMA, 263,* 530–536.

46. Harris, M. I. (1991). Epidemiological correlates of NIDDM in Hispanics, whites, and blacks in the US population. *Diabetes Care, 14*(Suppl. 3), 639–648.

47. Hayes-Bautista, D. (1992). Latino health indicators and the underclass model: From paradox to new policy models. In A. Furino (Ed.), *Health policy and the Hispanic* (pp. 32–47). Boulder, CO: Westview Press.

48. Haynes, S. G., Harvey, C., Montes, H., Nicken, H., Cohen, B. H. (1990). Patterns of cigarette smoking among Hispanics in the United States: Results from the HHANES 1982–1984. *Am J Public Health, 80*(Suppl.), 47–53.

49. Hazuda, H. P., Haffner, S. P., Stern, M. P., & Eifler, C. W. (1988). Effects of acculturation and SES on obesity and diabetes in Mexican Americans: The San Antonio Heart Study. *Am J Epidemiol, 128,* 1289–1301.

50. Higginbotham, J. C., Trevino, F. M., & Ray, L. A. (1990). Utilization of curanderos by Mexican Americans: Prevalence and predictors: Findings from HHANES 1982–84. *Am J Public Health, 80*(Suppl.), 32–35.

51. Hough, R. L., Landsverk, J., Karno, M., et al. (1987). Utilization of health and mental health services by Los Angeles Mexican Americans and non-Hispanic whites. *Arch Gen Psychiatry, 44,* 702–709.

52. Kaplan, M., & Marks, G. (1990). Adverse effects of acculturation: Psychological distress among Mexican American young adults. *Soc Sci Med, 31*(12), 1313–1319.

52a. Kato, P. M., Soto, R., Goldberg, R. B., & Sosenko, J. M. (1991). Comparison of the lipid profiles of Cubans and other Hispanics with non-Hispanics. *Arch Intern Med, 151,* 1613–1616.

53. Kehrer, B. H., & Wollin, C. M. (1979). Impact of income maintenance on low birthweight. *J Hum Resour, 12,* 434–462.

53a. LaCroix, A. Z., Haynes, S. G., Savage, D. D., & Havlik, R. J. (1989). Rose questionnaire angina among United States black, white and Mexican-American women and men. *Am J Epidemiol, 131,* 423–433.

54. Lewin-Epstein, N. (1991). Determinants of regular source of health care in black, Mexican, Puerto Rican, and non-Hispanic white populations. *Med Care, 29,* 543–557.

55. Lopez, S. (1981). Mexican-American usage of mental health facilities: Underutilization reconsidered. In A. Baron Jr. (Ed.), *Explorations in Chicano psychology* (pp. 139–164). New York: Praeger.

56. Madsen, W. (1964). Value conflicts in folk psychiatry in South Texas. In A. Kiev (Ed.), *Magic, faith and healing* (pp. 420–440). New York: Free Press.

57. Marin, G., Marin, B. V., & Padilla, A. M. (1982). Aspectos atribucionales de la utilización de servicios de salud. *Interam J Psychol, 16,* 78–89.

58. Markides, K. S., Levin, J. S., & Ray, L. A. (1985). Determinants of physician utilization among Mexican Americans: A three generations study. *Med Care, 23,* 226–246.

59. Markides, K. S., Ray, L., Stroup-Benham, C., & Trevino, F. (1990). Acculturation and alcohol consumption in the Mexican American population of the Southwestern United States: Findings from the HHANES, 1982–84. *Am J Public Health, 80*(Suppl.), 42–46.

60. Marks, G., Garcia, M., & Solis, J. (1990). Health risk behaviors of Hispanics in the United States: Findings from HHANES, 1982–84. *Am J Public Health, 80*(Suppl.), 20–26.

61. Maurer, J. D., Rosenberg, H. M., & Keemer, J. B. (1990). Deaths of Hispanic origin, 15 reporting states, 1979–1981. *Vital Health Stat, 20*(18), 5–16.

62. Mechanic, D. (1979). Correlates of physician utilization: Why do major multivariate studies of physician utilization find trivial psychosocial and organizational effects? *J Health Soc Behav, 20,* 387–396.

63. Mendoza, F., Ventura, S., Valdez, B., Castillo, R., Saldivar, L., et al. (1991). Selected measures of health status for Mexican-American, mainland Puerto Rican, and Cuban American children. *JAMA, 265,* 227–232.

64. Mitchell, B. D., Hazuda, H. P., Haffner, S. M., Patterson, J. K., & Stein, M. P. (1991). Myocardial infarction in Mexican-Americans and non-Hispanic whites: The San Antonio Heart Study. *Circulation, 83,* 45–51.

65. Mitchell, B. D., Stern, M. P., Haffner, S. M., Hazuda, H. P., & Patterson, J. K. (1990). Risk factors for cardiovascular mortality in Mexican Americans and non-Hispanic whites: The San Antonio Heart Study. *Am J Epidemiol, 131,* 423–433.

66. Moran, E. M. (1992). Epidemiological factors of cancer in California. *J Environ Pathol Toxicol Oncol, 11,* 303–307.

67. Mosciscki, E., Locke, B., Rae, D., & Boyd, J. H. (1989). Depressive symptoms among Mexican Americans: The Hispanic Health and Nutrition Examination Survey. *Am J Epidemiol, 130,* 348–360.

68. Muñoz, R. F. (1980). A strategy for the prevention of psychological problems in Latinos: Emphasizing accessibility and effectiveness. In R. Valle & W. Vega (Eds.), *Hispanic natural support systems: Mental health promotion perspectives* (pp. 85–96). Sacramento: California Department of Mental Health, Office of Prevention.

69. Muñoz, R. F., Ying, Y. W., Armas, R., Chan, F., & Gurza, R. (1986). The San Francisco depression prevention research project: A randomized trial with medical outpatients. In R. F. Muñoz (Ed.), *Depression prevention: Research directions* (pp. 199–216). Washington: Hemisphere.

70. National Center for Health Statistics. (1991). Advance report of final mortality statistics, 1988. *Mon Vital Stat Rep, 39*(4, Suppl. Health U.S.).

71. National Center for Health Statistics. (1992). Advance report of final mortality statistics, 1989. *Mon Vital Stat Rep, 80*(8, Suppl. 2).

72. National Center for Health Statistics. (1992). *Health, United States, 1991.* Hyattsville, MD: U.S. Public Health Service.

73. National Center for Health Statistics. (1993). Advance report of final mortality statistics, 1990. *Mon Vital Stat Rep, 40*(7, Suppl.).

74. National Center for Health Statistics. (1993, May 12). Personal communication with Lois Fingerhut.

75. National Institute on Drug Abuse. (1987). *Use of selected drugs among Hispanics: Mexican Americans, Puerto Ricans, and Cuban Americans. Findings from the HHANES.* Washington, DC: U.S. Department of Health and Human Services.

76. Neff, J. (1986). Alcohol consumption and psychological distress among U.S. Anglos, Hispanics, and blacks. *Alcohol Alcoholism, 21,* 111–119.

77. Nelson, M. (1992). Socioeconomic status and childhood mortality in North Carolina. *Am J Public Health, 82,* 1133–1136.

78. Nichaman, M. Z., & Garcia, G. (1991). Obesity in Hispanic Americans. *Diabetes Care, 14*(Suppl. 3), 691–694.

79. Padilla, E., Olmedo, E., & Loya, F. (1982). Acculturation and the MMPI performance of Chicano and Anglo college students. *Hisp J Behav Sci, 4,* 451–466.

80. Page, B. (1980). The children of exile: Relationships between the acculturation process and drug use among Cuban American youth. *Youth & Society, 11*, 431–447.

81. Pawson, I. G., Martorell, R., & Mendoza, F. E. (1991). Prevalence of overweight and obesity in U.S. Hispanic populations. *Am J Clin Nutr, 53*, 1522S–1528S.

82. Perez, R., Padilla, A. M., Ramirez, A., Ramirez, R., & Rodriquez, M. (1980). Correlates and changes over time in drug and alcohol use within a barrio population. *Am J Community Psychol, 6*, 621–636.

83. Polednak, A. P. (1992). Cancer incidence in the Puerto Rican–born population of Connecticut. *Cancer, 70*, 1172–1176.

84. Portes, A., & Bach, R. L. (1985). *Latin journey: Cuban and Mexican immigrants in the United States.* Berkeley: University of California Press.

85. Portes, A., & Rumbaut, R. G. (1990). *Immigrant America: A portrait.* Berkeley: University of California Press.

86. Rogler, L., Cortes, D., & Malagady, R. (1991). Acculturation and mental health status among Hispanics. *Am Psychol, 46*, 585–597.

87. Rubel, A. (1960). Concepts of disease in Mexican-American culture. *Am Anthropol, 62*, 795–814.

88. Ruiz, P., & Langrod, J. (1976). The role of folk healers in community mental health services. *Community Ment Health J, 12*, 392–404.

89. Sandoval, M. C. (1979). Santeria as a mental health care system: An historical overview. *Soc Sci Med, 13B*, 137–151.

90. Schick, F. L., & Schick, R. (1991). *Statistical handbook on U.S. Hispanics.* New York: Oryx Press.

91. Schur, C. L., Bernstein, A. B., & Berk, M. L. (1987). The importance of distinguishing Hispanic subpopulations in the use of medical care. *Med Care, 25*, 627–641.

92. Scopetta, M. A., King, O. E., & Szapocznik, J. (1977). *Relationship of acculturation, incidence of drug abuse, and effective treatment for Cuban Americans* (NIDA Final Report, Research Contract No. 271-75-4136). Bethesda, MD: National Institute on Drug Abuse.

93. Selik, R. M., Castro, K. G., & Papaionnou, M. (1988). Racial/ethnic differences in the risk of AIDS in the United States. *Am J Public Health, 78*, 1539–1545.

94. Selik, R. M., Castro, K. G., Papaionnou, M., & Ruehler, J. W. (1989). Birthplace and the risk of AIDS among Hispanics in the United States. *Am J Public Health 79*, 836–839.

95. Smith, G. D., & Egger, M. (1992). Socioeconomic differences in mortality in Britain and the United States. *Am J Public Health, 82*, 1079–1081.

96. Sorenson, S., & Golding, J. (1988). Suicide ideation and attempts in Hispanics and non-Hispanic whites: Demographic and psychiatric disorder issues. *Suicide Life Threat Behav, 18*, 205–218.

97. Stein, S. A., Fox, S. A., & Maturata, P. J. (1991). The influence of ethnicity, socioeconomic status, and psychological barriers on use of mammography. *J Health Soc Behav, 32*, 101–113.

98. Stern, M. P., Gaskell, S. P., Allen, C. R., Garza, V. Gonzalez, J. L., & Waldrop, R. H. (1982). Cardiovascular risk factors in Mexican Americans in Laredo, Texas: II. Prevalence and control of hypertension. *Am J Epidemiol, 113,* 556–562.

99. Stern, M. P., & Haffner, S. M. (1992). Type II diabetes in Mexican Americans: A public health challenge. In A. Furino (Ed.), *Health policy and the Hispanic* (pp. 57–75). Boulder, CO: Westview Press.

100. Stern, M. P., Knapp, J. A., Hazuda, H. P., Haffner, S. M., Patterson, J. K., & Mitchell, B. D. (1991). Genetic and environmental determinants of type II diabetes in Mexican Americans. *Diabetes Care, 14*(Suppl. 3), 649–654.

101. Sumaya, L. V. (1991). Major infectious diseases causing excess morbidity in the Hispanic population. *Arch Intern Med, 151,* 1513–1520.

102. Syme, L. S., & Berkman, L. F. (1976). Social class, susceptibility and sickness. *Am J Epidemiol, 104,* 1–8.

103. Szapocznik, J., & Kurtines, W. (1988). Acculturation, biculturalism and adjustment among Cuban Americans. In A. M. Padilla (Ed.), *Acculturation theory, model and some new findings* (pp. 139–159). Boulder, CO: Westview Press.

104. Torrey, E. F. (1972). The irrelevancy of traditional mental health services for urban Mexican-Americans. In M. Levitt & B. Rubenstein (Eds.), *On the urban scene* (pp. 19–36). Detroit: Wayne State University Press.

105. Trapido, E. J., McCoy, C. B., Strickman-Stein, N., Engel, S., Zavertnik, J. J., & Comerford, M. (1990). Epidemiology of cancer among Hispanic males: The experience in Florida. *Cancer, 65,* 657–662.

106. Trevino, F. M., Moyer, M. E., Valdez, R. B., & Stroup-Benham, C. A. (1992). Health insurance coverage and utilization of health services by Mexican Americans, Puerto Ricans, and Cuban Americans. In A. Furino (Ed.), *Health policy and the Hispanic* (pp. 158–170). Boulder, CO: Westview Press.

107. Trevino, R. M., & Moss, A. J. (1984). *Health indicators for Hispanic, black and white Americans* (Vital Health Statistics, Series 10, No. 148). Hyattsville, MD: National Center for Health Statistics.

108. Trotter, R. T., II. (1981). Remedios caseros: Mexican American home remedies and community health problems. *Soc Sci Med, 15B,* 107–114.

109. Trotter, R. T., II, & Chavira, J. A. (1981). *Curanderismo: Mexican American folk healing.* Athens: University of Georgia Press.

110. U.S. Bureau of the Census. (1991). *The Hispanic population in the United States: March 1990* (Current Population Report, Series P-20, No. 449). Washington, DC: U.S. Government Printing Office.

111. U.S. Bureau of the Census. (1991). *General, social and economic data* (U.S. Summary Table 152, PC80-1, No. 1).

112. U.S. Bureau of the Census. (1991). *Race and Hispanic origin, 1990* (Census Profile No. 2). Washington, DC: U.S. Department of Commerce.

113. U.S. Department of Health and Human Services. (1985). *Report of the Secretary's Task Force on Black and Minority Health: Vol. 2. Crosscutting issues in minority health.* Washington, DC: U.S. Government Printing Office.

114. U.S. Department of Health and Human Services. (1990). *Healthy people 2000: National health promotion and disease prevention objectives.* Washington, DC: U.S. Government Printing Office.

115. U.S. Department of Health and Human Services. (1986). *Report of the Secretary's Task Force on Black and Minority Health: Vol. 8. Hispanic health issues.* Washington, DC: U.S. Government Printing Office.

116. Vega, W. A., Gil, A., Warheit, G., Apospori, E., & Zimmerman, R. (1993). The relationship of drug use to suicide ideation and attempts among African American, Hispanic, and white Non-Hispanic male adolescents. *Suicide Life Threat Behav, 23,* 110–119.

117. Vega, W. A., Gil, A. G., & Zimmerman R. S. (1993). Patterns of drug use among Cuban-American, African-American, and white non-Hispanic boys. *Am J Public Health, 83,* 257–259.

118. Vega, W. A., Hough, R. L., & Miranda, M. R. (1985). Modeling cross-cultural research in Hispanic mental health. In W. A. Vega & M. R. Miranda (Eds.), *Stress and Hispanic mental health: Relating research to service delivery* (pp. 1–29) (DHHS Publication No. [ADM] 85-1410). Rockville, MD: National Institute of Mental Health.

119. Vega, W. A., Kolody, B., Hwang, J., & Noble, A. (1993). Prevalence and magnitude of perinatal substance exposures in California. *N Engl J Med, 329,* 850–854.

120. Vega, W. A., Kolody, B., Valle, R., & Weir, J. (1991). Social networks, social support, and their relationship to depression among immigrant Mexican women. *Hum Organ, 50,* 154–162.

121. Ventura, S. J., & Tappel, S. M. (1985). Childbearing characteristics of the US and foreign-born Hispanic mothers. *Public Health Rep, 100,* 647–652.

122. Wells, I. B., Hough, R. L., Golding, J. M., Burnam, M. A., & Karno, M. (1987). Which Mexican Americans underutilize health services? *Am J Psychiatry, 144,* 918–922.

123. Wilkinson, R. G. (1990). Income distribution and mortality: A "natural" experiment. *Sociol Health Illness, 12,* 1082–1084.

124. Wolfgang, P. E., Semeiks, P. A., & Burnett, W. S. (1991). Cancer incidence in New York City Hispanics, 1982–1985. *Ethn Dis, 1,* 263–272.

125. Wolinsky, F. D. (1978). Assessing the effects of predisposing, enabling and illness-morbidity characteristics on health service utilization. *J Health Soc Behav, 19,* 384–396.

126. Wood, P. R., Hidalgo, H. A., Prihoda, T. J., & Kromer, M. E. (1993). Hispanic children with asthma: Morbidity. *Pediatrics, 265,* 227–232.

CHAPTER FIVE

Segregation, Poverty, and Empowerment

Health Consequences for African Americans

Thomas A. LaVeist

The past three decades have brought important changes to America's racial landscape. Most notably, African Americans have gained control of the political and policymaking apparatus of many of America's major cities. Further, we have witnessed the development of a growing black middle class. These facts are undeniable. Their legacy, however, is uncertain.

Despite apparent advances, many problems persist. The data speak loudly to the existence among African Americans of greater social and health problems than among their white compatriots. African Americans have higher rates of unemployment, illiteracy, unwed and teen births, low birthweight, homicide, and infant mortality. In a 1985 essay, John McKnight labeled these facts "an inventory of health costs of powerlessness."[1] How can we reconcile these grim realities with recent black social, political, and economic gains? In other words, what are the health consequences of black social and political progress?

SOCIAL FACTORS AND INFANT MORTALITY

It has become the dominant view among medical sociologists and demographers that improvements in the general standard of living are the primary reason for the impressive declines in infant mortality in industrialized societies.

I am grateful to Sam Shapiro and Barbara Starfield for comments on earlier drafts of this manuscript. Data collection was supported by a grant from the Michigan Health Care Educational and Research Foundation, Inc. (Grant No. 027-SAP/87-04).

Observations of the effect of societal factors on mortality rates surfaced as early as the first decades of the twentieth century.[2] Studies demonstrating the impact of social forces on mortality can be found among the earliest works in sociology.[3] René Dubos's study of 1959 is perhaps most closely associated with this perspective.[4] However, numerous other examples exist in both the social and the health sciences literature.[5-12]

Based on his cross-national examination of the effects on mortality of improvements in the standard of living, Preston found a declining marginal return on increasing increments in standard of living.[13] Therefore, it would seem that further declines in mortality in industrialized societies are dependent on medical technology. However, Wise and colleagues' examination of more recent experiences in Boston suggests that, as medical technology approaches its maximum utility in reducing infant mortality, social factors will reclaim the central role in producing infant deaths.[14,15] It stands to reason that the most vulnerable populations would be most severely affected.

Since the United States began to collect race-specific data, the black infant mortality rate has consistently been reported to be double the white rate. This suggests that over the years African Americans have experienced consistent and invariant deprivation relative to whites. Figure 5.1 shows that, whereas infant mortality rates for both black and white Americans have declined since

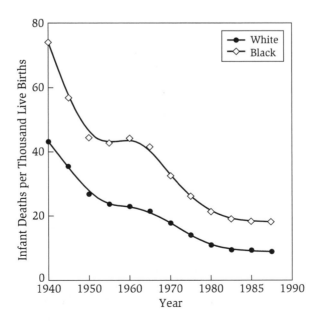

Figure 5.1 Black-White Disparity in Infant Mortality in the United States.

at least 1940, little progress has been achieved in reducing the black-white relative rate.

However, the relationship between race and infant mortality is more complex than the persistent 2:1 ratio displayed in Figure 5.1 would suggest because the spatial variation in the black-white infant mortality rate is also substantial.

Figure 5.2 shows the distribution of the black-white five-year infant mortality differential ratio (relative rate) aggregated over the years 1981 to 1985 for all U.S. cities of 50,000 or more that are at least 10 percent black. The analysis displayed in Figure 5.2 indicates that the degree of black-to-white relative disadvantage varies substantially across the cities. The figure shows a leptokurtic normal curve. The black-white infant mortality ratio ranges between .56 and 5.02, and in eight cities there is a higher infant mortality rate for whites than for blacks. Cities range from having an infant mortality rate that is lower among blacks than whites to having a rate that is more than triple among blacks as compared to whites. In one extreme outlier, Kenner, Louisiana, the black infant mortality rate is five times the white rate. (This outlier was excluded from the figure, but was included in all analysis.) The list of cities examined in this study,

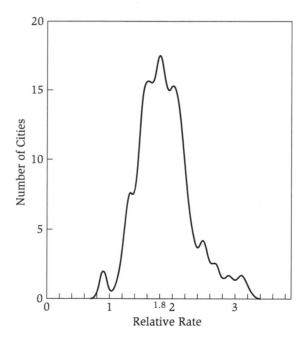

Figure 5.2 Black-White Relative Rate of Infant Mortality in U.S. Cities of 50,000, 1981–1985.

along with their infant mortality rates and black-white ratios, is displayed in the Appendix to this chapter.

Perhaps social factors in these cities have had a differential impact on African Americans and whites. If so, elucidating these factors may help to identify areas of potential for intervention. By successfully manipulating them, we may bring about a reduction in the current black-white disparity in infant mortality. I propose to examine three social factors: racial residential segregation, poverty, and black political empowerment.

RACIAL RESIDENTIAL SEGREGATION

. . . one Black, one White—separate and unequal.
—U.S. National Advisory Commission on Civil Disorders[16]

In its 1968 report to President Lyndon Johnson, the National Advisory Commission on Civil Disorders concluded, "Our nation is moving toward two societies, one Black, one White—separate and unequal."[16] More than two decades later there is reason to believe that we are no longer moving toward separation, but, rather, have arrived at the point where racial segregation has become an enduring feature of America's social arrangement[17] (see Table 5.1).

In 1987 the U.S. infant mortality rate ranked seventeenth internationally. However, when the U.S. black-white disparity is viewed in an international context, the rate for white Americans improves to twelfth and the African American rate drops to twenty-sixth. If America has indeed become two societies, then white American society is comparable to other industrialized countries, whereas black American society borders on being a Third World nation.

Yankauer was the first to establish empirically a link between racial segregation and health status. In his analysis of data from New York City in the 1940s, Yankauer observed that infant mortality rates, for both blacks and whites, were highest in the most severely segregated black neighborhoods.[18] The racial segregation–infant mortality finding has been replicated in more recent national studies. I demonstrated this relationship in an earlier study that analyzed large and midsized U.S. cities.[19] Although I found black infant mortality rates to be higher in highly segregated cities, I discovered that white rates were essentially unaffected by a city's level of segregation. Indeed, white rates dropped only slightly as segregation increased. Jiobu's path analysis of a somewhat smaller set of cities during the 1960s also demonstrated a link between segregation and infant mortality.[20]

Although the empirical link between segregation and mortality is fairly straightforward, the specific supporting mechanisms for this association are less

Table 5.1. International Comparisons of Infant Mortality Rates, 1986

Rank	Country	IMR
1	Sweden	7.0
2	Japan	7.1
3	Finland	7.6
4	Norway	8.1
5	Netherlands	8.2
6	Denmark	8.4
7	Switzerland	8.5
8	Australia	9.6
9	France	9.6
10	Spain	10.3
11	Singapore	10.8
12	*United States–white*	*11.0*
12	Canada	11.0
13	Belgium	11.7
14	Austria	11.9
14	New Zealand	11.9
17	*United States–total*	*12.1*
18	German Democratic Republic	12.3
19	Federal Republic of Germany	12.6
20	Italy	14.3
21	Israel	15.1
22	Jamaica	16.2
23	Czechoslovakia	16.8
24	Greece	17.9
25	Cuba	18.5
26	*United States–black*	*20.0*

Note: IMR = infant mortality rate.

direct. The body of research on this topic suggests the prevalence of a variety of problematic social conditions in highly segregated black communities. Previous research has established that segregated black urban communities are highly toxic environments,[21,22] which are not as well served by city services,[23,24] lack adequate medical services,[25] and have higher housing costs, thus leading to an inflated cost of living.[26] Thus, segregation can be viewed primarily as an easily quantifiable summary measure of differences in the material living conditions of black and white Americans.

POVERTY

The level of living of the masses of Negroes trapped in these
densely populated continuously deteriorating ghettoes [is] not
likely to keep pace with "the American way of life."
—Killian and Grigg[27]

Poverty is the best documented social risk factor for infant mortality. Empirical examples of the relationship between them can be found as early as the first decade of the twentieth century.[2] The sheer volume of research supporting a link between poverty or low socioeconomic status and infant mortality is impressive.[28-32] In fact, one author pronounced any further research on the relationship between poverty and infant mortality to be "a waste of time, money and effort, because the gross relationship [had] been established conclusively enough."[33]

It is axiomatic to state that poverty has been an enduring component of the African American reality. Indeed, some scholars have had difficulty distinguishing the line of demarcation between being black and being impoverished. Some researchers have used race as an indicator of poverty status. It has even been asserted, somewhat controversially, that black-white disparities in infant mortality (and health status in general) can be attributed solely to black-white disparities in socioeconomic status. Others have argued, however, that race is more complex. Status as an African American is not quite the equivalent of being a low-income white American. African Americans have cultural values and behaviors; because of racism, they are exposed to potential health risks that sustain race as a determinant of health status, irrespective of social class.

The resolution of this debate is best left for another occasion. However, for now, the establishment of two important facts is relevant: first, that socioeconomic status is an important social risk factor for infant mortality and, second, that poverty is more prevalent among African Americans than among white Americans.

POLITICAL POWER AS A STRATEGY FOR HEALTH

True liberation can be acquired and maintained only when the Negro people
possess power; and power is the product and flower of organization.
—A. Phillip Randolph[34]

Several scholars have speculated that political empowerment might have a beneficial impact on health status.[1,35,36] In a 1989 letter to the editor of the *Journal of the American Medical Association,* Braithwaite and Lythcott argued that race differentials in health status were outward manifestations of power differentials and asserted that the feelings of hopelessness and alienation from societal institutions impeded appropriate health and illness behaviors. This, they argued, resulted in poorer health status among African Americans.[35]

In an essay published in the *Canadian Journal of Public Health*, McKnight maintained that the traditional tools of public health have met with only limited success in improving the health status of disenfranchised groups.[1] Thus, because the highest indexes of poor health were found among groups with the least power, the social and political empowerment of these groups may lead to new remedies that are more effective in improving their health status.

My empirical examination supported the hypothesis that political power would affect health status.[36] Black postneonatal mortality rates were lower in cities where African Americans had higher levels of political power; white postneonatal mortality rates were not affected by the level of black political power. Therefore, black political power led to a narrowing of the postneonatal mortality gap between African Americans and whites. The theoretical link between black political power and black postneonatal mortality is shown in Figure 5.3. Tests to determine the mechanisms that create the observed association ruled out the most obvious explanation: that black elected officials might allocate resources in such a way as to benefit African Americans. Rather, the analysis led me to conclude that community organization is the common factor underlying the infrastructure that both facilitates greater black political power and improves the material conditions of African Americans' lives. These improved conditions in turn are manifested in lower black postneonatal mortality rates.

ASSESSING THE IMPACT OF SEGREGATION, POVERTY, AND POLITICAL POWER

The research literature contains support for each factor—segregation, poverty, and political power—as an important social predictor of health status. Yet how interrelated are these social phenomena in their impact on black-white

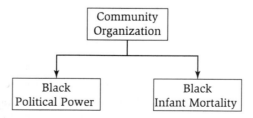

Figure 5.3 Schematic of the Relationship Between Black Political Power and Black Infant Mortality.

differentials? I will address this question through an empirical examination of data from cities throughout the United States. Cities were selected for the study that had a population in 1980 equal to or exceeding 50,000, at least 10 percent of which was African American. These selection criteria resulted in a population of 176 cities representing thirty-two states and all regions of the United States. Data for the analysis were derived from various published sources, including the National Center for Health Statistics, the U.S. Census Bureau, and the Joint Center for Political and Economic Studies.

Infant mortality rate is a long-standing general indicator of overall social and economic development, availability, and use of health services, health status of women of childbearing age, and quality of social and physical environment.[37] It has been applied for this purpose in studies conducted at various levels of analysis: international,[13] national,[38] state,[20,39] county,[40] and city.[41] The black-white disparity in infant mortality is computed by taking the ratio of black to white infant mortality rates for each city (relative rate). Five-year rates (1981–1985) are used in order to control for possible single-year variations in cities with few births or infant deaths.

Racial residential segregation is measured using the index of dissimilarity for 1980. The index is a measure of the degree of racial residential segregation based on a scale ranging from 0 (no segregation) to 100 (complete segregation). (See White[42,43] or Duncan and Duncan[44] for a complete empirical and conceptual assessment of this measure.) Poverty rates are based on the percentage of families whose income and family size indicated that their standard of living was below the federally determined poverty level at the time of the 1980 U.S. Census. Black political power is the ratio of the percentage of African Americans on the city council to the percentage of African Americans in the voting-age population for 1983–1984.[45–47]

FINDINGS

Figure 5.4 schematically displays the conceptual model that guided my analysis. I hypothesized that racial residential segregation was an exogenous variable with a causal link to both poverty and political power. Each variable was predicted to be directly related to the black-white disparity in infant mortality. Segregation, furthermore, was hypothesized to be both directly and indirectly associated with the black-white disparity in infant mortality.

To begin the analysis, I conducted a preliminary assessment of the general relationships among the variables by calculating unadjusted correlation coefficients. The results of this preliminary analysis, displayed in Table 5.2, show that residential segregation has a statistically significant association with each endogenous variable except white poverty. In cities with high levels of

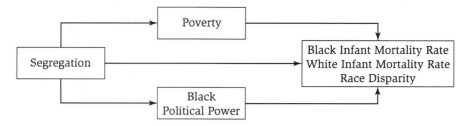

Figure 5.4 Infant Mortality Rate (IMR) Conceptual Model.

segregation, a larger proportion of the black population lives below the poverty level. However, a city's degree of segregation is not significantly related to white poverty.

A less deleterious consequence of segregation is reflected in the positive association between segregation and black political power, which indicates that African Americans are better able to achieve political power in highly segregated cities. This finding, which is consistent with Vedlitz and Johnson's analysis,[48] probably reflects the fact that most cities elect city council representatives by districts. Highly segregated cities more often contain districts that constitute majority black voting blocs, thus improving the likelihood of electing African American representatives. Because the measure of black political power is based on city council representation, this finding is to be expected.

The relationship between segregation and the black-white disparity in infant mortality replicates analysis published elsewhere.[18-20] The table indicates a conformation with the findings from these studies, which is that the disparity in black-white infant mortality rates tends to be greater in highly segregated cities.

Table 5.2 also shows that for both blacks and whites poverty is positively associated with black infant mortality. White poverty is also significantly inversely associated with the black-white disparity in infant mortality: that is, as

Table 5.2. Zero-Order Correlations

Endogenous Variable	Residential Segregation	Black Poverty	White Poverty	Black Political Power
Black poverty	.327***			
White poverty	−.066	.225***		
Black political power	.259***	.191**	.116	
Black infant mortality	.247***	.181**	.060	−.121*
White infant mortality	−.124*	.164*	.418***	.062
Race disparity in infant mortality	.305***	.047	−.153*	−.048

*$p \le .1$; **$p \le .05$; ***$p \le .01$.

the poverty rate of whites in a city climbs, the gap between black and white infant mortality rates narrows. This narrowing takes place because the white infant mortality rate is so adversely affected by white poverty rates. Finally, although the presence of black political power clearly reduces black infant mortality rates, the magnitude of the reduction is not enough to affect the black-white disparity significantly.

It is interesting to note three interrelated findings.

1. Black infant mortality is higher in highly segregated cities.
2. Black political power is greater in highly segregated cities.
3. Black infant mortality is lower in cities with greater black political power and higher in cities with high segregation.

These may, at first, appear to be contradictory findings; however, further analysis reveals that they are not. I have described elsewhere the modifying impact of black political power on the connection between segregation and black infant mortality.[49] In a highly segregated black community political empowerment can reduce (but not entirely eliminate) the negative consequences of segregation. This finding illustrates the importance of multivariate analysis. The preliminary bivariate (unadjusted) analysis presented in Table 5.2 is instructive; however, it is necessary to conduct multivariate analysis in order to determine if the relationships presented in Table 5.2 persist once the influence of other potentially confounding variables is taken into account.

Tables 5.3 and 5.4 present multivariate analysis to examine the relationships outlined in Figure 5.4. Table 5.3 assesses how segregation is related to black poverty, white poverty, and black political power. Control variables indicating

Table 5.3. OLS Regression Unstandardized Coefficients for Black Poverty, White Poverty, and Black Political Power Regressed on Segregation

Independent Variable	Black Poverty	White Poverty	Black Political Power
Constant	28.14	3.97	.025
Segregation	.165***	−.497	.012***
Log of population	−2.64**	.218	−.062
West	−5.492***	1.397**	.208
North Central	−2.032*	1.209***	.145*
Northeast	.092	3.134***	.083
R^2 (adjusted)	.20	.21	.09

Note: OLS = ordinary least squares.

*$p \leq .1$; **$p \leq .05$; ***$p \leq .01$.

Table 5.4. OLS Regression Unstandardized Coefficients for Black Infant Mortality, White Infant Mortality, and the Black-White Disparity in Infant Mortality

Independent Variable	Infant Mortality Rate		Black-White Disparity
	Black	White	
Constant	14.05	9.31	2.20
Segregation	.065**	−.032**	.012***
Black poverty	.075*		−.002
White poverty		.316***	−.034**
Black political power	−.238*	.093	.018
Log of population	−.197	.038	−.154
West	−2.648**	−.647	−.218*
North Central	1.718**	.976**	−.023
Northeast	.404	.207	−.018
R^2 (adjusted)	.11	.22	.10

Note: OLS = ordinary least squares; IMR = infant mortality rate.

$*p \leq .1; **p \leq .05; ***p \leq .01.$

the city's regional location and the natural log of its population are included in each model for two reasons: (1) the relationship between segregation and the dependent variables (poverty and black political power) may vary by region, or (2) the size of the city's population may influence the consequences of segregation on the dependent variables. By controlling for region and population it is possible to calculate the adjusted relationship between segregation and the dependent variables.

Table 5.3 shows that after adjusting for the effects of the other variables in the analysis (listed in the table) the relationship between segregation and poverty has not been affected. Although segregated cities tend to have higher levels of black poverty, white poverty rates are not significantly affected by segregation. Also, although African Americans in segregated cities suffer higher poverty rates, they are better able to attain political power. These findings are consistent with Table 5.2. Table 5.3 also shows that black urban poverty rates are lower in the West and the North Central region than they are in the South. However, white urban poverty rates are highest in the Northeast.

Are these relationships implicated in black infant mortality? The analyses displayed in Table 5.4 show that, after accounting for the effects of the other social factors on black infant mortality, the crude relationships displayed in Table 5.2 have not been eliminated. Black infant mortality is higher in very segregated cities and in cities where there is more black poverty. Black infant mortality rates are lower in cities where blacks have achieved greater political power. Regionally, black infant mortality rates are higher in the North Central part of the country and lower in the West compared to the South. It should also be noted that white poverty is far more strongly associated with white infant mortality than black poverty is with black infant mortality. The inverse association between segregation and white infant mortality suggests that whites benefit from segregation. However, the nonsignificant effect of black political power on white infant mortality suggests that black political gains have not come at the expense of whites.[36]

The model in Table 5.4 shows how the relationships between segregation, poverty, and black political empowerment extend to the black-white disparity in infant mortality. This model indicates that the zero-order associations summarized in Table 5.2 also hold up within multivariate analysis. The black-white gap in infant mortality is greater in more highly segregated cities. The disparity is smaller in cities with high rates of white poverty. However, black poverty and black political empowerment do not directly affect the black-white disparity in infant mortality. The analysis also shows that the black-white disparity in infant mortality is smaller in the West than in the South.

SUMMARY AND DISCUSSION

In spite of strong achievements in improving the chances of survival for infants born in the United States, there has been little success in reducing the national black-white differential in infant mortality. The black infant mortality rate has been reported consistently to be double the white rate. However, when the black-white infant mortality disparity is examined within smaller geographic units, a more complex relationship between race and infant mortality emerges. There is, indeed, substantial geographic variation in the degree of black to white relative disadvantage.

Three factors distinguished cities in this analysis: segregation, poverty, and black political empowerment. Because these are potentially malleable social factors, policy and other interventions have the potential to be effective. The association between segregation and the black-white disparity in infant mortality consists of a higher black infant mortality rate and a lower white infant mortality rate in highly segregated cities. Poverty is associated with both black and white infant mortality, but only white poverty is directly related to the differential in black-white infant mortality. Black infant mortality rates are lower in cities where blacks have gained a measure of political empowerment. However, the effect of this power on black infant mortality is not strong enough to significantly reduce the disparity in black-white infant mortality.

Previous findings indicate that, even among middle-class African Americans, race dictates access to neighborhoods whose resources (for example, schools, medical services, employment opportunities) are commensurate with level of income. They are excluded from neighborhoods where their white middle-class counterparts reside largely on the basis of race.[50] Villemez demonstrated that African Americans get a smaller return for their investments in human capital, such as quality of residence and education, than do whites.[51] Thus, black spatial mobility is artificially constrained. Structural barriers militate against the link between spatial and social mobility.[52,53]

The interplay between residential segregation and the political and social organization of cities produces structural constraints that limit black life chances.[50,54] Limitations on black spatial mobility constrain even the more affluent African Americans by restricting their access to employment opportunities,[55–58] relegating their children to inferior schools,[59,60] and exposing them to greater environmental health risks.[22,61] Thus, regardless of economic resources, many middle-income African Americans are forced to live in socio-environmental conditions that—although superior to those of low-income blacks—are not consistent with their economic status. This finding coincides with the stronger association between poverty and infant mortality among whites than blacks ($b = .375$, $\beta = .4$, $p < .001$ for whites and $b = .075$, $\beta = .12$, $p < .1$ for blacks).

My analysis suggests the importance of research to explore the city characteristics that lead to the variability in infant mortality rates displayed in Figure 5.2. In none of the models I have presented does the adjusted R^2 exceed 22 percent of variance explained. Future research is needed to examine the impact of other correlates of aggregate infant mortality on the black-white differential. Examples of these variables include access to medical technology, quality of housing,[31] overcrowded living conditions,[62] quality of medical care under Medicaid,[63] and exposure to air pollution.[64] Corman and Grossman concluded that the availability of abortion, of neonatal intensive care units, education, Medicaid, community health service projects, maternal nutrition programs, and family planning services has an impact on neonatal mortality rates at the county level.[40] However, the topic of black-white infant mortality differences has seldom been a primary concern in published reports.

We can learn important lessons from the characteristics that distinguish cities with a slight disparity in black-white infant mortality rates and cities from those in which a great gulf exists. Discovering more about these characteristics will help to guide policy and to inform intervention that may lead to reducing black-white disparities in infant mortality at the national level.

This line of research is still in the preliminary stages. Ecological data have their limitations, which means that it is of paramount importance to develop strong theory. An instructive line for future research—through qualitative investigations—would be an exploration of the specific mechanisms that link poverty, segregation, and political empowerment with infant mortality.

Notes

1. McKnight, J. L. (1985). Health and empowerment. *Can J Public Health,* *76*(Suppl.), 37–38.

2. Newsholme, A. (1910). *39th annual report of the Local Government Board* (England) (Report Cd 5312).

3. Durkheim, É. (1897/1951). *Suicide: A study in sociology.* New York: Free Press.

4. Dubos, R. (1959). *Mirage of health.* New York: Harper and Row.

5. Mckeown, T. (1976a). *The modern rise of population.* London: Edward Arnold.

6. Mckeown, T. (1976b). *The role of medicine: Dream, mirage or nemesis.* London: Nuffield Provincial Hospitals Trust.

7. Illich, I. (1975). *Medical nemesis: The exploration of health.* London: Chalder and Boyars.

8. McKinlay, J., McKinlay, S., & Beaglehole, R. (1988). Trends in death and disease and the contribution of medical measures. In H. E. Freeman & S. Levine (Eds.), *Handbook of medical sociology* (4th ed.). Englewood Cliffs, NJ: Prentice Hall.

9. McKinlay, J., McKinlay, S., & Beaglehole, R. (1989). A review of the evidence concerning the impact of medical measures on recent mortality and morbidity in the United States. *Int J Health Ser, 19,* 181–207.

10. McKinlay, J., & McKinlay, S. (1977). The questionable contribution of medical measures to the decline of mortality in the United States in the twentieth century. *Milbank Mem Fund Q/Health and Society, 55,* 405–428.

11. Rydell, L. H. (1976). Trends in infant mortality: Medical advances or socio-economic changes? *Acta Sociologica, 19,* 147–168.

12. Powles, J. (1973). On the limitations of modern medicine. *Science, Medicine and Man, 1,* 1–30.

13. Preston, S. (1975). The changing relation between mortality and level of economic development. *Population Studies, 29,* 231–248.

14. Wise, P. H. (1990). Poverty, technology and recent trends in the United States infant mortality rate. *Paediatr Perinat Epidemiol, 4,* 390–401.

15. Wise, P. H., First, L. R., Lamb, G. A., et al. (1988). Infant mortality increase despite high access to tertiary care: An evolving relationship among infant mortality, health care and socioeconomic change. *Pediatrics, 81,* 542–548.

16. U.S. National Advisory Commission on Civil Disorders. (1968). *Report of the National Advisory Commission on Civil Disorders.* Washington, DC: Author.

17. Massey, D. S. (1990). American apartheid: Segregation and the making of the underclass. *Am J Sociol, 96,* 329–357.

18. Yankauer, A. (1950). The relationship of fetal and infant mortality to residential segregation. *Am Sociol Rev, 15,* 644–648.

19. LaVeist, T. A. (1989). Linking residential segregation to the infant mortality race disparity. *Sociol Soc Res, 73,* 90–94.

20. Jiobu, R. M. (1972). Urban determinants of racial differentiation in infant mortality. *Demography, 9,* 603–615.

21. U.S. General Accounting Office. (1983). *Citing of hazardous waste landfills and their correlation with racial and economic status of surrounding communities.* Washington, DC: Author.

22. Bullard, R. D. (1983). Solid waste sites and the black Houston community. *Sociol Inq, 53,* 273–288.

23. Schneider, M., & Logan, J. R. (1982). Suburban racial segregation and black access to local public resources. *Soc Sci Q, 63,* 762–770.

24. Schneider, M., & Logan, J. R. (1985). Suburban municipalities: The changing system of intergovernmental relations in the mid-1970s. *Urban Affairs, 21,* 87–105.

25. Law, R. (1985). Public policy and health-care delivery: A practitioner's perspective. *Rev Black Polit Econ, 14,* 217–225.

26. Berry, B.J.L. (1976). Ghetto expansion and single-family housing prices: Chicago, 1968–1972. *J Urban Economics, 3,* 397–423.

27. Killian, L., & Grigg, C. (1964). *Racial crisis in America: Leadership in conflict.* Englewood Cliffs, NJ: Prentice Hall.

28. LaVeist, T. A. (1990). Simulating the effects of poverty on the race disparity in postneonatal mortality. *J Public Health Policy, 11,* 463–473.

29. Paneth, N., Wallenstein, S., Keily, J., & Susser, M. (1982). Social class indicators and mortality in low birth weight infants. *Am J Epidemiol, 116,* 364–375.

30. Gortmaker, S. (1979). Poverty and infant mortality in the United States. *Am Sociol Rev, 44,* 280–297.

31. Brooks, C. H. (1975). Path analysis of socioeconomic correlates of county infant mortality rates. *Int J Health Ser, 5,* 499–513.

32. Stockwell, E. G. (1962). Infant mortality and socio-economic status: A changing relationship. *Milbank Mem Fund Q, 40,* 101–111.

33. Anderson, O. W. (1958). Infant mortality and social and cultural factors: Historical trends and current patterns. In E. G. Jaco (Ed.), *Patients, physicians and illness.* Glencoe, IL.: Free Press.

34. Randolph, A. P. (1937). Quoted in Franklin, V. P. (1984). *Black self-determination: A cultural history of the faith of the fathers.* Westport, CT: Lawrence Hill.

35. Braithwaite, R. L., & Lythcott, N. (1989). Community empowerment as a strategy for health promotion for black and other minority populations. *JAMA, 261,* 282–283.

36. LaVeist, T. A. (1992). The political empowerment and health status of African Americans: Mapping a new territory. *Am J Sociol, 97,* 1080–1095.

37. Morris, M. D. (1979). *Measuring the condition of the world's poor: The Physical Quality of Life Index.* New York: Pergamon Press.

38. Cereseto, S., & Waitzkin, H. (1986). Economic development, political-economic system, and the physical quality of life. *Am J Public Health, 76,* 661–666.

39. Kleinman, J. C. (1986). State trends in infant mortality. *Am J Public Health, 76,* 681–688.

40. Corman, H., & Grossman, M. (1985). Determinants of neonatal mortality rates in the U.S.: A reduced form model. *J Health Economics, 4,* 213–236.

41. Altenderfer, M., & Crowther, B. (1949). Relationship between infant mortality and socio-economic factors in urban areas. *Public Health Rep, 64,* 331–339.

42. White, M. J. (1983). The measurement of spatial segregation. *Am J Sociol, 88,* 1008–1018.

43. White, M. J. (1985). Segregation and diversity measures in population distribution. *Population Index, 52,* 198–221.

44. Duncan, O. D., & Duncan, B. (1955). A methodological analysis of segregation indexes. *Am Sociol Rev, 20,* 210–217.

45. Karnig, A. K. (1976). Black representation on city councils. *Urban Affairs Q, 12,* 243–250.

46. Karnig, A. K. (1979). Black resources and city council representation. *J Politics, 41,* 134–149.

47. Robinson, T. P., & Dye, T. R. (1978). Reformism and black representation on city councils. *Soc Sci Q, 59,* 133–141.

48. Vedlitz, A., & Johnson, C. A. (1982). Community racial segregation, electoral structure and minority representation. *Soc Sci Q, 63,* 729–736.

49. LaVeist, T. A. (1988). *An ecological analysis of the effects of political inputs on health outcomes: The case of the black-white infant mortality disparity.* Unpublished Ph.D. dissertation, University of Michigan, Ann Arbor.

50. Massey, D. S., Condran, G. A., & Denton, N. A. (1987). The effects of residential segregation on black social and economic well-being. *Social Forces, 66,* 29–56.

51. Villemez, W. (1980). Race, class, and neighborhood: Differences in the residential return on individual resources. *Social Forces, 59,* 414–430.

52. Massey, D. S., & Mullan, B. P. (1984). Processes of Hispanic and black spatial assimilation. *Am J Sociol, 89,* 836–873.

53. Park, R. E. (1926). The urban community as a spatial pattern and a moral order. In E. W. Burgess (Ed.), *The urban community* (pp. 3–18). Chicago: University of Chicago Press.

54. Logan, J. R. (1978). Growth, politics and the stratification of places. *Am J Sociol, 84,* 404–416.

55. Deskins, D. R. (1988). Michigan's restructured automotive industry: Its impact on black employment. In F. S. Thomas (Ed.), *The state of black Michigan, 1988.* East Lansing: Michigan State University.

56. Cole, R. E., & Deskins, D. R. (1988). Racial factors in site location and employment patterns of Japanese auto firms in America. *California Management Review, 31,* 9–22.

57. Lewin-Epstein, N. (1985). Neighborhoods, local labor markets and opportunities for white and nonwhite youth. *Soc Sci Q, 66,* 163–171.

58. Parcel, T. (1979). Race, regional labor markets and earnings. *Am Sociol Rev, 44,* 262–279.

59. Farley, R. (1978). School integration in the United States. In F. D. Bean & W. P. Frisbie (Eds.), *The demography of racial and ethnic groups.* Orlando, FL: Academic Press.

60. Farley, R., & Taeuber, A. F. (1974). Racial segregation in the public schools. *Am J Sociol, 79,* 888–905.

61. Kitagawa, E. M., & Hauser, P. M. (1973). *Differential mortality in the United States.* Cambridge, MA: Harvard University Press.

62. Schwirian, K., & Lacreca, A. (1971). An ecological analysis of urban mortality rates. *Soc Sci Q, 52,* 574–587.

63. Brooks, C. H. (1978). Infant mortality in SMSAs before Medicaid: Test of a causal model. *Health Serv Res, 13,* 3–15.

64. Joyce, T. J., Grossman, M., & Goldman, F. (1989). An assessment of the benefits of air pollution control: The case of infant health. *J Urban Economics, 25,* 32–51.

Appendix

City Ratings in Five-Year Infant Mortality Race Disparity for All U.S. Cities of 50,000 or More and 10 Percent Black, 1981–1985

Rank	City	Total	Population		Infant Mortality	
			Black	White	Black	Ratio
1	Passaic, NJ	52,463	10,367	16.8	9.4	0.56
2	Fairfield, CA	58,099	7,175	12.3	7.3	0.59
3	Harrisburg, PA	53,264	23,234	23.4	15.2	0.65
4	Hawthorne, CA	56,447	7,530	10.8	8.5	0.79
5	Bossier City, LA	50,817	7,114	10.4	8.3	0.80
6	Daly City, CA	78,519	8,464	11.2	9.0	0.80
7	East St. Louis, IL	55,200	52,771	23.0	20.6	0.90
8	Cambridge, MA	95,322	10,409	9.9	8.9	0.90
9	Gary, IN	151,953	107,537	16.0	16.8	1.05
10	Elyria, OH	57,538	7,445	15.0	17.1	1.14
11	Oakland, CA	339,337	159,234	13.4	15.5	1.16
12	Lorian, OH	75,416	8,892	11.1	13.0	1.17
13	Fort Wayne, IN	172,196	25,063	13.4	16.7	1.25
14	Camden, NJ	84,910	45,028	16.7	20.9	1.25
15	Anderson, IN	64,695	8,870	13.4	16.8	1.25
16	Jersey City, NJ	223,532	61,954	16.2	20.4	1.26
17	Clarksville, TN	54,777	11,481	14.2	17.9	1.26
18	Lawton, OK	80,054	12,721	13.3	16.9	1.27
19	Asheville, NC	53,583	11,386	11.4	14.5	1.27
20	Kansas City, KS	161,087	40,826	13.3	17.0	1.28
21	Akron, OH	237,177	52,719	17.2	22.0	1.28
22	Chesapeake, VA	114,486	31,552	11.1	14.6	1.32
23	Baltimore, MD	786,775	431,151	12.5	16.5	1.32

Appendix (Continued)

Rank	City	Total	Population Black	Population White	Infant Mortality Black	Infant Mortality Ratio
24	Midland, TX	70,525	7,081	11.4	15.1	1.32
25	Alexandria, LA	51,565	24,653	13.1	17.4	1.33
26	Elizabeth, NJ	106,201	19,307	12.3	16.4	1.33
27	High Point, NC	63,380	17,803	15.1	20.3	1.34
28	New York, NY	7,071,639	1,784,124	12.1	17.0	1.40
29	Pontiac, MI	76,715	28,438	17.0	23.9	1.41
30	Long Beach, CA	361,334	40,732	11.4	16.3	1.43
31	Durham, NC	100,831	47,481	13.7	19.6	1.43
32	San Francisco, CA	678,974	86,414	10.2	14.6	1.43
33	Oak Park, IL	54,887	5,944	8.8	12.6	1.43
34	Daytona Beach, FL	54,176	17,705	13.3	19.1	1.44
35	New Haven, CT	126,109	40,153	14.6	21.1	1.45
36	Niagara Falls, NY	71,384	9,080	10.5	15.2	1.45
37	Louisville, KY	298,451	84,080	12.6	18.3	1.45
38	Port Arthur, TX	61,251	24,862	11.1	16.3	1.47
39	South Bend, IN	109,727	20,179	11.5	17.0	1.48
40	Portsmouth, VA	104,577	47,133	15.1	22.4	1.48
41	Houston, TX	1,595,138	440,257	11.1	16.5	1.49
42	Huntsville, AL	142,513	29,472	11.0	16.4	1.49
43	Birmingham, AL	284,413	158,223	11.8	17.6	1.49
44	Columbus, OH	564,871	124,880	11.2	16.8	1.50
45	Columbus, GA	169,441	57,884	12.2	18.3	1.50
46	Kansas City, MO	448,159	122,699	11.1	16.7	1.50
47	Denver, CO	492,365	59,252	10.5	15.8	1.50
48	Lansing, MI	130,414	18,075	12.2	18.5	1.52
49	Stamford, CT	102,453	15,552	9.5	14.5	1.53
50	Knoxville, TN	175,030	25,881	12.5	19.5	1.56
51	Beaumont, TX	118,102	43,237	11.2	17.5	1.56
52	Inglewood, CA	94,245	54,031	· 10.4	16.3	1.57
53	Newport News, VA	144,903	45,702	10.8	17.0	1.57
54	Atlanta, GA	425,022	282,912	12.4	19.6	1.58
55	Canton, OH	94,730	15,015	10.9	17.3	1.59
56	Irvington, NJ	61,493	23,429	11.4	18.1	1.59
57	Tulsa, OK	360,919	42,594	10.5	16.7	1.59
58	Galveston, TX	61,902	17,908	9.4	15.0	1.60
59	Carson, CA	81,221	23,879	10.9	17.4	1.60
60	Rochester, NY	241,741	62,332	11.3	18.1	1.60
61	Tallahassee, FL	81,548	25,981	12.7	20.4	1.61
62	Tuscaloosa, AL	75,211	26,376	11.2	18.1	1.62
63	Buffalo, NY	357,870	95,116	11.3	18.3	1.62

(*Continued*)

Appendix

City Ratings in Five-Year Infant Mortality Race Disparity for All U.S. Cities of 50,000
or More and 10 Percent Black, 1981–1985 (Continued)

			Population		Infant Mortality	
Rank	City	Total	Black	White	Black	Ratio
64	Oklahoma City, OK	403,213	58,702	12.6	20.5	1.63
65	Montgomery, AL	177,857	69,765	11.4	18.8	1.65
66	Toledo, OH	354,635	61,750	9.7	16.0	1.65
67	Sacramento, CA	275,741	36,866	9.1	15.1	1.66
68	Little Rock, AR	158,461	51,091	10.2	17.0	1.67
69	Paterson, NJ	137,970	47,117	10.3	17.2	1.67
70	Milwaukee, WI	636,212	146,940	10.6	17.8	1.68
71	Waterloo, IA	75,985	8,396	10.3	17.3	1.68
72	Aurora, IL	81,293	8,454	11.1	18.7	1.68
73	New Rochelle, NY	70,794	12,594	6.5	11.0	1.69
74	Chattanooga, TN	169,565	53,716	10.5	17.8	1.70
75	Philadelphia, PA	1,688,210	638,878	12.8	21.8	1.70
76	Tyler, TX	70,508	18,346	11.1	19.0	1.71
77	Warren, OH	56,629	10,273	8.7	14.9	1.71
78	Lake Charles, LA	75,226	28,556	7.8	13.4	1.72
79	Alexandria, VA	103,217	28,230	12.8	22.2	1.73
80	Jacksonville, FL	540,920	137,324	11.1	19.3	1.74
81	Mansfield, OH	53,927	8,580	13.1	22.8	1.74
82	Rockford, IL	139,712	18,372	10.3	18.1	1.76
83	Mount Vernon, NY	66,713	32,316	11.0	19.4	1.76
84	Norfolk, VA	266,979	93,987	12.7	22.4	1.76
85	Waco, TX	101,261	22,186	10.8	19.1	1.77
86	Charleston, WV	63,968	7,830	10.9	19.3	1.77
87	Omaha, NE	314,255	37,852	10.7	19.0	1.78
88	Peoria, IL	124,160	20,623	12.2	21.7	1.78
89	Shreveport, LA	205,820	84,627	10.1	18.1	1.79
90	Miami, FL	346,865	87,110	5.8	10.4	1.79
91	North Little Rock, AR	64,288	11,784	9.2	16.5	1.79
92	New Orleans, LA	557,515	308,136	10.7	19.2	1.79
93	Compton, CA	81,282	60,872	11.7	21.0	1.79
94	Greenville, SC	58,242	20,757	11.6	20.9	1.80
95	Virginia Beach, VA	262,199	26,291	11.5	20.8	1.81
96	Savannah, GA	141,390	69,267	11.8	21.4	1.81
97	Cleveland, OH	573,822	251,347	12.5	22.7	1.82
98	Macon, GA	116,896	52,054	10.9	19.9	1.83
99	Berkeley, CA	103,328	20,676	7.6	13.9	1.83
100	Providence, RI	156,804	18,546	10.2	18.7	1.83
101	Newark, NJ	329,248	191,743	12.2	22.7	1.86
102	Fayetteville, NC	59,507	24,338	12.3	22.9	1.86

Appendix (Continued)

Rank	City	Total	Population Black	Population White	Infant Mortality Black	Infant Mortality Ratio
103	Dallas, TX	904,078	265,594	9.5	17.7	1.86
104	Cincinnati, OH	385,457	130,467	9.9	18.6	1.88
105	Charleston, SC	69,510	32,419	12.4	23.3	1.88
106	Flint, MI	159,611	66,124	12.5	23.5	1.88
107	Hartford, CT	136,392	46,128	13.3	25.1	1.89
108	Springfield, MA	152,319	25,209	11.7	22.1	1.89
109	Bakersfield, CA	105,611	11,079	11.1	21.1	1.90
110	East Orange, NJ	77,690	64,654	9.5	18.1	1.91
111	Mobile, AL	200,452	72,568	8.8	16.8	1.91
112	Boston, MA	562,944	126,229	10.2	19.5	1.91
113	Fort Worth, TX	385,164	87,723	11.5	22.0	1.91
114	Orlando, FL	128,291	38,385	9.2	17.6	1.91
115	Tampa, FL	271,523	68,835	11.4	21.9	1.92
116	Wilmington, DE	70,195	35,926	14.4	27.9	1.94
117	Indianapolis, IN	700,807	152,626	11.5	22.3	1.94
118	Pasadena, CA	119,374	24,591	9.4	18.3	1.95
119	Decatur, IL	94,081	13,764	13.3	25.9	1.95
120	Nashville, TN	455,651	105,942	10.2	19.9	1.95
121	Grand Rapids, MI	181,843	28,602	10.8	21.3	1.97
122	Trenton, NJ	92,124	41,843	12.3	24.3	1.98
123	Springfield, IL	99,637	10,781	13.4	26.5	1.98
124	Los Angeles, CA	2,966,850	505,208	9.9	19.7	1.99
125	Charlotte, NC	314,447	97,627	9.4	18.8	2.00
126	Yonkers, NY	195,351	20,583	11.0	22.1	2.01
127	Lexington, KY	204,165	27,121	9.6	19.4	2.02
128	Winston-Salem, NC	131,885	52,952	9.1	18.4	2.02
129	Richmond, VA	219,214	112,357	11.6	23.5	2.03
130	Pine Bluff, AR	56,636	27,797	7.5	15.2	2.03
131	Las Vegas, NV	164,674	21,054	7.2	14.6	2.03
132	Chicago, IL	3,005,072	1,197,000	11.9	24.2	2.03
133	Austin, TX	345,496	42,118	8.2	16.7	2.04
134	St. Louis, MO	453,085	206,386	10.0	20.4	2.04
135	Detroit, MI	1,203,339	758,939	11.9	24.4	2.05
136	Norwalk, CT	77,767	10,755	7.6	15.8	2.08
137	Wichita, KS	279,272	30,200	10.1	21.0	2.08
138	North Charleston, SC	62,534	15,996	10.1	21.0	2.08
139	Gainesville, FL	81,371	16,787	11.3	23.5	2.08
140	Jackson, MS	202,895	95,357	8.4	17.5	2.08
141	Longview, TX	62,762	11,981	9.6	20.2	2.10
142	Lynchburg, VA	66,743	15,791	8.8	18.8	2.14

(*Continued*)

Appendix

City Ratings in Five-Year Infant Mortality Race Disparity for All U.S. Cities of 50,000
or More and 10 Percent Black, 1981–1985 (Continued)

Rank	City	Total	Population Black	White	Infant Mortality Black	Ratio
143	Pensacola, FL	57,619	19,458	5.4	11.6	2.15
144	Hampton, VA	122,617	42,070	10.5	22.6	2.15
145	Springfield, OH	72,563	12,394	12.8	27.7	2.16
146	St. Petersburg, FL	238,647	41,000	10.1	21.9	2.17
147	Dayton, OH	203,371	75,031	10.0	21.7	2.17
148	Albany, GA	74,059	35,178	9.6	20.9	2.18
149	Lafayette, LA	81,961	22,859	8.7	19.1	2.20
150	Washington, DC	638,333	448,229	10.8	24.0	2.22
151	Kalamazoo, MI	79,722	12,429	12.5	27.8	2.22
152	Pittsburgh, PA	423,938	101,813	11.6	25.9	2.23
153	Albany, NY	101,727	16,205	9.5	21.4	2.25
154	Youngstown, OH	115,436	38,556	10.5	23.7	2.26
155	Memphis, TN	646,356	307,702	9.6	22.0	2.29
156	Joliet, IL	77,956	15,607	10.7	24.8	2.32
157	Waterbury, CT	103,266	12,051	12.7	30.1	2.37
158	Champaign, IL	58,133	7,383	7.7	18.4	2.39
159	Greensboro, NC	155,642	51,373	8.3	20.0	2.41
160	Waukegan, IL	67,653	12,482	10.0	24.1	2.41
161	Bridgeport, CT	142,546	29,878	7.4	18.1	2.45
162	Pompano Beach, FL	52,618	9,071	7.0	17.2	2.46
163	Saginaw, MI	77,508	27,601	11.5	28.3	2.46
164	Columbia, SC	101,208	40,767	8.8	22.3	2.53
165	Racine, WS	85,725	12,610	7.6	19.7	2.59
166	Raleigh, NC	150,225	41,237	10.9	28.5	2.61
167	Roanoke, VA	100,220	22,028	13.2	35.4	2.68
168	Syracuse, NY	170,105	26,767	10.8	29.1	2.69
169	Evanston, IL	73,706	15,788	8.2	22.4	2.73
170	Wichita Falls, TX	94,201	10,409	10.1	28.5	2.82
171	Monroe, LA	57,597	27,992	6.3	17.8	2.83
172	Fort Lauderdale, FL	153,279	32,219	5.8	17.4	3.00
173	West Palm Beach, FL	63,305	17,599	7.3	22.1	3.03
174	Baton Rouge, LA	219,419	80,119	7.2	21.9	3.04
175	Cleveland Heights, OH	56,438	14,059	8.6	27.2	3.16
176	Kenner, LA	66,382	9,369	6.3	31.6	5.02

Note: A five-year aggregation is used because yearly fluctuations may be misleading when single years
are used.

PART TWO

CONCEPTUAL ISSUES IN THE STUDY OF RACE AND ETHNICITY

CHAPTER SIX

A Note on the Biological Concept
of Race and Its Application
in Epidemiologic Research

Richard Cooper

Racial differentials are a prominent feature of the epidemiology of mass disease in multiracial societies such as the United States. Although the concept of race may have a clear-cut practical meaning in many situations, its biological significance is often ambiguous. Analytic thinking in epidemiologic research generally proceeds on the assumption that at least some important proportion of the racial differential may be explained by population genetics. From that perspective it is disconcerting to recognize that anthropologists, in whose discipline the concept of race most naturally belongs, have arrived at the conclusion that human races in fact do not exist.[1-10] If it is true that "it is an error to believe that races are *things* . . . whose separate evolutionary development may be traced,"[1] then to what end is it justifiable to use the category of race in epidemiologic research? In an effort to address that question, this chapter has three purposes: (1) to argue against the biological concept of race, (2) to examine the shortcomings of the race concept in public health, and (3) to emphasize the social origins of racial differences.

RACE AND BIOLOGY: A HISTORICAL VIEW

The concept of race as applied to man was first introduced into the literature of biology by Buffon in 1749.[1] It was explicitly regarded as an arbitrary classification, serving only as a convenient label, not a definable scientific entity.

From the point of view of the biologist, the concept of race is an attempt to extend the taxonomic classification below the level of species. It shares the inherent weaknesses of the Linnaean system while introducing unique problems of its own.

Taxonomy is useful for two separate but interrelated reasons: it helps us understand evolution and provides a framework for examining present variation in plants and animals. Yet no zoological classification is absolute.[7-9] As Watt[7] points out: "From an evolutionary point of view taxonomy is arbitrary and static. Forcing the results of the dynamic and multiplex process of evolution into simple two-dimensional sets of pigeonholes cannot be done without losing information." For most biologists, use of race results in a net loss of information.

If consensus is any measure, defining the races of man has never been successfully accomplished.[1,10-13] It is important to emphasize that what is at stake here is not the possibility of designating groups of people that differ in some way. Human variation *is* self-evident; the existence of definable groups, or races, is not. The problem is twofold: Can we adequately describe human variability through the concept of race? Does this process help us understand the meaning of diversity within our species? Watt described this twofold requirement clearly:

> Human populations can be classified in ways that are broadly consistent with genetic affinities, just as they can be characterized by lists of "typical" traits or genes. However, they cannot be understood in those terms. Races as genetic groups can only really be understood in terms of the process by which they originated.[7]

The scientific purpose of the concept of race is therefore to give meaning to human variation, not merely to point out one or another aspect of that variation.[14] It goes without saying that race must at the same time delineate important and consistent genetic differences; it implies that a "package" of different genes, all of which ideally should be known, exists between groups. On both counts, historical efforts to use the race concept scientifically have ended in failure. Why?

First, geographic variation in gene frequency is mainly quantitative, or clinical, in nature. From Europe eastward across the Asian land mass, populations meld into one another. Circular phenomena also occur. That is, gene frequencies moving in one direction gradually change until they arrive back at the point of origin, where a sharp break may be observed. The problem of indistinct borders for racial groups might be solved by accepting several large races, such as two to five. However, the number of nonclassifiable groups will be great. On every continent there are isolated subpopulations that cannot be accommodated, such as the Pygmies, Kalahari Bushmen, Basques, and Lapps. Mass migration, old as well as recent, further blurs distinctions. The other extreme would be to reduce each population or "ethnic group," to a separate category. This is essentially the process of naming, not classifying, and is the approach taken by Dobzhansky et al.[12]

Second, human variation is primarily discordant, rather than concordant. That is, although two groups may be similar in skin color, they differ in other important features, such as height, blood type, or facial features. To classify on the basis of skin color arbitrarily assigns primary importance to that characteristic and forces all others to be ignored. Is there any reason to believe that variations in skin color subsume all, or any, biologically important human variation? The Masai, Pygmies of the African rain forest, inhabitants of southern India, Australian Aborigines, and natives of the Amazon delta are all dark skinned: are they members of the same race? Skin color in these groups probably reflects a common history of exposure to ultraviolet radiation, not a common racial origin. It is characteristic of this problem of race that although skin color is the most important single trait used in classification, it is the one least well suited to the purpose.

The solution to both these problems—clinical and discordant variation—lies in the use of multivariate analysis. No discrete "package" of gene differences has ever been described between two races—only relative frequencies of one or another trait. Simultaneous treatment of many continuous variables, not dichotomous categories, is the only appropriate method for studying human variation.[14] Only in this manner can we begin to manage the data that represent the entire range of variation across the species. This understanding is damaged, not assisted by, creation of arbitrary cutoff points.

Yet one might ask, is it not common practice in medicine and biology to divide a continuous distribution into discrete categories? Hemoglobin, blood pressure, and body mass index are all skewed normal distributions; yet we accept the validity of the concepts of anemia, hypertension, and obesity. For pathological conditions (such as hypertension), we have objective criteria (association with morbid sequelae), whereas for racial traits no such external reference system exists. The unusual case, such as sickle cell anemia, can easily be handled on its own merit without reference to a malfitting racial category. Just as single-gene abnormalities are recognized to be different from most diseases that require complicated gene-environment interaction, consistent difference in one gene between populations is rare and cannot express anything more than a minuscule proportion of the total potential variation.

A single trait, such as skin color, is not an adequate basis for characterizing human diversity. Variation in a single gene, such as that for sickle cell anemia, does not imply that populations that vary in that gene will vary in important ways for any other health condition. Transferring racial susceptibility from sickle cell anemia to cancer, for example, is an unjustified assumption. Discordant variation implies that unless two conditions can be shown to be linked, they should be assumed to be independent. Most public health analysis based on racial categories adopts this false analogy—that a "package" of genetic differences exists—and is thus fatally flawed.

Even if one could classify groups of people usefully by race, little would have been accomplished from the point of view of the anthropologist. As noted earlier, "Races as genetic groups can only really be understood in terms of the process by which they originated."[7] This point is central to my argument and deserves to be emphasized. It has been stated in a similar way by authors contributing to Montagu's work:

> Race has been considered as a concept of the Linnaean system of classification within which it is applied to groups of populations within a species. To apply a concept of the Linnaean system to a group of populations implies something about their revolutionary history.
>
> Race is a useful concept only if one is concerned with the kind of anatomical, genetic, and structural differences which were in time past important in the origin of races. . . . We may look backward to the explanation on the differences between people—then the concept of race is useful, but it is useful under no other circumstances, as far as I can see.[1]

Dobzhansky et al. also state:

> Race differences are then adaptations to diverse environments in different parts of the distribution area of the species. . . . Numerous racial differences between populations have originated and are being maintained by natural selection.[12]

Human variation is of interest to study primarily because adaptive value is assumed for the observed traits. Thus Coon[13] argued that the five races of man represent separate origins of the human species, with independent evolutionary histories. This position has been widely discredited.[1] The search for "pure" races is a false hope.[1,9] We do not have a history of man's wandering, nor will one ever be forthcoming. "It is an error to believe that races are *things* . . . whose separate evolutionary development may be traced."[1]

Although this limitation may be fatal for the anthropologist, it could still be argued that the epidemiologist needs a system that gives broad categories of gene distribution.[7] The epidemiologist presumably is not very much interested in the origin of genes. He or she wants to know only their present distribution and does not need to know anything about the "process by which they originated" to understand "races as genetic groups." Again, false analogy applies. Race is potentially useful *only* because it might tell us something about evolution. Man's health problems today are not in any major way a result of evolutionary history in the physical sense; it is cultural history that has produced the human disease burden. The genetic and evolutionary baggage purportedly contained in the concept of race is therefore of no interest to the epidemiologist either, except in the rarest of cases. The rare cases—for example, sickle cell anemia and skin cancer in white Australians—in no way justify the dominant role given to genetic explanations of between-race disease variation.

Despite these criticisms, the concept of race is still used routinely today by many biologists and anthropologists.[11-13] Is there any defensible application of the concept? Among the most prominent supporters of the race concept has been Theodosius Dobzhansky, who wrote in 1962 that "anthropologists are confronted with a diversity of human beings. . . . Race is the subject of scientific study and analysis simply because it is a fact of nature."[11] While acknowledging the views of critics, he maintained this position in the most recent edition of his influential textbook on evolution.[12] It is argued that "races, species, genera, and other categories are needed above all for the pragmatic purpose of communication."[12] It must be questioned, however, whether the concept of race that is being put forward bears much in common with its historical use. While concluding that "data gathered by anthropologists studying racial variation in mankind should not be underrated,"[12] Dobzhansky et al. offer a very limited rationale for continued use of the category. Race is returned to the status proposed by Buffon, a label of pure convenience. The number of races is to vary widely depending on the question being studied. Thus there may be "European" and "African" races on one occasion and, on another, "Nordics, Alpines, Mediterraneans, Armenoids, etc."[12] If one accepts this definition, it is hard to disagree with an earlier conclusion by these same authors: "Saying that a population is of such-and-such geographic origin is good enough."[12] An ever-changing label of convenience, based on "some criteria" and used in an ad hoc fashion to refer to different groups of traits, is what is proposed.

To name various population groups for the sake of comparing gene frequencies is not the same as creating a classification of *Homo sapiens* based on race. The "naming" process in effect denies the assumption that races have a structural relationship to each other, because of evolution, and that each category has systematic differences in a block, or package, of genes. In my view the use of the racial category implies that the groups differ in characteristics other than the primary one being compared. Otherwise, why not specify precisely the population and the trait? As we have argued, it is this assumption of consistent difference in many traits that is the essential failure of the race concept.

One final question must be addressed: how important is the potential racial variation? Glass has suggested that the number of gene differences between a West African and a native of Denmark, for example, may be very small indeed. He estimates that the "white race" differs characteristically—that is, on a population basis—by no more than six pairs of genes from the black.[15] Although others consider this estimate low, it serves to place this question in the proper context.[9] Typical variation within a population is orders of magnitude larger. Given the overall magnitude of potential variation, two persons of the same race could vary by thousands of genes. Lewontin has estimated that diversity between individuals in a population accounts for 85 percent of the total species variation, diversity within race accounts for 8.3 percent, and between-race diversity contributes only 6.3 percent.[16] Although consistent differences, such as in skin color, may tell us more about adaptive change than random, within-population variation, they will be overwhelmed by the weight of similarity when man is examined as a species. More recent consideration of "Haldane's dilemma" suggests that systematic variation between populations may be primarily due to genetic drift, rather than adaptation, thereby eliminating even the possible significance of racial differences from an evolutionary point of view.[12] At any rate there is no evidence, as noted earlier, that racial variation in disease is, in any but the most trivial way, genetic in origin. Different human populations exposed to similar environments are much more alike than different in their disease rates.

RACE CONCEPT AND PUBLIC HEALTH

The race concept is prominent in public health and medicine. The classic anthropological concept of race—in which the race label identifies a set of important genetic differences, however ill-defined—is used almost exclusively. The most obscure phenotypic variations, based on observations from small numbers of individuals with totally unknown genetic resemblance, are ascribed to "racial differences."[17] True genetic markers are rarely used, and the relationship between genotype and phenotype is almost universally ignored.

A common sequence of progress in understanding the cause of disease consists of replacing a genetic theory with an environmental explanation. Perhaps the most dramatic example is the story of a disorder known as kuru.[7] In 1959 a chronic progressive neurological disorder was described among the Fore people, a remote tribe in New Guinea. It occurred most commonly among women and young children, accounting for 90 percent of deaths among adult females in some villages. There was at first no evidence of contagiousness, since visitors were not affected and some Fore developed the disease years after they had left the endemic area. It clearly ran in families and appeared to be sex linked. On that basis it was assumed to be genetically determined, and a single-gene hypothesis was proposed.[7] Laws were considered to sterilize affected families. Further examination of local customs, however, demonstrated an alternative explanation. Burial rites for male relatives consisted of close contact with the corpse, with all tissues being cooked and eaten by women and young children. Subsequently, of course, a filterable viruslike particle was identified and a "slow virus" disease described. Thus a disease that was thought to be caused by a single gene and to be restricted to one racial group was finally recognized to be the result of an infection. Although both racial and sex linked, the determinants were purely social, not genetic. Kuru has now been eliminated from the Fore.

Racial differentials in virtually all diseases have been attributed to genetic factors. Common infectious diseases are no exception.[18-21] Classic studies on rheumatic fever in the last century from England clearly demonstrated the risk associated with poverty and crowding.[18] On the basis of a careful review of these data, Newsholme[20] concluded in 1895 that "the influence of heredity has been exaggerated" and "as to race there is no evidence." Nonetheless, in the United States rheumatic fever was a disease to which the Irish were considered racially susceptible, and it was linked to genes for red hair. As the Irish became more prosperous, the disease disappeared, only to recur in black migrants from the rural South to urban centers.[20] The incidence has now markedly decreased in that racial group as well. Today rheumatic fever in the United States is seen primarily among Latin American immigrants.

What is the central meaning of the race concept as it applies to public health? In public health and medical work, race is virtually never defined; that is, specific gene frequencies are rarely measured and the criteria for assignment to one or another race are not stated. One is even hard-pressed to find a classic or typical formulation of the race concept in medicine.

Recently a group of anthropologists addressed the race concept in public health directly, and their text serves as a useful reference point in this discussion. Rothschild, the editor, states the rationale for the book in the preface:

> Comparative ethnogenetics, a fresh field in which questions may be cultivated anew and unexpected insights harvested, may delineate some of the factors of evolutionary change. More importantly, knowledge of disease distribution . . . may . . . help to distinguish between the roles of exogenous and endogenous factors in causes and pathogenesis of these diseases.[22]

In the first chapter, entitled "The Biological Race Concept and the Diseases of Modern Man," Watt provides the theoretical framework for "comparative ethnogenetics." After reviewing the history of race, she takes the majority view of anthropologists: "Racial classifications by themselves have little explanatory value. . . . Physical anthropologists have abandoned race as a subject for research. . . . Race is no longer either a starting point for research on human evolution or an end."[7] (One wonders whether the editor read that last statement before he wrote that "comparative ethnogenetics . . . may delineate some of the factors of evolutionary change.") Although an intellectual corpse in anthropology, however, race is said by Watt to be vital for epidemiology: "When diseases are being related to genetic factors, . . . biological race is an easily applied general indicator of the genetic makeup of populations and individuals." More explicitly, the paradigm, says Watt, goes like this: "The race concept is a useful device where one may compare disease rates of genetically similar populations living in different environments and genetically different populations living in similar environments."[7]

Is it true that biological race is helpful in explaining disease variation? What are these genetic differences and similarities that are being identified? We almost never know. Are they important for the disease in question? Specific estimates are not available. In fact, infinitely more is to be learned by taking precisely the opposite approach from the one suggested by the ethnogeneticists. All humans, in terms of their susceptibility to all but the rarest of diseases, are genetically similar. Systematic variation in susceptibility has not been shown to fall along racial lines for any common disease. (Hypertension might be considered the most important single exception to this proposition and will be discussed subsequently.) Racial differences reflect different social environments, not different genes, even where two groups live side by side, as do blacks and whites in the United States. *Race does not mark in any important way for genetic traits; rather, it demonstrates beyond question the paramount role of the social causes.* We have much more to learn from that paradigm, rather than the one offered by ethnogenetics.

Blacks in the United States have age- and sex-specific mortality ratios that are 25 percent to 300 percent higher than those of whites. These ratios are likewise highly mobile over time. How can they be genetic? Age-adjusted death rates for blacks were 37 percent higher than for whites in the United States in 1977. The most common fatal illness for which we have a clear-cut racial-genetic explanation is sickle cell disease. In 1977 there were 80,000 excess deaths among blacks compared with whites; 277 deaths among blacks were coded to hemoglobinopathies, or 0.3 percent of the total excess. We must look for the explanation of the remaining excess mortality primarily in social causes.

ORIGINS OF RACE

If, as I have argued, the concept of race has no legitimate scientific claim to existence, why has it remained such a vital part of our cultural experience? Unlike outmoded concepts of evolution or the solar system, the concept of race is firmly held by the vast majority of people in our society, including, no doubt, most scientists; by the same token, the race concept retains a prominent role in the explanation of disease variation. Why is it so resilient? Why is it constantly being reincarnated in "new disciplines," such as comparative ethnogenetics and sociobiology? Clearly, the history of the race concept transcends any strictly scientific analysis. It must fulfill an important social need.

What are the historical origins of racism and the concept of race? The cultural anthropologists have responded to this question which so compellingly emerges from a critique of the biological literature. A very brief summary of their explanation is presented here. Boyd argues that although early societies had many forms of class and caste, "the concept of race, as an immutable physical entity as we now know it, probably did not exist."[9] Montagu[23] has been one of the more prominent exponents of the idea that the emergence of the African slave trade, the key to economic development in the seventeenth and eighteenth centuries, led to the invention of the modern concept of race. Blacks had to be branded as inferior in order to justify this barbaric practice. Although the slave trade was crucial in the origin of racism, a second development of this historical era had a more enduring effect. It was in America that the impact of slavery was felt most directly. The long-term needs of a growing multiracial society demanded the invention of institutionalized racism.

> The first Africans in Virginia, most historians agree, were classified as indentured servants. The status of "slave" simply did not yet exist. The low condition to which indentured servants were subjected signaled a form of labor organization unique to the New World. It was not possible to observe the European forms of labor organization and relations in a context where land was widely available and opportunities generally open. The large fortunes to be made from the cultivation of tobacco would simply not have been possible without forced servitude.
>
> It was into this world that Africans were brought in 1619. At first they were treated little differently from indentured servants, except perhaps in the length of their service. Details are obscure, but it appears that while some Africans served their entire lives, others earned freedom, at least in the period before 1660. Only after 1650 did laws and social practices distinguishing black workers from whites begin to appear in Virginia.[24]

With the arrival of greater numbers of white workers and the survival of many beyond the period of servitude, class conflict began to develop in the young colonies. In 1675, Nathaniel Bacon led a rebellion of poor and restless whites, aimed against the Indians, in direct violation of the orders of the colonial governor. The height of the rebellion was a march on Jamestown.[24] In the words of one historian, "For those with eyes to see, there was an obvious lesson in the rebellion. Resentment of an alien race might be more powerful than resentment of an upper class."[25] Slavery and its identification exclusively with people of color thus served two purposes: it provided both a tractable workforce for the plantation economy and a unifying impetus to white racism.

Racial divisions between blacks and poor whites were carefully cultivated.[26] Black-white marriages were outlawed and other social interactions were strictly limited. It is of interest that the most severe punishments for crossing the color line were reserved for whites, both free and indentured.[24] As Jordan has pointed out, if Englishmen held blacks in such low respect, why was it necessary to proscribe social interaction?[27] In fact, these laws were passed to prevent further racial mixing, not just to formalize existing social practices.

In addition to its political role, an economic function has been ascribed to racial divisions. Economists have been interested primarily in the "problem" of racial discrimination in the labor market. Conservative economists, such as Friedman,[28] tend to dismiss the issue. Other economists have argued that lower wages for blacks reflect economic loss taken by employers who must hire them. Supposedly lower productivity, which results from cultural inferiority, as well as dislike by both the employers and white coworkers for close contact with blacks, make it less desirable to hire blacks.[29] The conventional economic approach argues that racism is counterproductive in the economic sphere. Employers are said to lose profits, whereas white workers may gain by preferential access to better jobs. Conservative economists further argue that the free market will eventually eliminate racial discrimination and hire workers based only on qualifications.

Another view has recently emerged.[24,30-32] Racial discrimination is seen as a means of reducing labor costs by forcing minorities to take otherwise unacceptable jobs and by weakening the solidarity of the labor movement. Recent work by Reich[31] and others provides an important test of this theory. Reich bases his analysis on economic data from forty-eight metropolitan areas in the United States in 1960 and 1970. A measure of inequality, the ratio of black to white median income, is taken as an estimate of racism. After adjustment for a number of social factors (region, educational level, percent employment in industry, and so forth), Reich demonstrates that as black income goes down 10 percent, white income at the median falls by 1 percent. Likewise, the existence of racial differentials is not dysfunctional for the system; rather, it boosts profits. An additional important finding of this study, substantiated by several other economists, is the persistence over time of racial differences in income: "The median income of black families in 1978 remained at only 57 percent of that of white families. That is, the median income of blacks was at approximately the same relative level in the early 1950s."[31] A modest improvement in relative income occurred over the 1960s; beginning at 0.54 in 1964, the black-white ratio rose to a peak of 0.61 in 1969 and fell to 0.57 by 1977.[31] Historical trends in relative income are presented in Table 6.1.

In 1981 the median income of black families was 0.56; at the same time the education gap had narrowed to half a year.[33] As noted in a recent economic report, "The income gap between blacks and whites is less related to education than to job opportunities open to blacks."[34] Approximately $5 billion more would have been paid to black wage earners over the previous year if no white-black differential existed.[35] Clearly, racial divisions have economic value; this must in part explain why they have persisted.

**Table 6.1. Ratio of Nonwhite to White Median Income,
United States, 1945–1977**

Year	Nonwhite Families	Black Families	Nonwhite Males	Nonwhite Females
1945	0.56		n.a.	n.a.
1946	0.59		0.61	n.a.
1947	0.51		0.54	n.a.
1948	0.53		0.54	0.49
1949	0.51		0.49	0.51
1950	0.54		0.54	0.49
1951	0.53		0.55	0.46
1952	0.57		0.55	n.a.
1953	0.56		0.55	0.59
1954	0.56		0.50	0.55
1955	0.55		0.53	0.54
1956	0.53		0.52	0.58
1957	0.54		0.53	0.58
1958	0.51		0.50	0.59
1959	0.52		0.47	0.62
1960	0.55		0.53	0.70
1961	0.53		0.52	0.67
1962	0.53		0.49	0.67
1963	0.53		0.52	0.67
1964	0.56	0.54	0.57	0.70
1965	0.55	0.54	0.54	0.73
1966	0.60	0.58	0.55	0.76
1967	0.62	0.59	0.59	0.78
1968	0.63	0.60	0.61	0.79
1969	0.63	0.61	0.59	0.85
1970	0.64	0.61	0.60	0.92
1971	0.63	0.60	0.61	0.90
1972	0.62	0.59	0.62	0.95
1973	0.60	0.58	0.63	0.93
1974	0.64	0.60	0.63	0.92
1975	0.65	0.61	0.63	0.92
1976	0.63	0.59	0.63	0.95
1977	0.61	0.57	0.61	0.88

Note: n.a. = not available

SOCIAL CONTEXT OF RACE

If race is a category more defined by social than genetic characteristics, it should be possible to describe social variables that help explain differences in health status. It might even be argued that race assumes its functional role by providing the basis for assigning members of a racial group to a particular class status. Although it is true that interaction—that is, the effect of race on class standing—may be the major effect, the relationship cannot be understood on that basis alone, for at least two reasons. First, although socioeconomic variables may provide a partial explanation of mechanisms, they do not resolve the issue of causality. Second, race often makes an important impact on social status after equating income and education to the majority group.

Explaining racial differentials by education, income, and so forth, could in a casual sense be considered "overcontrol": race is not confounded by the other variables; it is antecedent to them. It is race that influences class standing. Furthermore, the "unadjusted" difference is the disease burden actually borne by blacks, and it is the "raw" facts that must be explained—and changed. An even more simplistic analytic error is sometimes made: biological variables, such as obesity, blood pressure (BP), smoking rates, and the like, are used to demonstrate why blacks have a health disadvantage. Clearly these are attributes, not causes. Ascribing inferior health status to exposure to a more dangerous social environment accepts as given precisely the thing to be explained.

An interesting exercise in examining the significance of socioeconomic status (SES) in racial differentials was recently undertaken in relation to homicide.[36] Homicide rates for blacks in the United States are seven times higher for males and five times higher for females. The social origins of this cause of death need not be elaborated. Based on the experience in Atlanta, Georgia, in 1971, the question was addressed, "Do blacks have a specific 'culture of violence'?" That is, for a similar set of social conditions, are rates higher among blacks than whites? After controlling for education, a sizable difference remained.[36] It was noted, however, that with identical education, blacks receive lower wages, and the effect of unemployment will also be hidden. Education and other measures of SES are not comparable across races. Substituting income further narrowed the gap, although it was not closed. Because of segregation, black purchasing power is also well below that of whites; for example, equal housing in a black neighborhood costs up to 30 percent more. The ability to buy uncrowded housing was then used to account for part of this social inequality. Using occupants per room as a direct estimate of purchasing power, the racial difference in domestic homicide rates disappeared altogether. In this analysis, of course, there was no absolute standard for comparing SES, and any variable chosen was necessarily arbitrary to some extent. Stepwise elimination of racial differences by more sensitive control of class standing, however, is an important theoretical consideration in research into potential environmental sources of health differentials.

An important example of this problem exists in the field of cardiovascular research. Hypertension represents the key potential exception to the proposition that racial differentials in common disease are social in origin. Although it is widely assumed that blacks are genetically predisposed to hypertension,[37] an environmental hypothesis is equally tenable. In the Hypertension Detection and Follow-Up Program data, BP differences between black and white females disappear with control for education and obesity.[38] The same is not true for males (black males being no more obese than white), and yet a clear social class gradient—as estimated by education—exists, which will sizably reduce the black-white gap for males as well.[39] Rates of hypertension for blacks with a college education were similar to those for whites who did not finish high school.[39] Earning capacity of black college graduates is almost identical to that of white high school graduates;[33] even use of more appropriate measures of income and purchasing power might eliminate these BP differences. Other unmeasured aspects of the social significance of race could also be playing a role. A more sophisticated approach to explaining racial differences in hypertension, as was attempted in relation to homicide, would be a useful test of the environmental hypothesis. In the absence of this test, it is distressing that genetic explanations have gained such widespread acceptance.

CONCLUSIONS

An explicit discussion of coronary heart disease (CHD) among blacks has not been attempted in this paper. It is obvious that cigarette use and nutritional factors, such as hypercholesterolemia and obesity, are determined primarily, if not exclusively, by social conditions. It is not the purpose of this paper, however, simply to reemphasize the point that social factors should be given primary importance. What is in need of clarification is the meaning of the concept of race.

The argument put forward here leads to three major conclusions: (1) In the biological sense there are no such things as races. Human variation does not occur in discrete packages. The appearance of a highly consistent pattern of differential mortality between races can be ascribed only to environmental (that is, social), not genetic, factors. (2) The concept of race itself is a social category. Whether it be Catholic in Ulster, Jew in Germany, Tamil in Sri Lanka, or black in the United States, the definition of a population subgroup is a result of economic and historical, not evolutionary, developments. (3) Health status of racial groups should be viewed within this context.

Blacks in the United States have a historically determined structural relationship to the social system. They do not represent a homogeneously distributed subsegment of the population, nor is there any indication that they are becoming so; black-white income ratios have not changed appreciably during this century. For all intents and purposes, black people in this society are imprisoned by institutional racism; this is the attribute of blackness which at bottom determines their health status. Although the character of the health disadvantage may evolve, for example, as a result of migration from the rural South to the urban North, the disadvantage itself is not likely to diminish until the intensity of racial discrimination is successfully reduced. The epidemiology of CHD among blacks in the United States has likewise been determined by these social conditions. Greater cigarette use, relative exclusion from preventive campaigns, bad nutrition, excess hypertension, and obesity are all important attributes of the contemporary experience of black Americans. Higher rates of CHD are to be anticipated.

Notes

1. Montagu, A. (Ed.). (1964). *The concept of race.* Toronto: Collier Macmillan, Canada.

2. Dobzhansky, T. (1973). *Genetic diversity and human equality.* New York: Basic Books.

3. Boyd. W. C. (1963). Genetics and the human race. *Science, 140,* 1057.

4. Woodward, V. (1981). *Heredity and human society.* Minneapolis: Burgess.

5. Chase, A. (1980). *The legacy of Malthus: The social costs of the new scientific racism.* Champaign, IL: University of Illinois Press.

6. Gossett, T. F. (1965). *Race: The history of an idea in America.* New York: Schocken Books.

7. Watt, E. S. (1981). The biological race concept and the diseases of modern man. In H. R. Rothschild (Ed.), *Biocultural aspects of disease* (pp. 3–22). New York: Academic Press.

8. Ehrlich, P. R., & Holm, R. W. (1964). A biological view of race. In A. Montagu (Ed.), *The concept of race* (pp. 153–197). Toronto: Collier Macmillan, Canada.

9. Boyd, W. C. (1950). *Genetics and the races of man* (pp. 186–209). Boston: Little, Brown.

10. Gould, S. J. (1979). *Ever since Darwin: Reflections in natural history.* New York: Norton.

11. Dobzhansky, T. (1962). Comment on Livingstone. *Curr Anthropol, 3,* 279.

12. Dobzhansky, T., Ayala, F. J., Stebbins, G. L., & Valentine, J. W. (1977). *Evolution.* San Francisco: Freeman.

13. Coon, C. S. (1962). *The origin of races.* New York: Knopf.

14. Barnicot, N. A. (1964). Taxonomy and variation in modern man. In A. Montagu (Ed.), *The concept of race* (pp. 180–227). Toronto: Collier Macmillan, Canada.

15. Glass, B. (1943). *Genes and the man.* New York: Columbia University Press.

16. Lewontin, R. C. (1972). Apportionment of human diversity. *Evol Biol, 6,* 381.

17. Dunn, F. G., Oigman, W., Sungaard-Riise, K., Messerli, P. H., Ventura, H., Reisin, E., & Frohlic, E. D. (1983). Racial differences in cardiac adaptation to essential hypertension determined by echocardiographic indexes. *J Am Coll Cardiol, 1,* 1348.

18. Paul, J. R. (1957). *The epidemiology of rheumatic fever.* New York: American Heart Association.

19. Stollerman, G. H. (1975). *Rheumatic fever and streptococcal infection.* New York: Grune & Stratton.

20. Newsholme, A. (1895). Milroy lectures: Rheumatic fever. *Lancet, 1,* 589, 657.

21. Wintrobe, S., et al. (1970). *Harrison's principles of internal medicine.* New York: McGraw-Hill, p. 865.

22. Rothschild, H. R. (Ed.). Preface. In *Biocultural aspects of disease.* New York: Academic Press.

23. Montagu, A. (1945). *Man's most dangerous myth: The fallacy of race.* New York: Columbia University Press.

24. The roots of racism. (1982). *Progressive Labor Magazine, 15*(3), 1–16.

25. Morgan, E. (1975). *American slavery, American freedom.* New York: Norton.

26. Bennet, L. (1966). *Before the Mayflower: A history of the Negro in America, 1619–1964.* Baltimore: Penguin Books.

27. Jordan, W. (1968). *White over black: American attitudes toward the Negro, 1550–1812.* Baltimore: Penguin Books.

28. Friedman, M. (1962). *Capitalism and freedom.* Chicago: University of Chicago Press.

29. Becker, G. (1957). *The economics of discrimination.* Chicago: University of Chicago Press.

30. Cherry, R. (1978). Economic theories of racism. In D. M. Gordon (Ed.), *Problems in political economy: An urban perspective* (pp. 170–182). Lexington, MA: Heath.

31. Reich, M. (1957). *Racial inequality: A political-economic analysis.* Princeton, NJ: Princeton University Press.

32. Tabb, W. (1971). Capitalism, colonialism, and racism. *Rev Radical Polit Econ, 3,* 90.

33. Gap in income between the races as large as in 1960, study finds. (1983, July 18). *New York Times,* p. 1.

34. *Dream deferred: The economic status of black Americans* (Working paper). (1983). Washington, DC: Center for the Study of Social Policy.

35. News release. (1983, August 1). Washington, DC: U.S. Department of Labor, Bureau of Labor Statistics.

36. Centerwall, B. S. (1982, June). *Race, socioeconomic status, and domestic homicide: Atlanta, 1971–1972.* Paper presented at the 1982 Society for Epidemiologic Research conference, Cincinnati.

37. Genetics, environment, and hypertension. (1983). *Lancet, 1,* 681.

38. Langford, H. G. (1981). Is blood pressure different in black people? *Postgrad Med J, 57,* 749.

39. Hypertension Detection and Follow-up Program Cooperative Group. (1977). Race, education and prevalence of hypertension. *Am J Epidemiol, 106,* 351.

CHAPTER SEVEN

Beyond Dummy Variables and Sample Selection

What Health Services Researchers Ought to Know About Race as a Variable

Thomas A. LaVeist

The analysis of race has a long history among health scientists in America.[1,2] Decades of research have revealed substantial race differences in morbidity, mortality, health and illness behavior, access and utilization of health services, and other issues of interest to health services researchers.[3,4] Due partly to these persistent research findings and partly to social convention, it has become standard practice to publish health and vital statistics stratified by race, to statistically control for race in multivariate analysis, and to exclude individuals from analysis on the basis of their race.[1] These conventions are routinely taught in graduate programs in health services research, medical sociology, biostatistics, epidemiology, and other allied health fields. However, rarely is the appropriateness of these conventions questioned. Moreover, it is only in the rare case that an investigator will provide an explicit justification for these practices. Yet there are serious problems with the operational definition, measurement, and conceptualization of race. These problems have gone largely ignored.

This chapter is an attempt to initiate a dialogue regarding the analysis of race in health services research. How is race defined? How might it best be measured? How should race be conceptualized? Similar dialogues have taken

I am grateful for helpful comments from Dr. Marsha Lillie-Blanton and Dr. Suzanne Orr, and from two anonymous reviewers on earlier drafts of this manuscript. An earlier version of this manuscript was delivered at the annual meeting of the Association of Health Services Research, Chicago, June 1992.

place in other disciplines.[1,5-8] There is growing interest in understanding the proper use of race in health research;[9-11] however, this literature has been developing without input from health services researchers. An understanding of the definition, measurement, and conceptualization of race is a prerequisite to the proper interpretation of research results regarding race. Such a dialogue is particularly appropriate for health services researchers because of the close ties between health services research and health policy development.

WHAT IS RACE?

Race is a social category, not a biological category. It is a concept that has changed over time and is variable across societies. Illustrative of this point is a comparison of the policies for assigning racial status in three societies: the United States, Japan, and Brazil. Table 7.1 displays a condensed version of the protocol, issued by the U.S. National Center for Health Statistics, and once used to assign racial status on birth certificates. As the table illustrates, a child could be assigned "white" only if both parents had been designated "white." However, in every other case, the race of the father determined the race of the child. Thus, the offspring of a Japanese male and a black female resulted in the designation "Japanese" on the child's birth certificate, and a union of a black male and a Japanese female resulted in a designation as a "black" child. However, the result of the mating between a white person and a person of any other racial/ethnic group resulted in a child who was a member of the nonwhite group, regardless of which parent was white. This policy was changed in 1989 so that children are now assigned the race of the mother, regardless of the race group the father claims.

Table 7.1. U.S. Policy for Assigning Racial Status on Birth Certificates, Prior to 1989

Father	Mother	Child
White	White	White
White	Black	Black
White	Japanese	Japanese
Black	White	Black
Black	Black	Black
Black	Japanese	Black
Japanese	White	Japanese
Japanese	Black	Japanese
Japanese	Japanese	Japanese

Source: National Center for Health Statistics.

Table 7.2 shows the racial classification scheme used in Japan until 1985. In that country a child was designated Japanese only if his or her father was Japanese. The official policy was that this scheme was to be followed without regard to the race or nationality of the mother. In 1985, the Japanese national legislature amended the constitution so that a person would be considered Japanese if either parent was Japanese.

The Brazilian classification scheme is outlined in Table 7.3. In that country interracial mating is handled by assigning the offspring to a third racial category, mulatto (a classification formerly used in the United States[12]). The Brazilians then divide mulattos into a set of subcategories on the basis of the relative lightness or darkness of the person's skin complexion.

These three countries over less than a decade produced five different policies for assigning racial status. What, then, is the biological relevance of race? Race is a concept that is determined fundamentally by political and social forces without regard to biogenetics or scientific rigor. It can be argued that the sociopolitical nature of race is not problematic for health research if what is being measured by a race dummy variable is commonly understood. There is a

Table 7.2. Japanese Policy for Assigning Racial Status on Birth Certificates, Prior to 1985

Father	Mother	Child
White	Japanese	White
Black	Japanese	Black
Japanese	White	Japanese
Japanese	Black	Japanese

Source: University of Michigan, Center for Japanese Studies.

Table 7.3. Brazilian Policy for Assigning Racial Status on Birth Certificates

Father	Mother	Child
White	White	White
White	Black	Mulatto*
Black	White	Mulatto
Black	Black	Black

*Mulatto is broken into fine distinctions based on physical characteristics: *Pretos* (black), *Preto Retinto* (dark black), *Cabra* (slightly less black), *Cabo Verde* (slightly less black), *Escuro* (lighter still), *Mulato Esuro* (dark mulatto), *Mulato Claro* (light mulatto), *Sararas, Moreno, Blanco de terra, Blanco.*

Source: Degler, C. N. (1971). *Neither black nor white: Slavery and race relations in Brazil and the United States.* New York: Macmillan.

generally held notion that consensus exists regarding the meaning of race. But is this notion based in reality?

In examining representative medical and allied health dictionaries for definitions of race, I found significant variability among their definitions. Some dictionaries defined race in entirely biological terms while others recognized the social and political aspects of race. *A Dictionary of Epidemiology* provides a terse definition that embraces the biological concept without providing rigorous biological guidelines for identifying individual races. This dictionary also does not acknowledge the social or political aspects of race. Race is defined as "persons who are relatively homogeneous with respect to biological inheritance."[13]

In *A Dictionary of Genetics* race is defined as a scientific, biogenetic concept, "a phenotypically and/or geographically distinctive subspecific group, composed of individuals inhabiting a defined geographic and/or ecological region, and possessing characteristic phenotypic and gene frequencies that distinguish it from other such groups."[14] The dictionary then adds a curious sentence that contradicts the implied scientific rigor of the first part of the definition. "The number of racial groups that one wishes to recognize within a species is usually arbitrary but suitable for the purposes under investigation."

The *International Dictionary of Medicine and Biology* views race as a biological concept that defies discrete categorization:

A subspecies or other division or subdivision of a species. Human races are generally defined in terms of original geographic range and common hereditary traits which may be morphological, serological, hematological, immunological, or biochemical. The traditional division of mankind into several well-recognized racial types such as Caucasoid (White), Negroid (Black), and Mongoloid (Yellow) leaves a residue of populations that are of problematical classification, and its focus on a limited range of visible characteristics tends to oversimplify and distort the picture of human variation.[15]

The *Psychiatric Dictionary* is in fundamental agreement with the *International Dictionary of Medicine and Biology*: "[T]he term race implies a blood related group with characteristic and common hereditary traits . . ."[16] Likewise, this dictionary does not embrace the most commonly accepted categories of human races: "Primary race or subspecies—the Caucasian, the Mongoloid, and the Negroid—are generalized racial types, hypothetical stocks, rather than living races." The *Psychiatric Dictionary* then goes on to advance the biological concept of "race disease": "Group of individuals susceptible to the same disease. . . . One might conceive, therefore, as well of a gastric ulcer race, a manic depressive race, a meningococcus susceptible race, or gall-bladder race, as of the present customarily accepted black, yellow or white divisions of mankind."

The Dictionary of Modern Medicine provides the most interesting but least informative definition of race I found among the dictionaries. This definition illustrates an attempt to incorporate the biological, political, and social conceptions of race, however unsuccessfully:

> An ethnic classification, subdivided in the U.S. into five categories, according to origin: (1) White, not Hispanic (Europe, North Africa, Middle East); (2) Black not Hispanic (Africa); (3) Hispanic; (4) American Native (Indians, Eskimos); (5) Asian and Pacific Islanders; stratification by race is of interest in several areas of medicine for a number of specific reasons. *Clinical Medicine:* Some HLAs are more common in certain racial groups and may be associated with particular diseases, thus helping to diagnose and manage difficult cases. *Public Policy:* The Civil Rights Act of 1964 mandated equality in employment and educational policy and knowledge of race favors minority candidates. *Transfusion Medicine:* Certain red cell antigens may be relatively uncommon in a particular race and knowledge of race reduces the labor required to find a suitable unit for transfusion. *Transplantation:* Human leukocyte antigens (HLA) differ somewhat according to race and may be used to identify potential recipients for organ transplantation.[17]

The first part of this definition is tautological in that it defines race as merely the sum of its categories as they are currently officially recognized by the U.S. government. The examples that are provided to demonstrate the relevance of race in medicine are also problematic. The explanations for clinical medicine, transfusion medicine, and transplantation refer to race differences in certain HLAs (and are addressed in the next section of this article). The explanation for public policy, however, addresses a politically charged issue, affirmative action. It is not clear how this example clarifies the meaning of race at either the theoretical or the practical level.

Dorland's Illustrated Medical Dictionary defines race more broadly:

> 1. an ethnic stock, or division of mankind; in a narrower sense, a national or tribal stock; in a still narrower sense, a genealogic line of descent; a class of persons of a common lineage. In genetics, races are considered as populations having different distributions of gene frequencies. 2. a class or breed of animals; a group of individuals having certain characteristics in common, owing to a common inheritance; a subspecies.[18]

The *Dorland's* definition attempts to incorporate ethnicity, nationality, tribe, and geneological lineage under race. In doing so, this definition exposes the most serious problem faced by American health researchers who are interested in conducting research on race. That is, in the United States the fine distinctions of ethnic, tribal, or national variations within race groups is obscured in favor of physical appearance. For example, ethnicity refers to cultural commonality; yet the descendants of Africans, Spaniards, and Indians share a common ethnic identity in the Dominican Republic. Are they all members of the same race group? Officially, in the United States, they are all regarded as Hispanic.

However, in daily social interaction in the United States, they would be regarded as black or white based on their appearance and their degree of acculturation into American society. Mexican, Cuban, and El Salvadoran immigrants to America are all categorized as Hispanic, obscuring their nationality and cultural differences.

Europeans from Southern Italy, Northern Ireland, and Southern France come from distinctly different cultural traditions, yet upon arrival in the United States they are categorized as white. Rarely is this source of variation considered in health research. The same can be said for Native Americans and Southeast Asians. The Yoruba of Brazil and Nigeria share a common ethnic/cultural heritage, yet they differ in nationality. Within the American cultural context they both would be regarded as black, thus adopting the health risks associated with that group.

In health services research, the race dummy variable (the most common method of measuring and conceptualizing race) is used to measure all of these: ethnicity, skin color, and nationality. This results in some degree of measurement error, but more important, the lack of conceptual clarity leaves a great deal of room for erroneous interpretations of research findings and consequently for ineffective public policy.

USES OF RACE IN HEALTH RESEARCH

Williams found that race is a frequently used variable in health services research.[19] In his analysis of the uses of race in *HSR: Health Services Research* he found that 64 percent of articles included race in their analysis. The most common use of race was as a binary (dummy) variable used as a control in regression analysis. This finding is consistent with analysis of practices in related fields, such as medical sociology[20] and epidemiology.[1]

Race is often conceptualized as a proxy for other (not measured) variables that are known or believed to correlate with race (for example, socioeconomic status, discrimination, cultural factors, unspecified biological differences among race groups, and so forth). But it seems logical that if race is a proxy for other factors such as biology or culture, then a need exists to find more creative ways to measure these other factors. If we are to learn how best to intervene in the various problems of concern to health services researchers (the impact of health services on the disease process, access to and utilization of health services, and the like), greater conceptual precision is necessary.

An example taken from the entry on race in *The Dictionary of Modern Medicine* serves to illustrate this point. It is suggested in that dictionary that some "human leukocyte antigens (HLAs) are more commonly found in certain racial groups."[17] Knowledge of HLA type is helpful in predicting rejection of transplanted organs. A researcher who is interested in specifying a regression model that would predict rejection of transplanted organs might specify the outcome of organ transplantation (rejected or not rejected) as the dependent variable and a race dummy variable as the independent variable. The researcher would find that, although this model explained some proportion of the variance in transplantation outcome, it did not fully explain the variance.

If the researcher would, next, specify a second model with the same variables and the addition of a second independent variable—HLA match between the organ donor and the organ recipient (good match or not good match)—the significant effect of the race dummy variable would reduce to nonsignificance and the HLA match variable alone would explain a very high proportion of the variance in rejection of organ transplantation. Thus, the relevant determinant of which organ transplantations are likely to be successful is HLA match. Race, then, is a less than fully satisfactory proxy for the biogenetic factor (HLA). Consequently, any policy that used race as the primary screen to determine who gains access to organs would be misguided.[21]

Moreover, from a statistical standpoint the simple inclusion of a race dummy variable in a regression model is inadequate if the objective is to develop interventions to affect race differences in a dependent variable. This approach merely allows the researcher to report on differences in the intercept without providing any information about the potential for differences in the effects of the independent variables on the dependent variable (the regression slopes). This approach simply produces adjusted means for the dependent variable for each race group. So a regression model that attempts to predict number of prenatal care visits as a function of health insurance status, age, and race (black or white) results in information on black-white differences in mean number of prenatal care visits adjusting for insurance status and age. A statistically significant coefficient for the race binary variable in such a model specification without further analysis often leads to such illogical, yet commonly published conclusions as "race is a significant determinant of prenatal care utilization." Such a conclusion eventually filters into medical and public health practice. Clearly, a person's skin color does not determine prenatal care utilization.

To explore more fully the effects of race in the analysis, it would be necessary to specify models separately for the groups being compared and to conduct a test for a statistically significant difference in the parameter estimates for the same variable across the two models. This has the equivalent effect of specifying a multiplicative interaction term between the race binary variable and each of the other independent variables. Thus, one could determine whether black-white differences existed in the effect of insurance status and age on number of prenatal care visits. Such knowledge is a minimum requirement if one is interested in the development of public health programs or policy to reduce race disparities in prenatal care utilization. This is but one example. There are many others.

A second common practice for dealing with race, among health services researchers and other health scientists, is to eliminate one race group in sample selection. At times there may be conceptual justification for doing this. From a practical standpoint the use of a racially homogeneous data set in secondary analysis may be unavoidable. But one should be careful not to attempt to generalize findings for such a data set as if it were representative.

In practice, justified examples of using race as a criterion in sample selection are rare. It is, however, common to find studies that examine, for example, the relationship between smoking and heart disease among white men. If it is the case that the physiological mechanisms that link smoking to heart disease differ by race, then it would be helpful to outline what those differences are. Otherwise, neither the use of race as a criterion in sample selection nor as a "control" variable in such a study is justified.

Definitional and conceptual problems aside, there are measurement problems with race that have not been adequately addressed. There are different methods of measuring race that are associated with the various sources of data typically used in health services research.[22,23] Race is assigned on the birth certificate based on a visual assessment of the birth mother (and there is reason to suspect that even this varies by hospital). Race is typically assigned on death certificates based on the visual inspection of the body by the funeral director. Telephone and mail surveys are respondent self-reports, and in face-to-face surveys race is typically assigned by the interviewer upon visually inspecting the respondent. Race assignment on patient discharge records is sometimes based on the respondent's self-report and at other times is assigned by the admitting intake receptionist; in medical records abstracts, race is usually obtained from the hospital admitting records. Each of these methods has an associated measurement error that has gone ignored.

A CONCEPTUAL MODEL OF RACE

What is race and how should one use it in research on health and health services? This question can be answered in two ways, theoretically and practically. The theoretical will be addressed in this section; the practical will be addressed in the next.

Traditionally, race is viewed as a combination of biological, cultural, and social (usually meaning socioeconomic status) characteristics of individuals. Researchers have traditionally made the implicit assumption of within-group homogeneity among these characteristics. I argue that rather than encompassing three *homogeneous* underlying factors (biology, culture, and social factors), the race dummy variable covers two *heterogeneous* underlying factors (societal factors and cultural/ethnic factors). Societal factors refer to factors that are external to the individual, for example, poor sanitation and other city services in many African American communities[24-28] or race differences in receiving quality medical care.[29-31] Cultural/ethnic factors refer to individual-level behavior—such as dietary practices, tobacco and alcohol use, or responses to stressful events—that can be linked to cultural norms. Thus, in the present formulation, race as it relates to health research is viewed as a complex multidimensional construct. Individuals are allowed to vary among the several components of the construct; thus, homogeneity is not assumed within groups. This construct is schematically represented in Figure 7.1.

The conceptual model specifies race as a latent factor of which the manifest indicator is most frequently color of skin. Skin color is a continuous variable (varying between light and dark skin). However, it is typically dichotomized. No specific guidelines exist for determining the point in the continuum at which the line of demarcation is drawn. Rather, this critical decision is typically left to societal interpretation. (This is certainly the case in most face-to-face surveys, as it is in daily interpersonal interactions.)

The process by which individuals assign racial status to others is called physiognomy (defined literally as the art of judging on the basis of appearance). As individuals are judged, they are assigned to categories that determine their level of exposure to external health risks. Thus, although black and white Hispanics share a common ethnicity, black Hispanics have fewer opportunities for access to mainstream societal resources than white Hispanics.[32] Therefore, black

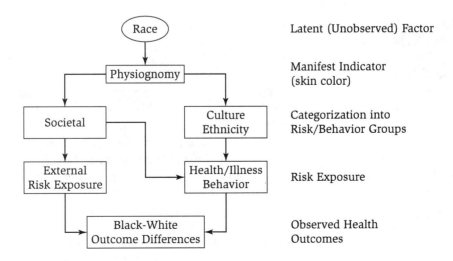

Figure 7.1 Conceptual Model of Race.

Hispanics have a societal health risk exposure profile that more closely resembles that of non-Hispanic blacks. However, one would expect the health and illness behaviors of black Hispanics to resemble more closely those of white Hispanics than of non-Hispanic blacks.

Individuals, too, identify themselves with a racial group (as is the case in mail or telephone surveys). Along with self-identification comes the acceptance of cultural norms and practices that have implications for health and illness behavior. Moreover, societal factors may also have an impact on health and illness behavior. For example, low socioeconomic status may constrain the dietary options of an individual or the nature of his or her employment, or travel distances may make it difficult to keep medical appointments or comply with medical regimens.

Finally, the consequences of these various factors—societally determined level of health risk exposure, culturally determined health and illness behavior, and the interaction between societal factors and health and illness behavior—combine to produce observed morbidity and mortality differentials across race groups.

SOME PRACTICAL CONSIDERATIONS IN THE USE OF RACE

Consideration of this multidimensional construct leads naturally to practical implications for health services researchers. First, we must acknowledge that what is measured by the race dummy variable is not culture, biology, values, or behavior. What is actually measured by the race variable is skin color. And, since this is the case, it is more productive to measure skin color more accurately. Where possible, color of skin should be measured as a continuous variable. In studies in which race is regarded as a measure of culture (for example, health services utilization or health and illness behavior), it may be less useful to specify race as a continuous variable. However, there is evidence to support the hypothesis that the degree of lightness or darkness of a person's skin may affect that person's level of exposure to health risks.[33] Klag et al. used a light meter to measure the relative lightness or darkness of his respondents' skin color.[34] However, this may be impractical in some data collections. Alternatively, one might code skin color as light, medium, or dark, based on the evaluation of a trained interviewer. In the case of nonblack groups, such as Asian Americans, the measurement of skin color is less relevant. It may be more relevant in this case to measure degree of acculturation into American culture.

Measuring race as a continuous variable may not be possible when using certain types of data (for example, hospital discharge data). However, it would be possible to indicate how race was measured in the data set. Was it measured by the interviewer's visual assessment of the respondent? Was it measured by the respondent's self-report? This is useful because as the model displayed in Figure 7.1 shows, societal health risk exposure is determined not by the respondent's self-identified race, but rather by the health risk group to which he or she is assigned—most frequently by others. On the other hand, the culturally determined health and illness behavior risks are determined by the respondent's self-identity. Ideally, one would have dual measures of race in the data set (one of them assigned by the interviewer and the second the respondent's self-report).

It would also be ideal to measure ethnic identifiers in addition to race. Differences in morbidity, mortality, and health and illness behavior within race groups are greatly understudied. Federal data sets routinely collect ethnic identification with regard to Hispanics; however, it would be beneficial to extend this practice to other groups by collecting country of origin, for instance, among whites, Asians, blacks, and Hispanics.

Researchers should consider carefully the appropriateness of statistically "controlling" for race in analysis. Scholars should consider, explicitly, how they are conceptualizing race before including the race dummy variable in a regression model to "control for race." In many cases this control is unnecessary, for example in a study of the relationship between smoking and heart disease; it is unnecessary to "control" for race unless there is a reason to expect that the physiological link between smoking and heart disease is different among racial groups. Moreover, any race differences in the frequency of underlying confounding factors (such as HLAs) would be better addressed by directly measuring the factor for which race is a proxy. If this is not possible, it would be important to clearly indicate the factor for which race is serving as a proxy, and any policy or practice implications to be derived from the research should be developed with this in mind.

Moreover, there is a need to develop more creative and precise measures of factors for which race is believed to be a proxy—such as culture.

When race is included in analysis as a control variable (justifiably or not), it is important to provide an interpretation of the findings. It is not sufficient to include race in a regression analysis as a control variable, obtain a statistically significant effect, and then not provide an interpretation of that finding.

When race differences are observed, it is necessary that investigators examine both the within-group and between-group variation to determine whether true race differences exist or if the observed differences are caused by variation within race groups. For example, it is likely that differences in dietary practices and in access to health care among African Americans living in rural South Carolina are more like those of whites living in rural Arkansas than they are like those of African Americans living in Detroit.

It is also necessary that investigators provide a theoretically grounded rationale for excluding respondents from their analysis because of their race. One recent study actually found an *increase* in this practice among epidemiologists.[1]

Such findings emphasize the importance of the recent policy changes at the National Institutes of Health. Investigators are now required to include women and minorities as study subjects in clinical research unless "compelling scientific or other justification" not to include them exists.

Health and public policy implications are particularly important for health services research. Ways in which one conceptualizes race have much to do with the development of policy and the eventual success of the policy. Biological determinism suggests that few of the interventions at the disposal of health services can be effective in reducing race-associated health differentials. A purely behavioral conceptualization suggests that all interventions should focus on modifying individuals' behaviors. A societal conceptualization of race differences suggests that all necessary changes are external to the individual.

In practice it seems most likely that some contributions of behavioral and social factors account for race differences in health status, health services utilization, and so forth. The multidimensional construct presented in this article allows for a case-specific conceptualization of race. In some cases the behavioral aspects of race (actually ethnicity) will be most important. In other cases the importance will fall to societal factors (factors external to the individual). Consequently, policy designed to improve race differentials in health status, health services utilization, access, and other issues of interest to health services researchers must also be case specific.

In short, health services researchers should treat the race variable with the same degree of caution and skepticism they bring to any other variable.

Notes

1. Jones, C. P., LaVeist, T. A., & Lillie-Blanton, M. (1991). "Race" in the epidemiologic literature: An examination of the *American Journal of Epidemiology,* 1921–1990. *Am J Epidemiol, 134*(10), 1079–1084.

2. Krieger, N. (1987). Shades of difference: Theoretical underpinnings of the medical controversy on black/white differences in the United States, 1830–1870. *Int J Health Serv, 17*(2), 259–278.

3. U.S. Department of Health and Human Services. (1985). *Report of the Secretary's Task Force on Black and Minority Health.* Washington, DC: U.S. Government Printing Office.

4. Braithwaite, R. L., & Taylor, S. E. (1992). *Health issues in the black community.* San Francisco: Jossey-Bass.

5. Leiberman, L. (1968). The debate over race: A study in the sociology of knowledge. *Phylon, 39*(4), 127–141.

6. Davis, J. E. (1992, Spring). Reconsidering the use of race as an explanatory variable in program evaluation. In *New Directions for Program Evaluation* (No. 53, pp. 55–67). San Francisco: Jossey-Bass.

7. Cooper, R., & David, R. (1986). The biological concept of race and its application to public health and epidemiology. *J Health Polit Policy Law, 11*(1), 97–116.

8. Zuckerman, M. (1990). Some dubious premises in research and theory on racial differences: Scientific, social and ethical issues. *Am Psychol, 45*(12), 1297–1303.

9. Cooper, R., Steinhauer, M., Miller, W., David, R., & Schatzkin, A. (1982). Racism, society and disease: An exploration of the social and biological mechanisms of differential mortality. *Int J Health Serv, 11*(3), 389–414.

10. Byrd, W. M. (1990). Race, biology and health care: Reassessing a relationship. *J Health Care Poor Underserved, 1*(3), 278–296.

11. Nelson, N. M. (1970). On racism in science. *N Engl J Med, 283*(11), 594–595.

12. Lee, S. M. (1993). Racial classification in the U.S. Census, 1890–1990. *Ethnic and Racial Studies, 16*(1), 75–94.

13. Last, J. M. (1988). *A dictionary of epidemiology* (2nd ed.). New York: Oxford University Press.

14. King, R. C., & Stansfield, W. D. (1990). *A dictionary of genetics.* London: Oxford University Press.

15. Becker, E. L., & Landav, S. I. (1986). *International dictionary of medicine and biology.* New York: Oxford University Press.

16. Campbell, R. J. (1981). *Psychiatric dictionary* (5th ed.). London: Oxford University Press.

17. Segen, J. C. (1992). *The dictionary of modern medicine.* Park Ridge, NJ: Parthenon.

18. Taylor, E. J. (1988). *Dorland's illustrated medical dictionary* (27th ed.). Philadelphia: W. S. Saunders.

19. Williams, D. R. (1992, June). The concept of race in health services research, 1966–1990. Paper delivered at the annual meeting of the Association for Health Services Research, Chicago.

20. LaVeist, T. A., Williams, D. R., Lillie-Blanton, M., & Jones, C. (1992, August 13–17). The uses of race in medical sociology: An analysis of the *Journal of Health and Social Behavior.* Delivered at the annual meeting of the American Sociological Association, Pittsburgh.

21. Kasiske, B. L., Neylan, J. F., Riggio, R. R., Danovitch, G. M., Kahana, L., Alexander, S. R., & White, M. G. (1991). The effect of race on access and outcome in transplantation. *N Engl J Med, 324*(5), 302–307.

22. Hahn, R. A., Mulinare, J., & Teutsch, S. M. (1992). Inconsistencies in coding of race and ethnicity between birth and death in U.S. infants. *JAMA, 267*(2), 259–263.

23. Frost, F., & Shy, K. K. (1980). Racial differences between linked birth and infant death records in Washington state. *Am J Public Health, 70*(9), 974–976.

24. LaVeist, T. A. (1989). Linking residential segregation to the infant mortality race disparity. *Sociol Soc Res, 73*(2), 90–94.

25. LaVeist, T. A. (1992). The political empowerment and health status of African Americans: Mapping a new territory. *Am J Sociol, 97*(4), 1080–1095.

26. LaVeist, T. A. (1993). Segregation, poverty and empowerment: Health consequences for African Americans. *Milbank Q, 71*(1), 41–64.

27. Bullard, R. D. (1983, Spring). Solid waste sites and the black Houston community. *Sociol Inq, 53,* 273–288.

28. U.S. General Accounting Office. (1983). *Citing of hazardous waste landfills and their correlation with racial and economic status of surrounding communities* (RCED-83-168). Washington, DC: U.S. Government Printing Office.

29. Ford, E., Cooper, R., Castaner, A., Simmons, B., & Mar, M. (1989). Coronary arteriography and coronary bypass survey among whites and other racial groups relative to hospital-based incidence rates for coronary artery disease: Findings from NHDS. *Am J Public Health, 79*(4), 437–439.

30. Yergen, J., Flood, A. B., LoGerfo, J. P., & Diehr, P. (1987). Relationship between patient race and the intensity of hospital services. *Med Care, 25*(7), 592–603.

31. Gittelsohn, A. M., Halpern, J., & Sanchez, R. L. (1991). Income, race and surgery in Maryland. *Am J Public Health, 81*(11), 1435–1440.

32. Denton, N. A., & Massey, D. S. (1989). Racial identity among Caribbean Hispanics: The effects of double minority status on residential segregation. *Am Sociol Rev, 54*(5), 790–808.

33. Keith, V. M., & Herring, C. (1991). Skin tone and stratification in the black community. *Am J Sociol, 97*(3), 760–778.

34. Klag, M. J., Whelton, P. K., Coresh, J., Grim, C. E., & Kuller, L. H. (1991). The association of skin color with blood pressure in U.S. blacks with low socioeconomic status. *JAMA, 265*(5), 599–602.

CHAPTER EIGHT

The Bell Curve

On Race, Social Class, and Epidemiologic Research

Carles Muntaner
F. Javier Nieto
Patricia O'Campo

In a recently published book entitled *The Bell Curve: Intelligence and Class Structure in American Life* (henceforth *The Bell Curve*),[1] the late Harvard professor of psychology Richard Herrnstein and Heritage Foundation researcher Charles Murray claim that the position of U.S. citizens in the country's class structure is, to a significant extent, the consequence of inherited differences in "g," a general factor of intelligence that is measured by intelligence quotient (IQ) tests. Furthermore, these differences in "g" are responsible for racial differences in class position (that is, some racial groups inherently have more or less "g"). Using a series of regression analyses of data from the National Longitudinal Survey of Youth, which include a proxy for IQ as an independent variable, Herrnstein and Murray suggest that inherited differences in "g" are responsible for black-white differences in behaviors such as crime and having children out of wedlock. The explanations put forward by Herrnstein and Murray regarding the fact that poverty disproportionately affects blacks in the United States (that is, reflecting inherited differences in "g") has made race the center of the controversies surrounding the book.[2]

The aim of the present commentary is to briefly review the limitations of *The Bell Curve* claims with regard to racial differences in intelligence and health outcomes and to establish a parallel between the epistemological stance of the book

---

The authors thank Gary L. Oates for his comments on earlier versions of this manuscript.

regarding race and mainstream epidemiologic research. Herrnstein and Murray claim that several conclusions regarding racial differences in tests of cognitive ability are "beyond significant technical dispute" (p. 22).[1] Chief among their conclusions are that IQ tests are not biased against ethnic or racial groups and that racial differences in cognitive ability are substantially heritable. The main but unstated assumption behind these conclusions is that the variable "race," as operationalized in social science and epidemiologic studies (that is, "black," "white"), has a fundamentally biological interpretation.

CURRENT CONTEXT OF "BIOLOGICAL DETERMINISM"

The debate regarding the inheritance of racial differences in IQ is a long-standing academic battle that has sporadically surfaced in the broader public domain over the past several decades. In the late 1960s and early 1970s, similar arguments to those advanced by *The Bell Curve* were advanced by Jensen,[3] Eysenck,[4] and Herrnstein[5] himself. Efforts at debunking the claims of hereditarian explanations for racial differences in IQ measures[6-10] were not successful enough to thwart this research program altogether.

Thus, although *The Bell Curve* has been launched to reach a nonacademic readership,[2,11] its assumptions regarding the operationalization and interpretation of the variable race are frequently found in the academic world,[12,13] including public health.[14] *The Bell Curve* represents an effort to reach large audiences, but its views are in many cases shared by standard research publications working in the "biological determinist" paradigm. For example, *The Bell Curve* defends research in developmental psychology that includes the extension of inherited racial differences in cognitive ability to brain size, rate of sexual maturation, length of the menstrual cycle, penis size, infant mortality, and mental health.[15]

The research program on biological determinism is also represented in the recent history of epidemiology and public health. An extreme and rare instance is the enduring opposition to considering smoking as a major risk factor for lung cancer and cardiovascular disease, coupled with the attempt to explain away the risk attributed to cigarette smoking in terms of inherited personality traits differentially distributed among racial groups.[16] A more prevalent case of biological determinism appears in the studies on the inheritance of cognitive abilities as an explanation for the different location of minorities in the social structure as well as their undermining of welfare policies aimed at improving the health of African Americans.[17]

Given the increasing skepticism among biologists and anthropologists surrounding the use of race as a biological category,[18,19] its use in epidemiology and public health as an implicit biological category should be reexamined.[20,21]

In biology and anthropology, the resiliency of the biological determinist research program has been explained by the influence of the broader social environment in defining what constitutes worthwhile research.[7,19,22] In contrast, in epidemiology and public health, the "falsifiability criterion" toward scientific knowledge prevails.[23,24] Consequently, in epidemiology, cautious calls for additional studies allow the perpetuation in major biomedical forums of hypotheses of race as a biological category predisposing to illness, even when more realistic alternative mechanisms have been suggested[18–21] and even tested.[25,26]

Our attempt is not to censor the authors' version of biological determinism. One of the ethical principles of scientific conduct is tolerance for the test of hypotheses and the use of methods that one dislikes.[27] Nevertheless, as the sociology and history of science have shown, decisions about basic assumptions guiding research are social phenomena not understandable by simply monitoring the empirical progress of a given field.[22] The scientific community determines in part the acceptability of hypotheses for inquiry, publication, and continued funding through a social process in which certain assumptions are uncritically accepted even in the face of empirical refutation.[28] In the biomedical fields, including epidemiology, one such assumption is that racial labels such as "black" and "white" classify human beings into groups with genetic homogeneity for health outcomes.[20,29,30]

RELEVANCE TO EPIDEMIOLOGIC RESEARCH

Significance of Causal Assumptions Underlying the Use of the Variable Race

Race is widely used in biomedical research, often without any explicit indication of the theoretical construct that its use implies.[20] Even basic pathophysiological mechanisms shared by different animal species are systematically studied in humans separately by race without a clear rationale. The underlying and often unstated assumption, however, is that racial differences are mainly genetically determined, which in turn can lead to conclusions that could have profound public health implications, as in the following examples.

Race-Specific Standards for Hematologic Parameters

Without any evidence from genetic studies, the observation that blacks tend to have a lower leukocyte count than whites, for example, led scientists to the conclusion that "neutropenia is probably a normal genetically determined characteristic" in people of African descent (p. 1023).[31] Similarly, African Americans have been reported to have lower hemoglobin values than whites even after "controlling for socioeconomic differences."[32] However, this study, as well as many other epidemiologic studies, does not in fact adequately control for socioeconomic confounders. If racial differences persist after stratification or adjustment by surrogates of socioeconomic position and other risk factors, no matter how imperfect or partial these surrogates are, investigators often conclude that a genetic factor must be playing a role. A basic methodological principle, that is, that adjusting for an imperfect surrogate of a suspected confounder leads to imperfect adjustment (residual confounding), is unfortunately rarely invoked.

Clearly, despite criticism of the genetic hypothesis to explain racial differences in hematologic parameters,[33] the majority of scientists take at face value the "normality" of lower hemoglobin and neutrophil values in blacks. Moreover, some researchers recommend separate hematologic reference values for blacks[34] without concern for the biological plausibility of the mechanisms linking skin color to hematologic parameters (that is, the philosophy of pragmatism).

Race-Specific Birthweight Distributions

A second example of implicit genetic determinism involves arguments regarding the potential genetic origins of low birthweight in infants from different racial/ethnic groups. Since the 1940s, recommendations for race-specific standards for black and white infants to define low birthweight have been published,[35–37] and more recently differences in birthweight distributions between white and Asian infants have been studied.[38] The proposals for race-specific standards have been fueled by the consistent finding that low birthweight blacks, as defined with the <2,500 g cutoff, have lower perinatal mortality than white counterparts.[39] The subject has been recently revived after the application of statistical models that separately fit the population distribution of birthweight[40] and birthweight-specific mortality for blacks and whites.[41] The result is standardized and different birthweight distributions for blacks and whites. These models eliminate the "apparent paradox" of better survival in small black babies since with these standardized distributions, blacks generally have greater perinatal mortality.[39,42] These results have been interpreted as suggesting that the differences in population distributions of birthweight are genetically determined.[39] However, the authors did not take full advantage of the information that was available on social class, such as maternal education.[39] The main argument here is not derived from biological theory but is statistical (that is, their model fits the apparent paradox of better survival in small black babies as compared with white babies). However, the predominant factors causing low birthweight and prematurity may differ because of unmeasured social exposures determined by class position and racial discrimination, with different severity in terms of mortality. The mechanical use of the variable race precludes an understanding of why black immigrants show much lower low birthweight rates than U.S.-born blacks, why black-white differences in low birthweight rates are not evident in other nations, or why paternal race does not affect the birthweight distribution of those born to white mothers and black fathers.[43-45] Although adjustment of birthweight to population-specific weight standards underscores racial differences in preterm delivery,[46] the assumption or suggestion that such a relevant risk factor might be genetically linked to skin color[38,39] promotes a biological notion of race, providing justification for more research on the biology of race and making direct examination of race-associated social deprivation secondary.

Racial Differences in Blood Pressure

A third example of implicit biological determinism is hypertension, in which an elevated prevalence is still observed in blacks after adjustment for education or income levels.[47,48] The genetic origin of the elevated risk of hypertension in blacks is taken for granted in epidemiology and medicine. In a recent review by Cooper and Rotimi,[47] the weakness and inconsistencies of this prevalent dogma are highlighted. Critical psychosocial aspects of the lifelong experience of racial discrimination are not taken into account. For example, black women who respond passively to the experience of racial discrimination are more likely to have high blood pressure than those who respond actively when faced with discrimination.[25] Studies have also suggested that denial of the experience of racial discrimination and acceptance of its associated belief system, in addition to the direct experience of discrimination in the workplace, produce adverse effects on blood pressure.[20]

Although the role of racial discrimination as a possible determinant of hypertension has been emphasized by a few epidemiologists,[29] most investigators continue searching for biological mechanisms that would explain an increased genetic susceptibility in blacks. Increased susceptibility to sodium or sodium retention is a popular one, although the results are far from consistent.[49] Even if some populations had a higher sensitivity to sodium, this most likely would represent a phenotypic difference.[47] Speculative historical hypotheses (for example, Middle Passage) of this suspected racial susceptibility to salt intake have been discredited.[47] For example, one may challenge such hypotheses by noting the impropriety of using solely U.S. samples to make inferences about white and black races.[26]

As the hypertension research illustrates, the disregard for racial discrimination as an explanation for racial inequalities in health is matched by the lack of evidence supporting genetic explanations. The consideration that a specific phenotypic trait such as skin color is a marker for an increased susceptibility to a wide variety of diseases and pathophysiological traits must be justified. Skin color is mostly a reflection of a common history of exposure to ultraviolet radiation, and its use for characterizing a discrete "package" of genetic material has been by now widely discredited in anthropological research.[19,29,47,50] Since the 1950s, it has been known that human biological characteristics affected by migration selection or drift are distributed in geographic gradations or clines such as those for facial features, hair texture, epidermal melanin, ABO alleles, which do not correlate.[19] For example, the gene codes for type B blood increase in frequency from west to east across Europe and Asia, reflecting migrations out of Asia, whereas epidermal melanin is distributed in a decreasing pattern from the equator to northern latitudes in response to selection for protection against ultraviolet-B radiation. Thus, discordant patterns of heterogeneity falsify descriptions of populations as if they were genotypically or even phenotypically homogeneous (that is, biological races[19]). Furthermore, 85 percent of human genetic variation is found within human populations rather than between the major populations socially labeled as "races."[51] Therefore, according to the "received view" in physical anthropology and evolutionary biology,[19,30] biological races appear to be the outcome of social perception.

SUGGESTIONS FOR EPIDEMIOLOGIC RESEARCH

Now is the time for social explanations to constitute the first hypotheses when looking at racial inequalities in health. Different racial/ethnic groups might have different social experiences that affect health. Examples of this are presented in Table 8.1, which is a summary of discrimination mechanisms that might operate as cumulative exposures over the lifetime. It has been empirically demonstrated, for example, that African Americans are less likely to receive a mortgage loan than whites of similar education and income level[52] and are systematically denied access to middle- and upper-income housing developments.[53] In addition, minority students with the same academic achievements as their white peers are less likely to be included in accelerated tracks in the public school system,[54] and minority defendants with identical socioeconomic positions as white defendants are subjected to a harsher administration of justice.[55] These are examples of differential life experiences that are not accounted for by the standard surrogates of social class.

Another form of implicit biological determinism in epidemiology takes place when researchers use individual-level categories (for example, occupation, race, gender) without an explicit statement of the theory that might explain differences in health outcomes associated with these categories. Thus, some researchers may adopt a pragmatic approach to social epidemiology[56] and conclude that "education" is the preferred social stratification predictor of health. This practice leaves the explanation of what determines education to the reader's implicit theory of causality.[57] Because people in general have a tendency toward attributing people's behavior to intrinsic properties of those people,[57] biological determinism becomes a likely explanation among biomedically trained scholars in particular.[7] This mechanism might be even more compelling when scholars use

Table 8.1. Mechanisms of Discrimination Experienced Differently by Race/Ethnic Groups with Potential Health Significance over the Life Span, by Mode of Social Interaction, According to Published Sources

Discrimination		
Economic	Political	Cultural
Access to goods and services (for example, loans, health insurance, health care, justice, schooling)	Political rights (for example, civil rights, desegregation, democratic representation, empowerment)	Belief systems (for example, stereotypes, attitudes, beliefs and depiction of groups by media, firms, and government)
Myers[63]	Fraser[2]	Williams et al.[20]
Darity et al.[65]	Jacoby and Glauberman[11]	Krieger et al.[21]
Barbarin[67]	Mann[55]	Lott and Maluse[62]
Residential segregation (for example, housing, environmental exposures)		Greenwald and Banaji[68]
Massey et al.[64]		Swim et al.[69]
Brown[66]		Ruggiero and Taylor[70]
Access to labor markets (for example, schooling, training, employment, promotions, primary labor markets) (that is, "good jobs" with benefits); wages and salaries; workplace hazards; and psychosocial environment		Lerner[75]
		James[72]
		Judd et al.[73]
Turner et al.[52]		
Oakes[54]		
Darity et al.[65]		
Barbarin[67]		
Reich[71]		

categories such as race and gender, which have a long history of biologically determinist folk psychology.[58]

The views presented in *The Bell Curve* are one extreme in what can be conceived as a continuum of racial discriminatory views that permeate all research including medical and public health. Most epidemiologists and public health practitioners probably find the arguments of *The Bell Curve* outrageous.

However, many epidemiologists continue to use the variable race uncritically and with little attention to theory.[20,29,59] That is, they fail to consider possible social determinants of racial inequalities in health, including mechanisms originating from exposure to multiple forms of racial discrimination.[20] Even though considering racial and ethnic minorities to be inherently more susceptible to hypertension, leukopenia, and low birthweight may seem more acceptable than considering them more prone to low performance in "cognitive ability" tests, the rationale for these inferences does not differ essentially from the rationale behind the conclusions of *The Bell Curve*.

Sociologists routinely spell out their assumptions and mechanisms in their studies of the determinants of poverty (for example, culture of poverty, biological determinism, social change, and social class[60]). The adoption of similar standards would certainly help the theoretical development of the use of race and social class in epidemiologic research. Even more desirable would be the replacement of topologies such as race or occupation for mechanisms (for example, exposure to racism, racial identity, work-related stresses) and exposures[20] or social processes including not only economic inequality and power asymmetries[60] but also cultural relations[61] (see Table 8.1[62-73]).

The history of the twentieth century has provided evidence that only a short time is required for beliefs about the biological origin of differences in class structure to be translated into policy and that these social policies can have devastating consequences.[9,74,75] The success of the ideas endorsed by *The Bell Curve* and similar efforts in shaping public health policy will partially depend on the energy with which they are discredited in epidemiologic forums, on methodological and empirical[13,76] as well as ethical grounds.

Notes

1. Herrnstein, R. J., & Murray, C. (1994). *The bell curve: Intelligence and class structure in American life.* New York: Free Press.

2. Fraser, S. (Ed.). (1995). *The bell curve wars: Race, intelligence, and the future of America.* New York: Basic Books.

3. Jensen, A. R. (1969). How much can we boost IQ and scholastic achievement? *Harvard Educ Rev, 39,* 1–123.

4. Eysenck, H. J. (1971). *The IQ argument: Race, intelligence and education.* New York: Library Press.

5. Herrnstein, R. J. (1973). *I.Q. in the meritocracy.* Boston: Atlantic–Little Brown.

6. Gould, S. J. (1981). The hereditarian theory of IQ: An American invention. In S. J. Gould, *The mismeasure of man* (pp. 146–233). New York: Norton.

7. Lewontin, R. L., Rose, S., & Kamin, L. J. (1984). IQ: The rank ordering of the world. In R. L. Lewontin, S. Rose, L. J. Kamin, *Not in our genes: Biology, ideology and human nature* (pp. 83–129). New York: Pantheon Books.

8. Kamin, L. J. (1974). *The science and politics of IQ.* Potomac, MD: Erlbaum.

9. Chorover, S. L. (1979). *From genesis to genocide.* Cambridge, MA: MIT Press.

10. Schiff, M., & Lewontin, R. C. (1986). *Education and class: The irrelevance of IQ genetic studies.* London: Clarendon Press.

11. Jacoby, R., & Glauberman, N. (eds.). (1995). *The bell curve debate: History, documents, opinions.* New York: Random House.

12. Bouchard, T. J., & Dorfman, D. D. (1995). Two views of the bell curve. *Contemp Psychol, 40,* 415–421.

13. Hauser R. M., Taylor H. F., & Duster, T. (1995). Symposium: The bell curve. *Contemp Sociol, 24,* 149–161.

14. LaVeist, T. A. (1994). Beyond dummy variables and sample selection: What health services researchers ought to know about race as a variable. *Health Serv Res, 29,* 3–16.

15. Rushton, J. P. (1989). Population differences in susceptibility to AIDS and evolutionary analysis. *Soc Sci Med, 28,* 1211–1220.

16. Eysenck, H. J. (1991). Were we really wrong? *Am J Epidemiol, 133,* 429–433.

17. Jackson, J. F. (1993). Human behavioral genetics, Scarr's theory and her views on interventions: A critical review and commentary on their implications for African American children. *Child Dev, 64,* 1318–1332.

18. Gould, S. J. (1977). Why we should not name human races: A biological view. In S. J. Gould, *Ever since Darwin* (pp. 231–236). New York: Norton.

19. Lieberman, L., & Jackson, F. L. (1995). Race and three models of human origin. *Am Anthropol, 97,* 231–242.

20. Williams, D. R., Lavizzo-Mourey, R., & Warren, R. C. (1994). The concept of race and health status in America. *Public Health Rep, 109,* 26–41.

21. Krieger, N., Rowland, D. L., Herman, A. A., et al. (1993). Racism, sexism, and social class: Implications for studies of health, disease, and well-being. *Am J Prev Med, 9*(Suppl. 6), 82–122.

22. Kuhn, T. S. (1962). *The structure of scientific revolutions.* Chicago: University of Chicago Press.

23. Sober, E. (1987). Optimist/pessimist. *Behav Brain Sci, 10,* 87–88.

24. Greenland, S. (Ed.). (1987). *Evolution of epidemiologic ideas: Annotated readings on concepts and methods.* Newton Falls, MA: Epidemiologic Resources.

25. Krieger, N. (1990). Racial and gender discrimination: Risk factors for high blood pressure? *Soc Sci Med, 30,* 1273–1281.

26. Dressler, W. (1991). Social class, skin color, and arterial blood pressure in two societies. *Ethn Dis, 1,* 60–77.

27. Bunge, M., & Ardila, R. (1987). *Philosophy of psychology.* Berlin: Springer Verlag.

28. Lakatos, I., & Musgrave, R. (1970). *Criticism and the growth of knowledge.* New York: Cambridge University Press.

29. Cooper, R., & David, R. (1986). The biological concept of race and its application to public health and epidemiology. *J Health Polit Policy Law, 11,* 97–116.

30. Cavalli-Sforza, L. L., Menozzi, P., & Piazza, A. (1994). Scientific failure of the concept of human races. In L. L. Cavalli-Sforza (Ed.), *The history and geography of human genes.* Princeton, NJ: Princeton University Press.

31. Shaper, A. G., & Lewis, P. (1971). Genetic neutropenia in people of African origin. *Lancet, 2,* 1021–1023.

32. Garn, S. M., Ryan, A. S., & Abraham, S. (1980). The black-white difference in hemoglobin levels after age, sex, and income matching. *Ecol Food Nutr, 10,* 69–70.

33. Jackson, R. T. (1990). Separate hemoglobin standards for blacks and whites: A critical review of the case for separate and unequal hemoglobin standards. *Med Hypotheses, 32,* 181–189.

34. Reed, W. W., & Diehl, L. F. (1991). Leukopenia, neutropenia, and reduced hemoglobin levels in healthy American blacks. *Arch Intern Med, 151,* 501–505.

35. Anderson, N. A., Brown, E. W., & Lyon, R. A. (1943). Causes of prematurity: III. Influence of race and sex on duration of gestation and weight at birth. *Am J Dis Child, 65,* 523–534.

36. Brown, E. W., Lyon, R. A., & Anderson, N. A. (1945). Causes of prematurity: IV. Influence of maternal illness on the incidence of prematurity: Employment of a new criterion of prematurity for the Negro race. *Am J Dis Child, 70,* 314–317.

37. Rooth, G. (1980). Low birthweight revisited. Lancet, *1,* 639–641.

38. Wen, S. W., Kramer, M. S., & Usher, R. H. (1995). Comparison of birth weight distributions between Chinese and Caucasian infants. *Am J Epidemiol, 141,* 1177–1187.

39. Wilcox, A. J., & Russell, I. T. (1986). Birthweight and perinatal mortality: III. Towards a new method of analysis. *Int J Epidemiol, 15,* 188–196.

40. Wilcox, A. J., & Russell, I. T. (1983). Birthweight and perinatal mortality: I. On the frequency distribution of birthweight. *Int J Epidemiol, 12,* 314–318.

41. Wilcox, A. J., & Russell, I. T. (1983). Birthweight and perinatal mortality: II. On weight-specific mortality. *Int J Epidemiol, 12,* 319–325.

42. Wilcox, A. J., & Russell, I. T. (1990). Why small black infants have a lower mortality rate than small white infants: The case for population-specific standards for birth weight. *J Pediatr, 116,* 7–10.

43. Rowland Hogue, C. J., & Hargraves, M. A. (1993). Class, race, and infant mortality in the United States. *Am J Public Health, 83,* 9–12.

44. Collins, J. W., & David, R. J. (1993). Race and birthweight in biracial infants. *Am J Public Health, 83,* 1125–1129.

45. Kleinman, J. C., Fingerhut, L. A., & Prager, K. (1991). Differences in infant mortality by race, nativity status, and other maternal characteristics. *Am J Dis Child, 145,* 194–199.

46. Wise, P. (1993). Confronting racial disparities in infant mortality: Reconciling science and politics. *Am J Prev Med, 9*(Suppl. 6), 7–16.

47. Cooper, R., & Rotimi, C. (1994). Hypertension in populations of West African origin: Is there a genetic predisposition? *J Hypertens, 12*, 215–227.

48. Hypertension Detection and Follow-up Program Cooperative Group. (1977). Race, education and prevalence of hypertension. *Am J Epidemiol, 106*, 351–361.

49. Madhavan, S., & Alderman, M. H. (1994). Ethnicity and the relationship of sodium intake to blood pressure. *J Hypertens, 12*, 97–103.

50. Harris, M. (1989). *Our kind: The evolution of human life and culture.* New York: Harper Perennial.

51. Lewontin, R. L. (1973). The apportionment of human diversity. *Evol Biol, 6*, 381–397.

52. Turner, M. A., Fix, M., & Struyk, R. Y. (1991). *Opportunities denied, opportunities diminished: Racial discrimination in hiring* (Urban Institute Report No. 91-9). Washington, DC: Urban Institute.

53. *Baltimore Neighborhoods Inc. and Fenwick-Shaffer* v. *Winchester Homes.* (1993). Baltimore City Circuit Court Civil Action Suit No. 90066002/CC1:0092.

54. Oakes, J. (1982). Classroom social relationships: Exploring the Bowles and Gintis hypothesis. *Sociol Educ, 55*, 197–212.

55. Mann, C. R. (1993). *Unequal justice: A question of race.* Bloomington: Indiana University Press.

56. Winkleby, M. A., Jatulis, D. E., Frank, E., et al. (1992). How education, income and occupation contribute to risk factors for cardiovascular disease. *Am J Public Health, 82*, 816–820.

57. Nisbett, R., & Ross, L. (1980). *Human inference: Strategies and shortcomings of social judgment.* Englewood Cliffs, NJ: Prentice Hall.

58. Kitcher, P. (1985). *Vaulting ambition: Sociobiology and the quest for human nature.* Cambridge, MA: MIT Press.

59. Jones, C. P., LaVeist, T. A., & Lillie-Blanton, M. (1991). "Race" in the epidemiologic literature: An examination of the *American Journal of Epidemiology, 1921–1990. Am J Epidemiol, 134*, 1079–1084.

60. Wright, E. O. (1994). *Interrogating inequality.* London: Verso.

61. Lamont, M. (1992). *Money, morals and manners: The culture of the French and American upper middle class.* Chicago: University of Chicago Press.

62. Lott, B., & Maluse, D. (Eds.). (1995). *The social psychology of interpersonal discrimination.* New York: Guilford Press.

63. Myers, S. L. (1993). Measuring and detecting discrimination in the post–civil rights era. In J. H. Stanfield & R. M. Dennis (Eds.), *Race and ethnicity in research methods.* Newbury Park, CA: Sage.

64. Massey, D. S., Gross, A. B., & Shibuya, K. (1994). Migration, segregation, and the geographic concentration of poverty. *Am Sociol Rev, 59*, 425–445.

65. Darity, W., Guilkey, D., & Winfrey, W. (1995). Ethnicity, race, and earnings. *Econ Lett, 47,* 401–408.

66. Brown, P. (1995). Race, class, and environmental health: A review and systematization of the literature. *Environ Res, 69,* 15–30.

67. Barbarin, O. A. (1981). Community competence: An individual systems model of institutional racism. In O. A. Barbarin, P. R. Good, O. Martin Pharr, et al. (Eds.), *Institutional racism and community competence.* Rockville, MD: National Institute of Mental Health.

68. Greenwald, A. G., & Banaji, M. R. (1995). Implicit social cognition: Attitudes, self-esteem, and stereotypes. *Psychol Rev, 102,* 4–27.

69. Swim, J. K., Aikin, K. J., Hall, W. S., et al. (1995). Sexism and racism: Old fashioned and modern prejudices. *J Pers Soc Psychol, 68,* 199–214.

70. Ruggiero, K. M., & Taylor, D. M. (1995). Coping with discrimination: How disadvantaged group members perceive discrimination that confronts them. *J Pers Soc Psychol, 68,* 826–838.

71. Reich, M. (1981). *Racial inequality.* Princeton, NJ: Princeton University Press.

72. James, S. A. (1993). Racial and ethnic differences in infant mortality and low birth weight: A psychosocial critique. *Ann Epidemiol, 3,* 130–136.

73. Judd, C. M., Park, B., & Ryan, C. S., et al. (1995). Stereotypes and ethnocentrism: Diverging interethnic perceptions of African American and white American youth. *J Pers Soc Psychol, 69,* 660–681.

74. Kelves, D. J. (1985). *In the name of eugenics.* New York: Knopf.

75. Lerner, R. M. (1992). *Final solutions: Biology, prejudice, and genocide.* University Park: Pennsylvania State University Press.

76. Hauser, R. M., & Carter, W. Y. (1995, August). *The Bell Curve as a study of social stratification.* Paper presented at the annual meeting of the American Sociological Association, Washington, DC.

CHAPTER NINE

Latino Terminology

Conceptual Bases for Standardized Terminology

David E. Hayes-Bautista
Jorge Chapa

The search continues for an appropriate generic term for persons of different kinds of Latin American origin or descent, living in the United States. Numerous articles published by many journals have continued to use different terminologies and operationalization methodologies. As pointed out earlier,[1] there is no commonly accepted term nor method for defining and counting such a group. This chapter offers an epistemological and conceptual basis for terminology and methodology, which may serve as a basis for standardization. The term of reference that is offered is "Latino," to be applied to all persons of that soon-to-be-described background, irrespective of ethnicity (Hispanic or non-Hispanic), language (Spanish, Portuguese, or other), or race (mestizo, Indian, Asian, black, or white). The grounds for the choice of the term "Latino" will be given, as will some suggestions for operationalization.

AN ANALYSIS OF TERMINOLOGY

It should be a given that before an item is categorized and named, some rational basis for the categorization and subsequent terminology should exist. In the case of Latinos, the rational bases have been confused, hence the confusion of terms. What is there about a Latino that makes him or her so? Is it a language, a surname, a mythical ancestor from Spain, or is it the fact of origin in a country of Latin America? In our present analysis, the only element among these that is shared by all Latinos is the last one: origin in a Latin American country. As we examine the different bases that have been used for classification of Latinos, we shall see that country of origin is the major, indisputable, clear-cut characteristic. Further, we shall appreciate why the Latin American countries are different from countries of origin in Europe, and hence why Latinos should be the object of policy considerations that were not given to European immigrants and their descendants.

Historically, three different epistemological bases have been used for the categorization of Latinos, hence three very different types of terminologies. Over time, these different bases have been confused with one another, until we have arrived at the present-day dilemma.

The major conceptual basis historically used for the identification of Latinos has been political and geographic. This basis was pronounced in the Monroe Doctrine in 1823 and continues to the present. The use of this basis has resulted in the identification of the nationality of individuals from countries in Latin America. However, it was and continues to be confused with a racial categorization, purporting to identify a racially distinct group. Although in a formal sense the racial categorization has not been used since about 1940, it still forms a large part of everyday "man in the street"[2] perceptions of Latinos. Since 1940, new synthetic measures, derived from what has been termed a "cultural" basis, have been used as a sort of euphemism. This last basis has been extremely arbitrary, misleading, and deceptive. Let us see how these different bases have had their influence over time, in order to understand better this chapter's opening assertion that the only "real" basis for terminology, hence the most accurate, is related to and derived from national origin.

THE MONROE DOCTRINE AND NATIONAL IDENTIFICATION

The young republic of the United States, huddled on the eastern coast of the continent, followed with some interest the struggle for independence of the former colonies of European powers in the rest of the hemisphere. While the Europeans bickered among themselves about the proper disposition of formerly Spanish holdings (as shown so clearly in the Polignac Memorandum of 1823, in which France pledged not to attempt to incorporate such holdings into its own imperial ambitions), the United States announced the doctrine (later to be called the Monroe Doctrine) which fixed the U.S. relationship to the rest of the hemisphere in no uncertain terms. The Monroe Doctrine declared that the entire hemisphere was in the U.S. sphere of influence, and that the principle of nonintervention by European powers applied to all former colonies of all European powers, not just those of Spain.

The formal definition of residents of Latin America was initially fixed by national citizenship: that is, an inhabitant of Mexico was a Mexican, and of Venezuela, a Venezuelan. No other formal racial, ethnic, cultural, or other meaning was implied.

MANIFEST DESTINY AND THE EMERGENCE OF RACE

However, the inhabitants of Latin America (particularly Mexico) stood astride the path of manifest destiny. The annexation of other peoples and the incorporation of foreign territories were bound up in a process through which a national identification was supplanted by a racial one—one in which the conquered race was relegated to a lower social level than that of the conquering race.

We may examine the situation of California as a case in point. The popular image of Mexicans living in California was in many ways fixed by the accounts of "Yankee" travelers and adventurers written between 1820 to 1847. By the time of the Mexican War and the Gold Rush of 1849, North American arrivals to California had already formed an image of a "race" with peculiar attributes (p. 14).[3] Richard Henry Dana, a proper Bostonian visiting California in 1835, described the Mexicans of California as "an idle, thriftless people" (p. 59).[4] The inhabitants were described by other observers at best as a "proud, indolent people doing nothing but riding after herds from place to place" (p. 187);[5] and at worst as having a "dull, suspicious countenance, the small twinkling, piercing eyes, the laxness and filth of a free brute, using freedom as a mere means of animal enjoyment, dancing and vomiting as occasion and inclination appears to require" (pp. 356–357).[6]

The racial attitude was forcefully stated in 1836 by William H. Wharton, who agitated for American possession of Texas by writing that "God will forbid . . . Texas . . . should be permanently benighted by . . . the rapine of Mexican misrule. The Anglo-American race are destined to be forever proprietors of this land" (p. 2).[7]

By armed force, the United States defeated Mexico in a war that was divisive in the United States itself. Abraham Lincoln openly debated the conduct of the war, and a major participant, Ulysses S. Grant, then a lieutenant, wrote later when president, "To this day I regard the (Mexican) war as one of the most unjust ever waged by a stronger against a weaker nation" (p. 313).[8] Shortly thereafter, the northern half of Mexico was incorporated into the United States by the conclusion of the Mexican War. The Treaty of Guadalupe Hidalgo, which ended the hostilities, pronounced the rights of a nationality group, the former citizens of Mexico who were now living in the United States. No mention of race was made in the official documents.

However, the large numbers of miners arriving from the United States during the Gold Rush of 1849 clashed with the Mexicans who had been living for generations in California, and the dominant group (the forty-niners), prepared by their readings of the early Yankee accounts of the native people, quickly saw these former citizens of Mexico in terms of race. One miner described the lynching of a Mexican woman in 1851, using a racial category: "in keeping with the characteristics of her race, Juanita had a quick passion" (p. 204).[9] In 1854, a resident of Los Angeles described the execution of a Mexican "who . . . had killed one of his own race, about a woman" (p. 104).[10]

FROM NATIONALITY TO RACE: THE GREASERS

In the nineteenth century, "greaser" was a term commonly used in a racial sense to describe the former Mexican citizens living in recently acquired territories. Initially, in Texas, New Mexico, Arizona, and early California, "greaser" was used exclusively to describe Mexicans.[11] However, after the arrival of other Latin Americans, especially in the gold fields of California, the term "greaser" was applied to all persons of Latin American origin. Indeed, the perceptions of non-Latinos about non-Mexican-origin Latinos in early California provide some clues about the current search for terminology and method.

By 1850, there were four distinctly different Latino groups, categorized by nationality, in California: the "Californios" (originally born in Mexican territory, but by then putatively citizens of the United States), Mexicans (largely miners from the northern Mexican state of Sonora who had immigrated after 1848), Peruvians, and Chileans (both also from the mining centers there). These Latin Americans of different nationality groups saw themselves as quite distinct from each other. However, mining society tended to see them all as one race or people, generally lumping them all together under the term "greaser." For policy purposes they were treated as one group. One of the first pieces of legislation passed by the new state was a "Foreign Miners" tax, aimed at excluding Latin American miners (the "foreigners") from claiming rights in the gold fields. The native-born Californios were considered foreigners for this purpose, in spite of being legally citizens.[12]

Irrespective of the intra-Latino differences seen by the Latinos themselves, in the eyes of the everyday North American inhabitant of California, and in the eyes of some early laws, all Latinos were seen to be identical and were dealt with as one "race."

This perception of all Latinos as a single group in California was repeated at a national level.

THE U.S. LATIN AMERICAN EMPIRE

U.S. designs on Latin American territory antedated the Monroe Doctrine. As early as 1811, John Quincy Adams expressed an opinion that it would only be a matter of time until "by the law of political gravitation" Cuba would become a part of the United States (p. 903).[8] The digestion of Mexican territories was slowed a bit by the Civil War, but toward the end of the nineteenth century, political sentiment in this country called for a further expansion into Latin American territories. In order to justify doing so, Latin Americans as persons were continuously cast as belonging to a less advanced and different race; thus, the confusion of race for nationality continued on a larger scale.

President Ulysses S. Grant proposed annexing the Dominican Republic during his term. The Republican Party platform for 1895, developed for William McKinley, contained provisions for the purchase and annexation of the Danish West Indies and for the construction of a canal across Nicaragua, in an American zone (p. 904).[8]

After the Spanish-American War—the "splendid little war," as John Hay described it—the U.S. flag flew over Cuba and Puerto Rico. Henry Cabot Lodge announced that the United States had acquired "rightful supremacy in the Western Hemisphere." In the space of a very few years, U.S. troops had carried out further operations in Mexico, Nicaragua, and Haiti, and U.S. "diplomacy" had meddled with Colombia to suddenly produce the new republic of Panama, which promptly granted the United States a concession to build a canal.

Theodore Roosevelt developed the "Roosevelt corollary" to the Monroe Doctrine, which not only warned Europe against intervention in Latin America but also unabashedly reserved the right of U.S. intervention. Roosevelt wrote that when a nation "knows how to act with decency . . . it need fear no interference from the United States. . . . But brutal wrongdoing, or an impotence that results in a general loosening of the ties of civilized society, may finally require intervention by some civilized nation, and in the Western Hemisphere the United States cannot ignore this duty" (p. 912).[8]

Although the formal relations expressed were political, in most common usage there was a careless and casual inference that the other nations in the Western Hemisphere were populated by a different race. This line between national identity and race was quite faint, and crossed many times, as evident in Roosevelt's claim that in dealing with Latin American publics he would "show those Dagos they will have to behave decently" (p. 911).[8] In the working assumptions of the general North American public, the "race" of Latin Americans was a reality, and it was the antithesis of the civilized U.S. population.

FORMAL CONFUSION OF RACE FOR NATIONALITY

We see this confusion of race for nationality reflected in the terminology and methodology used by various public health and other official agencies in the early twentieth century. Reflecting in part a national debate over immigration and national origin quotas, the Los Angeles County Health Department began compiling statistics for Latinos of Mexican origin. As early as 1916, death and infant mortality statistics were reported for "white" and "Mexican." Epistemologically, we may appreciate now that a racial category (white) was compared to a national origin category (Mexican). By 1921, statistics for nursing services were presented for "White, Mexican and Other (Negro, Oriental)" (p. 46).[13]

In this irrational process, something was considered inherent in persons of Mexican national origin that could be passed on to succeeding generations. A study of tuberculosis done in 1924 in Los Angeles County separated out the "Mexican" from the "total" population. Then, in a curious way, the Mexican population was further subdivided into "Mexican" and "non-citizen Mexican" (p. 4).[14] In terms of birth and citizenship, this was an impossibility. If interpreted literally, this would mean that citizenship was somehow passed from parent to child, hence one could speak of Mexicans being born in the United States. The intent, however, was to trace a perceived racial group, using a term of national origin as identifier.

In 1929, Governor Young of California appointed the Mexican Fact Finding Committee to gather data for policy purposes. In its final report, the committee noted that Mexicans were racially distinct from whites in that "the bulk of immigration from Mexico into the United States is from the pure Indian or the Mestizo stocks of the Mexican population" (p. 24).[13]

A flurry of sociological studies done on the plight of Latinos in Southern California around that era adopted the confused race/nationality terminology, vide the titles of some of these works:

- "The Mexican Housing Problem in Los Angeles"[15]
- "The Mexicans in Los Angeles"[16]
- "The Mexican in Los Angeles from the Standpoint of the Religious Forces of the City"[17]

The leading document of the time was a study by Emory Bogardus titled *The Mexican in the United States,* which announced itself as a study in race relations and constantly referred to Mexicans as a racial group.[18]

This confusion of race for nationality was given formal approval by the U.S. Bureau of the Census. The earliest standardized censuses, from 1820 to 1860, included three racial categories: White, Negro (Free or Slave), and Other. In 1860, Indian and Chinese were added, and Japanese in 1870. Reflecting the need to track the influence of immigration, from 1860 on separate items asked about country of birth.[19] Those born in Mexico could be identified by this procedure.

The growth of the Mexican population after 1910 led to the policy attention just mentioned, which required better statistics than had been captured in earlier censuses.

For the 1930 Census, a new category was added to the race/color question, which gave formal acceptance to using nationality for race. The coding instructions for the race/color entry stipulated that ". . . all persons born in Mexico, or having parents born in Mexico, who are definitely not white, Negro, Indian, Chinese or Japanese, should be returned as Mexican (Mex)" (p. 52).[20] A nationality was formally recognized as a race.

So entrenched had this confusion of race for nationality become that at least one major Latino organization, the League of United Latin American Citizens, saw itself as representing a racial group. The articles of incorporation of that group included such statements as, "We solemnly declare once for all to maintain sincere and respectful reverence for our racial origin, of which we are proud" (p. 365).[21]

This confusion seeped into health policy work. A study issued in 1938 by the California Bureau of Child Hygiene conveniently managed to stereotype Mexicans as a separate racial group by such statements as, "There seems to be no understanding in the Mexican mind of a binding contract between patient and doctor" (p. 38).[22] This same report casually spoke of "American born Mexicans," and at one point mentioned that "a total of 1,726 Mexican births occurred in San Bernardino county."

Clearly, while a term of nationality ("Mexican") was used, the implication was that Mexicans were a race apart. This perception was not limited to Mexican-origin Latinos. A national poll conducted in 1940 by the Office of Public Opinion Research turned up racial categorization of Latin Americans by the general public. A national sample was asked to select words from a list that to them best described the "people of Central and South America." The term chosen as number one by 80 percent of the respondents was "dark skinned." The next five words chosen as descriptors were, in descending order: "quick tempered," "emotional," "religious," "backward," "lazy." Positive descriptors were rarely selected. Less than 15 percent of the sample chose any of the following words: "intelligent," "honest," "brave," "generous," "progressive," "efficient" (p. 502).[23] It is evident that a popular perception of the inhabitants of Latin American countries as a very distinct people, with all the characteristics of a race, had emerged as a result of over a century of U.S.–Latin American interaction.

Domestic policy regarding Latinos, especially Mexicans, was at worst viciously exclusionary, as seen in the massive roundups and deportations of Mexican-looking persons (including many citizens) during the Depression, the segregation of Mexicans into separate schools, and the denial of service in private institutions. Signs reading "No Mexicans Allowed" were not uncommon up through the 1950s; for a poignant recounting, the film *Chulas Fronteras* provides excellent material. At best, policy adopted a "white man's burden" tone, reluctantly dealing with the problem of an ignorant, dirty, and uneducated population. Latinos were identified as a race apart; they had been treated as such ever since the pronouncement of the Monroe Doctrine.

THE ERA OF CULTURAL EUPHEMISMS

The Disappearance of Identifiers

By 1930, records in California and the Southwestern United States often showed a category which utilized the terminology of nationality but which carried with it the explicit implication of race. By the end of World War II, both categories had been formally done away with and were replaced by a series of jumbled euphemisms.

By a series of policy decisions at both judicial and executive levels, which are not clear, Mexicans suddenly ceased to be a race apart and were declared to be "white." Coding instructions for the 1940 Census stipulated that "Mexicans were to be listed as White, unless they were definitely Indian or some race other than White" (p. 61).[20] This had the result of Latino identifiers suddenly disappearing from sight. The Census of 1950 reported that there were three major races: white, Negro and Other. "Persons of Mexican birth or ancestry who are not definitely Indian, or of other non-white race were classified as white" (p. 2).[24]

As recently as 1958, official California State publications had to explain that Mexicans were then considered white. The *Statistical Abstract* for that year, in reporting deaths by race (which included white, Negro, Indian, Chinese, Japanese, and other), explained starkly that "White includes Mexican."[25]

While the Mexican-origin Latino population had disappeared from statistics, Latinos had not disappeared from everyday social reality. The need to gather data about this group led to the adoption of many different identifiers.

Spanish Surname

For the 1950 Census, an ex post facto approximation of the Mexican-origin Latino was developed by matching the returns from the five Southwestern states to a master list of Spanish surnames. This group became known as the "white person of Spanish surname," which has served as denominator in many studies since then.

Birthplace

Meanwhile, the Puerto Rican Latino population living on the mainland increased greatly in the 1950s, and data were needed about them. The 1960 Census instructed that upon observation by the enumerator, "Puerto Ricans, Mexicans or other persons of Latin [sic] descent would be classified as 'White' unless they were definitely Negro, Indian, or some other race." The Spanish surname criterion was used to approximate the Mexican-origin population in the five Southwestern states. In New York state only, a question was asked about birthplace, with three possible answers: "United States," "Puerto Rico," "Elsewhere."

By utilizing these two variables, surname and birthplace, the two Latino groups were supposed to have been approximated.

Spanish Language

The political ferment among Latino groups in the 1960s demanded ever better data. In an attempt to capture an improved enumeration, the 1970 census adopted a hodgepodge composite approach (p. 70).[20] The "Spanish heritage population" was defined as

- Those with a Spanish surname *or* Spanish language, in the five Southwestern states.
- Those with Puerto Rican birth or parentage, in the three middle Atlantic states.
- Those with Spanish language, in the remaining forty-two states (pp. 2–3).[26]

Epistemologically, three different variables were being combined: surname and/or language (cultural) and birthplace/parentage (nationality). These were applied differentially across the country.

In terms of race, these persons were considered to be white. Indigenous attempts by respondents to be categorized as other-than-white were overridden by instructions to the enumerator. "Chicano," "La Raza," "Mexican-American," and "Brown" were to be changed to white (p. 75).[20]

Spanish Origin

In an attempt to reconcile the differing variables, a 5 percent sample of the 1970 Census was asked to respond to questions on nationality, which was given a cultural label: "Spanish origin." "Respondents were asked if they were of Mexican, Puerto Rican, Cuban, Central or South American, or other Spanish origin or descent" (p. 8).[26] The data from a national origin question appeared to be the best available, and it became the denominator to which the cultural denominators were compared.

HISPANIC

A new category was created by executive fiat in the 1970s. The federal Office of Management and Budget (OMB) developed a new term with a new methodology: "Hispanic." This term had not been used in earlier counts. The term was operationalized as, "A person of Mexican, Puerto Rican, Cuban, Central or South America or other Spanish culture or origin, regardless of race."[27]

Epistemologically, this definition is a mixture of a culturally derived term ("Hispanic") operationalized partially by nationality and partially by culture, and partially not operationalized at all by the extremely open-ended phrase "other Spanish . . . origin." While this combination has been useful to examine the Latino population in the aggregate, it has been noted that it is less than useful in studying the social mobility of higher income, higher education Latinos, for the degree of error introduced can be quite large.[1] In the policy arena, particularly in the area of affirmative hiring and admission practices, this combination of bases presents an essentially unbounded universe, which has resulted in situations that can only be described as utter confusion:

- An organization that promotes ties between Spain and the United States, the Spanish American Heritage Association, declared in 1980 that "[a] Hispanic person is a Caucasian of Spanish ancestry. The Mexican American and Puerto Rican are not Caucasians of Spanish ancestry, and therefore are not Hispanic."[28]

- The U.S. Department of Transportation published regulations in 1980 that attempted to interpret the OMB definition. These regulations define Hispanics as those from Mexico, the Caribbean, and Central and South America. Explicitly excluded were people from Spain and Portugal.[28]

- In 1985, as reported in "S.F. Debates: Are Spaniards Hispanic?" a Spanish woman demanded that the San Francisco Human Rights Commission apply affirmative action benefits to Spanish individuals. Her claim to benefits was that "When . . . they look at the name, they're going to think that I'm Latina. It's many of the Latin Americans who are privileged."[29]

Many similar confusing acts committed in the attempt to define who is "Hispanic" and why have been commented upon previously.[1]

The 1980 Census used a modified version of "Spanish/Hispanic" as the term of reference. It was operationalized by a combination of nationality and culture. The choices for respondents to select from were Mexican, Mexican American, Chicano, Puerto Rican, Cuban, other Spanish/Hispanic.[30]

This last choice—other Spanish/Hispanic—introduces a tautology that has led to problems in response. Is a Spaniard Hispanic? By this definition, yes. Let us follow out some further problems. Is a Cape Verdean Hispanic? Is a Filipino Hispanic? Is a Brazilian Hispanic? Is a Brazilian identical to a Cape Verdean? Are both identical to a Portuguese? These and other questions emerge when an unclear conceptual basis is used to classify and name groups. How, indeed, are Latinos to be described?

LATINO: THE PREFERRED TERM OF REFERENCE

The conceptual and epistemological grounds for selecting a term and opera-tionalizing it should be clear by now. The major social fact linking the United States to Latin America is political and geographic, reflected in the historical links, defined by the Monroe Doctrine, to the various countries in the Western Hemisphere. No other country, or set of countries, has had this same sustained type of linkage. Analytically, there is no such thing as a Latin American race. Yet many individuals and officials, for 162 years and more, have behaved as if such a "race" existed. The euphemisms (surname, language, "Hispanic") are diffuse and imprecise and do not address the major dynamic that has created the perceptions and policies applied to Latin Americans in the United States. The term of reference has to respect the diverse national origins and the waves of population movement from Latin America for over four centuries.

The generic term that best fits these criteria is "Latino." This term is derived from "Latin America" and, as such, preserves the flavor of national origin and political relationship between the United States and Latin America (other terms used to refer to this region tend to be divisive, such as Indo-America, Spanish America, or Ibero-America). Latino is culturally neutral, with respect to Latin American cultures. A Brazilian is as much a Latin American as a Mexi-can. It is also racially neutral, an important strength when one considers that 51.9 percent of the Mexican-origin population in California in 1980 described itself racially as "other"; a smaller percentage, 47.7 percent, described itself as "white" (p. 18).[30] It is quite evident from such responses that such terms as "white, Hispanic," or "white person of Spanish surname" would not be accept-able descriptors to the majority of the Latino population that considers itself nonwhite.

Despite its masculine "o" ending, the term "Latino" is sex neutral. By the rules of Spanish orthography, all collective terms (nouns, pronouns, and adjec-tives) when used in reference to a grouping containing both sexes, utilize the masculine ending. The term "Hispanic," when used in Spanish, is similarly declined ("Hispano"). Thus, the term "Latino" refers to both sexes, irrespective of endings.

Perhaps most important, the term "Latino" has been, in the authors' experi-ence, the term that most Latinos find least objectionable. An example of this may be seen in the American Public Health Association itself. When, in the early 1970s, a group of Mexican-origin and Puerto Rican–origin Latinos met to form a caucus, the proposal to call the group the Chicano Caucus was vetoed by the Puerto Ricans, and the proposal to call it the Boricua Caucus was vetoed by the Mexicans. Both groups rejected outright the title Hispanic Caucus, with many imprecations, commenting further that no one present was a

Spaniard. After years of debate, the name Latino Caucus was chosen, in large part because it was considered the least objectionable of all the alternatives. In the authors' experience while researching various Latino groups, the most common term of reference used, with only very minor exceptions, is nationality. Latinos, particularly of the immigrant generation, define themselves in relation to country of origin ("I am a Mexican"; "I am a Brazilian"; "I am a Chilean") before making any other identification as to race, language, culture, or personal lineage.

This desire to maintain a national origin identity is very strong. The *Los Angeles Times* undertook investigative reporting among the growing Mexican and non-Mexican Latino population in Southern California precisely to determine what term would best fit these different groups. The first major finding was that most Latinos in that region vigorously rejected the term "Hispanic." This is seen in numerous editorials—in newspapers both large and small, in English and Spanish—with titles such as

- "Don't Call Us Hispanics"[31]
- "Latino, si—Hispanic, no"[32]
- "Hispanic—una subdivision de 'Latinos'?"[33]

The second finding by the *Times* was that most respondents viewed "Latino" to be an adequate, appropriate, and acceptable self-description that expressed to their own satisfaction their desire to maintain a sense of national origin while yet expressing links between them. As a result of this effort, the style guide of the *Los Angeles Times* states:

- *Latino* is the preferred umbrella term for all Spanish-surnamed groups in the United States.
- Use *Chicano* as an abbreviated synonym for Mexican American unless it is established that the individual prefers the latter. A reporter should establish the preference rather than make an assumption.[34]

Respecting the desire of Latinos not to be categorized as Hispanic, an unwritten editorial policy holds that the term "Hispanic" will be used only when directly quoting someone who uses the term.[35]

IDENTITY AND TERMINOLOGY

The question of Latin American identity is one that has long been debated in Latin America itself. For 300 years, from 1521 until independence in 1821, Latin American identity was defined in terms of the major colonial powers. For example, Mexico, prior to independence, was called New Spain, and there was no terminology problem. New Spain was Spanish, and the identity of Indians, mestizos, and blacks was a nonissue. However, upon achieving independence, largely in the early nineteenth century, two schools of thought arose. One held that the only commonality in Latin American identity was the legacy of Spanish language and institutions. The other held that Latin American identity was to be found in its Indian past. The "Hispanistas" and the "Indigenistas" were also representative of political groups—the Hispanistas being identified with largely conservative, wealthy land-owning groups, while the Indigenistas claimed to be the voice of the poor, landless peasant. Civil wars, revolutions, and insurrections have been fought under the banner of Hispanism or Indigenism, with perhaps the bloodiest being the Mexican Revolution of 1910 to 1917 (which the Indigenistas won) and the subsequent bloody Cristero Revolt. In academia, literature, music, and the plastic arts, the philosophical struggle continues over whether Latin America is basically Spanish (or, more grandly, "Iberian") or is Indian. Even the terminology used to refer to the region reflects this 160-year debate: the Hispanistas use terms such as "Hispano America" or "Ibero-America," while Indigenistas will claim terms such as "Indo-America."

And yet, given the U.S. presence since 1823, both groups unhesitatingly use the term "America Latina" or "Latinoamerica" to refer to the region. To refer to people, ideas, or products from that area, "Latino Americano" is shortened to "Latino," and there is no confusion as to what is meant. While the term "Latin" may be used by a few analysts to refer to Mediterranean Europe, the term "Latino" is not: in everyday usage, it refers to things Latin American. In the best epistemological, perhaps hermeneutic sense, the term means what its users intend it to mean. While a very narrow reading of dictionaries (whether Webster's or the Real Academia) may try to include Italians, French, and Rumanians as "Latins," no stretching of commonplace usage could include such peoples as Latinos, a notion which would be rejected by Latinos and Rumanians alike. Such similar narrow readings of dictionaries such as the Real Academia define Chicano as having its roots in *chicaneria* (literally, chicanery), an etymology which has been rejected by numerous Chicano scholars.

The current debate over terminology for Latinos in the United States continues this 160-year-old conflict, sometimes verbal, sometimes armed, over Latin American identity. Only now it is further recognized in Latin America that a major element in current Latin American identity is the relation to the United States, and that whatever directions the identity debate takes, it has to include the powerful presence and influence of that northern colossus.[36]

In sum, we propose using a nationality derived term "Latino," to describe a geographically derived national origin group that has been constantly and consistently viewed and treated as a racial group, in both individual and institutional interaction, while in the United States.

OPERATIONALIZATION

The term "Latino" should be used uniformly to refer to persons residing in the United States whose nationality group, or the country in which the person or the person's parents or ancestors were born, is a Latin American country in the Western Hemisphere. Excluded from the term Latino would be persons of Spanish, Portuguese, Cape Verdean, or Filipino origin. Included would be non-Hispanic Latin Americans, such as Brazilians, Guyanese, and so forth, all of whom fell under the sweep of the Monroe Doctrine.

The term "Latino" is a generic one. It should be recognized that there are vast differences between Latino groups of different national origin. Given the importance of immigration to the current explosive growth of the Latino population, it is imperative that the specific national origin of any Latino group studied be specified. The few recent studies that have investigated the social and economic characteristics of "Hispanic" subgroups have found that the differences are often greater than the similarities (p. 3),[37] (pp. 1–5).[38] There are also differences between U.S.-born and foreign-born Latinos. We strongly suspect that the same is true of direct health variables as well. For research, policy, and programmatic purposes, it is important to know if one is working with Mexican- or Cuban-origin Latinos. Thus, we propose that the term "Latino" always carry a national origin modifier, for example, "Mexican-origin Latino." Only when speaking of a mixed Latino population (such as the entire Latino population of the United States) should the term be used without a modifier.

Some special attention should be given to Latinos of New Mexico. Northern New Mexico has been populated for nearly 400 years by pockets of Mexican-origin persons. For centuries this group has referred to itself by terms such as "Hispano" and "Manito." These terms identify the "*patria chica,*" or regional identity, of such individuals and are similar to other *patria chica* terms used in the rest of Mexico: those from Guadalajara call themselves Tapatios, those from Vera Cruz are Jarochos, and those from Mexico City are proud to be Chilangos. The Manitos or Hispanos share a fairly homogeneous and distinctive history. New Mexico is also currently experiencing a rapid influx of immigrants from Mexico, with a different history and experience. Some have felt that the Manitos are indeed pure Spanish and hence can only be referred to as Hispanic. It should be pointed out that the confusion of nationality for race is continued by this line of reasoning. The first church built in Santa Fe was constructed by Indians from Tlaxcala, Mexico, most of whom stayed there and became part of the Latino population. Attempts to idealize or identify strictly Spanish ancestry founder upon the rocks of reality. Furthermore, in the authors' experience with northern New Mexicans, they use a variety of reference terms, including Raza, Chicano, Mexican American, Hispano, Manito, and Latino. The major Spanish language radio station in that region, broadcasting from Española, New Mexico, proudly calls itself Radio Mexicana. The Manitos or Hispanos are Latinos, although their unique depth of history should be preserved in identifiers. We suggest that the term "Mexican-origin Latino" apply when speaking of both the recent and ancient Mexican-origin groups, and the term "New Mexican Hispano Latino" be used when referring exclusively to the northern New Mexican group, with the understanding that "Hispano" is a term of *patria chica* identity and does not refer to either racial or cultural origin.

National origin is fairly easily and reliably captured. The "Hispanic" category of the 1980 Census consists of four major national origin subgroups and one residual category: Mexican, Puerto Rican, Cuban, Central or South American, and Other Spanish. The first four of these reflect populations that can be defined unambiguously by the researcher. For example, it is possible for a researcher to specify that he or she will include as part of the target population only respondents who have either one parent or two grandparents of one particular subgroup. This is roughly the procedure that was followed in the screening interview for the National Chicano Survey.[39] Members of the first three groups rank very high in terms of consistency of self-identification. The Other Spanish category ranks among the lowest.[40,41] This consistency of response suggests that it is possible to meaningfully identify members of this group by nationality.

To summarize, there are three items of information that need to be utilized when referring to Latino populations.

- The generic term "Latino"
- Nationality subgrouping: Mexican-origin, Cuban-origin, Brazilian-origin, and so forth
- Nativity: U.S.-born or foreign-born

The first two items should always be specified when indicating a particular Latino group. The third item need not always be specified, but it must be discovered during the initial stages of any research regarding a Latino population.

A great deal of health research has been done on the basis of administrative and other records that did not ascertain Latino national origin. The surname of the individual named on these records has often been used as the basis for attributing membership in one Latino group or another. When a Latino population has been approximated on the basis of a cultural euphemism (surname or language), the method should be alluded to after the term Latino, so as to caution the reader that a mixture of bases is taking place. Thus, "Latino (Spanish surname)" or "Latino (Spanish language)" allows the reader to know the synthetic bases used for approximating the Latino population under study. Research based on identifying individuals with Spanish surnames can, strictly speaking, be generalized only to the Spanish surname population. As already indicated, the members of this group can vary greatly by region, sex, marital status, and the exact composition of the surname list.[42]

The Latino population living in the United States is in a phase of defining itself, both vis-à-vis the United States and vis-à-vis the different national origin subgroups. An emergent identity seems to be in the making[43] that transcends the Spanish language to embrace all Latin American–origin elements. The term "Latino" reflects this process.

THE REVERSE ANGLE: ANGLO OR WHITE

Concern has been raised about the identification of non-Latino, nonblack, non-Asian populations in the United States. This population has at times been called the "white" population. In the Southwestern United States, Latinos have commonly used the cultural term "Anglo" to refer to non-Latinos. Further into Latin America, cultural/racial terms such as "Caucasian," "Saxon," and "Yankee" may be used. More often, a nationality term, "North American," is used, but this term may be applied to blacks and Asians of North American citizenship as well as to whites.

The style guide of the *Los Angeles Times*[34] provides the following instruction to its reporters on this topic:

In general, use the word *white* to refer to the majority group in our society. *Anglo* may be used as a synonym for white in stories that deal exclusively with whites and Chicanos, especially, for example, if the Chicanos involved use the term *Anglos* themselves. In Los Angeles school desegregation stories, use *white, black* and *Chicano.*

Probably the most neutral term would be a redundancy: "white, non-Latino." The redundancy will be necessary for a number of years to clear up the confusion sown by the inaccurate but widely used terms "white, Hispanic" and "white person of Spanish surname." Some Latinos see themselves as nonwhite, some as white, but nearly all see themselves as somehow connected to Latin America. Most whites do not see themselves as related to Latin America. The term "white, non-Latino" allows a clear definition of what is intended, without offending too many sensibilities.

CONCLUSION

We have provided here a conceptual basis for developing and operationalizing a standard terminology to refer to persons of Latin American origin or descent. In our analysis, the major trait shared by all Latin American countries is not language, race, or culture, but is political—the unilaterally imposed Monroe Doctrine. This political linkage has colored North American views of persons from the Latin American region, and has formed the basis for domestic policy adopted regarding them. Given this we conclude that

- "Latino" is the most appropriate term of reference to use to refer to persons of Latin American origin or descent residing in the United States.

- It should be recognized that the term reflects nationality and not language, race, or culture.

- The term should be applied only to persons whose descent or origin lies in Western Hemisphere countries. Persons of Spanish national ancestry outside the Western Hemisphere should not be considered Latino.

Certainly this presentation will not be the last word on this topic: it is our intention to provide a framework for further discussion, debate, and thought.

Notes

1. Hayes-Bautista, D. E. (1980). Identifying "Hispanic" populations: The influence of research methodology on public policy. *Am J Public Health, 70,* 353–356.

2. Schutz, A. (1973). *Collected papers, Vol. 1: The problem of social reality.* The Hague: Martinus Nijhoff.

3. Pitt, L. (1968). *The decline of the Californios.* Berkeley: University of California Press.

4. Dana, R. H., Jr. (1840). *Two years before the mast: A personal narrative of life at sea.* Boston: Bates and Lauriat.

5. Camp, C. (Ed.). (1928). *James Clyman: American frontiersman, 1792–1881: His own reminiscences and diaries.* San Francisco: California Historical Society.

6. Farnham, T. J. (1844). *Travels in the Californias and scenes in the Pacific Ocean.* New York: Saxton and Miles.

7. de Leon, A. (1983). *They called them greasers: Anglo attitudes toward Mexicans in Texas, 1821–1900.* Austin: University of Texas Press.

8. Herring, H. (1968). *A history of Latin America.* New York: Knopf.

9. Coy, O. C. (1929). *Gold days.* Sacramento, CA: Powell.

10. Bell, H. (1881). *Reminiscences of a ranger, or, early times in Southern California.* Los Angeles: Yarnell, Caystile and Mathes.

11. McWilliams, C. (1968). *North from Mexico.* New York: Greenwood.

12. Peterson, R. H. (1975). *Manifest destiny in the mines: A cultural interpretation of anti-Mexican nativism in California, 1848–1853.* San Francisco: R&E Associates.

13. Young, C. C. (1930). *Mexicans in California: Report of the Mexican Fact Finding Committee.* Sacramento: California State Printing Office.

14. California State Bureau of Tuberculosis. (1925). *A statistical study of sickness among the Mexicans.* Sacramento: California State Printing Office.

15. Fuller, E. (1920). The Mexican housing problem in Los Angeles. In *Studies in Sociology, I.* Los Angeles: Southern California Sociological Society.

16. The Mexicans in Los Angeles. (Sept. 15, 1920). *Survey,* p. 715.

17. Oxnam, G. B. (1921). The Mexicans in Los Angeles from the standpoint of the religious forces of the city. *Ann Am Acad Polit Soc Sci,* pp. 130–133.

18. Bogardus, E. S. (1934). *The Mexican in the United States.* Los Angeles: University of Southern California Press.

19. U.S. Bureau of the Census. (1975). *Historical statistics of the U.S.: Colonial times to 1970* (2 vols.). Washington, DC: U.S. Government Printing Office.

20. U.S. Bureau of the Census. (1979). *Consistency of reporting of ethnic origin in the current population survey* (Technical Paper No. 31). Washington, DC: Author.

21. Moquin, W. (1971). *A Documentary history of the Mexican Americans.* New York: Bantam.

22. California Bureau of Child Hygiene. (1938). *Maternal and child health among the Mexican groups in San Bernardino and Imperial Counties.* Sacramento: California State Department of Public Health.

23. Cantril, H. (Ed.). (1951). *Public opinion, 1935–1946.* Princeton, NJ: Princeton University Press.

24. U. S. Bureau of the Census. (1952). *1950 Census of the population: Tracted cities, California* (Bulletin P-D28). Washington, DC: U.S. Government Printing Office.

25. Senate Fact Finding Committee on Commerce and Economic Development. (1958). *California statistical abstract.* Sacramento: California State Printing Division.

26. Siegel, J. S., & Passel, J. S. (1979). *Coverage of the Hispanic population of the United States in the 1970 Census: A new sociological analysis* (Current Population Reports, Special Studies, No. 82). Washington, DC: U.S. Bureau of the Census.

27. *Federal Register, 43*(87) (1978, May 4), p. 19269.

28. Langley, R. (1980). Hispanics: It's all a matter of classification. *Arizona Republic.*

29. Smith, R.S.F. (1985). S.F. Debates: Are Spaniards Hispanics? *San Francisco Chronicle.*

30. U.S. Bureau of the Census. (1982). *Persons of Spanish origin by state, 1980* (Supplementary Report PC80-S1-7). Washington, DC: U.S. Government Printing Office.

31. del Olmo, F. (1981, May 1). "Don't call us Hispanics." *Los Angeles Times.*

32. del Olmo, F. (1981, October 25). "Latino, si—Hispanic, no." *Los Angeles Times.*

33. Casparius, R. (1986, January 14). "Hispanic—una subdivision de 'Latinos'?" *Los Angeles La Opinion.*

34. Los Angeles Times. (n.d.). *Style Guide.* Los Angeles: Author.

35. F. del Olmo, personal communication with the authors, 1986.

36. Monsivais, C. (1982). *Amor perdido.* Mexico City: Era.

37. Jaffe, A. J., & Cullen, R. M. (1980). *The changing demography of Spanish America.* New York: Academic Press.

38. Borjas, G., & Tienda, M. (1985). *Hispanics in the U.S. economy.* New York: Academic Press.

39. Arce, C. (1979). *Screening questionnaire for the National Chicano Survey.* Ann Arbor: University of Michigan, Institute for Survey Research. Mimeograph.

40. U.S. Bureau of the Census. (1975). *Comparison of persons of Spanish surname and persons of Spanish origin in the United States* (Technical Paper No. 38). Washington, DC: Author.

41. Howard, C. A., Sumil, J. M., Buechley, R. W., Schrag, S. D., & Key, C. R. (1982). Survey research in New Mexico Hispanics: Some methodological issues. *Am J Epidemiol, 117,* 27–34.

42. Passel, J. S., & Word, D. L. (1980, April). *Constructing the list of Spanish surnames for the 1980 Census: An application of Baye's Theorem.* Paper presented at the annual meeting of the Population Association of America, Denver, CO.

43. Padilla, F. M. (1984, Summer). On the nature of Latin ethnicity. *Soc Sci Q, 65*(2).

PART THREE

RACIAL AND ETHNIC
DISPARITIES IN HEALTH CARE

CHAPTER TEN

Racial and Ethnic Differences in Access to Medical Care

Robert M. Mayberry
Fatima Mili
Elizabeth Ofili

In 1985, the Department of Health and Human Services (DHHS) released the *Report of the Secretary's Task Force on Black and Minority Health* (sometimes referred to herein as the Task Force Report).[1-8] This landmark report represented the first time DHHS had made a concerted effort among its agencies and programs to raise the awareness of the health of racial and ethnic minorities in the United States and the relative poor health of minority groups compared to the majority white population. The Task Force Report was the culmination of work, which began in 1984, of a primary group of eighteen senior scientists and officials within DHHS, charged by DHHS secretary Margaret M. Heckler with the responsibility of studying the persistent health disparity between white Americans and African, Hispanic, Native, and Asian Americans. Dr. Thomas E. Moore, deputy director of the National Institutes of Health, was appointed chairman of the task force, and experts from the nonfederal community were invited to consult with primary task force members in exploring the magnitude of health disparities and why these disparities continued to exist given the steady improvement in overall health in the United States. Acknowledging that health disparity was complex and influenced by many behavioral, social, economic, cultural, biological, and environmental factors, the task force further affirmed that the interaction of these factors on health status is "poorly understood for

Support for this article was provided by the Henry J. Kaiser Family Foundation (Grant No. 97-4501).

the general population and even less so for minorities." Existing sources of data were one obvious problem in attempting to understand dimensions of health disparity by race and ethnicity. More data existed on African Americans, although still insufficient; data for other ethnic groups, such as Hispanic and Asian subgroups and Native Americans, were very limited and often lacking.

Nevertheless, it was apparent based on the available information at the time the task force began its work that African Americans, Hispanics, Native Americans, and some Asian and Pacific Islander groups, relative to white Americans, were not benefiting equally from the cumulative scientific knowledge and advanced medical capacity to diagnose, treat, and cure disease. And while the primary emphasis of the Task Force Report was health status differences by race and ethnicity, access, availability, and utilization of health services were discussed, albeit in a limited manner, as contributing factors to health status and the health disparity gap between minority and nonminority populations. The task force observed that gross indicators of access and utilization of services, such as the number of annual visits to a physician, had narrowed as a result of the major insurance programs of Medicaid* and Medicare.† However, the report indicated that racial and ethnic groups continued to have poorer access to quality health care services and different patterns of utilization relative to white Americans, including a lower use of preventive services, a greater likelihood of not having a usual source of care, and a greater likelihood of being uninsured.

Since the release of the Task Force Report, along with its recommendations for eliminating disparities in health status, there has been an increased awareness of and sensitivity to minority health issues and a proliferation of studies and reports attempting to investigate further racial and ethnic differences in health status, access to services, and outcomes. This article presents our review of the literature on racial and ethnic differences in health care services from 1985 to the present. Particularly important among the task force recommendations that helped to guide our literature review is the call for the DHHS to adopt and foster a research agenda to investigate factors affecting minority health, specifically factors in the health care setting that influence diagnosis and treatment of racial and ethnic minorities.

---

*The Medicaid program became law in 1965 as a jointly funded cooperative venture between the federal and state governments to assist states in the provision of adequate medical care to eligible needy persons. Medicaid is the largest program providing medical and health-related services to America's poorest people. It covers approximately 36 million individuals, including children, the elderly, and people who are eligible to receive federally assisted income maintenance payments.

†The Medicare program is the nation's largest health insurance program, covering approximately 39 million Americans. The program, administered by the Health Care Financing Administration (HCFA), provides health insurance to people age sixty-five and older and those who have permanent kidney failure and certain people with disabilities. Medicare was established by Congress in 1965.

NEW CONTRIBUTION

We critically reviewed the published research since 1985 to describe further the nature of racial and ethnic differences in access to preventive, diagnostic, and therapeutic services as well as how far research in these areas in the intervening years has advanced the understanding of these disparities. A main purpose of this review and synthesis of the health services research literature was to better understand the contributing factors for these disparities in access to health care services and to highlight areas that may be most productive in future investigations that aim to reduce disparities in access to health care between ethnic minorities and the majority white population.

METHODS

We searched the MEDLINE database for studies conducted in the United States and published in peer-reviewed journals during the period from 1985 through October 1999. We chose the year 1985 to coincide with the release of the Report of the DHHS Secretary's Task Force on Black and Minority Health. We initially searched the literature, with the assistance of experienced librarians, using the key words *racial stocks, ethnic groups, United States, health services accessibility, barriers to care, utilization, treatment,* and *diagnosis.* We then conducted a second search specific to key patient conditions or health service areas, such as cancer, cardiovascular disease and stroke, diabetes, infant mortality, child health, HIV and AIDS, mental health, psychiatric disorders, emergency care, preventive services, and health services utilization. Hard copies of all abstracts that indicated that a purpose of a study was access to screening, diagnostic care, and therapeutic care by race and ethnicity were retrieved, and each abstract was reviewed by at least two health outcomes research scientists for relevance to the topic. Hard copies of relevant articles were then retrieved and further reviewed. In instances of disagreement, the article was reviewed by a third or fourth research scientist, and any disagreement was resolved through consensus.

Articles selected for final inclusion in this review were those that (1) indicated that a primary purpose of the study was variation in medical care access by race and ethnicity, (2) contained original findings, (3) presented actual quantitative and comparative data, and (4) met general and acceptable principles of scientific research. Each article had to specify the racial or ethnic groups being compared, and any that lumped "minorities" into a single category for comparison to whites, for example, were excluded. With regard to Hispanics and Asians, our preference would have been to include only articles that indicated specific ethnicities, such as Mexican, Puerto Rican, or Cuban Americans and Japanese, Chinese, Korean, and so on. We allowed articles to remain in the review with broader categories of Hispanics or Latinos and Asians or Pacific Islanders. With regard to scientific research, the article had to state a clear research question or purpose and define clearly the research methods, data sources, and data collections and analytical procedures. We considered certain articles to be sentinel because they reported original findings of disparities in access to medical care (or a lack thereof) or they provided unique insights that helped to explain previously published findings.[‡] Review articles were not considered in our synthesis.

After this literature review process, articles were categorized by major subheadings to coincide with major subject areas of the Task Force Report: heart disease and stroke, cancer, diabetes, and infant and child care. Other subheadings in this review are HIV/AIDS, specifically chosen because of the sufficient body of literature and the impact on minority communities, and mental health, as a reasonable subheading for a broad and substantial body of literature on care access by race/ethnicity. We also addressed the substantial body of literature on particular types of primary, rehabilitative, long-term, and emergency care, under the subheading of health services, since it did not fit within the health condition subheadings.

Our purpose in this review is not to present information extensively and laboriously from the nearly 400 articles that were reviewed. Instead, we will present results from published articles that clearly indicate the nature of the disparities in access to care by race and ethnicity, represent the body of literature for the subheadings, and especially, provide clues to explaining the observed racial and ethnic disparities in access to care. Under each subheading, we present the results from selected published articles (usually with accompanying explanatory comments and interpretation), provide a general critique of the body of literature, and where appropriate, suggest general areas for future investigations, based on study findings, that may be most productive in helping to explain racial and ethnic differences in access to health care services.

FINDINGS

Our review of the health services literature over the past decade and a half since the release of the Task Force Report revealed significant differences in access to medical care by race and ethnicity within certain disease categories and types of health services. Most studies have varied in their attempts to control for possible explanatory variables—most important are SES (or some surrogate

---

[‡]Free copies of the commissioned report (No. 1526), which includes annotated sentinel articles, are available on the Kaiser Family Foundation Web site (www.kff.org) or through the publication request line at 800-656-4533.

measure of social and economic status), insurance coverage, stage or severity of disease, comorbidities, and type and availability of health care services. In some cases, when important variables are controlled, racial and ethnic disparities in access are reduced and may even disappear under certain circumstances. Nonetheless, the literature shows that racial and ethnic disparities persist in significant measure for several disease categories and service types. Findings are irrefutably consistent for certain areas (invasive cardiac care), require careful interpretation in some areas (cancer and HIV/AIDS), and are muddled in other areas (mental health). In specific health care settings (diabetes care) and under certain circumstances, no racial and ethnic disparities are observed. Altogether, findings from the published literature raise many questions about equity and fairness in health care delivery.

REVIEW BY HEALTH CONDITION

Heart Disease and Stroke

The 1985 *Report of the Secretary's Task Force on Black and Minority Health* documented the excess cardiovascular disease mortality burden, especially for stroke, among African Americans relative to whites as well as the higher rate among African Americans of nonfatal stroke.[4] Death rates from coronary heart disease were similar among black and white men, but among women, blacks had a higher mortality as well as incidence rate. While the data were more sparse for other ethnic groups, the Task Force Report indicated lower death rates for heart disease among Hispanic, Native American, and some Asian Americans compared to white and African Americans. The Task Force Report also noted the importance of access to care for cardiovascular disease and documented that African Americans made fewer physician office visits, were more likely to be seen in hospital clinics and emergency rooms, were less likely to be seen by a cardiovascular specialist, and were less likely to undergo coronary arteriography and coronary bypass surgery than were white Americans.

Since that time, researchers have repeatedly documented racial and ethnic differences in access to invasive diagnostic and therapeutic interventions for heart disease and stroke. Study findings have consistently indicated that African Americans are less likely to receive pharmacological therapy, diagnostic angiography and catheterization, and invasive surgical treatments for heart disease and stroke relative to white Americans with similar clinical disease characteristics. The magnitude of the observed black-white differences often varies due to differences in the age and gender distributions of the study populations, data sources used in the investigations (such as hospital discharge, claims-based, or registry data), and other factors such as primary diagnosis of interests, diagnostic specificity or mix of participants included in the study, severity of disease, and comorbidities as well as study designs and analytical approaches used to estimate access disparity. Given the amazing consistency of findings of the numerous studies, it is highly unlikely that observed racial and ethnic differences are spurious. Equally unlikely is that these consistently observed differences are explained by known factors related to access to invasive cardiac procedures, such as disease severity.

Two major factors are important in assessing the use and appropriateness of invasive cardiac procedures: access to the cardiologist for comprehensive invasive diagnostic evaluation and disease severity, which is the strongest predictor of treatment selection. These studies that include only angiographically confirmed diagnoses and account for some measure of disease severity are particularly informative in understanding racial and ethnic differences in cardiac care, since these major factors can no longer be considered explanatory if ethnic differences remain in study analytical results. One of the earlier studies by Maynard et al.[9] is particularly noteworthy in that it not only documented differences by race in the receipt of invasive cardiac procedures for patients with coronary disease confirmed by angiography but also alluded to other factors beyond diagnostic evaluation, such as appropriate use of surgical treatment and possible patient refusal. In this study of patients enrolled from July 1974 to May 1979 in fourteen clinics in the United States and one clinic in Canada, African Americans were less likely than whites (47 percent versus 59 percent) to be recommended for bypass surgery—accounting for other sociodemographic factors such as age, gender, and occupational status, and clinical factors, including disease severity. Furthermore, African American patients who were recommended for bypass surgery were also less likely to have surgery (81 percent versus 90 percent), which resulted in the overall bypass surgery rate in this study of 38 percent among blacks and 58 percent among whites. The differences between surgery recommendation and having surgery indicate other complex care decision-making factors, including patient's preference or aversion, which may be related to the observed racial disparity in surgical treatment. It is also interesting to note that only 1 percent of blacks compared to 12 percent of whites who were recommended for nonsurgical treatment had surgery, indicating perhaps an overuse of surgery in this study population, particularly for whites.

Albeit limited to a single institution, Peterson et al.[10] at the Duke University Medical Center in North Carolina published one of the more comprehensive studies of black-white difference in cardiac care, accounting for more potentially explanatory variables and exploring many of the complex issues in clinical decision making as well as appropriateness of therapeutic procedures. Among patients diagnosed between 1984 and 1992 with obstructive coronary disease whose status and disease severity was angiographically defined, blacks were 32 percent less likely to have had coronary bypass surgery and similarly less likely to have any revascularization procedure. These differences were not explained by other demographic variables, such as age and gender, smoking status, comorbidities, disease severity, and insurance status. Of further note, black-white differences for bypass surgery were greater among patients with severe disease than among patients without severe disease and most pronounced among patients expected to survive for more than one year.

Hannan et al.[11] extended the analysis of ethnic differences even further by specifically accounting for appropriateness as well as necessity of bypass surgery. Among patients with angiographically confirmed coronary artery disease admitted in 1994 to 1996 to mostly urban New York hospitals, African Americans and Hispanics were similarly less likely (36 percent and 40 percent, respectively) than non-Hispanic whites to undergo bypass surgery when the procedure was judged to be appropriate, that is, when expected health benefits exceeded negative consequences of surgery. African Americans were 37 percent less likely to undergo bypass surgery than whites when the procedure was judged to be necessary, that is, surgery was appropriate and the physician was obligated to recommend the procedure. (Hispanics were as likely as whites to undergo surgery when surgery was judged necessary.) Disease severity (measured by three-vessel disease and left main disease) was the strongest predictor of access to bypass surgery; age and insurance status but not gender were also predictors.

Most studies exploring racial and ethnic differences in cardiac care were not limited to angiographically confirmed subjects but rather generally investigated differences in diagnostic and therapeutic procedures. Weitzman et al.[12] published study findings of patients hospitalized for myocardial infarction who were admitted between January 1987 and December 1991 to twenty-two participating acute care, teaching and nonteaching community hospitals in four states (North Carolina, Mississippi, Maryland, and Minnesota). While there was an indication of a racial difference for angiography, the results demonstrated significant differences for percutaneous transluminal coronary angioplasty, coronary artery bypass graft surgery, and thrombolytic therapy. Blacks were 50 to 60 percent less likely to have had angioplasty, 60 to 70 percent less likely to have had bypass surgery, and 50 percent less likely to have had thrombolytic therapy, accounting for age, gender, comorbidity, geography, and availability of cardiac catheterization facilities. Other studies had previously shown the lower likelihood of these cardiac care procedures for African Americans relative to whites.[13-17] The black-white differences in access to invasive cardiac procedures are less consistent or the association is less strong for thrombolytic therapy, catheterization, or angioplasty versus the difference for bypass surgery.[10,18,19]

Most studies have compared African Americans to whites, but some studies have investigated disparities for other ethnic Americans. Results may be less consistent for Hispanics and, in general, may not be observed for Asians.[20] Ramsey et al.[21] found no significant difference for bypass surgery and marginal differences for angioplasty between Mexican American and non-Hispanic whites in Corpus Christi, Texas. Goff et al.[22] in Corpus Christi found 43 percent less likelihood of thrombolytic therapy for Mexican Americans among myocardial infarction patients. Mickelson, Blum, and Geraci,[23] at a Veterans Administration (VA)§ medical center, found Hispanics to be 71 percent less likely to receive thrombolytic therapy. Canto et al.[20] found a marginal difference between Asians and Pacific Islanders and whites for thrombolytic therapy among acute myocardial infarction patients but no significant differences for angiography, angioplasty, or bypass. This study also found no significant difference in invasive procedures between Native Americans and whites.

Black-white differences in access to cardiac care, on the other hand, are observed for the many populations studied, including Medicare beneficiaries[24-29] and military veterans receiving care in the VA hospitals.[23,30-33]

In addition to the above-mentioned disease diagnoses, black-white differences in access to care have also been documented for other cardiovascular conditions, including congestive heart failure[34] and peripheral artery diseases.[35] Among low-income veterans with stroke or transient ischemic attacks who were less likely to have supplemental care outside the VA health care systems, African Americans were significantly less likely than whites to receive cerebral arteriography (53 percent less likely) and subsequent carotid endarterectomy (72 percent less likely).[36] Racial differences in access to heart transplantation have also been documented, with African Americans less likely to receive transplants even after controlling for prognosis following transplantation, clinical and demographic factors, income, and distance to a transplant center.[37] African Americans and Hispanics have also been observed to be less likely than whites to be screened for cholesterol level and diagnosed with hypercholesterolemia, even after controlling for insurance coverage, SES, and number of visits.[38]

The degree to which racial and ethnic disparities exist in invasive cardiac procedures is influenced by insurance status, with the greatest differences found among the uninsured and Medicaid population and the smallest disparities among the privately insured.[11,13,18] Among the uninsured, African Americans were half as likely to undergo angiography and one-third as likely to undergo bypass surgery compared to uninsured whites, even after adjusting for comorbidities.[13] Moreover, even within the VA health care system, which is

---

§To minimize the effect of insurance status, many studies in our review confined their study populations to individuals covered by specific health care programs, in this case, the U.S. Department of Veterans Affairs (VA). About 10 percent of 27 million veterans use the VA's system of inpatient, outpatient, and community-based services each year; if veterans are eligible for services, the care is free. Compared to other hospitals, VA facilities are more likely to be large, located in urban areas, and serve more chronic psychiatric patients. VA users are more likely to be African American, male, older, poor, less educated, underemployed, and without family support, and more likely to have worse health conditions, besides lacking other health insurance coverage.

mandated to provide inpatient care to all eligible veterans free of charge, investigators have found racial differences in the treatment of cardiac and stroke patients.[31,33,39] On the other hand, Mirvis and Graney[40] found that the likelihood of cardiac catheterization and bypass surgery among VA patients with coronary diseases was greater for African Americans than for whites if a cardiac catheterization laboratory and cardiac surgical program were present at the local VA facility.

In contrast, one study showed that racial and ethnic differences in access can be mitigated by a universally accessible system. Specifically, Taylor et al.[41] studied 1,441 military patients seeking care for acute myocardial infarction in the Department of Defense (DoD) health care system** and found no racial differences in the rate of cardiac catheterization or revascularization after controlling for age, gender, cardiovascular risk factors, and clinical characteristics. However, whites were more likely than nonwhites to be considered for cardiac catheterization within six months of the initial hospital discharge.

The strength and weaknesses of each individual study vary, and there are methodological considerations in assessing the validity of findings. We have alluded to variables that were accounted for in published studies and thought to at least partially explain the observed racial/ethnic difference, including severity of disease and other factors related to access to cardiac care, such as insurance status. The methodological inadequacy of an individual study may be a relatively moot point in the context of the body of literature that gives consistent findings and in which one study, often the more recent study, may overcome the specific failing of a previous investigation. As mentioned earlier, studies in which the primary diagnosis is specific and disease status and severity of disease are well defined, such as angiographically, represent more refined investigations[10,11,25] compared to other studies in which diagnoses are not angiographically confirmed or include mixed and otherwise nonspecific cardiovascular disease diagnoses.[17]

Of course, studies conducted in specific locales, such as urban settings, or statewide studies have limited generalizability to different geographic locations, which may differ according to resources availability and population characteristics. Yet, despite varying locations of previous investigation, study results are almost invariably consistent.

The lack of SES indicators in the study of racial and ethnic differences in health care is a common refrain among researchers. Nearly all the studies of

---

**The Department of Defense guarantees free access to health care services to all active duty and retired military personnel and their dependents. Approximately 9 million people are served through a large, nationwide, staff-model managed care plan that operates military hospitals and free-standing clinics and directly employs physicians and other providers. Care at these facilities is free to beneficiaries.

racial and ethnic differences in access to cardiac care reviewed lacked SES information and were not able to evaluate the relative influence of education, for instance, and insurance status. The argument regarding SES is valid because SES, of which income and education are components, is related to care-seeking behavior, lifestyle, and other behavioral factors. The argument, however, may be overblown in regard to access to cardiac care, in which the individual has presented himself for medical care for a major or threatening event of heart attack or stroke. The more salient factor at this point is insurance coverage.

The 1999 study by Daumit et al.[42] helps to address SES and particularly insurance status in relation to catheterization and revascularization procedures in a seven-year longitudinal study of African American and white patients with new-onset end-stage renal disease (ESRD), who are at high risk of cardiovascular disease and who are eligible for Medicare insurance. This study also represents the exception in that it accounted for several SES variables (that is, level of education, marital status, employment status, and type of employment) and type of insurance in its analysis. Among ESRD patients, African Americans were 29 percent less likely to have had catheterization, 52 percent less likely to have had coronary angioplasty, and 44 percent less likely to have had bypass surgery during follow-up, even accounting for SES and insurance. However, among the subgroup of patients who were Medicare insured before the onset of ESRD and whose insurance status remained unchanged, there was no racial difference for cardiac procedure rates (all procedures combined) at follow-up.

The investigation by Peterson et al.[10] of racial differences in cardiac care access among angiographically confirmed coronary artery disease patients did not have specific information on SES factors but did include type of insurance, which is a surrogate for SES, in its analyses. However, insurance status was not a significant predictor of treatment selection in multivariate analyses, most likely due to the fact that 96 percent of whites and 87 percent of African Americans had private or Medicare insurance. If the "other" category of insurance (not defined by the authors) included mostly uninsured or Medicaid-insured African Americans, the 32 percent difference in the rate of bypass surgery for African Americans relative to whites is a conservative estimate.[13] While this study also alluded to appropriateness and necessity of surgical treatment in cardiac care, Hannan et al.[11] specifically addressed these two important issues and also found disparity in bypass surgery rates for African Americans relative to whites when the procedure was appropriate (a 36 percent rate deficit) and necessary (a 37 percent rate deficit). In contrast, the results of a study by Leape et al.[43] found no racial/ethnic differences in revascularization procedure rates, but revascularization rates varied according to whether patients received the procedure on-site or off-site at participating hospitals. This study, however, with a smaller study sample did not distinguish between angioplasty and bypass surgery (the two procedures were lumped together) and did not define coronary disease diagnoses as specifically as Hannan et al.,[11] including as study subjects all patients with "suspected atherosclerosis." A previous study from Los Angeles by Laouri et al.[44] is consistent with Hannan et al.'s findings.[11] Among angiographically confirmed disease, African Americans were 51 percent less likely to undergo coronary bypass surgery and 80 percent less likely to undergo angioplasty when the procedures were considered necessary. Laouri et al.[44] further accounted for the site in which the procedures were performed (public versus private hospital), which may explain the magnitude of differences in this and the Hannan et al. study,[11] which were conducted in different geographic locations.

Another important factor that has been explored in recent studies is the patient's refusal of or aversion to invasive procedures.[11,39] The black-white differences in aversion rates tend to be small relative to the black-white differences in procedure rates[39] and, at best, could only partially explain the procedure rate difference. Only 5 to 10 percent of patients refused revascularization according to interviews with the cardiologists,[43] whereas the physician made the decision not to recommend bypass surgery 90 percent of the time among patients who did not undergo surgery.[11]

Studies that found greater racial/ethnic disparities among the uninsured and Medicaid populations compared to privately insured groups indicate that financial factors modify the effect of race/ethnicity on medical care access and suggest areas of research that may be very productive. Investigations that distinguish the features of health care systems where racial and ethnic differences in access to care are diminished (for example, DoD) relative to others (for example, VA) would significantly advance our understanding of these disparities in regard to organizational and financial structures, since these systems also differ in accessibility (for example, universal or equal), care management, and perhaps quality. Studies focusing on decision making by patients and physicians regarding cardiac diagnostic and therapeutic procedures would also be helpful. Such studies may reveal racial and ethnic differences in patients' and physicians' preferences for various cardiac procedures as well as the impact of physician-patient interactions on patients' decisions whether to receive such interventions. Studies that attempt to understand the psychosocial basis for higher aversion rates for invasive procedures may shed additional light on access disparities.

Cancer

The Task Force Report indicated that the poorer cancer survival rates observed for racial and ethnic Americans, particularly African Americans, may be due in part to delay in the detection of cancer and differences in the availability of various treatment options.[3] The data available to the task force were generally limited to cancer mortality and incidence rates; data on access to medical care by race and ethnicity were scarce and virtually unavailable for Asian, Hispanic, and Native Americans. Since the release of the Task Force Report, numerous investigators have attempted to confirm the task force findings and to determine the extent to which race and ethnicity affect access to screening and diagnostic and therapeutic interventions for various types of cancer. The results have been somewhat inconsistent.

With respect to breast cancer screening, earlier surveys showed racial disparities, but the gap appears to be narrowing,[45,46] at least for women younger than age sixty-five.[47] National survey results from 1992 indicate that white and African American women had similar rates of mammography and clinical breast exams[47-49] but also that Hispanic women were screened far less frequently.[50-52] Also, elderly African American women had lower mammography use rates than their white counterparts despite the initiation of Medicare reimbursement for screening mammograms in 1991.[53,54]

As observed for breast cancer, African American women were not disadvantaged in screening for cervical cancer, with similar rates among whites and African Americans (92 percent) but a somewhat lower rate among Hispanics (84 percent).[49] Indeed, after controlling for socioeconomic factors including age, income, education, marital status, urbanicity, and source of care, African American women were 2.7 times more likely than white women to have had a Pap test, but Hispanic women remained 20 percent less likely than white women to have had a Pap test. The higher rate of Pap testing among African Americans was previously documented.[55]

Screening is associated with several individual and population characteristics, including education or awareness level, health care utilization patterns and preferences, and cultural differences.[49,55] Other factors, such as income and having a usual source of care, rather than race and ethnicity, may be predictors of breast and cervical screening.[49,56] Having no source of care was the strongest predictor for breast and cervical cancer screening, even stronger than education level, and women in health maintenance organizations (HMOs) may be more frequently screened than women with other types of insurance.[55] Among older women who were Medicare insured, the number of primary care visits was a predictor of mammography but did not explain the observed black-white differences in mammography screening.[47] While the exact constellation of these factors may not be known with certainty in predicting cancer screening, national public awareness and early detection programs as well as community-based initiatives have incorporated knowledge of predictors in intervention efforts and contributed significantly to overall improvement in cancer screening and narrowing of the disparity gap.

In contrast to cancer screening, most studies, although not all, have documented racial and ethnic differences in the stage of cancer at diagnosis, with African Americans and Hispanics more likely to be diagnosed at advanced stages.[57-64] For example, with respect to breast cancer in women younger than age forty, a study of women from the Metropolitan Detroit Cancer Surveillance System during a nine-year period found that African Americans were more likely to be diagnosed with remote disease than were whites (6 versus 4 percent, respectively);[63] the difference was even greater for women older than eighty (21 versus 13 percent, respectively). The proportion of patients diagnosed with metastatic stage prostate cancer was 35.4 percent for African Americans and 22.2 percent for whites, according to data from the population-based Connecticut cancer registry.[62] Significantly, a study within the DoD health system, which ensures universal access for all beneficiaries, found no racial differences in stage of breast cancer at diagnosis.[64] However, this was not true for prostate cancer; 26 percent of black and 12 percent of white, military, active duty personnel, dependents, and retirees had distant metastases at diagnosis according to the DoD tumor registry data of newly diagnosed prostate cancer cases between 1973 and 1994.[61] The findings among DoD beneficiaries are not clearly explained. For breast cancer, equal frequency of screening may explain the lack of differences in breast cancer stage at diagnosis for black and white women. The black-white prostate cancer stage differences were crude or unadjusted and did not account for the possibility of age differences among blacks and whites and the increased risk of prostate cancer among younger African American men.

Research findings are not entirely consistent with regard to ethnic differences in cancer treatment. Early studies of breast cancer patients from the mid-1980s using data from the Surveillance, Epidemiology, and End Results (SEER) program of the National Cancer Institute reported crude or unadjusted racial differences in surgical treatment of breast cancer.[65] Later SEER studies, however, revealed that African American, Hispanic, and white breast cancer patients received various treatments at similar rates.[66] Satariano, Swanson, and Moll,[67] at the SEER program Metropolitan Detroit Cancer Surveillance System, also found no racial difference for early-stage breast cancer treatment and noted that hospital size was the strongest predictor of partial mastectomy for African American women. On the other hand, a study of women with ovarian cancer revealed that white women were more likely to receive a combination of chemotherapy and surgical intervention, while African Americans were more often treated with chemotherapy alone.[68] Moreover, African American women were twice as likely as whites to receive inappropriate treatment and had poorer survival rates, even after controlling for age, residential area, income, and cancer care facility.

Ball and Elixhauser[69] specifically investigated black-white differences in treatment procedures for patients hospitalized with colorectal cancer. Using 1987 discharge data from a representative sample of more than 500 acute care hospitals in the United States participating in the Hospital Cost and Utilization Project, this study of men and women indicated that African Americans were less likely to receive major therapeutic procedures for colorectal cancer (colon resection, total cholecystectomy, colonoscopy, or bronchoscopy). Accounting for patient demographic characteristics (including insurance status), comorbidities, therapeutic complications, and hospital characteristics, African Americans with primary tumor and no metastasis were 41 percent less likely than similar whites to receive a major therapeutic treatment for colorectal cancer, whereas African Americans with metastasis were 27 percent less likely to receive a major treatment. In contrast, racial disparities in access to treatment for colorectal cancer were not observed for veterans treated nationwide at VA medical centers.[70] The study of patients with prostate cancer in the universally accessible DoD health care system revealed no racial disparities in waiting time for treatment, treatment methods, or survival rates.[61]

One of the most compelling studies regarding the black-white disparity in cancer treatment was recently published by Bach et al.[71] Among Medicare beneficiaries sixty-five years of age and older with early stage, non-small-cell lung cancer, a surgically treatable condition, the rate of surgery was lower among black than among white patients diagnosed between 1985 and 1993. The 17 percent less likelihood for African Americans to have undergone surgical resection was not due to comorbidity factors, age, gender, median income of residence area, geographic region, or type of Medicare insurance (managed care versus indemnity coverage).

Perhaps one of the most disturbing studies of cancer patients found significant racial differences in the adequacy of pain management.[72] Specifically, in a study of elderly nursing home residents with cancer, African Americans were 63 percent more likely than whites to receive no pain medication, accounting for gender, marital status, severity of illness, and cognitive performance.

Many of the cancer studies have significant data limitations. Often, cancer studies have relied on crude and incomplete measures of type of treatment provided and do not take into account comorbidities and other factors that influence treatment decisions. Therefore, the appropriateness of treatment cannot be determined. The specific chemotherapeutic agents and therapy amount and schedule are not evaluated in these studies, nor is stage-specific indication for treatment. Furthermore, the extent of disease, such as lymph node involvement and tumor size, may not have been compared among study subjects. Oftentimes, only the treatment delivered or planned as the first course is recorded in the medical record, and the comprehensiveness of treatment cannot be evaluated.[62] While surgery is an inpatient procedure, radiation treatment may be performed on an outpatient basis and is more difficult to document. In other words, these study results reflect only general patterns of cancer treatment and clinical management.

Observations of racial differences in access to cancer treatment in earlier studies may be explained by specific indications for cancer treatment (such as cancer stage at diagnosis, tumor histology, and coexisting medical conditions), which is information that was often not available to researchers. Future studies should focus on the quality and appropriateness of cancer treatments to further explore possible disparities in cancer treatment. Racial differences in cancer stage at diagnosis is another unexplored area that may be partially explained by access to advanced cancer screening and diagnostic services. Cultural factors that may delay diagnosis and treatment for some ethnic groups should also be explored.

Diabetes

Racial and ethnic differences in medical care for diabetes have not been consistently documented since the release of the Task Force Report, and the published peer-reviewed literature on access to care by race and ethnicity was somewhat limited for this common condition. We identified four relevant articles: two were conducted in HMO settings,[73,74] one is a nationally representative cross-sectional survey conducted in 1989,[75] and the fourth is a study of national Medicare claims data for 1992 and 1993.[76] In the study of an HMO population in 1996, no racial disparities were found in patient and physician adherence to accepted diabetes management guidelines.[73] Another HMO study from 1997 found no racial differences in laboratory test frequency or results, but after adjusting for insulin use and socioeconomic variables, African Americans were found to have poorer glycemic control than were whites.[74]

Other studies have also indicated no racial or ethnic variation in certain aspects of diabetes care but have revealed differences in methods of diabetes control and patient education.[75] Specifically, African Americans were more likely to be treated with insulin but less likely to receive daily injections or to self-monitor their blood glucose levels. Also, while African Americans were more likely than other groups to receive patient education, the median number of hours of instruction was lower. In studies looking at complications from diabetes mellitus among Medicare beneficiaries, the findings revealed that African Americans with diabetes were 30 percent less likely than their white counterparts to have an eye care visit,[76] a disparity potentially related to quality of preventive care.

The results of two HMO studies that found little or no racial differences in diabetes care access may be explained by the fact that study subjects were all privately insured patients in equally accessible health care systems. That black and white patients had similar primary care visits supports this interpretation of equal access for this study population.[74] There were weaknesses to the study that found racial differences in eye care visits.[76] The study could only account for the SES factor—that is, income and education—using county-level and not individual-level data, and did not account for insurance type. Accounting for individual-level data on SES factors might have indicated different results, most likely a greater black-white difference if African Americans were disproportionately in the low income and education as well as insurance strata.

Future research should attempt to identify ways to improve diabetes control by targeting ethnic minority groups as well as their health care providers. Emphasis should be given to identifying factors among ethnic groups that have an impact on the effectiveness of glycemic control efforts, including adherence to diabetes care guidelines.

HIV/AIDS

Our review of the HIV/AIDS literature of the past fourteen years reveals the existence of significant racial and ethnic disparities in access to HIV/AIDS diagnostic services and therapy, although in some settings these disparities were not found. Moore et al.[77] found that race was the strongest predictor of the receipt of drug therapy, with African Americans 41 to 73 percent less likely than whites to receive particular drug agents. Racial differences remained even after controlling for age, sex, mode of HIV transmission, insurance, residence, income, and education. The receipt of drug therapy was also found to be positively related to being white, having insurance, and having a college education.[78]

In contrast to the studies just referenced, Bennett et al.[79] found no racial or ethnic differences in African American, Hispanic, Asian, and white VA patients in the timing of bronchoscopy or receipt of timely drug therapy. Among non-VA patients, racial differences appeared, with African Americans and Hispanics more likely than whites to die in the hospital and less likely to receive a timely diagnostic bronchoscopy. However, after controlling for insurance and admitting hospital characteristics, these racial differences lacked statistical significance for African Americans and were smaller for Hispanics. Nonetheless, a recent national survey of adults infected with HIV indicated that African Americans and Latinos (Hispanics) were less likely to receive adequate care for their disease relative to whites, based on several measures including antiviral therapy and adjusting for multiple confounding variables including age, gender, education, and insurance coverage.[80] The sample in this study included only 71 percent of eligible respondents, and those with poor access may have been underrepresented. The study also relied on self-reported data, including medication information, for which the reliability was unknown. Nevertheless, African Americans showed deficits in four of six access-to-care measures, and Latinos showed deficits in three of six access measures. These study results indicate the need to identify barriers to HIV/AIDS therapy that are not accounted for by insurance and education status.

Infant and Child Health Services

Prenatal Care. The Task Force Report noted racial differences in rates of infant mortality and low birthweight and highlighted the importance of assuring early and continuous prenatal care for ethnic Americans.[6] Since the release of the Task Force Report, these disparities in health outcomes persist, and racial and ethnic gaps in prenatal care continue. The racial and ethnic disparities in the receipt and sufficiency of prenatal care are well documented.[81,82] Several studies have indicated that white women enter prenatal care earlier than Hispanic and African American women and are more likely to receive health behavior advice regarding their pregnancies.[83,84] Further analyses have shown differences within the Hispanic population, with Cuban American women more likely to obtain adequate prenatal care than Puerto Ricans and Hispanic women of Mexican and Central/South American origin.[85]

As we have seen for other health care areas, the health care system, particularly the DoD, may reduce racial and ethnic disparities in access to care. Smaller racial differences were observed in prenatal care utilization in military women compared to civilian women.[86] Among military women, African Americans were 21 percent less likely than white women to initiate prenatal care in the first trimester of pregnancy; among civilian women, they were 49 percent less likely to initiate prenatal care early in pregnancy.

Studies have also indicated that African American infants were admitted to neonatal intensive care units (NICUs) more than 2.5 times as frequently as white infants.[87] This disparity was not driven by the greater frequency of low-birthweight infants among African Americans but rather due to the higher rates of neonatal complications and death. The specific content of prenatal care among racial and ethnic minorities has also been investigated in several studies. African American women are less likely to receive health behavior advice about such items as smoking cessation and alcohol use from their prenatal care providers.[84] In investigation of the use of prenatal care technologies among racial and ethnic groups,[88] African Americans were less likely than whites to receive amniocentesis and ultrasound but not tocolysis. The results of a study of practice variation in high-risk pregnancies also showed no racial differences in receipt of tocolysis, a widely accepted treatment for premature labor, but also found that African American and Latino women were significantly less likely than white women to receive corticosteroid therapy, a less accepted treatment for this condition.[89] Furthermore, tocolysis varied by clinical factors such as multiple births, coexisting conditions such as diabetes, and by early stage of labor, whereas receipt of corticosteroid therapy varied by hospital site, indicating that discretionary factors influence treatment decisions.

The results in general indicate that the use and type of prenatal care differs for black and Hispanic women compared to white women, at least for certain content items. However, there are inherent limitations in these investigations. All the previous studies are limited to assessing a few prenatal care content items that are available in the data sources used. While finding differences among blacks and whites in prenatal care advice for smoking and alcohol use, the study did not find racial differences for advice for the other two items, drug use and breast feeding.[84]

Furthermore, the research on health education provided during pregnancy was based on self-reports from a national survey, and the reliability of the responses was unknown. The reliability of information is also an issue for the national study, which used only birth certificate data to assess variation in amniocentesis and ultrasound.[88] Study results varied. For example, in a cohort study of all single live births at a teaching hospital, African American women were more likely than whites to receive a prenatal ultrasound examination.[90] Furthermore, receipt of an ultrasound was inversely related to education, and was less frequent among privately insured patients. Others have also found that certain prenatal care services vary by SES factors, that is, marital status and education, more than by race,[91] which may help to explain the variation in these study results reported. Also, related to the issue of whether race or other factors are more predictive of care access, LaVeist, Keith, and Gutierrez[92] showed that racial/ethnic difference in certain measures of prenatal care were explained by private insurance, clinic availability, and travel distance.

Immunization. Immunization rates among racial and ethnic groups have improved in recent years, and the gap between ethnic minority and white children has narrowed. Several studies from the early and mid-1990s documented low immunization rates among minority children.[93] In a study of low-income children in Los Angeles, only 70 percent of Latino children and 53 percent of African American children were up-to-date for vaccinations at three months, and even fewer—only 43 percent of Latino and 26 percent of African American children—were up-to-date at two years of age.[94] From 1994 to 1995, the National Immunization Survey found similar disparities in racial and ethnic immunization rates in twenty-eight urban centers.[95] However, by 1996, survey findings showed that immunization rates for minority children ages nineteen to thirty-five months approached or exceeded the 90 percent national objective for coverage, and the gap between white children and African American and Hispanic children had narrowed.[93] Moreover, researchers have found that disparities in vaccination rates are linked to socioeconomic variables such as insurance status and family characteristics rather than to race or ethnicity per se, with urban areas less well vaccinated.[96]

Children's Health. In general, minority children appear to have poorer access to health care services than do white children—but this pattern is also highly linked to economic status. Study findings have shown that poor, nonwhite children had longer waiting times and fewer visits at doctors' offices and were more likely to use the emergency room for primary care.[82,97–100] Furthermore, study findings indicate that African American and Hispanic children were less likely to receive prescription medications and had fewer medications in general than did white children, even after adjusting for socioeconomic factors, including mother's education, insurance coverage, usual source of medical care, health conditions, and number of physician visits.[101]

African American children were observed to use emergency departments as their usual source of care at twice the frequency of white children.[100] Besides ethnicity, significant demographic risk factors for routine use of emergency departments by children included having a single parent, having a mother with less than a high school education, being poor, and living in an urban setting. Polynesian children (that is, Hawaiians, Samoans, and other Pacific Islanders) were more likely to seek emergency care at pediatric emergency departments than were whites and African Americans.[102] Frequent users of emergency departments did not appear to lack medical care resources as measured by immunization rates, insurance, and a primary care physician, suggesting that sociocultural factors are related to the use of emergency services for routine care.

Asthma Care. Racial differences in patterns of care for children with asthma have also been observed. Among Medicaid beneficiaries, African American children with asthma were more likely to make emergency room visits for care, less likely to make primary care office visits, and equally likely to have a prescription filled relative to white children.[103] Another study of Medicaid enrollees found that African American children who had been hospitalized for asthma had significantly fewer primary care visits following hospitalization than did their white counterparts.[104] Incidentally, similar patterns of care have also been observed for African Americans and white adults with asthma.[105] While both studies were among children with similar insurance coverage (that is, Medicaid), administrative claims-based data do not include measures of disease severity.

Further studies should focus on causes of adverse pregnancy outcomes and evaluate prenatal care quality and the specific content of services as well as attempt to explain the reasons for lower-quality prenatal care rendered to minority women. Identifying social and cultural determinants of early initiation of prenatal care, especially among low-income women, would improve the effectiveness of intervention programs. Evaluation of previous and ongoing programs to improve immunization coverage for inner-city communities would enhance future interventions. Regarding asthma care, sociocultural variables should be explored in explaining racial and ethnic differences in the use of primary care services and the proclivity for using emergency departments as a primary source of care.

Mental Health

As with some other disease categories, studies of the use of mental health services by racial and ethnic minorities have yielded mixed results. Racial and ethnic disparities have been noted in outpatient services, inpatient admissions, and drug therapy, although the findings have not been consistent and their implications are not understood.[106,107]

No differences in psychiatric hospitalization rates or inpatient hospital days by race and ethnicity were observed among insured federal employees, based on a national database of administrative claims, whereas age, residence, hospital bed availability, and insurance plan option were predictive.[106] In a study of inpatient and outpatient services of the Los Angeles County mental health system, race and ethnicity did not have a consistent pattern related to number of treatment sessions, treatment modality, treatment settings, and the therapist's professional discipline, although SES status, primary language, and diagnosis were related to the type and amount of treatment services used.[108] The study by Padgett et al.,[106] which lacked diagnostic data on the nature and severity of the mental health problems, indicates some of the methodological limitations of many of these studies.

Inpatient and outpatient diagnoses also varied by race and ethnicity, although the patterns were not consistent.[108] African Americans were more than six times as likely as whites to receive a diagnosis of alcohol or substance abuse, whereas whites were nearly four times as likely to receive a diagnosis of a personality disorder.[109] Interestingly, African Americans with high SES were more than three times as likely as their white counterparts to be tested for alcohol or substance abuse, suggesting a provider's biased perception of African Americans. Various researchers have shown that African Americans and Asians were more likely than whites to be diagnosed with an organic or psychotic disorder such as schizophrenia, while Hispanics were less likely to be so diagnosed.[109-111]

This body of literature is particularly muddled regarding access to mental health care by race and ethnicity. Future investigations should focus on differential diagnoses and treatment among racial and ethnic groups to determine if misdiagnoses are occurring. Furthermore, studies should determine whether variation in inpatient and outpatient services exists and for what reasons, as well as the appropriateness of service utilization.

Review by Health Service

In addition to reviewing the literature on access to medical services by health condition, we also reviewed studies that looked at access to particular types of services—specifically, primary, rehabilitative, and long-term services. There is obviously a good deal of overlap in the two bodies of literature, and herein, we discuss only those significant works that did not fit within our health condition structure.

In general, studies of access to health services find health insurance and poverty status to be the strongest determinants,[112] but often, race and ethnicity were found to have an independent effect as well. Study findings have consistently indicated that adolescent and adult African Americans and Hispanics were less likely than whites to have any physician contact in the past year, even after accounting for income and health status.[113] African Americans who did have physician contact reported fewer visits than whites and less satisfaction with the physicians' treatment.[114] Moreover, in one study limited to Medicare beneficiaries, African Americans were found to have lower use of ambulatory and preventive services than were whites, even after adjusting for income.[115]

In looking at hospital services, studies have documented lower access among African Americans and other minorities even after taking into account differences in health status, source of payment, and site of hospitalization.[116] Racial and ethnic minorities were less likely than whites to receive a wide range of procedures, including dialysis, arterial catheterization and cardiac bypass, endoscopy, bronchoscopy, cesarean section, and organ transplantation.[117,118] While African Americans were less likely to receive some procedures, they were significantly more likely to receive an inpatient service for organ removal (bilateral orchiectomy) or (lower limb) amputation, accounting for age, gender, and income.[115] Moreover, studies of Medicare beneficiaries found that African Americans had less access to technologically advanced procedures and rehabilitation services than did whites.[119]

Many studies have examined the relationship between race and ethnicity and the routine use of emergency rooms. Disparities in use of the emergency care department among African American, white, and Hispanic ambulatory adult patients have been explained by differences in age, health insurance coverage, having a regular source of care, and having barriers to health care.[120] Although African Americans and whites were observed to use hospital emergency rooms at the same rate, marital status was a unique determinant of use for African Americans, and gender, education, insurance, employment status, and region of residence were unique determinants for whites.[121] Even within the emergency department, services may vary by race and ethnicity. In a unique study among persons seen at an emergency department for long-bone fractures, Hispanics were found to be twice as likely as non-Hispanic whites with the similar fractures to receive no pain medication.[122] In multivariate analyses, adjusting for patient characteristics (including insurance), severity of injury, physician characteristics (including specialty), and possible ethanol intoxication, the risk of receiving no pain medication was more than seven times that of whites.

Racial and ethnic disparities have also been documented in the use and types of posthospital services. For example, discharge planning for African American patients compared to whites was less likely to involve a nursing home placement and more likely to use formal services in the home, which the authors attributed to differences in cultural preference.[123] In addition, for those African Americans who did seek nursing home placement, discharge delays from the hospital were longer than for whites regardless of clinical and demographic characteristics.[123]

The studies varied widely in source of data and potentially explanatory variables available for analysis. In some cases, only age and gender were accounted for.[119,124] In other instances, surrogates of SES were accounted for,[115] and in some instances, major factors such as insurance status, comorbidities, and diagnostic information were also accounted for.[125]

This is a broad body of literature that raises several issues, which to date have not been adequately addressed. Future studies are needed to understand why racial and ethnic disparities in access to various health care services exist. Studies should assess ethnic differences in patient preferences, medical knowledge, health beliefs and perception of illness, satisfaction with health care, compliance with prescribed medication, and availability of social, economic, and caregiving support. Studies that examine the appropriateness of care according to presenting signs and symptoms will also help to clarify this body of literature. Whether barriers exist, such as shortages, lack of financial resources and/or insurance, language, discrimination, and cultural attitudes and expectations of medical care, have not been extensively investigated. Also, future studies should attempt to understand the bases for racial differences in patients' use of specialty care providers and utilization of specialized procedures. Finally, future research should also focus on the level of cultural competency of providers, physicians' attitudes toward minority patients, the effect of race on physicians' treatment decisions, the effect of patient-physician discordance on clinical decisions, and institutional decision-making policies.

DISCUSSION

Our review of the literature over the past fifteen years revealed that racial and ethnic minorities often do not have access to health services at the same rate as do whites. The reasons for these disparities are varied, complex, and in general, poorly understood at this point. In fact, our understanding of the health care disparities by race and ethnicity has advanced very little since the 1985 release of the DHHS *Report of the Secretary's Task Force on Black and Minority Health*. And while we do not know why these disparities exist, it is clear from the entire literature that disparities in access to health care are not adequately explained by insurance, income or other measures of SES, comorbidities, severity of disease at diagnosis, availability of services, or patient preferences. That these disparities exist in some areas, such as cardiac care, cancer surgical treatment, and HIV/AIDS therapy, and not in other areas, such as diabetes care and cancer screening, suggests that the cost of care is an important consideration in clinical decisions for ethnic minority groups. Study findings that suggest the disparity is reduced for privately insured patients may also be an indication of payment-conscious clinical decisions.

That racial and ethnic disparities in treatment are not found in the universally accessible DoD health care system suggests that clinical decisions are related to consideration of the importance of human capital and perhaps that uniformity in care delivery eliminates racial and ethnic disparities. On the other hand, racial and ethnic disparities are observed among patients for whom care is equally accessible, such as patients in the VA system and Medicare and Medicaid beneficiaries, and suggest that potentially equal access to care does not reduce inequities. And yet, under special circumstances within these care systems, racial and ethnic disparity is eliminated (for example, long-term care for ESRD patients who have Medicare coverage).[42]

For cardiac care, a straightforward explanation of access disparity seems reasonable; ethnic minorities, particularly African Americans, are denied access to invasive procedure more so than are whites. That is, the physician does not recommend the procedure as often for African Americans. The presumed reason not to recommend bypass surgery is the physician's best judgment, based on the patient's clinical condition.[11] One may then assume that the variation in the rates of cardiac recommendation and procedures between black and white patients is due to real differences in clinical disease or fallibility of diagnostic information on which the physician makes a decision. The fallibility of diagnostic information seems a less likely explanation.[126] However, the aggressiveness of the diagnostic evaluation in explaining racial disparity in cardiac care has not been investigated.[10] There are unknown and subjective factors related to clinical decision making that have resulted in a lower rate of admission to coronary triage[126] and lower catheterization rates[127] for African Americans. These subjective factors may also explain the lower rates of recommendation and subsequent invasive coronary surgery for African Americans.

A similar explanation for observed racial and ethnic disparities in cancer treatment is precluded because of the lack of data on appropriateness of treatment and quality of previous investigations. At best, the current research provides a general indication that African Americans and other ethnic minorities may have lower access to diagnostic tests and may be less likely to receive major therapeutic interventions on a timely basis. Furthermore, when there is general agreement on the appropriateness of treatment—for example, surgical resection for early stage, non-small-cell lung cancer—African Americans are less likely to be treated.[71] Study results among patients in the universally accessible DoD health care system[61] and among veterans treated nationwide at VA medical centers[70] again suggest that equality in access and uniformity in the delivery of services reduce racial disparity in cancer treatment.

Moreover, the reasons ethnic minorities may be diagnosed with cancer at more advanced stages are poorly understood and seldom explored in the current literature. While equal or universal access to diagnostic services may provide some answers, other explanations must be sought. Researchers beginning to investigate this issue have found that patient delay in seeking treatment as well as certain cultural beliefs that discourage women from seeking care may play an important role in the stage at which breast cancer is diagnosed.[75] Whatever the basis for the disparity, however, stage of cancer at diagnosis is the primary explanatory factor for racial differences in cancer survival rates.[58] Consequently, further investigations aimed at understanding racial and ethnic disparities in the timeliness of diagnosis hold great potential for improving cancer survival rates for minorities. These investigations must recognize the intersection of personal factors (screening frequency), preventive behavior (symptom recognition and care-seeking behavior), and aggressiveness of diagnostic evaluation to more fully understand the nature of racial disparities in care.[128] Little is known about ethnicity-specific cultural factors for Asian subgroups, Hispanic subgroups, Native Americans, and African Americans related to cancer diagnosis as well as treatment.[129]

While younger African American women appear to have achieved equivalent or even superior access to certain screening services, Hispanic women continue to lag behind. That older African American women have lower mammography screening rates than do white women also provides challenges for explaining disparities in certain subgroups of the population. Immunization coverage in children is also indicative of disparities in subgroups, such as urban minorities. Cancer screening and childhood immunizations are preventive services in which the effectiveness and benefits are proven. Herein may lie a greater commonality between cancer screening and immunization services. They represent the interrelationships of SES, culture, belief, and behavior. But more important, national efforts by the public and private sectors as well as community-based initiatives have resulted in closing (breast and cervical cancer screening) or narrowing (childhood immunization) the racial/ethnic gap.

Racial and ethnic variation in access to health services may be affected by numerous other variables that were not consistently considered in the existing literature. Numerous investigators have found that health insurance and SES are the greatest predictors of access to health care but do not fully account for the observed disparities by race and ethnicity. Other important factors include the age at onset and duration of disease, severity of disease and symptoms, coexisting conditions, physical and psychological characteristics, geographic location, family and social supports, and the type of hospital where care is received.[22,24] And while studies of racial and ethnic disparities in access to care have not consistently adjusted for these important factors, the published literature routinely indicates significant variation in access to primary, rehabilitative, and long-term care services by race and ethnicity.

Despite the limitations described above, the literature documents well poorer access to medical care among racial and ethnic minorities for several disease groups and types of health services. Indeed, the literature has generally documented racial differences in access to primary care services, prenatal care, and various high-tech diagnostic and therapeutic procedures. In addition, racial differences in the receipt of mental health services have been documented. For this area of research, it is difficult to discern clear patterns of racial and ethnic differences in diagnosis and treatment. Also, with respect to treatment for HIV/AIDS, African Americans have been shown to be significantly less likely to receive particular drug agents, even after controlling for various socioeconomic factors.

It is also significant that several studies showed that racial and ethnic differences in access to medical treatment are reduced or absent under universally accessible systems such as the DoD health care system, the VA medical system (for some disease conditions), and in HMOs.[130] Nonetheless, even under the theoretically universal access system offered by the VA, studies have shown that racial and ethnic disparities persist.[31]

The lack of racial and ethnic difference in diabetes care may be related to the setting of care and the nature of care. In general, difference in care among blacks and whites were not found in HMO settings. Diabetes care is also provided by primary care physicians. Patient education and self-management are significant components and less costly to the medical care system.

In sum, the literature shows that racial and ethnic minorities frequently do not have the same access to medical treatment and other health services as the majority white population. This is particularly true for African Americans, and the differences observed between blacks and whites in access to care are not due to the fact that African Americans have been studied more.[11] The magnitude of these disparities is related to socioeconomic and insurance status but also to other factors that are ill defined and difficult to quantify. The history of medical care in the United States is replete with examples of discriminatory practices that denied ethnic minorities access to services based on skin color. Thus, the medical care system of the past is correctly described as a racist institution, and the legacy of racism should not be minimized. Clearly, the patient's race, but specifically skin color, influence physician decision making, whether it is overt prejudice or subconscious perceptions. Nonetheless, in a nation that prides itself on having the best health care system in the world, racial and ethnic disparities in access to medical care require greater public attention and further scrutiny to correct the critical injustice they create.

Future investigations that further document disparity by race and ethnicity will provide little to advance our understanding in this area. Focused studies that explore the reasons for racial and ethnic disparities in access to health services will be most helpful in reducing racial and ethnic disparities in access to care. Much of the current literature has focused on African American versus white comparisons and to a much lesser degree on Hispanics and other minority groups; future work should attempt to discern the particular factors important to improving access for these groups as well.

Other important areas of research should include analyses of the impact of financial barriers, organizational barriers, and physician and patient decision making on racial and ethnic differences in access to specific health services. Intragroup versus intergroup comparisons may be a productive approach to discern why, for instance, some African Americans achieve access while others do not. The intragroup comparison study approach is particularly important because it seems apparent that some, if not most, persons within an ethnic group have access to quality care. The effort to distinguish why some members of a particular ethnic group have access to services while others do not may reveal some of the sociocultural factors that distinguish the ethnic minority group from the white majority population and may provide the opportunity to identify unique within-group factors that could lead to improved access for these populations.

Notes

1. U.S. Department of Health and Human Services. (1985). *Report of the Secretary's Task Force on Black and Minority Health: Vol. 1. Executive summary.* Washington, DC: U.S. Government Printing Office.

2. U.S. Department of Health and Human Services. (1985). *Report of the Secretary's Task Force on Black and Minority Health: Vol. 2. Crosscutting issues in minority health: Perspectives on national health data for minorities, minority access to health care, health education and information, minority and other health professionals serving minority communities.* Washington, DC: U.S. Government Printing Office.

3. U.S. Department of Health and Human Services. (1986). *Report of the Secretary's Task Force on Black and Minority Health: Vol. 3. Cancer.* Washington, DC: U.S. Government Printing Office.

4. U.S. Department of Health and Human Services. (1986). *Report of the Secretary's Task Force on Black and Minority Health: Vol. 4. Cardiovascular and cerebrovascular diseases.* Washington, DC: U.S. Government Printing Office.

5. U.S. Department of Health and Human Services. (1986). *Report of the Secretary's Task Force on Black and Minority Health: Vol. 5. Homicide, suicide, and unintentional injuries.* Washington, DC: U.S. Government Printing Office.

6. U.S. Department of Health and Human Services. (1986). *Report of the Secretary's Task Force on Black and Minority Health: Vol. 6. Infant mortality and low birthweight.* Washington, DC: U.S. Government Printing Office.

7. U.S. Department of Health and Human Services. (1986). *Report of the Secretary's Task Force on Black and Minority Health: Vol. 7. Chemical dependency, diabetes.* Washington, DC: U.S. Government Printing Office.

8. U.S. Department of Health and Human Services. (1986). *Report of the Secretary's Task Force on Black and Minority Health: Vol. 8. Hispanic health issues, survey of the non-federal community, inventory of DDHS program efforts in minority health.* Washington, DC: U.S. Government Printing Office.

9. Maynard, C., Fisher, L. D., Passamani, E. R., & Pullum, T. (1986, December). Blacks in the Coronary Artery Surgery Study (CASS): Race and clinical decision making. *Am J Public Health, 76,* 1446–1448.

10. Peterson, E. D., Shaw, L. K., DeLong, E. R., Pryor, D. B., Califf, R. M., & Mark, D. B. (1997, February 13). Racial variation in the use of coronary-revascularization procedures: Are the differences real? Do they matter? *N Engl J Med, 336,* 480–486.

11. Hannan, E. L., Ryn, M. V., Burke, J., Stone, D., Kumar, D., Arani, D., Pierce, W., Rafii, S., Sanborn, T. A., Sharma, S., Slater, J., & DeBuono, B. A. (1999). Access to coronary artery bypass surgery by race/ethnicity and gender among patients who are appropriate for surgery. *Med Care, 37*(1), 68–77.

12. Weitzman, S., Cooper, L., Chambless, L., Rosamond, W., Clegg, L., Marcucci, G., Romm, F., & White, A. (1997, March 15). Gender, racial, and geographic differences in the performance of cardiac diagnostic and therapeutic procedures for hospitalized acute myocardial infarction in four states. *Am J Cardiol, 79,* 722–726.

13. Carlisle, D. M., Leake, B. D., & Shapiro, M. F. (1995, March). Racial and ethnic differences in the use of invasive cardiac procedures among cardiac patients in Los Angeles County, 1986 through 1988. *Am J Public Health, 85,* 352–356.

14. Ford, E., Cooper, R., Castaner, A., Simmons, B., & Mar, M. (1989, April). Coronary arteriography and coronary bypass survey among whites and other racial groups relative to hospital-based incidence rates for coronary artery disease: Findings from NHDS. *Am J Public Health, 79,* 437–440.

15. Gillum, R. F. (1987, May). Coronary artery bypass surgery and coronary angiography in the United States, 1979–1983. *Am Heart J, 113,* 1255–1258.

16. Hannan, E. L., Kilburn, H. J., O'Donnell, J. F., Lukacik, G., & Shields, E. P. (1991). Interracial access to selected cardiac procedures for patients hospitalized with coronary artery disease in New York State. *Med Care, 29*(5), 430–441.

17. Wenneker, M. B., & Epstein, A. M. (1989, January 13). Racial inequalities in the use of procedures for patients with ischemic heart disease in Massachusetts. *JAMA, 261,* 253–257.

18. Giles, W. H., Anda, R. F., Casper, M. L., Escobedo, L. G., & Taylor, H. A. (1995, February 13). Race and sex differences in rates of invasive cardiac procedures in U.S. hospitals: Data from the National Hospital Discharge Survey. *Arch Intern Med, 155,* 318–324.

19. Maynard, C., Litwin, P. E., Martin, J. S., Cerqueira, M., Ho, M. T., Kennedy, J. W., Cobb, L. A., Schaeffer, S. M., Hallstrom, A. P., & Weaver, W. D. (1991, January 1). Characteristics of black patients admitted to coronary care units in metropolitan Seattle: Results from the Myocardial Infarction Triage and Intervention Registry (MITI). *Am J Cardiol, 67,* 18–23.

20. Canto, J. G., Taylor, H. A., Rogers, W. J., Sanderson, B., Hilbe, J., & Barron, H. V. (1998, November 1). Presenting characteristics, treatment patterns, and clinical outcomes of non-black minorities in the National Registry of Myocardial Infarction, 2. *Am J Cardiol, 82,* 1013–1018.

21. Ramsey, D. J., Goff, D. C., Wear, M. L., Labarthe, D. R., & Nichaman, M. Z. (1997). Sex and ethnic differences in use of myocardial revascularization procedures in Mexican Americans and non-Hispanic whites: The Corpus Christi Heart Project. *J Clin Epidemiol, 50*(5), 603–609.

22. Goff, D. C., Nichaman, M. Z., Ramsey, D. J., Meyer, P. S., & LaBarthe, D. R. (1995, May). A population-based assessment of the use and effectiveness of thrombolytic therapy: The Corpus Christi Heart Project. *Ann Epidemiol, 5,* 171–178.

23. Mickelson, J. K., Blum, C. M., & Geraci, J. M. (1997, April). Acute myocardial infarction: Clinical characteristics, management and outcome in a metropolitan Veterans Affairs medical center teaching hospital. *J Am Coll Cardiol, 29,* 915–925.

24. Allison, J. J., Kiefe, C. I., Centor, R. M., Box, J. B., & Farmer, R. M. (1996, December). Racial differences in the medical treatment of elderly Medicare patients with acute myocardial infarction. *J Gen Intern Med, 11,* 736–743.

25. Ayanian, J. Z., Udvarhelyi, I. S., Gatsonis, C. A., Pashos, C. L., & Epstein, A. M. (1993, May 26). Racial differences in the use of revascularization procedures after coronary angiography. *JAMA, 269,* 2642–2646.

26. Gatsonis, C. A., Epstein, A. M., Newhouse, J. P. Normand, S.-L., & McNeil, B. J. (1995). Variations in the utilization of coronary angiography for elderly patients with an acute myocardial infarction: An analysis using hierarchical logistics regression. *Med Care, 33,* 625–642.

27. Goldberg, K. C., Hartz, A. J., Jacobsen, S. J., Krakauer, H., & Rimm, A. A. (1992, March 18). Racial and community factors influencing coronary artery bypass graft surgery rates for all 1986 Medicare patients. *JAMA, 267,* 1473–1477.

28. McBean, A. M., Warren, J. L., & Babish, D. (1994, February). Continuing differences in the rates of percutaneous transluminal coronary angioplasty and coronary artery bypass graft surgery between elderly black and white Medicare beneficiaries. *Am Heart J, 127,* 127–287.

29. Udvarhelyi, S., Gatsonis, C., Epstein, A. M., Pashos, C. L., Newhouse, J. P., & McNeil, B. J. (1992, November 11). Acute myocardial infarction in the Medicare population: Process of care and clinical outcomes. *JAMA, 268,* 2530–2536.

30. Mirvis, D. M., Burns, R., Gaschen, L., Cloar, F. T., & Graney, M. (1994, November 1). Variation in utilization of cardiac procedures in the Department of Veterans Affairs Health Care System: Effect of race. *J Am Coll Cardiol, 24,* 1297–1304.

31. Peterson, E. D., Wright, S. M., Daley, J., & Thibault, G. E. (1994, April). Racial variation in cardiac procedure use and survival following acute myocardial infarction in the Department of Veterans Affairs. *JAMA, 271,* 1175–1180.

32. Sedlis, S. P., Fisher, V. J., Tice, D., Esposito, R., Madmon, L., & Steinberg, E. H. (1997). Racial differences in performance of invasive cardiac procedures in a Department of Veterans Affairs medical center. *J Clin Epidemiol, 50,* 899–901.

33. Whittle, J., Conigliaro, J., Good, C. B., & Lofgren, R. P. (1993, August 26). Racial differences in the use of invasive cardiovascular procedures in the Department of Veterans Affairs Medical System. *N Engl J Med, 329,* 656–658.

34. Philbin, E. F., & DiSalvo, T. G. (1998, July 1). Influence of race and gender on care process, resource use, and hospital-based outcomes in congestive heart failure. *Am J Cardiol, 82,* 76–81.

35. Brothers, T. E., Robison, J. G., Sutherland, S. E., & Elliott, B. M. (1997, February). Racial differences in operation for peripheral vascular disease: Results of a population-based study. *Cardiovasc Surg, 5,* 26–31.

36. Oddone, E. Z., Horner, R. D., Monger, M. E., & Matchar, D. B. (1993, December 27). Racial variations in the rates of carotid angiography and endarterectomy in patients with stroke and transient ischemic attack. *Arch Intern Med, 153,* 2781–2786.

37. Ozminkowski, R. J., Friedman, B., & Taylor, Z. (1993). Access to heart and liver transplantation in the late 1980s. *Med Care, 3*(11), 1027–1042.

38. Naumburg, E. H., Franks, P., Bell, B., Gold, M., & Engerman, J. (1993). Racial differentials in the identification of hypercholesterolemia. *J Fam Pract, 36*(4), 425–430.

39. Oddone, E. Z., Horner, R. D., Diers, T., Lipscomb, J., McIntyre, L., Cauffman, C., Whittle, J., Passman, L. J., Kroupa, L., Heaney, R., & Matchar, D. (1998). Understanding racial variation in the use of carotid endarterectomy: The role of aversion to surgery. *J Natl Med Assoc, 90*(1), 25–33.

40. Mirvis, D. M., & Graney, M. J. (1998, April 15). Impact of race and age on the effects of regionalization of cardiac procedures in the Department of Veterans Affairs Health Care System. *Am J Cardiol, 81,* 983–987.

41. Taylor, A. J., Meyer, G. S., Morse, R. W., & Pearson, C. E. (1997, October). Can characteristics of a health care system mitigate ethnic bias in access to cardiovascular procedures? Experience from the Military Health Services System. *J Am Coll Cardiol, 30,* 901–907.

42. Daumit, G. L., Herman, J. A., Coresh, J., & Powe, N. R. (1999, February 2). Use of cardiovascular procedures among black persons and white persons: A 7-year nationwide study in patients with renal disease. *Ann Intern Med, 130,* 173–182.

43. Leape, L. L., Hilborne, L. H., Bell, R., Kamberg, C., & H. Brook, R. (1999, February 2). Underuse of cardiac procedures: Do women, ethnic minorities, and the uninsured fail to receive needed revascularization? *Ann Intern Med, 130,* 183–192.

44. Laouri, M., Kravitz, R. L., French, W. J., Yang, I., Milliken, J. C., Hilborne, L., Wachsner, R., & Brook, R. H. (1997, April). Underuse of coronary revascularization procedures: Application of a clinical method. *J Am Coll Cardiol, 29,* 891–897.

45. Ackermann, S. P., Brackbill, R. M., Bewerse, B. A., Cheal, N. E., & Sanderson, L. M. (1992). Cancer screening behaviors among U.S. women: Breast cancer, 1987–1989, and cervical cancer, 1988–1989. *Morbid Mortal Wkly Rep, 41,* 17–25.

46. Breen, N., & Kessler, L. (1994). Changes in the use of screening mammography: Evidence from the 1987 and 1990 National Health Interview surveys. *Am J Public Health, 84,* 62–67.

47. Burns, R. B., McCarthy, E. P., Freund, K. M., Marwill, S. L., Schwartz, M., Ash, A., & Moskowitz, M. A. (1996, August 1). Black women receive less mammography even with similar use of primary care. *Ann Intern Med, 125,* 173–182.

48. Frazier, E. L., Jiles, R. B., & Mayberry, R. (1996). Use of screening mammography and clinical breast examinations among black, Hispanic, and white women. *Prev Med, 25,* 118–125.

49. Martin, L. M., Calle, E. E., Wingo, P. A., & Heath, C.W.J. (1996). Comparison of mammography and Pap test use from the 1987 and 1992 National Health Interview surveys: Are we closing the gaps? *Am J Prev Med, 12,* 82–90.

50. Arbes, S. J., & Slade, G. D. (1996, September). Racial differences in stage at diagnosis of screenable oral cancers in North Carolina. *J Public Health Dentistry, 56,* 352–354.

51. Perez-Stable, E. J., Sabogal, F., & Otero-Sabogal, R. (1995). Use of cancer-screening tests in the San Francisco Bay Area: Comparison of Latinos and Anglos. *J Natl Cancer Inst Monographs, 1995*(18), 147–153.

52. Tortolero-Luna, G., Glober, G. A., Villarreal, R., Palos, G., & Linares, A. (1995). Screening practices and knowledge, attitudes, and beliefs about cancer among Hispanic and non-Hispanic white women 35 years old or older in Nueces County, Texas. *J Natl Cancer Inst Monograms, 1995*(18), 49–56.

53. Hoffman-Goetz, L., Breen, N. L., & Meissner, H. (1998, Winter). The impact of social class on the use of cancer screening within three racial/ethnic groups in the United States. *Ethn Dis, 8,* 43–51.

54. Preston, J. A., Scinto, J. D., Ni, W., Wang, Y., Galusha, D., Schulz, A. F., & Petrillo, M. K. (1997, November). Mammography underutilization among older women in Connecticut. *J Am Geriatr Soc, 45,* 1310–1314.

55. Harlan, L. C., Bernstein, A. B., & Kessler, L. G. (1991, July). Cervical cancer screening: Who is not screened and why? *Am J Public Health, 81,* 885–890.

56. Kirkmam-Liff, B., & Kronefeld, J. J. (1992). Access to cancer screening services for women. *Am J Public Health, 82,* 733–735.

57. Bentley, J. R., Delfinoa, R. J., Taylor, T. H., Stowe, S., & Anton-Culver, H. (1988). Differences in breast cancer stage at diagnosis between non-Hispanic white and Hispanic populations, San Diego County 1988–1993. *Breast Cancer Res Treat, 50,* 1–9.

58. Eley, J. W., Hill, H. A., Chen, V. W., et al. (1994, September 28). Racial differences in survival from breast cancer: Results of the National Cancer Institute Black/White Cancer Survival Study. *JAMA, 272,* 947–954.

59. Mayberry, R. M., Coates, R. J., Hill, H. A., Click, L. A., Chen, V. W., Austin, D. F., Redmond, C. K., Fenoglio-Preiser, C. M., Hunter, C. P., Haynes, M. A., Muss, H. B., Wesley, M. N., Greenberg, R. S., & Edwards, B. K. (1995, November). Determinants of black/white differences in colon cancer survival. *J Natl Cancer Inst, 87,* 1686–1693.

60. Mettlin, C. J., Murphy, G. P., Cunningham, M. P., & Menck, H. R. (1997). The National Cancer Data Base report on race, age, and region variations in prostate cancer treatment. *Cancer, 80,* 261–266.

61. Optenberg, S. A., Thompson, I. M., Friedrichs, P., Wojcik, B., Stein, C. R., & Kramer, B. (1995, November 22–29). Race, treatment, and long-term survival from prostate cancer in an equal-access medical care delivery system. *JAMA, 274,* 1599–1605.

62. Polednak, A. P., & Flannery, J. T. (1992, October 15). Black versus white racial differences in clinical stage at diagnosis and treatment of prostatic cancer in Connecticut. *Cancer, 70,* 2152–2158.

63. Satariano, W. A., Belle, S. H., & Swanson, G. M. (1986, July). The severity of breast cancer at diagnosis: A comparison of age and extent of disease in black and white women. *Am J Public Health, 76,* 779–782.

64. Zaloznik, A. J. (1995). Breast cancer stage at diagnosis: Caucasians versus Afro-Americans. *Breast Cancer Res Treat, 34,* 195–158.

65. Bain, R. P., Greenberg, R. S., & Whitaker, J. P. (1986). Racial differences in survival of women with breast cancer. *J Chronic Disease, 39,* 631–642.

66. Farrow, D. C., Hunt, W. C., & Samet, J. M. (1992, April 23). Geographic variation in the treatment of localized breast cancer. *N Engl J Med, 326,* 1097–1101.

67. Satariano, E. R., Swanson, G. M., & Moll, P. P. (1992, February). Nonclinical factors associated with surgery received for treatment of early-stage breast cancer. *Am J Public Health, 82,* 195–198.

68. Parham, G., Phillips, J. L., Hicks, M. L., Andrews, N., Jones, W. B., Singleton, H. M., & Menck, H. R. (1997, August 15). The National Cancer Data Base report on malignant epithelial ovarian carcinoma in African-American women. *Cancer, 80,* 816–826.

69. Ball, J. D., & Elixhauser, A. (1996). Treatment differences between blacks and whites with colorectal cancer. *Med Care, 34,* 970–984.

70. Dominitz, J. A., Samsa, G. P., Landsman, P., & Provenzale, D. (1998, June). Race, treatment, and survival among colorectal carcinoma patients in an equal-access medical system. *Cancer, 82,* 2312–2320.

71. Bach, P. B., Cramer, L. D., Warren, J. L., & Begg, C. B. (1999, October 14). Racial differences in the treatment of early-stage lung cancer. *N Engl J Med, 341,* 1198–1205.

72. Bernabei, R., Gambassi, G., Lapane, K., et al. (1998). Management of pain in elderly patients with cancer. *JAMA, 279,* 1877–1882.

73. Martin, T. L., Selby, J. V., & Zhang, D. (1995, August). Physician and patient prevention practices in NIDDM in a large urban managed-care organization. *Diabetes Care, 18,* 1124–1132.

74. Wisdom, K., Fryzek, J. P., Havstad, S. L., Anderson, R. M., Dreiling, M. C., & Tilley, B. C. (1997, June). Comparison of laboratory test frequency and test results

between African-Americans and Caucasians with diabetes: Opportunity for improvement. *Diabetes Care, 20,* 971–977.

75. Cowie, C. C., & Harris, M. I. (1997, February). Ambulatory medical care for non-Hispanic whites, African-Americans, and Mexican-Americans with NIDDM in the U.S. *Diabetes Care, 20,* 142–147.

76. Wang, F., & Javitt, J. C. (1996, November). Eye care for elderly Americans with diabetes mellitus: Failure to meet current guidelines. *Ophthalmology, 103,* 1744–1750.

77. Moore, R. D., Stanton, D., Gopalan, R., & Chaisson, R. E. (1994, March 17). Racial differences in the use of drug therapy for HIV disease in an urban community. *N Engl J Med, 330,* 763–768.

78. Graham, N. M., Jacobson, L. P., Kuo, V., Chmiel, J. S., Morgenstern, H., & Zucconi, S. L. (1994). Access to therapy in the Multicenter AIDS Cohort Study, 1989–1992. *J Clin Epidemiol, 47,* 1003–1012.

79. Bennett, C. L., Horner, R. D., Weinstein, R. A., Dickinson, G. M., Dehovitz, J. A., Cohn, S. E., Kessler, H. A., Jacobson, J., Goetz, M. B., Simberkoff, M., Pitrak, D., George, L., Gilman, S. C., & Shapiro, M. F. (1995, August 7–21). Racial differences in care among hospitalized patients with pneumocystis carinii pneumonia in Chicago, New York, Los Angeles, Miami, and Raleigh-Durham. *Arch Intern Med, 155,* 1586–1592.

80. Shapiro, M. F., Morton, S. C., McCaffrey, D. F., Senterfitt, J. W., Fleishman, J. A., Perlman, J. F., Athey, L. A., Keesey, J. W., Goldman, D. P., Berry, S. H., & Bozette, S. A. (1999, June 23–30). Variations in the care of HIV-infected adults in the United States: Results from the HIV Cost and Services Utilization Study. *JAMA, 281,* 2305–2375.

81. Alexander, G. R., & Cornely, D. A. (1987). Racial disparities in pregnancy outcomes: The role of prenatal care utilization and maternal risk status. *Am J Prev Med, 3,* 254–261.

82. Moore, P., & Hepworth, J. T. (1994). Use of perinatal and infant health services by Mexican-American Medicaid enrollees. *JAMA, 272,* 297–304.

83. Balcazar, H., Cole, G., & Hartner, J. (1992). Mexican-Americans' use of prenatal care and its relationship to maternal risk factors and pregnancy outcome. *Am J Prev Med, 8*(1), 1–7.

84. Kogan, M. D., Alexander, G. R., Kotelchuk, M., & Nagey, D. A. (1992). Relation of content of prenatal care to the risk of low birth weight. *JAMA, 271,* 13405.

85. Albrecht, S. L., & Miller, M. K. (1996). Hispanic subgroup differences in prenatal care. *Soc Biol, 43,* 38–58.

86. Barfield, W. D., Wise, P. H., Rust, F. P., Rust, K. J., Gould, J. B., & Gortmaker, S. L. (1996, October). Racial disparities in outcomes of military and civilian births in California. *Arch Pediatr Adolesc Med, 150,* 1062–1067.

87. Langkamp, D. L., Foye, H. R., & Roghmann, K. J. (1990, July). Does limited access to NICU services account for higher neonatal mortality rates among blacks? *Am J Perinatol, 7,* 227–231.

88. Brett, K. M., Schoendorf, K. C., & Kiely, J. L. (1994). Differences between black and white women in the use of prenatal care technologies. *Am J Obstet Gynecol, 170,* 41–46.

89. Bronstein, J. M., Cliver, S. P., & Goldenberg, R. L. (1997, February). Practice variation in the use of interventions in high-risk obstetrics. *Health Ser Res, 32,* 825–839.

90. Moore, R.M.J., Kaczmarek, R. G., & Hamburger, S. (1990). Prenatal ultrasound: Are socially disadvantaged groups afforded equal access? *J Health Care Poor Underserved, 1,* 229–236.

91. Hansell, M. J. (1991, August). Sociodemographic factors and the quality of prenatal care. *Am J Public Health, 81,* 1023–1028.

92. LaVeist, T. A., Keith, V. M., & Gutierrez, M. L. (1995). Black/white differences in prenatal care utilization: An assessment of predisposing and enabling factors. *Health Ser Res, 30,* 43–58.

93. Centers for Disease Control and Prevention. (1997, October 17). Vaccination coverage by race/ethnicity and poverty level among children aged 19–35 months—United States, 1996. *Morbid Mortal Wkly Rep, 46,* 963–968.

94. Wood, D., Donald-Sherbourne, C., Halfon, N., Tucker, M. B., Ortiz, V., Hamlin, J. S., Duan, N., Mazel, R. M., Grabowsky, M., Brunell, P., & Freeman, H. (1995, August). Factors related to immunization status among inner-city Latino and African-American preschoolers. *Pediatrics, 96,* 295–301.

95. Centers for Disease Control and Prevention. (1996). National, state, and urban area vaccination coverage levels among children aged 19–35 months—United States, July 1994–June 1995. *Morbid Mortal Wkly Rep, 45,* 508–513.

96. Moore, P., Hepworth, J. T., & Fenlon, N. (1996). Indicators of differences in immunization rates of Mexican American and white non-Hispanic infants in a Medicaid managed care system. *Public Health Nurse, 13,* 21–30.

97. Cornelius, L. J. (1993). Barriers to medical care for white, black and Hispanic American children. *J Natl Med Assoc, 85*(4), 281–288.

98. Flores, G., Bauchner, H., Feinstein, A. R., & Nguyen, U.-S.D.T. (1999, July). The impact of ethnicity, family income, and parental education on children's health and use of health services. *Am J Public Health, 89,* 1066–1071.

99. Fleischer, A. B., Feldman, S. R., & Bradham, D. B. (1994, January). Office-based physician services provided by dermatologists in the United States in 1990. *J Invest Dermatol, 102,* 93–97.

100. Halfon, N., Newacheck, P. W., Wood, D. L., & St. Peter, R. F. (1996). Routine emergency department use for sick care by children in the United States. *Pediatrics, 98,* 28–34.

101. Hahn, B. A. (1995). Children's health: Racial and ethnic differences in the use of prescription medications. *Pediatrics, 95,* 727–732.

102. Yamamoto, L. G., Zimmerman, K. R., Butts, R. J., Amaya, C., Lee, P., Miller, N. L., Shirac, L. K., Tanaka, T. T., & Leung, F. K. (1995). Characteristics of frequent pediatric emergency department users. *Pediatr Emerg Care, 11,* 340–346.

103. Lozano, P., Connell, F. A., & Koepsell, T. D. (1995, August). Use of health services by African-American children with asthma on Medicaid. *JAMA, 274,* 469–473.

104. Ali, S., & Osberg, J. S. (1997). Differences in follow-up visits between African American and white Medicaid children hospitalized with asthma. *J Health Care Poor Underserved, 8,* 83–98.

105. Murray, M. D., Stang, P., & Tierney, W. M. (1997). Health care use by inner-city patients with asthma. *J Clin Epidemiol, 50,* 167–174.

106. Padgett, D. K., Patrick, C., Burns, B. J., & Schlesinger, H. J. (1994). Ethnic differences in use of inpatient mental health services by blacks, whites, and Hispanics in a national insured population. *Health Ser Res, 29,* 135–153.

107. Snowden, L. R., & Cheung, F. K. (1990). Use of inpatient mental health services by members of ethnic minority groups. *Am Psychol, 45,* 347–355.

108. Flaskerud, J. H., & Hu, L. T. (1992). Racial/ethnic identity and type of psychiatric treatment. *Am J Psychiatry, 149,* 379–384.

109. Chung, H., Mahler, J. C., & Kakuma, T. (1995). Racial differences in treatment of psychiatric inpatients. *Psychiatry Ser, 46,* 586–591.

110. Leo, R. J., Barayan, D. W., Sherry, C., Michalek, C., & Pollock, D. (1997). Geropsychiatric consultation for African-American and Caucasian patients. *Gen Hosp Psychiatry, 19,* 216–222.

111. Strakowski, S. M., Shelton, R. C., & Kolbrener, M. L. (1993). The effects of race and comorbidity on clinical diagnosis in patients with psychosis. *J Clin Psychiatry, 54,* 96–102.

112. Guendelman, S., & Schwalbe, J. (1986, October). Medical care utilization by Hispanic children: How does it differ from black and white peers? *Med Care, 24,* 925–937.

113. Bartman, B. A., Moy, E., & D'Angelo, L. J. (1997). Access to ambulatory care for adolescents: The role of a usual source of care. *J Health Care Poor Underserved, 8,* 214–226.

114. Blendon, R. J., Aiken, L. H., Freeman, H. E., & Corey, C. R. (1989). Access to medical care for black and white Americans: A matter of continuing concern. *JAMA, 261,* 278–281.

115. Gornick, M. E., Eggers, P. W., & Reilly, T. W. (1996). Effects of race and income on mortality and use of services among Medicare beneficiaries. *N Engl J Med, 335,* 791–799.

116. Carlisle, D. M., Valdez, R. B., & Shapiro, M. F. (1995). Geographic variation in rates of selected surgical procedures within Los Angeles County. *Health Ser Res, 30,* 27–42.

117. Abrams, J., & Nathan, H. (1991). Recipient race does not influence waiting time for a cadaveric renal transplant: One organ procurement organization's experience. *Transplant Procedure, 23,* 2607–2609.

118. Gonwa, T. A., Morris, C. A., Mai, M. L., Husberg, B. S., Goldstein, R. M., & Klintmalm, G. B. (1991). Race and liver transplantation. *Arch Surgical, 126*(9), 1141–1143.

119. Baron, J. A., Barrett, J., Katz, J. N., & Liang, M. H. (1996, January). Total hip arthroplasty: Use and select complications in the U.S. Medicare population. *Am J Public Health, 86,* 70–72.

120. Baker, D. W., Stevens, C. D., & Brook, R. H. (1996). Determinants of emergency department use: Are race and ethnicity important? *Ann Emerg Med, 28,* 677–682.

121. White-Means, S. I., & Thornton, M. C. (1989). Nonemergency visits to hospital emergency rooms: A comparison of blacks and whites. *Milbank Q, 67,* 35–37.

122. Todd, K. H., Samaroo, N., & Hoffman, J. R. (1993, March 24–31). Ethnicity as a risk factor for inadequate emergency department analgesia. *JAMA, 269,* 1537–1539.

123. Falcone, D., & Broyles, R. (1994, Fall). Access to long-term care: Race as a barrier. *J Health Polit Policy Law, 19,* 583–595.

124. Escarce, J. J., Epstein, K. R., Colby, D. C., & Schwartz, J. S. (1993, July). Racial differences in the elderly's use of medical procedures and diagnostic tests. *Am J Public Health, 83,* 948–954.

125. Giacomini, M. K. (1996, June 10). Gender and ethnic differences in hospital-based procedure utilization in California. *Arch Intern Med, 156,* 1217–1224.

126. Johnson, P. A., Lee, T. H., Cook, E. F., Rouan, G. W., & Goldman, L. (1993, April 15). Effect of race on the presentation and management of patients with acute chest pain. *Ann Intern Med, 118,* 593–601.

127. Schulman, K. A., Berlin, J. A., Harless, W., Kerner, J. F., Sistrunk, S., Gersh, B. J., Phil, D., Dube, R., Taleghani, C. K., Burke, J. E., Williams, S., Eisenberg, J. M., & Escarce, J. J. (1999, February 25). The effect of race and sex on physicians' recommendations for cardiac catheterization. *N Engl J Med, 340,* 618–626.

128. Hunter, C. P., Redmond, C. K., Chen, V. W., et al. (1993, July 14). Breast cancer: Factors associated with stage at diagnosis in black and white women: Black/White Cancer Survival Study Group. *J Natl Cancer Inst, 85,* 1129–1137.

129. Lannin, D. R., Matthews, H. F., Mitchell, J., Swanson, M. S., Swanson, F. H., & Edwards, M. S. (1998, June 10). Influence of socioeconomic and cultural factors on racial differences in late-stage presentation of breast cancer. *JAMA, 279,* 1801–1807.

130. Clancy, C. M., & Franks, P. (1997, December). Utilization of specialty and primary care: The impact of HMO insurance and patient-related factors. *J Fam Pract, 45,* 500–508.

CHAPTER ELEVEN

Disparities in Health Care by Race, Ethnicity, and Language Among the Insured

Findings from a National Sample

Kevin Fiscella
Peter Franks
Mark P. Doescher
Barry G. Saver

Racial and ethnic disparities in various aspects of health care have been extensively documented but remain poorly understood. Minority race or ethnicity has been linked to a lower likelihood of having a regular source of care, fewer physician visits, and lower total health care expenditures.[1,2] Previous studies have shown that black patients receive less appropriate management of congestive heart failure and pneumonia,[3] poorer quality of hospital care,[4] fewer pediatric prescriptions,[5] fewer admissions for chest pain,[6] lower-quality prenatal care,[7] less smoking cessation counseling,[8] and less preventive care, including fewer mammograms and influenza vaccinations among the elderly.[9,10]

Although disparities in health care for ethnic minorities other than black patients have received less attention, available evidence suggests that Hispanic Americans are also affected. Compared with non-Hispanic white patients, Hispanic patients receive fewer mammograms, Papanicolaou tests, and influenza vaccinations,[11] less prenatal care,[11] fewer cardiovascular procedures,[12] and less analgesia for metastatic cancer,[13] trauma,[14] and childbirth.[15] However, relatively

Funded by the Robert Wood Johnson Foundation through the Changes in Healthcare Financing and Organization Initiative. Also, the authors thank the *Medical Care* editor and anonymous reviewers for their helpful suggestions.

few studies have specifically examined the contribution of language and access barriers to these disparities.

In this study, we used the Andersen-Newman behavioral model[16,17] to examine the effect of race, ethnicity, and English fluency on health care use using national data. We hypothesized that adjustment for predisposing factors (sociodemographic characteristics) would reduce disparities, that adjustment for need factors (health status and smoking) would increase disparities, and that further adjustment for enabling factors (health insurance, regular source of care, income, and phone access) would again reduce disparities.

MATERIALS AND METHODS

Data Source

Data are from the Community Tracking Study (CTS) Household Survey conducted in 1996 and 1997.[18] It is a telephone survey of 60,446 persons representing the U.S.-housed, noninstitutionalized population. Sixty communities were randomly selected using stratified sampling with probability in proportion to population size to ensure representation of the U.S. population. Although random-digit dialing was used to select most households, a small sample was also included to represent households without phones; these respondents were provided cellular phones for the interviews. The survey was conducted in both English and Spanish, depending on the preference of the respondent. Mathematica Policy Research (Princeton, NJ) produced a Spanish version of the survey. After translation from English to Spanish, a second translator reviewed the survey. Any differences between the two translations were reconciled between the two independent translators, both of whom were members of the American Translators Association. Mathematica Policy Research validated the Spanish versions of the questions using in-house researchers whose native language is Spanish. Survey data included sociodemographic characteristics, health insurance, use, health status, and preventive health services. Analyses for this study were confined to adults eighteen to sixty-four years old with insurance (private or Medicaid), thus excluding 8,607 subjects and yielding a total of 31,003 participants. The overall CTS Household Survey response rate was 65 percent. Question response rates exceeded 99 percent for the independent variables of primary interest, race and ethnicity, and for each of the dependent measures.

Primary Independent Variables

Race. Race was classified as "white," "black," or "other," based on self-reports. Because "other" comprises an unknown mixture of Asians and Pacific Islanders,

American Indians and Native Alaskans, and others, we excluded this category (1,894 subjects) from the analysis.

Ethnicity. Ethnicity was classified as Hispanic or non-Hispanic, based on self-reports. Data regarding ethnicity or race were missing for sixty-three subjects.

Language. Hispanic patients were further classified as primarily English speaking or Spanish speaking, depending on the language in which the survey was conducted. Fifty-one subjects were excluded because the survey language was not reported.

Predisposing Factors

Demographic Characteristics. Demographic characteristics included age (nineteen to twenty-nine, thirty to forty-four, or forty-five to sixty-four years), sex, marital status (married or not), household size, and community size (large metropolitan region, >200,000 persons; small metropolitan region, <200,000 persons; or nonmetropolitan region), and education (less than high school, high school degree or equivalent, some college, or college degree or degrees).

Need Factors. We used self-reported health status as a proxy for need. Health status was assessed using the Medical Outcomes Study Short Form 12-item (SF-12) health survey. The SF-12 provides two summary scores, one for physical health (range, 10–70; mean 36 in the entire CTS sample) and one for mental health (range, 9–72; mean 38 in the entire CTS sample), and has been shown to be reliable and valid compared with the well-established, longer SF-36.[19,20] Data were imputed by CTS personnel for 1,624 subjects.

Respondents were asked whether they currently smoked, formerly smoked, or never smoked. Smoking status data were missing for 1,205 subjects.

Enabling Factors. Having a regular source of care was a dichotomous variable ("Is there a place you usually go when you are sick, or need advice about your health?").

Type of health care insurance (Medicaid or private) was assessed. Adults with Medicare or other publicly funded insurance besides Medicaid were excluded.

Health maintenance organization (HMO) coverage was assessed, and membership was determined by the response to a survey item asking whether the patient's insurance plan was an HMO or not.

Household income levels were grouped by percentages of the poverty level for 1996 (<100%, 100%–199%, 200%–299%, 300%–399%, ≥400%).

Telephone access was a dichotomous variable ("Was there any time during the past 12 months when you did not have a working telephone in your household for 2 or more weeks?").

Dependent Variables

We used standard dichotomous measures for medical, mental health, and preventive health services use.

Physician Visit. The physician visit measure was based on a report of at least one physician visit in the past year (all adults). There were no missing or imputed data for this variable.

Mental Health Visit. The mental health visit measure was based on a report that the respondent had "seen or talked to a mental health professional such as a psychiatrist, psychologist, psychiatric nurse, or clinical social worker" in the past year (all adults). Data were imputed for fifty-two subjects.

Mammography. Respondents were asked whether they had received a mammogram in the past year (women >50 years). Twenty-six subjects were excluded because of missing data.

Influenza Vaccination. Respondents were asked whether they had received an influenza vaccination in the past year (adults >55 years). Thirty-seven subjects were excluded because of missing data.

Analysis

To account for the complex design of the CTS Household Survey,[18] analyses were conducted using SUDAAN.[21] The impact of race, ethnicity, and language was examined using a series of logistic regression models for each use measure. The first model is unadjusted, and the second model adds predisposing factors (age, sex, marital status, family size, and education). The third model adds need factors, and the last model adds enabling factors (family income, usual source of care, telephone access, type of health insurance, and community size). In each model, non-Hispanic white adults serve as the reference category. (For each dependent measure, models 1 to 3 excluded less than 1 percent of respondents, and model 4 excluded approximately 5 percent of respondents because of survey item nonresponse.) Interaction terms were assessed for the possibility of effect modification between race or ethnicity and the covariate's income, education, and type of insurance coverage. To better reflect the effect sizes of race, ethnicity, and language, the odds ratios obtained from the logistic regression analyses were transformed to relative risks using the method of Zhang and Yu.[22]

RESULTS

In Table 11.1, we summarize key characteristics of the five groups. Compared with the four minority groups, non-Hispanic white patients tended to be older, married, and less likely to live in a large metropolitan area. They were more

Table 11.1. Sample Characteristics by Race, Ethnicity, and Language

Characteristic	White $N = 25,289$	Hispanic, English-Speaking $N = 1,652$	Hispanic, Spanish-Speaking $N = 746$	Black $N = 3,316$
Age, years				
18–29	21.3% (0.4%)	30.8% (1.3%)	27.9% (3.0%)	26.3% (0.8%)
30–44	42.3% (0.4%)	43.1% (1.5%)	44.8% (5.0%)	44.3% (1.0%)
45–64	36.4% (0.5%)	26.1% (1.3%)	27.2% (6.9%)	29.4% (1.0%)
Male sex	49.1% (0.2%)	48.8% (1.2%)	50.9% (2.6%)	42.3% (0.8%)
Marital status, single	31.5% (0.6%)	41.7% (1.5%)	37.4% (2.3%)	58.9% (1.3%)
Mean family size	2.7 (0.03)	2.8 (0.05)	3.1 (0.2)	2.4 (0.04)
Community size				
Large metropolitan	70.4% (1.9%)	90.8% (2.2%)	93.7% (2.4%)	77.1% (5.0%)
Small metropolitan	6.7% (0.5%)	2.0% (0.6%)	0.9% (0.7%)	6.9% (1.0%)
Rural	22.9% (1.8%)	7.2% (2.0%)	5.5% (2.2%)	16.0% (5.3%)
Medicaid insurance	3.3% (0.3%)	8.7% (1.2%)	19.5% (3.2%)	16.5% (1.5%)
HMO member	42.3% (0.6%)	61.1% (1.6%)	58.6% (2.8%)	52.6% (1.9%)
Current smoker	25.5% (0.5%)	20.3% (1.0%)	17.0% (1.8%)	26.1% (1.2%)
Health status*				
PCS12 score, mean	51.4 (0.1)	50.9 (0.3)	48.8 (0.5)	49.1 (0.3)
MCS12 score, mean	52.6 (0.1)	51.2 (0.3)	51.3 (0.5)	51.2 (0.3)
Income as percentage of poverty				
<100%	12.0% (0.3%)	19.8% (1.6%)	41.9% (5.0%)	27.4% (1.6%)
100–199%	15.0% (0.5%)	21.6% (1.7%)	35.9% (2.4%)	24.2% (1.1%)
200–399%	36.1% (0.5%)	33.9% (2.0%)	17.2% (3.4%)	30.0% (1.4%)
≥400%	37.0% (0.6%)	24.7% (1.4%)	5.0% (1.2%)	18.5% (1.2%)
Education				
Less than high school	7.3% (0.3%)	15.5% (1.8%)	52.9% (6.2%)	15.8% (1.0%)
High school/GED	33.5% (0.5%)	34.4% (1.7%)	24.7% (1.6%)	39.0% (1.2%)
Some college	29.5% (0.6%)	28.5% (1.3%)	14.2% (2.2%)	28.1% (1.1%)
College degree	29.8% (0.5%)	21.7% (2.3%)	8.3% (3.8%)	17.1% (1.0%)
No usual source of care	9.8% (0.3%)	12.9% (1.0%)	18.2% (1.6%)	11.6% (0.8%)
No telephone in household	2.2% (0.2%)	3.3% (0.7%)	5.5% (1.2%)	5.1% (0.7%)
Physician visit in past year	78.7% (0.3%)	77.2% (1.1%)	61.0% (2.1%)	78.9% (0.9%)
Mental health visit in past year	8.1% (0.2%)	8.7% (0.9%)	4.0% (0.9%)	6.9% (0.6%)
Mammogram in past year (women ≥50 years)	35.4% (0.8%)	45.0% (4.9%)	27.0% (4.4%)	40.1% (2.9%)
Influenza vaccine in past year (adults ≥55 years)	37.6% (1.0%)	32.3% (4.4%)	11.0% (3.6%)	27.3% (2.9%)

Note: Data are percentage or mean (*SE*). HMO = health maintenance organization; PCS12 = physical health status; MCS12 = mental health status; GED = Graduate Equivalency Diploma.

*Higher scores on the PCS12 and the MCS12 indicate better health status.

likely to be privately insured and to report better physical and mental health. They also had higher income and education levels, and were more likely to have a usual source of care and a telephone in the household.

Table 11.2, model 1, shows unadjusted relative risk ratios comparing use for each of the five groups. English-speaking Hispanic patients did not differ

Table 11.2. Effect of Predisposing, Need, and Enabling Factors on Racial-, Ethnic-, and Language-Related Health Care Use

Health Service	Model 1	Model 2	Model 3	Model 4
Physician visit				
Hispanic: English speaking	0.94 (0.84–1.04)	0.95 (0.84–1.07)	0.95 (0.84–1.07)	0.94 (0.83–1.07)
Hispanic: Spanish speaking	0.77 (0.72–0.83)	0.81 (0.73–0.87)	0.79 (0.72–0.85)	0.84 (0.77–0.92)
Black	1.01 (0.93–1.09)	1.01 (0.92–1.10)	0.94 (0.85–1.03)	0.97 (0.89–1.07)
Mental health				
Hispanic: English speaking	1.07 (0.89–1.30)	1.01 (0.82–1.23)	0.93 (0.75–1.15)	0.85 (0.66–1.07)
Hispanic: Spanish speaking	0.50 (0.32–0.76)	0.46 (0.30–0.72)	0.42 (0.28–0.65)	0.38 (0.23–0.59)
Black	0.86 (0.72–1.03)	0.68 (0.56–0.81)	0.59 (0.49–0.71)	0.48 (0.39–0.57)
Mammogram (age ≥50 years)				
Hispanic: English speaking	1.27 (1.03–1.52)	1.20 (0.95–1.46)	1.21 (1.02–1.48)	1.20 (0.92–1.49)
Hispanic: Spanish speaking	0.74 (0.41–1.11)	0.61 (0.39–0.90)	0.61 (0.39–0.91)	0.51 (0.29–0.81)
Black	1.13 (0.97–1.30)	1.00 (0.84–1.18)	0.96 (0.80–1.14)	0.96 (0.81–1.13)
Influenza vaccination (age 55–64 years)				
Hispanic: English speaking	0.87 (0.66–1.11)	0.93 (0.71–1.18)	0.94 (0.71–1.18)	0.94 (0.71–1.19)
Hispanic: Spanish speaking	0.30 (0.15–0.52)	0.36 (0.18–0.69)	0.35 (0.17–0.67)	0.37 (0.17–0.75)
Black	0.73 (0.58–0.87)	0.79 (0.63–0.96)	0.78 (0.63–0.96)	0.78 (0.63–0.96)

Note: Data are relative risk (95% CI). Model 1 is adjusted for race/ethnicity; model 2 adds age, sex, marital status, family size, and education; model 3 adds smoking, mental health status, and physical health status; model 4 adds insurance type, health maintenance organization status, usual source of care, telephone access, and income.

significantly from non-Hispanic white patients in the likelihood of having a physician visit, mental health visit, or influenza vaccination, but were more likely to have had a mammogram. In contrast, Spanish-speaking Hispanic patients were significantly less likely than non-Hispanic white patients to have had a physician visit (*RR*, 0.77; 95% CI, 0.72–0.83), mental health visit (*RR*, 0.50; 95% CI, 0.32–0.76), or influenza vaccination (*RR*, 0.30; 95% CI, 0.15–0.52). Black patients were significantly less likely than non-Hispanic white patients to have had an influenza vaccination (*RR*, 0.73; 95% CI, 0.58–0.87), but did not significantly differ in the likelihood of having a physician visit, mental health visit, or mammogram.

Table 11.2, models 2 to 4, shows the effects for each group after adjustment for predisposing, need, and enabling factors. After adjusting for predisposing factors, English-speaking Hispanic patients did not differ significantly from non-Hispanic white patients in any measure. The likelihood of having a physician visit did change with adjustment. The relative risk for any visit with a mental health provider steadily declined with each successive adjustment, but did not reach statistical significance. The relative risk for mammography decreased slightly and was no longer statistically significant after adjustment for predisposing factors, and showed little change with additional adjustment. Similarly, the relative risk of influenza vaccination decreased slightly after adjustment for predisposing factors and then showed little change with further adjustment.

After adjustment for predisposing factors, Spanish-speaking Hispanic patients were significantly less likely than non-Hispanic white patients to have had a physician visit, visit with a mental health provider, mammogram, or influenza vaccination. The relative risk of having had a physician visit decreased slightly with adjustments for predisposing and enabling factors, but increased slightly with adjustment for need factors. For mental health visits, the relative risk ratios became more pronounced with each additional adjustment, and a similar pattern was observed for mammography. For influenza vaccination, adjustment for predisposing factors reduced the relative risk ratios slightly, but there was little change with additional adjustments.

The picture for black patients was mixed. For any physician visit, there was no evidence of a statistically significant difference, though the relative risk decreased after adjusting for need factors. With adjustment for predisposing factors, black patients were significantly less likely to have had any visit with a mental health provider (*RR*, 0.68; 95% CI, 0.56–0.81), and the likelihood of doing so decreased further with additional adjustment for need and enabling factors, and remained statistically significant. There was no evidence of a significant relation between receipt of mammography and black ethnicity compared with non-Hispanic white ethnicity. African Americans were significantly less likely than non-Hispanic white patients to report receiving an influenza vaccination, an effect that did not change appreciably with adjustment.

DISCUSSION

Using data from a large, nationally representative survey, we examined the associations of race, ethnicity, and English fluency on the likelihood of having a physician visit, mental health visit, mammogram, or influenza vaccination. We observed significant differences in health care use for English fluency and race, and examined how these associations were altered by accounting for predisposing, need, and enabling factors.

Among Hispanic patients, crude and adjusted findings differed sharply according to English fluency. After adjustment for predisposing factors, English-speaking Hispanic patients displayed a use pattern similar to non-Hispanic white patients. In contrast, Spanish-speaking Hispanic patients had a significantly lower likelihood than non-Hispanic white patients of having had a physician visit, visit with a mental health provider, influenza vaccination, or mammogram. Adjustment for need and enabling factors did not appreciably alter these findings.

Previous studies have shown that Hispanic patients have lower health care use than white patients, including fewer physician visits[23] and lower use of outpatient mental health services,[24] mammography,[11,25] and influenza vaccinations.[26] Our findings based on insured, nonelderly adults suggest that the Hispanic disparity in use is largely confined to Spanish-speaking Hispanic patients. These results are consistent with previous studies suggesting that lack of English fluency is associated with reduced health care use.[27-30] For example, using data from the National Hispanic Health and Nutrition Examination Survey, Solis et al.[31] reported that English fluency, but not ethnic self-identification, predicted having had a physical, dental, eye, or breast examination, or a Papanicolaou test. However, disparities in the care between Hispanic patients and non-Hispanic patients were not assessed. Weinick and Krauss[29] examined the effect of English fluency on ethnic disparities in pediatric use and found that these disparities were eliminated after adjusting for language fluency. Recently, Jacobs et al.[32] showed that professional interpreter services increased the delivery of health care to patients with limited English fluency. Our study adds to this growing literature by showing that language fluency (or closely associated factors, such as acculturation[33,34]) is the primary contributor to ethnic disparities in access to studied types of care among insured, nonelderly Hispanic adults.

Black patients also had a significantly lower likelihood of having received an influenza vaccination, which was not explained by adjustment for predisposing, need, or enabling factors. Furthermore, racial differences in the likelihood of having had a visit with a mental health provider became statistically significant after adjusting for predisposing factors and remained significant after further adjustment for need and enabling factors. There were no racial differences in the likelihood of having had a physician visit or mammogram.

The racial disparity in influenza vaccination is consistent with findings from the Behavioral Risk Factor Surveillance Survey among elderly respondents, but this finding was not explained by any of the factors included in our model. Other factors, such as patient preference or physician bias, may explain this disparity. However, data from the Medicare Current Beneficiary Survey show no racial difference in reasons for not obtaining influenza vaccinations.[35]

Racial and ethnic differences in mental health use have not been adequately studied using large, national samples. However, regional studies of privately insured adults suggest that black patients and Hispanic patients have lower use of outpatient mental health services than non-Hispanic white patients.[24,27] Whether the lower likelihood of having a visit with a mental health provider among black patients is attributable to differences in the patient's perceived need, attitudes toward mental care, or physician referral bias cannot be assessed with these data.

These findings should be tempered by the limitations of the study. First, these data are derived exclusively from self-report and are subject to bias. Previous studies suggest that respondents tend to underestimate the time interval since they received a particular service,[36–38] and use of preventive services is consistently found to be overreported when subjected to medical record confirmation.[39] Studies of the effect of race, ethnicity, education, and language on self-reported accuracy of preventive care have shown mixed results.[38,40]

Second, use of dichotomized measures of physician visits and mental health visits may have reduced our ability to detect differences between groups. Furthermore, we were unable to distinguish primary care from specialist visits. Previous studies have suggested that minorities, even those with health insurance, have reduced access to specialists,[41] particularly in fee-for-service systems.[42]

Third, we did not assess the impact of access barriers (for example, travel time, waiting time, out-of-pocket expenses). Although it is likely that some access barrier factors contribute to racial and ethnic disparities in care, Spanish-speaking parents cite language fluency as the foremost access barrier to health care for their children.[30]

Finally, the CTS sampling strategy may limit the generalizability of the findings to U.S. Spanish-speaking Americans. Most of the communities sampled were large metropolitan areas. As Table 11.1 shows, few Hispanic patients surveyed resided in small metropolitan areas. This finding suggests that Hispanic patients residing in small communities in the West and Southwest may have been excluded from the sample. Thus, our findings may not generalize to this group. In addition, the survey's marginal response rate (65 percent) may limit generalizability of the findings.

In summary, we observed significant associations of race and language fluency with health care use in a national sample of insured, nonelderly adults. Most of these associations were not explained by traditional factors that are commonly measured in large surveys like the CTS. Improved understanding of the salience of race and English fluency to health care use is needed if the ambitious goal of Healthy People 2010 to eliminate racial and ethnic disparities in health status is to be achieved.

Notes

1. Fiscella, K., Franks, P., & Clancy, C. M. (1998). Skepticism toward medical care and healthcare utilization. *Med Care, 36,* 180–189.

2. Centers for Disease Control and Prevention. (1998). Demographic characteristics of persons without a regular source of medical care: Selected states, 1995. *JAMA, 279,* 1603.

3. Ayanian, J. Z., Weissman, J. S., & Chasan-Taber, S., et al. (1999). Quality of care by race and gender for congestive heart failure and pneumonia. *Med Care, 37,* 1260–1269.

4. Kahn, K. L., Pearson, M. L., Harrison, E. R., et al. (1994). Healthcare for black and poor hospitalized Medicare patients. *JAMA, 271,* 1169–1174.

5. Hahn, B. A. (1995). Children's health: Racial and ethnic differences in the use of prescription medications. *Pediatrics, 95,* 727–732.

6. Johnson, P. A., Lee, T. H., Cook, E. F., et al. (1993). Effect of race on the presentation and management of patients with acute chest pain. *Ann Intern Med, 118,* 593–601.

7. Kogan, M. D., Kotlechuck, M., & Johnson, S. (1993). Racial differences in late prenatal care visits. *J Perinatol, 13,* 14–21.

8. Doescher, M. P., & Saver, B. G. (2000). Physicians' advice to quit smoking: The glass remains half empty. *J Fam Pract, 49,* 543–547.

9. Gornick, M. E., Eggers, P. W., Reilly, T. W., et al. (1996). Effects of race and income on mortality and use of services among Medicare beneficiaries. *N Engl J Med, 335,* 791–799.

10. Burns, R. B., McCarthy, E. P., Freund, K. M., et al. (1996). Black women receive less mammography even with similar use of primary care. *Ann Intern Med, 125,* 173–182.

11. Collins, S. C., Hall, A., & Neuhaus, C. (1999). *U.S. minority health: A chartbook.* New York: The Commonwealth Fund.

12. Carlisle, D. M., Leake, B. D., & Shapiro, M. F. (1995). Racial and ethnic differences in the use of invasive cardiac procedures among cardiac patients in Los Angeles County, 1986 through 1988. *Am J Public Health, 85,* 352–356.

13. Cleeland, C. S., Gonin, R., Baez, L., et al. (1997). Pain and treatment of pain in minority patients with cancer: The Eastern Cooperative Oncology Group Minority Outpatient Pain Study. *Ann Intern Med, 127,* 813–816.

14. Todd, K. H., Samaroo, N., & Hoffman, J. R. (1993). Ethnicity as a risk factor for inadequate emergency department analgesia. *JAMA, 269,* 1537–1539.

15. Hueston, W. J., McClaflin, R. R., Mansfield, C. J., et al. (1994). Factors associated with the use of intrapartum epidural analgesia. *Obstet Gynecol, 84*, 579–582.

16. Andersen, R., Lion, J., & Anderson, O. (1976). *Two decades of health services research: Social survey trends in use and expenditures.* Cambridge, MA: Harvard University Press.

17. Andersen, R. M. (1995). Revisiting the behavioral model and access to medical care: Does it matter? *J Health Soc Behav, 36*, 1–10.

18. Kemper, P., Blumenthal, D., Corrigan, J. M., et al. (1996). The design of the community tracking study: A longitudinal study of health system change and its effects on people. *Inquiry, 33*, 195–206.

19. Ware, J. E., Jr., Kosinski, M., & Keller, S. D. (1996). A 12-item short-form health survey: Construction of scales and preliminary tests of reliability and validity. *Med Care, 34*, 220–233.

20. Jenkinson, C., Layte, R., Jenkinson, D., et al. (1997). A shorter form health survey: Can the SF-12 replicate results from the SF-36 in longitudinal studies? *J Public Health Med, 19*, 179–186.

21. Research Triangle Institute. (2000). *SUDAAN. Professional software for Survey Data Analysis, ver 7.56.* Research Triangle Park, NC: Research Triangle Institute.

22. Zhang, J., & Yu, K. F. (1998). What's the relative risk? A method of correcting the odds ratio in cohort studies of common outcomes. *JAMA, 280*, 1690–1691.

23. Forrest, C. B., & Whelan, E. M. (2000). Primary care safety-net delivery sites in the United States: A comparison of community health centers, hospital outpatient departments, and physicians' offices. *JAMA, 284*, 2077–2083.

24. Padgett, D. K., Patrick, C., Burns, B. J., et al. (1994). Ethnicity and the use of outpatient mental health services in a national insured population. *Am J Public Health, 84*, 222–226.

25. Calle, E. E., Flanders, W. D., Thun, M. J., et al. (1993). Demographic predictors of mammography and Pap smear screening in U.S. women. *Am J Public Health, 83*, 53–60.

26. Mark, T. L., & Paramore, L. C. (1996). Pneumococcal pneumonia and influenza vaccination: Access to and use by U.S. Hispanic Medicare beneficiaries. *Am J Public Health, 86*, 1545–1550.

27. Scheffler, R. M., & Miller, A. B. (1989). Demand analysis of mental health service use among ethnic subpopulations. *Inquiry, 26*, 202–215.

28. Derose, K. P., & Baker, D. W. (2000). Limited English proficiency and Latinos' use of physician services. *Med Care Res Rev, 57*, 76–91.

29. Weinick, R. M., & Krauss, N. A. (2000). Racial/ethnic differences in children's access to care. *Am J Public Health, 90*, 1771–1774.

30. Flores, G., Abreu, M., Olivar, M. A., et al. (1998). Access barriers to health care for Latino children. *Arch Pediatr Adolesc Med, 152*, 1119–1125.

31. Solis, J. M., Marks, G., Garcia, M., et al. (1990). Acculturation, access to care, and use of preventive services by Hispanic patients: Findings from HHANES 1982–84. *Am J Public Health, 80*(Suppl.), 11–19.

32. Jacobs, E. A., Lauderdale, D. S., Meltzer, D., et al. (2001). Impact of interpreter services on delivery of health care to limited-English-proficient patients. *J Gen Intern Med, 16,* 468–474.

33. Wells, K. B., Hough, R. L., Golding, J. M., et al. (1987). Which Mexican-Americans underutilize health services? *Am J Psychiatry, 144,* 918–922.

34. Hubbell, F. A., Chavez, L. R., Mishra, S. I., et al. (1996). Beliefs about sexual behavior and other predictors of Papanicolaou smear screening among Latinas and Anglo women. *Arch Intern Med, 156,* 2353–2358.

35. Centers for Disease Control and Prevention. (1999). Reasons reported by Medicare beneficiaries for not receiving influenza and pneumococcal vaccinations—United States, 1996. *Morbid Mortal Wkly Rep, 48,* 886–890.

36. Bowman, J. A., Sanson-Fisher, R., & Redman, S. (1997). The accuracy of self-reported Pap smear utilisation. *Soc Sci Med, 44,* 969–976.

37. Paskett, E. D., Tatum, C. M., Mack, D. W., et al. (1996). Validation of self-reported breast and cervical cancer screening tests among low-income minority women. *Cancer Epidemiol Biomarkers Prev, 5,* 721–726.

38. Zapka, J. G., Bigelow, C., Hurley, T., et al. (1996). Mammography use among sociodemographically diverse women: The accuracy of self-report. *Am J Public Health, 86,* 1016–1021.

39. Warnecke, R. B., Sudman, S., Johnson, T. P., et al. (1997). Cognitive aspects of recalling and reporting health-related events: Papanicolaou smears, clinical breast examinations, and mammograms. *Am J Epidemiol, 146,* 982–992.

40. Newell, S. A., Girgis, A., Sanson-Fisher, R. W., et al. (1999). The accuracy of self-reported health behaviors and risk factors relating to cancer and cardiovascular disease in the general population: A critical review. *Am J Prev Med, 17,* 211–229.

41. Blustein, J., & Weiss, L. J. (1998). Visits to specialists under Medicare: Socioeconomic advantage and access to care. *J Health Care Poor Underserved, 9,* 153–169.

42. Clancy, C. M., & Franks, P. (1997). Utilization of specialty and primary care: The impact of HMO insurance and patient-related factors. *J Fam Pract, 45,* 500–508.

PART FOUR

WHY DISPARITIES EXIST

CHAPTER TWELVE

Black-White Differences in the Relationship of Maternal Age to Birthweight

A Population-Based Test of the Weathering Hypothesis

Arline T. Geronimus

African American infants are more likely than white infants to be born preterm or low birthweight, and on average face twice the risk of death.[1] These differentials have persisted for decades, despite general and race-specific declines.[2] Closing this gap remains a high-priority national public objective.[3] However, the processes that result in this differential remain poorly understood.[4,5] Many biobehavioral and medical risk factors have been identified, including maternal age, hypertension, anemia, and tobacco use during pregnancy.[4-8] However, few investigators conceptualize these risk factors as part of a theory-based causal process linking social background factors to the biological mechanisms through which they are associated with poor birth outcome. An implicit but largely untested assumption is that risk factors operate the same way across populations; study of interaction effects is undeveloped.[9] The importance of returning to basic research approaches—even ones that may question the universal validity of previously identified risk factors—is highlighted by recent observations and research findings. For example,

Funding for this research came from the National Institute of Child Health and Human Development, Grant No. HD24122-05. I am grateful to John Bound for statistical consultation, helpful discussions, and comments on earlier drafts, and to Marianne Hillemeier and Lisa J. Neidert for research and computer programming assistance. An earlier version of this paper was presented at the May 1993 workshop "Preterm Delivery and Other Pregnancy Outcomes Among Black Women," at the Centers for Disease Control, Atlanta.

Schoendorf and colleagues[10] note that the size of the racial disparity in poor birth outcome is often *greater* among mothers with few traditional risk factors than it is among others. In addition, clinical pregnancy risk-screening protocols based on traditional risk factors have been shown to have poor predictive validity, especially when applied to certain socioeconomic or ethnic subpopulations.[11,12] These findings suggest the importance of moving beyond the identification of specific "risk factors" apart from their social context and to consider the possibility that the effects of specific demographic or behavioral risk factors may not be invariant across populations.[13-15] In doing so, it is useful to consider psychosocial mechanisms that may vary across populations and heterogeneity within the African American population, as well as taking race comparative approaches.[15,16]

One traditional risk factor that merits reconsideration is maternal age. Maternal age has conventionally been seen as an important determinant of birth outcome and has most often been thought to represent a mother's biological or psychosocial preparedness for childbearing. Young maternal age, or teenage childbearing, has been a source of particular concern. However, the magnitude of the U.S. black-white disparity in neonatal mortality has been observed to widen with increasing maternal age, because risk among black infants *increases* between the late teens and the twenties, while risk for white infants *decreases* between these maternal ages.[13,17,18] Geronimus[18] proposed the "weathering" hypothesis, namely that the effects of social inequality on the health of populations may compound with age, leading to growing gaps in health status through young and middle adulthood that can affect fetal health. This hypothesis suggests that maternal age be reexamined as being not only a developmental indicator but also a reflection of the ways in which social inequality, racial discrimination, or race bias in exposures to psychosocial or environmental hazards may, on a population level, affect differentially the health of black and white women who will become mothers, not only in absolute terms, but also interactively with each other and cumulatively as women age.

Specific to the African American population, Geronimus[18] hypothesizes that the health status of women may begin to deteriorate in detectable ways in young adulthood as a response to perpetual social and environmental insult or prolonged active coping with stressful circumstances. Such insult may have negative implications for a woman's health or health behaviors and for the health of her infant should she become a mother. Descriptive research provides indirect evidence consistent with this hypothesis. Among women of reproductive age, prevalence rates of health and behavioral characteristics that can complicate pregnancy are excessive among U.S. blacks compared to whites and the increase in prevalence rates with age is more rapid among blacks. Such patterns of increase among women characterize biomedical risk factors, such as hypertension; behavioral risks, such as smoking; and risks that result from environmental exposures, such as circulating blood lead levels.[18] However, it has yet to be determined whether these differential health trajectories among *nonpregnant* women accurately characterize women's health during pregnancy or explain the differential maternal age patterns of poor birth outcome. Furthermore, research to date has described national black or white averages. If social inequality affects the health of young adult women differentially, then one would expect to see variation in maternal age trajectories of poor birth outcome among African American women with respect to social class.

In the current paper we test two working hypotheses that follow from the weathering perspective. Data constraints preclude a complete test of the theory, but based on the theory, one would predict that the following would be the case:

1. The black-white disparity in low or very low birthweight rates and in maternal health-related determinants will widen with maternal age.

2. Among black mothers, the increase with maternal age in low or very low birthweight rates will be more rapid among members of low socioeconomic groups compared to others. Differential prevalence of adverse maternal health characteristics will help explain any social gradient in the effects of maternal age on birthweight.

DATA AND ANALYTIC APPROACH

We analyze all black and white singleton first births to Michigan residents aged fifteen to thirty-four in 1989 ($N = 54{,}888$, representing 96 percent of all 1989 Michigan black and white first births), using linked birth and infant death certificate data combined with information from the 1980 Census on the socioeconomic characteristics of the maternal residential area. We limit the sample to first births to control for the potentially confounding effects of maternal age and parity on the risk of poor birth outcome, and to fifteen- to thirty-four-year-olds due to the infrequency and extreme selectivity of first births to women at younger or older ages.

The birth certificate revisions implemented in 1989 provide enhanced maternal health information compared to vital statistics from earlier years, including, for the first time, data on tobacco usage during pregnancy.[19] We have appended census information on the mean income of the maternal residential zip code area to each birth record as a proxy for maternal socioeconomic status. We chose this measure of socioeconomic group for theoretical and practical reasons. The measure of socioeconomic status that is available on the birth certificate, maternal education, is not reliably recorded. In addition, it is unsuitable for a study of the relationship of maternal age to birth outcome because it is correlated with age (for example, fifteen-year-olds have not had the opportunity to complete their educations) and with age at first birth (fertility timing and educational attainment can be jointly determined). Further, geographically based measures more clearly match the construct implied by weathering, since they can encompass race bias in environmental exposures or in other health-related correlates of residential segregation.

When we began this investigation, data from the 1980 Census were the most recent available. Thus, we matched information to the birth record that described the 1980 economic characteristics of the mother's current (1989) zip code area. Findings from a validation study suggest that using census data removed by as much as a decade from the primary data to which they are appended does not materially affect regression results.[20] This is because the relative ranking of geographic units typically remains stable over time, even in the face of some change in absolute income levels. That is, extremely poor areas typically remain poor.

The multilevel nature of the data introduces a potential complication to statistical inference. Because we observe more than one birth in a given zip code, not all observations are independent. Such nonindependence may imply that estimated confidence intervals will underestimate the actual sampling variability. However, using replication methods,[21] we find, in this case, such biases to be negligible.

To test the research hypotheses, we describe maternal age patterns of low birthweight (LBW) (<2,500 grams) and very low birthweight (VLBW) (<1,500 grams) and of the prevalence of maternal health characteristics that are proximate determinants of poor birth outcome. We test models by estimating multivariate multinomial logistic regressions of the effects of maternal age, socioeconomic group, and maternal health characteristics during pregnancy on birthweight. By exponentiating the coefficients on the explanatory variables in specific regressions, we provide estimates of the relative odds of VLBW or LBW relative to a normal weight baby (2,500 to 3,999 grams). We estimate models separately for blacks and whites. To test the second set of hypotheses, we include socioeconomic status (SES) × Maternal Age Interactions. We define the explanatory variables as follows:

Maternal age. Maternal age is coded in single years as a continuous variable.

Racial identification. We code race as black or white according to the race of the mother.

SES. To proxy economic status, we construct a variable from 1980 Census files that represents the average family income in the zip code area. For all analyses, income values are transformed into their natural logarithms.

Maternal health characteristics. Smoking is measured as tobacco use during pregnancy (coded as 1 if *yes,* 0 if *no*). A separate category of those missing information on smoking behavior during pregnancy is maintained in the analyses. *Hypertension* includes dummy variables for mothers with either chronic hypertension or pregnancy-induced hypertension. Records with no information on medical risk factors are placed in a separate "missing" category. *High risk* is a variable that indicates a woman had an excess number of prenatal care visits, given the duration of her pregnancy. We include this as a maternal health characteristic because it indicates that in the clinician's judgment the course of the pregnancy required a more intensive regimen of medical attention than normally recommended. In models where multiple maternal risk factors are controlled, we include a variable, *total conditions,* representing a tally of all medical risk factors, both previous and pregnancy-induced conditions. Pregnancy-induced conditions include occurrences of nonhypertensive pregnancy-related disorders (diabetes, hydramnios/oligohydramnios, incompetent cervix, Rh sensitization, uterine bleeding). Previous conditions include occurrences of other medical conditions (cardiac disease, lung disease, genital herpes, anemia, hemoglobinopathy, renal disease). The total conditions variable also includes counts of those for whom some "other" condition was noted.

Prenatal care access. To control for prenatal care receipt we use the Kotelchuck Adequacy of Prenatal Care Utilization index (APNCU).[22] In the APNCU, the total number of prenatal visits reported is compared to the number which would be expected based on American College of Obstetricians and Gynecologists standards, given the date care began and the date of delivery. The proportion of observed to expected visits is then scaled (0–49% of expected = inadequate; 50–79% = intermediate; 80–109% = adequate; 110 + = adequate plus). We include those with missing information in the inadequate category. To control for prenatal care access, we include two dummy variables indicating whether the mother was coded as having either inadequate or intermediate care. The omitted category thus includes those with at least adequate care (the proportion of observed to expected visits is at least 80).

As implied above, we use information on the extent of prenatal care to measure access to care and pregnancy risk status. We do so because variation in prenatal care receipt occurs because women vary in their access to care and because women who perceive themselves or are perceived by physicians to be high risk may receive more care than others. Because obstetrics standards for adequate care apply to all women, regardless of their underlying health, we assume that whether a woman receives less than adequate care is largely a function of access rather than of perceived risk. Once we control for whether or not a woman has received at least adequate care, we view variation in whether or not she received adequate plus care as being a function of risk status. In general, this approach appears reasonable in light of the observed data. For example, black mothers are more likely than white to be in the inadequate care category or in the adequate plus category, suggesting that black women may have less access to care than white but, once in care, receive an intensive regimen because of worse health.

RESULTS

In Tables 12.1 and 12.2 observed rates of LBW or VLBW and of adverse maternal health characteristics, respectively, are reported by race and age of mother. For blacks, the maternal age patterns of rates of LBW or VLBW are upwardly sloping, with mothers aged fifteen to nineteen experiencing the *lowest* rates of poor birth outcome. Among whites, mothers in their teens and thirties experience slightly elevated rates of poor birth outcome compared to white women in their twenties. As a function of these different maternal age patterns, the size of the excess rate of LBW and VLBW for African Americans relative to whites is higher in the twenties and thirties than in the teens.

Table 12.2 shows that maternal age patterns of smoking also vary by race. Rates of smoking during pregnancy increase among African American mothers from the teens through the thirties, while rates for whites decrease. African American mothers in their teens and early twenties are less likely to smoke during pregnancy than are their white counterparts, but they are more likely to smoke during pregnancy by the latter half of the twenties than are whites. For both blacks and whites, the rates of hypertension during pregnancy are higher among older compared to younger mothers, but the increase in hypertension prevalence is steeper among blacks. Similarly, the percentage of mothers who are high risk increases with age among both blacks and whites, but more steeply for blacks. There is a 14.5 percentage point rise between the ages of fifteen to nineteen and thirty to thirty-four for blacks, but only a 7 percent rise for whites. The black-white gap increases accordingly.

In Table 12.3, we report the distribution of black or white mothers by maternal age who reside in areas with mean family incomes below the black median. Within either racial group younger mothers are more likely to live in socioeconomically disadvantaged areas than older mothers. Within each age group black

Table 12.1. Rates (per 100) and Rate Ratios of Low Birthweight and Very Low Birthweight by Maternal Age, African American and White Singleton First Births, Michigan, 1989

Maternal Age	N		LBW Rates and Rate Ratios			VLBW Rates and Rate Ratios		
	Black	White	Black	White	Black/White	Black	White	Black/White
15–19	5,244	8,992	11.6	6.3	1.8	2.7	1.2	2.3
20–24	3,384	14,415	12.4	5.0	2.5	2.9	0.8	3.6
25–29	1,482	14,541	14.0	4.9	2.9	3.6	0.6	6.0
30–34	608	6,172	17.8	6.2	2.9	6.1	1.2	5.1
Total	10,718	44,120	12.5	5.4	2.3	3.1	0.9	3.4

Table 12.2. Rates (per 100) and Rate Ratios of Smoking, Hypertension, and High Medical Risk During Pregnancy by Maternal Age, African American and White Singleton First Births, Michigan, 1989

	Rates		Rate Ratios
Maternal Age	Black	White	Black/White
Smoking			
15–19	7.4	33.7	0.2
20–24	14.6	24.2	0.6
25–29	17.3	15.3	1.1
30–34	20.9	15.0	1.4
Total	14.9*	21.9	0.7
Hypertension			
15–19	5.9	5.3	1.1
20–24	6.6	6.1	1.1
25–29	8.6	6.8	1.3
30–34	9.5	7.7	1.2
Total	7.5*	6.4	1.1
High risk			
15–19	29.0	20.9	1.4
20–24	33.4	24.1	1.4
25–29	36.5	25.4	1.4
30–34	43.5	27.9	1.6
Total	35.0*	24.4	1.4

Note: Smoking = tobacco use during pregnancy. "Hypertension" = chronic or pregnancy-associated hypertensive disease. "High risk" = receiving an excess number of prenatal visits, given the duration of pregnancy. See the text for more detailed definitions.

*Standardized to the white age distribution.

Table 12.3. Percentage of Mothers Living in Zip Codes with Mean Family Incomes Below African American Median,* by Race and Age, Singleton First Births, Michigan, 1989

	Black	White
Maternal Age	Percent Below	Percent Below
15–19	56.5	26.1
20–24	51.2	21.2
25–29	45.2	12.5
30–34	42.5	10.5

*$20,215.

mothers are far more likely than white to live in such areas. These differences are statistically significant ($p < .001$). Thus, the effects on poor birth outcome of maternal age or race are potentially confounded by socioeconomic group.

MULTINOMIAL LOGISTIC MODELS

For blacks the estimated effect of maternal age on LBW or VLBW is positive, statistically significant, and of substantial magnitude. For example, twenty-five-year-old black mothers experience 28 percent increased odds of low birthweight and a 70 percent increased odds of VLBW relative to fifteen-year-old black mothers. In contrast, among whites maternal age is not significantly related to VLBW or LBW. In Table 12.4 we report odds ratios for the effect on LBW and VLBW of postponing childbirth from age fifteen to age twenty-five, controlled

Table 12.4. Odds (95% Confidence Intervals) of Low Birthweight or Very Low Birthweight for Mothers Aged 25 Relative to Mothers Aged 15, Adjusted for Maternal Health Characteristics, African American or White Singleton First Births, Michigan, 1989

	African Americans	
Adjusting for	Low Birthweight	Very Low Birthweight
Prenatal care	1.32 (1.14, 1.53)	1.78 (1.41, 2.26)
Smoking*	1.21 (1.04, 1.41)	1.66 (1.30, 2.12)
High blood pressure*	1.29 (1.12, 1.50)	1.73 (1.36, 2.19)
High risk*	1.30 (1.13, 1.52)	1.75 (1.38, 2.22)
All conditions*†	1.17 (1.00, 1.36)	1.55 (1.21, 1.97)

	Whites	
Adjusting for	Low Birthweight	Very Low Birthweight
Prenatal care	1.03 (0.93, 1.14)	0.94 (0.75, 1.19)
Smoking*	1.15 (1.04, 1.28)	1.01 (0.80, 1.28)
High blood pressure*	1.01 (0.91, 1.12)	0.91 (0.72, 1.15)
High risk*	1.04 (0.94, 1.15)	0.96 (0.76, 1.20)
All conditions*†	1.11 (1.00, 1.23)	0.90 (0.72, 1.14)

*Prenatal care is also controlled in these models.

†Maternal health characteristics controlled include hypertensive disease (chronic or pregnancy associated), smoking, diabetes, hydramnios/oligohydramnios, incompetent cervix, Rh sensitization, uterine bleeding, cardiac disease, lung disease, genital herpes, anemia, hemoglobinopathy, renal disease, and other conditions.

for prenatal care receipt and adjusted for specific maternal health characteristics. Among blacks, when only prenatal care receipt is controlled, twenty-five-year-old mothers are estimated to experience 32 percent greater odds of LBW and 78 percent greater odds of VLBW than fifteen-year-old mothers. Controlling for smoking reduces this increase in the odds of LBW by one-third and in the odds of VLBW by 15 percent. Controlling for either hypertension or high-risk status accounts for only a small share (5 to 10 percent) of the increased odds of LBW or VLBW with advancing maternal age. Controlling for all of the measured maternal health characteristics reduces the increased odds of LBW almost by half, and the effect of maternal age is no longer statistically significant. For VLBW, the increased odds with older maternal age are reduced by 30 percent when all measured health characteristics are controlled, but the maternal age effect remains sizeable and statistically significant.

For whites we estimated linear and curvilinear functions of the effects of maternal age on poor birth outcome. For ease of presentation, we report results from the linear regressions, but in both cases we find little evidence of any effect of postponing childbirth on the risk of LBW or VLBW. However, controlling for smoking during pregnancy strengthens the (small) positive relationship between maternal age and the odds of LBW among whites. The estimated age effect becomes statistically significant and implies a fivefold increase in the odds of LBW when childbirth is postponed from age fifteen to twenty-five.

Although the unadjusted estimates suggest very different maternal age patterns of LBW or VLBW for blacks and whites, when all measured maternal health characteristics are controlled the racial difference in the effects on LBW of postponing childbearing from age fifteen to twenty-five narrows by 80 percent and is statistically insignificant. The difference in VLBW narrows by 20 percent, but remains substantial.

HETEROGENEITY AMONG AFRICAN AMERICANS

To illustrate the implications of the study findings for differences in weathering among blacks by socioeconomic group (that is, to address our second working hypothesis), we calculated selected odds ratios by LBW or VLBW from models including SES × Maternal Age Interactions. We limit this exercise to African Americans also because, using these data, there is no evidence of important maternal age or SES × Maternal Age Effects among whites.

Estimated odds ratios among African Americans by socioeconomic group (low, average, or high) for selected maternal ages relative to age fifteen are shown for LBW in Table 12.5, and for VLBW in Table 12.6. The final bank of columns in each table lists the odds ratios (low SES versus high SES) of LBW or VLBW at selected maternal ages. The top half of each table shows odds ratios

Table 12.5. Selected Odds Ratios (95% Confidence Intervals) of Low Birthweight by Maternal Age and Socioeconomic Status, Unadjusted and Adjusted for Maternal Health Characteristics, African American Singleton First Births, Michigan, 1989

	Odds Ratios (CIs) for Selected Maternal Ages Relative to Age 15			Odds Ratios Low SES/High SES	
Maternal Age	Low SES*	Average SES†	High SES‡	Maternal Age	Low/High
15/15	1.00 (1.00, 1.00)	1.00 (1.00, 1.00)	1.00 (1.00, 1.00)	15	0.85 (0.65, 1.10)
16/15	1.06 (1.04, 1.08)	1.03 (1.01, 1.04)	1.00 (0.97, 1.02)	16	0.90 (0.71, 1.14)
20/15	1.33 (1.19, 1.48)	1.14 (1.05, 1.23)	0.99 (0.88, 1.11)	20	1.14 (0.97, 1.34)
25/15	1.76 (1.42, 2.18)	1.30 (1.11, 1.52)	0.97 (0.77, 1.23)	25	1.53 (1.27, 1.85)
30/15	2.33 (1.69, 3.22)	1.48 (1.17, 1.87)	0.96 (0.67, 1.36)	30	2.06 (1.51, 2.82)
34/15	2.92 (1.94, 4.40)	1.64 (1.22, 2.21)	0.95 (0.60, 1.48)	34	2.62 (1.70, 4.02)

	Odds Ratios (CIs) for Selected Maternal Ages Relative to Age 15 Adjusted for Maternal Health Characteristics§			Odds Ratios Low SES/High SES Adjusted for Maternal Health Characteristics	
Maternal Age	Low SES*	Average SES†	High SES‡	Maternal Age	Low/High
15/15	1.00 (1.00, 1.00)	1.00 (1.00, 1.00)	1.00 (1.00, 1.00)	15	0.87 (0.67, 1.14)
16/15	1.04 (1.02, 1.07)	1.02 (1.00, 1.03)	0.99 (0.97, 1.02)	16	0.92 (0.72, 1.16)
20/15	1.23 (1.11, 1.37)	1.09 (1.01, 1.18)	0.97 (0.86, 1.09)	20	1.11 (0.95, 1.31)
25/15	1.52 (1.23, 1.89)	1.19 (1.01, 1.39)	0.93 (0.74, 1.18)	25	1.42 (1.17, 1.73)
30/15	1.88 (1.36, 2.60)	1.29 (1.02, 1.63)	0.90 (0.63, 1.28)	30	1.82 (1.32, 2.50)
34/15	2.22 (1.48, 3.35)	1.38 (1.03, 1.86)	0.87 (0.56, 1.37)	34	2.21 (1.43, 3.43)

*The typical pattern of odds ratios for black mothers living in zip code areas with mean incomes in the bottom 20% of mean incomes of all zip codes where black study mothers reside (median income = $15,812).

†The typical pattern of odds ratios for black mothers living in zip code areas with mean incomes at the median of mean incomes of all zip code areas where black study mothers reside (median income = $20,215).

‡The typical pattern of odds ratios for black mothers living in zip code areas with mean incomes in the top 20% of mean incomes for all zip code areas where black study mothers reside (median income = $25,606).

§Maternal health characteristics and prenatal care are controlled in these models.

Table 12.6. Selected Odds Ratios (95% Confidence Intervals) of Very Low Birthweight by Maternal Age and Socioeconomic Status, Unadjusted and Adjusted for Maternal Health Characteristics, African American Singleton First Births, Michigan, 1989

Maternal Age	Odds Ratios (CIs) for Selected Maternal Ages Relative to Age 15				Odds Ratios Low SES/High SES	
	Low SES*	Average SES†	High SES‡		Maternal Age	Low/High
15/15	1.00 (1.00, 1.00)	1.00 (1.00, 1.00)	1.00 (1.00, 1.00)		15	0.93 (0.59, 1.46)
16/15	1.07 (1.04, 1.11)	1.06 (1.03, 1.08)	1.04 (1.01, 1.08)		16	0.96 (0.63, 1.44)
20/15	1.43 (1.20, 1.70)	1.32 (1.17, 1.48)	1.22 (1.02, 1.46)		20	1.08 (0.82, 1.44)
25/15	2.04 (1.43, 2.90)	1.74 (1.37, 2.20)	1.49 (1.05, 2.12)		25	1.27 (0.95, 1.69)
30/15	2.91 (1.71, 4.93)	2.29 (1.61, 3.26)	1.82 (1.07, 3.08)		30	1.48 (0.93, 2.36)
34/15	3.86 (1.98, 7.55)	2.85 (1.83, 4.46)	2.13 (1.09, 4.16)		34	1.68 (0.88, 3.20)

Maternal Age	Odds Ratios (CIs) for Selected Maternal Ages Relative to Age 15 Adjusted for Maternal Health Characteristics§				Odds Ratios Low SES/High SES Adjusted for Maternal Health Characteristics	
	Low SES†	Average SES†	High SES‡		Maternal Age	Low/High
15/15	1.00 (1.00, 1.00)	1.00 (1.00, 1.00)	1.00 (1.00, 1.00)		15	0.94 (0.60, 1.49)
16/15	1.06 (1.02, 1.10)	1.05 (1.02, 1.07)	1.04 (1.00, 1.07)		16	0.96 (0.64, 1.46)
20/15	1.32 (1.10, 1.57)	1.25 (1.10, 1.42)	1.19 (1.00, 1.42)		20	1.04 (0.78, 1.39)
25/15	1.74 (1.22, 2.47)	1.57 (1.21, 2.02)	1.42 (1.00, 2.02)		25	1.15 (0.86, 1.55)
30/15	2.29 (1.35, 3.88)	1.96 (1.34, 2.87)	1.69 (1.00, 2.87)		30	1.28 (0.79, 2.05)
34/15	2.85 (1.46, 5.57)	2.35 (1.45, 3.81)	1.94 (1.00, 3.80)		34	1.38 (0.72, 2.67)

*The typical pattern of odds ratios for black mothers living in zip code areas with mean incomes in the bottom 20% of mean incomes of all zip codes where black study mothers reside (median income = $15,812).

†The typical pattern of odds ratios for black mothers living in zip code areas with mean incomes at the median of mean incomes of all zip code areas where black study mothers reside (median income = $20,215).

‡The typical pattern of odds ratios for black mothers living in zip code areas with mean incomes in the top 20% of mean incomes for all zip code areas where black study mothers reside (median income = $25,606).

§Maternal health characteristics and prenatal care are controlled in these models.

unadjusted for maternal health characteristics, while the bottom half shows odds ratios adjusted for maternal health characteristics.

The odds of LBW among blacks increase with maternal age, but the pattern is not uniform with respect to socioeconomic group. The increase is more dramatic for women in the lower SES category than at the median; while in the high-SES category, there is essentially no change with maternal age in the odds of low birthweight. Among those in the lower SES category, by age twenty, black mothers experience 1.33 times the odds of LBW as black fifteen-year-old mothers; by age thirty, the odds are 2.33 times larger than at age fifteen; and by age thirty-four the odds are almost three times the odds at age fifteen. Adjusting for the measured maternal health conditions accounts for a noteworthy share of the increase in the low-SES group. For example, 37 percent of the odds ratio for ages 34/15 is accounted for by maternal health characteristics.

Looking at the final bank of columns, we see the gap between low-SES mothers and high-SES mothers in their odds of LBW is estimated to be three times larger for thirty-four-year-old mothers than for those age fifteen. At age thirty-four, 25 percent of the excess odds of LBW experienced by mothers in low-SES areas compared to those in high-SES areas is accounted for by the measured maternal health characteristics.

The patterns for VLBW show that for all SES categories the odds of VLBW increase with age, but that the increase is most dramatic in the lowest SES category, where the odds increase almost fourfold between ages fifteen and thirty-four. Adjusting for maternal health characteristics accounts for 35 percent of this odds ratio. At age thirty-four, 44 percent of the difference between residents of low-SES and residents of high-SES areas is accounted for by such adjustment. However, in the comparisons between low- and high-SES areas, the point estimates approach statistical significance at the older maternal ages, but the confidence intervals are large and, unlike in the case of LBW, the null hypothesis of no difference cannot be rejected at the 0.05 level. (This imprecision may be the product of small sample sizes for VLBW or measurement error in the SES proxy).

SUMMARY AND DISCUSSION

Among African American mothers in Michigan, but not among white mothers, maternal age is statistically significantly and positively related to the odds of LBW and VLBW. The relationship between advancing maternal age and poor infant outcome is stronger among black mothers in low socioeconomic groups than in others, with a notable share of this interaction effect explained by the measured maternal health characteristics. These findings are consistent with the theoretical perspective that among the socioeconomically disadvantaged, black women's health deteriorates more rapidly over the young adult ages than does the health of the advantaged, and contributes to their increasing risk with age of low and very low birthweight. While the study design cannot provide a direct test of the mechanisms that link socioeconomic group to poor maternal health, the fact that this pattern is more pronounced among members of low socioeconomic groups than on average suggests these groups' adverse health characteristics may be related to hardships associated with social inequality.

On average, rates of maternal health characteristics that are risk factors for poor birth outcome increase with age more rapidly among black compared to white mothers. Moreover, almost all of the maternal age dimension to black-white differences in the odds of LBW is explained by these adverse maternal health characteristics. Such findings suggest an important social dimension to black-white differences in rates of poor birth outcome that is mediated through differences in the health or health behaviors of young women.

Among whites, there is little evidence to suggest weathering. Several factors may explain this. In Michigan, white mothers of any age are much less likely than blacks to live in very low SES areas. Even among teen mothers, almost three-quarters of whites live in areas with family incomes above the black median. This suggests the possibility that few whites may be exposed to the same degree of health insult as blacks. Methodologically, it raises the question whether the census-based approach for measuring socioeconomic group is adequate for the study of disadvantaged whites. Alternatively, important contributors to weathering that may differentially affect blacks and whites may not be captured by income variables alone. Lower purchasing power at specific incomes among blacks, racism, and race bias in exposures to childbearing hazards are examples of reasons why African Americans may exhibit greater evidence of weathering than whites.[14,23] The differential maternal age patterns of smoking between blacks and whites also help explain why the findings are consistent with weathering among blacks, but not whites, at least for patterns of LBW. As we later discuss, whether smoking should be thought of as an isolatable risk factor or also as a symptom of or response to underlying social processes is itself open to question and merits further investigation.

Due to data constraints, the effects of deteriorating maternal health on poor birth outcome among low-SES African Americans may be underestimated. First, underreporting of adverse health conditions on birth certificates is likely to be excessive among black or socioeconomically disadvantaged mothers relative to others.[19] The effect of differential underreporting would be to dampen estimated differences in risk by race or socioeconomic status. To mitigate this limitation, we controlled for prenatal care receipt in all models that included maternal health characteristics. However, our approach to using the prenatal care information may itself result in downward-biased estimates of the effects of maternal health characteristics on birth outcome. To the degree that obtaining adequate care will reflect not only access, but also the propensity of mothers in ill health to seek medical care, including prenatal care, in the model may represent overcontrol. To the extent that receipt of adequate plus care represents not only need but also access, the association between poor health and birth outcome may be understated.

Among African Americans, the maternal age and social gradients in risk appear to be more severe for VLBW than for LBW and less about them is explained by the measured maternal health characteristics. Given the estimated severity of these gradients for VLBW, the fact the VLBW infants account for over 60 percent of the black-white disparity in infant mortality,[24] and these infants' disproportionate risk of early childhood morbidity and functional impairment,[25] determining whether these findings imply that VLBW and LBW have different etiologies with respect to maternal health characteristics and socioeconomic disadvantage is important. Progress in answering this question must await further analysis with larger samples or better measures. It may be that the information on maternal health characteristics was less reliable for mothers of VLBW infants than for others, because of their greater likelihood of being from low socioeconomic groups or of experiencing preterm birth. While unable to shed clear light on the mechanisms, the study findings do indicate that contrary to conventional wisdom, the odds of VLBW among African American women in Michigan are substantially higher among older compared to younger mothers, especially in low socioeconomic groups.

As is true nationally, black and white women in Michigan have different fertility timing distributions, with blacks relatively more likely to experience early first births and whites more likely to experience births at relatively older ages. Thus, differential selection into age at first birth may provide an alternative interpretation of the results. However, if the age patterns of maternal health characteristics reflected only such selection, one would expect to find qualitatively different age patterns of adverse health characteristics among the population of reproductive age women as a whole. This is not the case. In national samples, the prevalence of hypertension and of cigarette smoking follows the same age patterns by race among nonpregnant women of reproductive age as those observed in this study population of mothers.[18]

The maternal age-race smoking patterns showing older black mothers to be more apt to smoke during pregnancy than black teen mothers are also consistent with those found in a national sample of mothers[17] and in a hospital sample in Baltimore.[26] In part, these patterns may represent cohort effects, as smoking prevalence among teenagers appears to have decreased in recent years.[27] While absolute proportions of women smoking by given ages may have changed over time, the general differential age patterns of smoking by race have been confirmed across cohorts.[18]

The extent to which smoking during pregnancy explains the differential maternal age patterns of LBW or VLBW between blacks and whites is notable. Black mothers are more likely to smoke at older ages than at younger ones, and smoking accounts for one-third of the estimated maternal age effect on LBW and 15 percent of the effect for VLBW. The lack of an overall maternal age affect among whites appears to be due to the greater prevalence of cigarette smoking among white teen mothers relative to older mothers. Once smoking is accounted for, the odds of bearing LBW babies are statistically significantly lower among younger white mothers than among older ones.

Taken at face value, these results suggest that reducing cigarette smoking among white teen or older black mothers could greatly diminish the differential maternal age patterns of low birthweight, highlighting the need for age-appropriate antitobacco interventions. Many antitobacco interventions target youth or are school based.[28] However, among black women, additional components of an effective antitobacco strategy to target young adults are necessary.

From the weathering conceptual perspective, it is also important to learn what psychosocial processes result in different age patterns of smoking among black and white women or mothers. One might wonder whether in a social or cultural context, smoking uptake among black women in their twenties has a rationale. One speculation is that excessive rates of smoking among African American women in their twenties and early thirties may be indicative of excessive rates of psychosocial stress to which smoking may be a response.[18] Advertising strategies by tobacco companies targeting female, working-class, and minority audiences may also augment the chances that African American women use smoking as one way to alleviate stress.[29] The structural sources of the stress, the stress itself, or the physical toll taken by actively coping with stress over a prolonged period may be unobserved factors that also contribute to the maternal age patterns of poor birth outcome among African Americans.[15,18] If this were the case, the smoking coefficient could be capturing some of these effects as well as any effects of smoking per se. Qualitative or survey research strategies may be critical sources of information on these or alternative possibilities.

Unlike smoking or all adverse health characteristics combined, accounting only for the specific risk factor of hypertension or high-risk status does not alter the estimated maternal age effect appreciably. The lack of explanatory power attributed to hypertension or to being high risk is surprising. It may reflect general or differential underreporting of medical conditions on birth certificates.[19] For example, hypertension prevalence rates for the study population are noticeably lower than national averages for reproductive-age women.[30] In addition, because we control for prenatal care receipt in our models and define high risk according to intensive prenatal care receipt, it may be due to the fact that current prenatal care regimens are able to avert the worst sequelae of these risks, but are not as effective in addressing the risk imposed by smoking. That is, the effects of the health conditions are most appropriately interpreted as estimates of their effects *given adequate prenatal care.* These effects may understate the contribution of these health conditions to poor birth outcome among the medically underserved.

The study findings also contribute to ongoing discussion of the relationship of older maternal age to birth outcome. Berkowitz et al.[31] found that among predominantly white, private patients at a tertiary hospital, advanced maternal age was associated with a somewhat higher rate of pregnancy and delivery complications but not with a statistically significantly increased rate of poor neonatal outcome. The current study results raise questions about the generalizability of these results to socioeconomically disadvantaged African American women or to women who do not give birth at tertiary centers. Overall, these findings suggest limitations to the conceptual approach that treats maternal age as if it represents primarily a universal developmental process rather than also being reflective of social processes that either affect selection into age at first birth or the impact of social inequality on women's health over time—that is, with age. For example, the results suggest that whether older maternal age is higher or lower risk than younger maternal age varies by race and socioeconomic status. In addition, maternal age appears to be a marker for different health and behavioral risk profiles in different populations. Of interest, the populations in which early births are most common are those where early births are the lowest risk, raising questions about the social construction of teen childbearing as a universally deleterious behavior.[18,32,33]

Clinically, these findings raise questions about the validity of routine clinical screening protocols that apply demographic risk characteristics uniformly to estimate risk status in pregnancy. The findings suggest the potential importance of targeting clinical interventions to the needs of socioeconomically disadvantaged African American primiparous women in their twenties and early thirties as one means to reduce the racial disparity in low and very low birthweight and infant mortality. More fundamentally, the study findings suggest the importance of comprehensive prevention strategies to improve the general health of socioeconomically disadvantaged women before they become pregnant, perhaps with special emphasis on smoking prevention and cessation, and of social change strategies that reduce social inequalities that affect health.

Notes

1. U.S. Department of Health and Human Services. (1985). *Report of the Secretary's Task Force on Black and Minority Health: Vol. 1. Executive summary.* Washington, DC: U.S. Government Printing Office.

2. Wise, P. H., & Pursley, D. M. (1992). Infant mortality as a social mirror. *N Engl J Med, 326,* 1558.

3. U.S. Public Health Service. (1991). *Healthy people 2000: National health promotion and disease prevention objectives: Full report, with commentary* (DHHS Pub. No. (PHS) 91-50212). Washington, DC: U.S. Government Printing Office.

4. Baldwin, W. (1986). Half empty, half full: What we know about low birth weight among blacks. *JAMA, 255,* 86.

5. Hogue, C.J.R. (1989). Preterm delivery: Can we lower the black infant's first hurdle? *JAMA, 262,* 548.

6. Burrow, G. N., & Ferris, T. F. (Eds.). (1988). *Medical complications during pregnancy* (3rd ed.). Philadelphia: W. B. Saunders.

7. Kleinman, J. C., & Kessel, S. S. (1987). Racial differences in low birthweight: Trends and risk factors. *N Engl J Med, 317,* 749.

8. Institute of Medicine. (1985). *Preventing low birthweight.* Washington, DC: National Academy Press.

9. Eberstein, I. W. (1989). Demographic research on infant mortality. *Soc Forum, 4,* 409.

10. Schoendorf, K. C., Hogue, C.J.R., Kleinman, J.C., & Rowley, D. R. (1992). Mortality among infants of black compared with white college-educated parents. *N Engl J Med, 326,* 1522.

11. Institute of Medicine and National Research Council. (1982). *Research issues in the assessment of birth settings.* Washington, DC: National Academy Press.

12. Molfese, V. J. (1989). *Perinatal risk and infant development: Assessment and prediction.* New York: Guilford Press.

13. Geronimus, A. T. (1986). The effects of race, residence, and prenatal care on the relationship of maternal age to neonatal mortality. *Am J Public Health, 76,* 1416.

14. David, R. J., & Collins, J. W. (1991). Bad outcomes in black babies: Race or racism? *Ethn Dis, 1,* 236.

15. James, S. A. (1993). Racial and ethnic differences in infant mortality and low birth weight: A psychosocial critique. *Ann Epidemiol, 3,* 130.

16. Ahmed, F. (1989). Urban-suburban differences in the incidence of low birthweight in a metropolitan black population. *J Natl Med Assoc, 81,* 849.

17. Geronimus, A. T., & Korenman, S. (1992). Maternal youth or family background? On the health disadvantages of infants with teenage mothers. *Am J Epidemiol, 137,* 213.

18. Geronimus, A. T. (1992). The weathering hypothesis and the health of African-American women and infants: Evidence and speculations. *Ethn Dis, 2,* 207.

19. Buescher, P. A., Taylor, K. P., Davis, M. H., & Bowling, J. M. (1993). The quality of the new birth certificate data: A validation study in North Carolina. *Am J Public Health, 83,* 1163.

20. Geronimus, A. T., Bound, J., & Neidert, L. (1993). *On the validity of using census geocode characteristics to proxy economic status* (Research Report No. 93-269). University of Michigan, Population Studies Center.

21. Wolter, K. M. (1985). *Introduction to variance estimation.* Berlin: Springer.

22. Kotelchuck, M. (1994). Adequacy of Prenatal Care Utilization index: Its U.S. distribution and association with low birthweight. *Am J Public Health, 84,* 1486.

23. Williams, D. R., Lavizzo-Mourey, R., & Warren, R. C. (1994). The concept of race and health status in America. *Public Health Rep, 109,* 26.

24. Iyasu, S., Becerra, J. E., Rowley, D. L., & Hogue, C.J.R. (1992). Impact of very low birthweight on the black-white infant mortality gap. *Am J Prev Med, 8,* 271.

25. McCormick, M. C., Brooks-Gunn, J., Workman-Daniels, K., Turner, J., & Peckham, G. J. (1992). The health and developmental status of very low-birth-weight children at school age. *JAMA, 267,* 2204.

26. McCarthy, J., & Hardy, J. (in press). Age at first birth and birth outcomes. *J Adolesc.*

27. U.S. Department of Health and Human Services. (1989). *Reducing the health consequences of smoking: 25 years of progress: A report of the Surgeon General* (DHHS Publication No. (CDC) 89-8411). Atlanta: Centers for Disease Control, Center for Chronic Disease Prevention and Health Promotion, Office of Smoking and Health.

28. U.S. Public Health Service. (1990). *Promoting health/preventing disease: Year 2000 objectives for the nation.* Washington, DC: U.S. Government Printing Office.

29. Davis, R. (1987). Current trends in cigarette advertising and marketing. *N Engl J Med, 316,* 725.

30. Geronimus, A. T., Andersen, H. F., & Bound, J. (1991). Differences in hypertension prevalence among U.S. black and white women of childbearing age. *Public Health Rep, 106,* 393.

31. Berkowitz, G. S., Skovron, M. L., Lapinski, R. H., & Berkowitz, R. L. (1990). Delayed childbearing and the outcome of pregnancy. *N Engl J Med, 322,* 659.

32. Blaxter, M. (1983). Health services as a defense against the consequences of poverty in industrialized societies. *Soc Sci Med, 17,* 1139.

33. Phoenix, A. (1991). *Young mothers?* Cambridge, UK: Polity Press.

CHAPTER THIRTEEN

Immigration and the Health of Asian and Pacific Islander Adults in the United States

W. Parker Frisbie
Youngtae Cho
Robert A. Hummer

The Asian and Pacific Islander population more than doubled in the United States during the 1980s (growth rate, 107.8 percent), making it the fastest growing race/ethnic group, followed by Hispanics (growth rate, 53 percent).[1] Rapid growth continues, with another doubling predicted by the U.S. Census Bureau by 2009.[2,3] Three-fourths of the Asian and Pacific Islander population growth has been due to immigration.[4] While notable from a strictly demographic standpoint, the heavy concentration of immigrants in the Asian and Pacific Islander population may have health implications that are particularly crucial. Evidence exists that the health of white and Hispanic immigrants is superior to that of their U.S.-born coethnics, and similar findings are beginning to appear regarding black immigrants. A lower mortality risk has been observed for immigrants compared with their U.S.-born counterparts, whether the comparisons are of adult mortality or of infants born to mothers distinguished according to nativity.[5-11]

Unfortunately, studies of the health of Asian and Pacific Islander immigrants based on nationally representative data are rare. Compared with other U.S. minorities, there has generally been little research on the Asian and Pacific Islander population, which has been described as "one of the most poorly

The authors gratefully acknowledge the support provided for this research by the National Institute of Child Health and Human Development (Grant RO1 HD36249). The authors also thank Starling G. Pullum for her insightful comments and computing assistance.

understood minorities [whose] health problems and health care needs have not been adequately recognized or addressed" (p. 26).[12,13] Furthermore, because of a lack of data sets large enough to enable intraethnic distinctions to be made in multivariate analyses, most previous research has analyzed the Asian and Pacific Islander population as an undifferentiated whole, masking the high degree of heterogeneity known (or suspected) to exist across national origin groups with respect to socioeconomic status, immigrant status, health status, and cultural characteristics.[14,15]

The feasibility of studying the health of *specific* Asian and Pacific Islander groups has been enhanced materially now that data generated by the National Health Interview Survey (NHIS) from 1992 onward have recently become available for research. An "advance data" report[3] based on these new data (pooled for 1992–1994) appeared in a 1998 publication of the U.S. Department of Health and Human Services; these data indicated that Asian and Pacific Islander sub-populations are dissimilar with respect to health conditions as well as socio-economic and demographic characteristics. However, the purpose of advance reports is to provide timely descriptions, not to model outcomes. A later study, which pooled 1986–1994 NHIS data but did not analyze specific Asian and Pacific Islander groups, indicated that the Asian and Pacific Islander population as a whole was very similar to whites with regard to the sex-specific and age-adjusted percentages in poor or fair health.[16] Neither of these highly informative studies investigated the impact of immigration on health.

The great diversity within the Asian and Pacific Islander population is associated with two different immigrant streams. The first is from countries that already have relatively large populations in the United States—consisting of, for example, Chinese, Filipinos, Japanese, Koreans, and, increasingly, Asian Indians—who tend on average to be highly educated and skilled (even when compared with the white majority).[17] The second stream consists of lower socioeconomic status groups and includes large numbers of refugees from Southeast Asian countries such as Vietnam.[4] Asians and Pacific Islanders in the former group seem to be healthier on average than those in the latter group,[3] and important differences within as well as between these two migration streams are almost certain to exist. It is quite likely, then, that immigrant status (both whether persons are foreign born or U.S. born [nativity] and time spent in the United States since immigration [duration]) is crucial to understanding health variations in the Asian and Pacific Islander population.

Prior research suggests two explanations for the health and mortality advantages of foreign-born persons: positive selection of immigrants and cultural "buffering." The first explanation hypothesizes that migration is selective of healthier and more robust persons.[9,18] The second suggests that compared with the United States, other cultures (at least Hispanic cultures) are more likely to be characterized by norms and values proscribing risky behaviors (for example, smoking, abuse of alcohol or drugs) and promoting healthy behaviors, including stronger familial and social support networks and better nutrition.[7,8,19,20] These hypotheses should be viewed as complementary rather than competing; that is, if positive selection does play a prominent role, immigrants—if all other relevant factors do not change—should be healthier than the native born. In addition, if the cultural interpretation is also valid, not only would immigrants be healthier but their advantage would also erode over time as acculturation to U.S. society proceeded. In other words, the validity and complementarity of the two propositions would be supported by the observation that immigrants are healthier than their U.S.-born counterparts and that, among immigrants, there is a gradient such that health declines with duration in this country.[21] To test the two hypotheses, the number of years an immigrant has been in the United States must be included in analytical models.

Accordingly, the primary objective of our research was to examine the effect of immigrant status (both nativity and duration) on the health of Asians and Pacific Islanders by constructing models in which national origin was covariate. This examination enabled us to test the two hypotheses and to provide, to our knowledge, the first assessment of immigrant status on variation in multiple indicators of health across specific Asian and Pacific Islander adult populations, taking into account the effects of immigrant status.

MATERIALS AND METHODS

Data were drawn from the NHIS data pooled for 1992–1995, the earliest and latest dates for which the information necessary for this analysis was available. Roughly 49,000 households, yielding approximately 125,000 persons of all ages, are included in the NHIS each year, and information is gathered about each person's health and sociodemographic characteristics.[22] The large size and consistency of the NHIS is especially important for calculating nationally representative health estimates for relatively small populations, in that these estimates can be made across multiple years of data collection.[22,23] Response rates are excellent, ranging from 96 to 98 percent. Throughout our study, we applied weights provided by the National Center for Health Statistics to take into account both sampling characteristics and nonresponse, as described in detail elsewhere.[24]

With the exception of family income, the amount of missing data for all variables included in this study was negligible. Income information was missing for about 17 percent of respondents. To evaluate the possibility of bias introduced by the missing income data, parallel regressions were performed in which income was first included and then excluded; the result was that no changes in our conclusions were required whether the cases for whom income was missing were included or not. Hence, following previous research, we included a missing category in the variable for operationalization of income.[11,25] SUDAAN software was used to produce standard errors and confidence intervals appropriate to the survey design.[26]

We focused on the health of persons aged twenty-five years or older, which yielded a sample of 8,249 Asians and Pacific Islanders plus more than 208,000 whites, with the latter included in the descriptive analysis only (for reasons mentioned below). Following presentation of descriptive results, the greatest attention was given to the relation between immigrant status and health indicators, adjusting for the effects of covariates shown or hypothesized to affect health status. Net effects were estimated by using logistic regression and were reported in the form of odds ratios (ORs); significance levels and confidence intervals were computed by using Wald statistics.[27] The white majority was not included in the regression models because of the likelihood that the much larger size of that group would overwhelm and obfuscate the associations involving Asians and Pacific Islanders. However, all multivariate models were reestimated with whites first included in and then omitted from the regression analysis, and the general conclusions regarding the impact of immigrant status remained the same.

From 1992 through 1995, the NHIS enabled ten specific Asian and Pacific Islander populations to be identified. In our study, we distinguished eight groups: Chinese, Filipino, Asian Indian, Japanese, Korean, Vietnamese, Pacific Islander, and Other Asians. It was possible to identify Hawaiians, Guamanians, and Samoans separately, but these groups taken separately represented too few cases for multivariate modeling and so were combined with other even smaller Pacific Islander populations. Even so, the number of Pacific Islanders was so small that we could draw only tentative conclusions for that group. The Other Asian category is a residual that allows no further race/ethnic subdivisions. Refugee groups from Southeast Asia (for example, Cambodia and Laos) make up a nonnegligible portion of this category.

The immigration variable was divided into four categories: native born; immigrant, duration zero to four years; immigrant, duration five to nine years; and immigrant, duration ten years or more. This specification is similar to that used in the 1998 National Center for Health Statistics advance data report[3] as well as in other publications (for example, the article by LeClere, Jensen, and Biddlecom[28]). Most crucial perhaps is the five-year duration cut point, because five years must elapse before an immigrant to the United States can obtain citizenship (spouses of citizens may become naturalized within three years). The advance data report also identified immigrants residing in the United States for less than one year and for more than fifteen years. However, the small number of cases in the former category prevented its use in our multivariate analysis, and our ancillary research (not shown) made it clear that the effects associated with residence of fifteen years or more were quite similar to those obtained when duration was top-coded at ten years.

We focused on three health outcomes. The first was respondent-reported health assessment, for which the possible responses were *poor, fair, good, very good,* and *excellent.* Following recent research,[16] we collapsed this measure into two categories: (1) poor and fair, and (2) good, very good, and excellent. Also of interest was whether the normal daily activities of adults were limited by disability, and we drew on the NHIS "activity limitation status" item to distinguish those persons with some activity limitation from those with no limitation. We also included information on the annual number of days spent in bed because of illness. Spending even one day in bed suggests an illness of at least modest severity, and being bedridden for a week or more would appear to indicate a more serious condition. All of the health items were based on self-reports, which have repeatedly been demonstrated to be both useful indicators of actual health status and predictors of mortality risk.[16,29,30]

We also examined the effects of Asian and Pacific Islander group membership and immigrant status on the annual number of visits to a physician and a measure of regular access to health care. Although the issue of access was not the primary focus of our research, for more than a decade there has been concern about whether the Asian and Pacific Islander population is inadequately served by the U.S. health care system.[12,30] Particularly relevant for our present purposes was the possibility that immigrants may be especially underserved[27,31] and that duration of residence may affect immigrant access to medical care.[27,28] Providing a substantive interpretation of variation in physician visits is complicated, because this variable plausibly can be viewed as either a proxy measure of health status or an indicator of access to health care, or both. Physician visits were divided into three categories: none, one or two, and three or more. Many persons in excellent health may elect to have regular preventive examinations, but several visits to a physician in any one year could also indicate health problems. It might be reasonable to view three or more visits to a physician in a year as a marker for some degree of ill health, one or two visits as normal access, and no visits as indicative of inadequate access. Unfortunately, the conceptual problem remains the same: that is, such an approach quickly leads to the confounding of health status with access to health care. Thus, we also included a direct indicator of access to health care (from data available in NHIS supplements for 1993–1995) that drew upon the item that inquired whether respondents had a usual person/place for medical care. Responses indicating one or more regular sources of care were coded "yes," those who reported no regular source were coded "no," and cases for whom data were missing were omitted. Health status was controlled in multivariate models when the effects of immigrant status on physician visits and regular source of medical care were estimated.

The associations of interest were adjusted by using a wide range of variables, including sex, age, marital status, living arrangement, family size, educational level, family income, and employment status, each of which has been demonstrated to have important effects on the health of adults or to be useful as a control when estimating the effects of other variables on health.[4,14,16,17,28,31] As evident in the tables that follow, measurement of the control variables was conventional and straightforward.

RESULTS

Heterogeneity of the Asian and Pacific Islander Population

Table 13.1 documents the great diversity in demographic and socioeconomic characteristics of the Asian and Pacific Islander populations and compares this population with non-Hispanic whites (hereafter referred to as whites). As shown, the family income of Japanese respondents exceeded that of all other groups, including whites, but the Chinese, Filipinos, Koreans, and especially Asian Indians surpassed the Japanese (and whites) in the proportion with a college degree. Vietnamese and Other Asians were the most disadvantaged with respect to education and income. Given our focus on persons aged twenty-five years or older, the variation in age was quite large. Mean age ranged from forty years for Asian Indians and Other Asians to almost fifty years for Japanese. Divorce and separation were uncommon among Asians and Pacific Islanders, ranging from a low of 2 percent among Asian Indians to 10 percent among Pacific Islanders (and whites). As might be expected on the basis of their recent history of war and immigration, Vietnamese were more likely than other Asian and Pacific Islander groups to live with a person other than a spouse and to have the largest mean family size (4.4 members per family compared with the low average of 2.7 and 2.8 for whites and Japanese, respectively). Obviously, then, it was necessary to adjust for these differences before we could specify the effect of immigrant status on the health of Asian and Pacific Islander populations.

Distributions of Immigration Status and Outcome Variables

The age-adjusted immigrant status of the Asian and Pacific Islander groups (Table 13.2) corresponded well with that anticipated on the basis of the immigration history of these populations. The proportion of U.S.-born Asian Indians, Koreans, and Vietnamese was very low (5.5 percent or less). Approximately 60 percent of Pacific Islanders and Japanese were U.S. born, which is not surprising given the fact that many Pacific Islanders (for example, Hawaiians) are U.S. citizens at birth and that substantial numbers of second- and later-generation Japanese Americans already resided in this country at the beginning of World War II.[32] Only very small proportions of whites were immigrants. There were only moderate differences in the proportions of medium- and long-term Asian and Pacific Islander immigrants (durations of five to nine and ten or more years, respectively). The largest proportions of very recent immigrants

Table 13.1. Distributions of Demographic and Socioeconomic Status Characteristics of Adults, by National Origin,
National Health Interview Survey, 1992–1995 Combined

Characteristic	White	Japanese	Chinese	Filipino	Korean	Asian Indian	Pacific Islander	Vietnamese	Other Asian
Sex (%)									
Male	47.9	41.5	48.8	41.9	42.1	56.5	50.9	50.2	47.3
Female	52.1	58.5	51.2	58.1	57.9	43.5	49.1	49.8	52.7
Age (mean) (years)	48.9	49.6	44.0	44.9	42.4	40.2	44.3	40.9	40.1
Marital status (%)									
Married	72.6	68.9	76.1	75.8	79.6	83.5	70.4	73.1	75.9
Widowed	8.3	8.4	5.0	5.6	5.1	3.2	4.8	4.0	4.5
Divorced or separated	9.7	7.4	3.8	5.4	5.1	2.0	9.9	5.6	6.8
Never married	9.4	15.2	15.2	13.2	10.2	11.3	14.9	17.3	12.8
Living arrangement (%)									
Live alone	15.4	14.3	8.7	5.2	8.9	6.6	8.9	2.7	6.2
Live with relative or nonrelative	13.0	18.5	19.3	23.5	14.2	13.8	21.9	27.6	20.5
Live with spouse	71.6	67.2	72.1	71.3	76.9	79.5	69.3	69.8	73.3
Mean family size (no. of persons)	2.7	2.8	3.4	4.0	3.2	3.5	3.9	4.4	4.0

(Continued)

Table 13.1. Distributions of Demographic and Socioeconomic Status Characteristics of Adults, by National Origin, National Health Interview Survey, 1992–1995 Combined (Continued)

Characteristic	White	Japanese	Chinese	Filipino	Korean	Asian Indian	Pacific Islander	Vietnamese	Other Asian
Educational level (%)									
Less than high school	16.4	9.1	18.3	11.0	12.1	10.5	18.5	28.0	32.0
High school graduate	38.4	31.4	22.8	19.5	28.0	16.8	47.9	30.5	27.3
Some college	20.8	24.0	13.7	21.5	18.9	13.1	23.4	18.5	17.6
College or more	24.5	35.5	45.3	48.1	41.0	59.5	10.2	23.1	23.1
Family income (%)									
<$10,000	5.8	3.0	7.3	3.2	5.7	4.5	5.1	9.7	8.6
$10,000–$19,999	13.2	6.5	12.3	8.9	11.9	11.8	12.0	15.3	20.5
$20,000–$34,999	21.7	15.5	17.0	17.8	22.8	17.3	20.4	15.9	26.2
≥$35,000	43.1	56.9	44.5	55.6	35.4	52.9	50.5	37.3	29.3
Data missing	16.2	18.2	18.9	14.5	24.2	13.4	12.1	21.8	15.4
Employment status (%)									
Employed	64.6	63.0	66.9	75.3	65.6	72.3	70.1	64.7	64.2
Unemployed	2.4	1.6	2.6	2.8	2.1	2.9	2.7	2.6	4.4
Not in labor force	33.0	35.5	30.6	21.9	32.4	24.9	27.2	32.7	31.4
All persons (no.)	208,393	1,015	1,965	1,753	773	997	264	785	697

Note: Except for rounding error, percentages sum to 100.0%; age and family size were measured as continuous variables.

Table 13.2 Age-Adjusted Percentage Distributions of Migration Status and Health Status of Asians and Pacific Islanders, by National Origin, National Health Interview Survey, 1992–1995 Combined

	White	Japanese	Chinese	Filipino	Korean	Asian Indian	Pacific Islander	Vietnamese	Other Asian
Migration status (%)									
0–4 years	0.5	10.4	19.1	14.5	15.4	21.7	4.7	27.1	12.0
5–9 years	0.4	3.6	16.5	16.9	19.4	24.2	4.7	15.7	14.5
≥10 years	3.7	25.2	51.1	58.2	59.7	51.6	28.4	53.9	61.1
U.S. born	95.5	60.8	13.3	10.4	5.5	2.5	62.2	3.3	12.4
Self-reported health status (%)									
Poor or fair	13.0	8.2	11.4	11.9	17.0	14.4	21.1	24.2	17.6
Good, very good, or excellent	87.0	91.8	88.6	88.1	83.0	85.6	78.9	75.8	82.4
Activity limitation (%)									
Yes	20.4	12.0	10.3	14.4	11.3	13.2	23.3	17.4	16.0
No	79.6	88.0	89.7	85.6	88.7	86.8	76.7	82.6	84.0
Annual bed days (%)									
≥7	13.2	10.9	7.9	11.2	11.0	13.5	21.2	12.9	10.4
1–6	29.8	31.6	23.8	28.8	22.2	24.7	28.3	25.9	25.3
None	56.9	57.6	68.3	60.0	66.7	61.8	50.5	61.2	64.3

(Continued)

Table 13.2 Age-Adjusted Percentage Distributions of Migration Status and Health Status of Asians and Pacific Islanders, by National Origin, National Health Interview Survey, 1992–1995 Combined (Continued)

	White	Japanese	Chinese	Filipino	Korean	Asian Indian	Pacific Islander	Vietnamese	Other Asian
Annual physician visits (%)									
≥3	40.8	36.9	30.1	32.6	30.8	36.8	38.7	40.6	38.6
1 or 2	36.4	38.0	36.0	42.1	32.8	33.9	36.1	33.4	28.8
None	22.7	25.1	33.8	25.3	36.4	29.4	25.2	26.0	32.6
Access to health care* (%)									
No	12.5	12.3	23.4	10.0	25.2	19.9	12.5	14.5	20.1
Yes	87.5	87.7	76.6	90.0	74.8	80.1	87.5	85.5	79.9
All persons (no.)	208,393	1,015	1,965	1,753	773	997	264	785	697

Note: Except for rounding error, percentages sum to 100.0%.

*National Health Interview Survey Access to Health Care Supplement, 1993–1995 combined.

were from Vietnam, India, and China, among whom one-fifth to one-fourth had been in the United States for less than five years.

Table 13.2 also shows the age-adjusted percentages of persons in various health status categories. By far the poorest conditions were found among Vietnamese and Pacific Islanders, who reported their health to be fair or worse in 24.2 and 21.1 percent of the cases, respectively. All other Asian and Pacific Islander populations reported a health status that was fairly similar, and sometimes superior, to that of whites. The latter finding was consistent with most previous research[3] and suggested that there was little analytical leverage to be gained by making whites the reference group in the logistic regression analysis that followed. Asians and Pacific Islanders appeared to be less affected by activity limitations than whites were. Only Pacific Islanders, at 23.3 percent, exceeded the level of limitations reported by whites, while the proportions in the other groups ranged fairly narrowly between 10.3 and 17.4 percent.

Over one-fifth of Pacific Islanders reported a week or more spent in bed annually, a figure about 8 percentage points higher than that for whites, Asian Indians, and Vietnamese and approximately twice as high as the proportion for other Asian and Pacific Islander populations. Only 50.5 percent of Pacific Islanders had zero bed days; in other groups, the range was from about 57 percent (Japanese and whites) to 68.3 percent (Chinese). The modal category for annual physician visits was three or more for whites and for five of the Asian and Pacific Islander groups (around 40 percent for all six groups). For Japanese, Chinese, and Filipinos, one or two visits was the most frequent response. Only among Koreans was zero visits to a physician the mode. The Chinese and Koreans were least likely to have regular access to health care. Roughly three-fourths of adults in these two groups reported a regular source of medical care as compared with 80 to 90 percent for each of the other groups.

Cross-tabulations were constructed of health variables, by immigrant status, for the entire Asian and Pacific Islander population taken as a whole (not shown; data available from the authors upon request) because the conclusions from these cross-tabulations were identical to those that emerged from the unadjusted (baseline) models (Tables 13.3 and 13.4). In any event, it was the net or adjusted associations that were of primary interest.

Effects of Immigrant Status and National Origin on Health

Baseline Model. As shown in the top panel of Table 13.3, which presents the analysis of the unadjusted association between immigrant status and health of the Asian and Pacific Islander population *considered as a whole,* immigrants were significantly less likely than their U.S.-born counterparts to have activity limitations or to report any bed days. In the unadjusted model, immigrants were *more* likely to report that their health was only poor or fair. Although the associations were not statistically significant, this finding was inconsistent with those that immigrants are much less at risk of activity limitations and of being

Table 13.3 Odds Ratios for the Effects of Immigrant Status on the Health of Asian and Pacific Islanders (n = 8,249), National Health Interview Survey, 1992–1995 Combined

	Self-Reported Health, Fair or Poor		Activity Limitation, Yes		Bed Days			
					1-6 Days		≥1 Week	
	OR†	95% CI†	OR	95% CI	OR	95% CI	OR	95% CI
Unadjusted model								
Immigrant status (U.S. born)								
0–4 years	1.06	0.83, 1.35	0.56**	0.42, 0.73	0.62**	0.51, 0.75	0.51**	0.39, 0.68
5–9 years	1.11	0.82, 1.50	0.60**	0.43, 0.83	0.68**	0.55, 0.85	0.50**	0.38, 0.66
≥10 years	1.20	0.97, 1.48	0.76***	0.62, 0.92	0.75***	0.63, 0.90	0.67***	0.55, 0.80
Intercept	-2.23**		-1.84**		-0.53**		-1.45**	
-2 log-likelihood	4.17		29.73**		62.17***			
Adjusted model‡								
Immigrant status (U.S. born)								
0–4 years	0.69*	0.49, 0.96	0.45**	0.33, 0.62	0.61**	0.51, 0.74	0.45**	0.32, 0.64
5–9 years	0.94	0.63, 1.42	0.65**	0.46, 0.93	0.70**	0.55, 0.87	0.51**	0.35, 0.74
≥10 years	0.95	0.66, 1.37	0.73***	0.60, 0.90	0.77**	0.64, 0.91	0.68**	0.53, 0.87

National origin (Japanese)

	OR	CI	OR	CI	OR	CI	OR	CI
Chinese	1.52*	1.06, 2.18	0.90	0.68, 1.21	0.84	0.67, 1.05	0.74	0.51, 1.07
Filipino	1.72**	1.15, 2.59	1.56**	1.17, 2.08	1.14	0.92, 1.42	1.20	0.89, 1.62
Korean	2.62**	1.75, 3.92	1.15	0.75, 1.74	0.82	0.59, 1.13	0.89	0.58, 1.36
Asian Indian	1.75*	1.07, 2.87	1.54*	1.08, 2.20	0.93	0.71, 1.22	1.24	0.83, 1.84
Pacific Islander	2.72**	1.91, 3.88	2.02*	1.17, 3.47	1.09	0.78, 1.53	2.08*	1.04, 4.15
Vietnamese	3.46**	2.19, 5.47	1.79**	1.23, 2.61	1.14	0.82, 1.59	1.38	0.93, 2.05
Other Asian	1.97**	1.28, 3.05	1.44	0.84, 2.44	0.98	0.76, 1.27	1.00	0.65, 1.54
Intercept	−5.29***		−4.59**		1.05**		−1.64**	
Chi-square test (−2 log-likelihood ratio)	671.77**		770.93**		568.53**			

Note: Reference category for self-reported health status is *good, very good, excellent;* for activity limitations, *none;* and for bed days, *none.* Other reference categories are in parentheses.

*$p < .05$; **$p < .01$.

†OR = odds ratio; CI = confidence interval.

‡Model adjusted for sex, age, marital status, living arrangement, family size, educational level, family income, and employment status.

ill enough to require bed rest. A likely explanation for this ambiguity is that the heterogeneity demonstrated to exist within the larger Asian and Pacific Islander population (Tables 13.1 and 13.2) obfuscated the associations.

Multivariate Models of Health Status. Controlling for demographic and socioeconomic diversity, and including Asian and Pacific Islander subgroup membership as a covariate, resolved most of the ambiguity. Results from the fully adjusted model (bottom panel of Table 13.3) showed that, compared with U.S.-born adults, Asian and Pacific Islander immigrants were more, not less, likely to report that their health was good or better. This finding, coupled with the diminution of the effect among those who had been in the United States for a brief period of time, was consistent with both the migration selectivity and acculturation hypotheses. The odds ratios pertaining to activity limitations provided even stronger support for the validity and complementarity of these hypotheses. Immigrants who had resided in the United States for all three durations studied were at significantly less risk of limitations in their daily activities than were Asians and Pacific Islanders born in the United States, and there was a monotonic increase in the odds ratios (OR = 0.45, OR = 0.65, and OR = 0.73) as duration increased from zero to four, to five to nine, to ten years or more, respectively, indicating that the greater the number of years immigrants had lived in the United States, the more similar they became to Asian and Pacific Islanders who were U.S. born. This perfectly consistent pattern was also evident with regard to bed days.

The differentials in health status among Asian and Pacific Islander subgroups, net of the effects of immigrant status and a large number of other factors (listed in both the text and in the stub column of Table 13.3), were also quite striking. Compared with the Japanese, *all* other Asian and Pacific Islander populations reported a greater risk of poor or fair health. By far the highest risk was observed for the Vietnamese (OR = 3.46), but the odds ratios for Koreans, Pacific Islanders, and Other Asians approached or exceeded 2.0. As would be expected on the basis of respondent-assessed health, except for the Chinese, activity limitations tended to be more prevalent among all other Asian and Pacific Islander groups than among the Japanese. Nevertheless, after adjustment for immigrant status and other potential determinants of activity limitations, the odds ratios for the Chinese (OR = 0.90) and Koreans (OR = 1.15) differed only slightly from that of the reference group regarding this outcome. Regarding bed days, the only statistically significant difference across Asian and Pacific Islander populations in the full model was that Pacific Islanders were more likely to have spent a week or more sick in bed (twice as likely as the Japanese).

Multivariate Models of Physician Visits and Medical Care Access

Baseline Model. The first panel of Table 13.4 presents estimates of the effects of immigrant status on annual physician visits and regular access to medical

Table 13.4. Odds Ratios for the Effects of Immigrant Status and National Origin on Physician Visits and Access to Health Care, National Health Interview Survey: for Physician Visits, 1992–1995 Combined; for Health Care, 1993–1995 Combined

| | Annual Visits to Physician | | | | Access to Health Care[†] Number | |
| | 1 or 2 Times | | ≥3 Times | | | |
	OR[‡]	95% CI[‡]	OR	95% CI	OR	95% CI
		Unadjusted model				
Duration (U.S. born)						
0 to <5 years	0.68**	0.56, 0.82	0.45**	0.37, 0.55	4.11**	2.64, 6.40
5 to <10 years	0.64**	0.51, 0.80	0.45**	0.36, 0.58	3.31**	2.06, 5.29
≥10 years	0.94	0.79, 1.13	0.64**	0.54, 0.75	1.40	0.90, 2.18
Intercept	0.35***		0.44***		−2.12**	
−2 log-likelihood	117.22**				206.53**	
		Adjusted model§				
Duration (U.S. born)						
0 to <5 years	0.77*	0.60, 0.98	0.52**	0.41, 0.68	3.48**	2.27, 5.32
5 to <10 years	0.72*	0.56, 0.93	0.54**	0.40, 0.74	2.72**	1.75, 4.22
≥10 years	0.94	0.74, 1.20	0.62**	0.48, 0.78	1.41	0.93, 2.14
National origin (Japanese)						
Chinese	1.01	0.81, 1.27	1.08	0.82, 1.42	1.35	0.91, 1.99
Filipino	1.47**	1.14, 1.89	1.28	0.97, 1.68	0.58*	0.37, 0.91
Korean	0.71*	0.54, 0.95	0.69*	0.50, 0.95	1.87**	1.21, 2.87
Asian Indian	1.10	0.84, 1.44	1.37	0.98, 1.93	1.21	0.74, 1.97
Pacific Islander	1.11	0.83, 1.49	0.99	0.63, 1.55	1.16	0.64, 2.09
Vietnamese	1.22	0.86, 1.72	1.48*	1.06, 2.05	0.83	0.48, 1.45
Other Asian	0.96	0.66, 1.39	1.15	0.80, 1.65	1.46	0.82, 2.58
Intercept	0.33		−0.78**		−1.78**	
Chi-square test (−2 log-likelihood ratio)	2,239.61**				566.69**	

Note: Reference category for physician visits is *none* and for health care access is *yes.* All other reference categories are in parentheses.

*p < .05; **p < .01.

[†]For this model, which is based on a National Health Interview Survey supplement, N = 4,755; for all other models, N = 8,249.

[‡]OR = odds ratio; CI = confidence interval.

§Model adjusted for health condition, activity limitation, bed days, sex, age, marital status, living arrangement, family size, educational level, family income, and employment status.

care, unadjusted and without distinction by national origin, for Asians and Pacific Islanders. Compared with the native born, physician visits were less common among immigrants. Foreign-born adults who had been in the United States for less than ten years were also three to four times more likely to have no regular source of medical care. For immigrants of long duration, only the odds ratio for three or more physician visits was significant. However, before drawing conclusions about access to health care, we constructed models that adjusted for health status as well as socioeconomic and demographic variables.

Multivariate Model. Controlling for health and the other variables listed in the stub column of Table 13.4 modestly reduced the influence of the effect of immigrant status on physician visits and regular access to medical care, but the pattern and levels of significance of the associations remained the same. Immigrants of all durations continued to be significantly less likely to have made three or more visits to a physician in the past year, and with the exception of long-term residents, they were also significantly less likely to report one or two annual visits. In the adjusted model, the odds of having no regular source of medical care remained strikingly large for immigrants who had resided in the United States for less than ten years. Thus, it appears that immigrants tend to be underserved compared with U.S.-born Asians and Pacific Islanders. In the adjusted model, just as for health status per se, immigrant use of health care began to more closely resemble conditions among the U.S.-born adults as duration increased. Regarding health status, while this pattern indicated a worsening of the immigrants' situation, for both regular access to medical care and physician visits the pattern suggested an improvement.

Only a few significant differences were found across Asian and Pacific Islander national origin groups with regard to physician visits and having a regular source of medical care, but those differences that did emerge were notable. Vietnamese and Koreans provided a striking contrast. The odds of visiting a physician three or more times were 50 percent higher for Vietnamese. Conversely, Koreans were significantly less likely to visit a physician at all. Again, the results with respect to medical care were consistent in that the odds ratio for Koreans having no regular care was almost 90 percent higher (OR = 1.87), whereas the odds ratio for Vietnamese was less than unity (but not statistically significant). A plausible explanation for the opposite positions of the Koreans and Vietnamese concerns differences in health insurance coverage. Examination of several Asian populations has shown that Koreans are the most likely to have no medical insurance of any type; specifically, 45.3 percent of Koreans in that study were not covered *at all*, while fully 40 percent of Vietnamese were covered by *public* health insurance, perhaps because of a heavy concentration of refugees in that population.[33]

DISCUSSION

Much previous research has concluded that Asians and Pacific Islanders are on average healthier compared with the general U.S. population. This conclusion has been challenged on the grounds that until very recently, no data sets existed that were either large enough or rich enough to support rigorous analysis of the diverse groups constituting the Asian and Pacific Islander population.[34] Furthermore, when investigating the health of Asians and Pacific Islanders, it is necessary to consider not only the high degree of heterogeneity across subpopulations but also the fact that immigration has played a dramatic role in the rapid growth of this minority. Accordingly, we used the most recent data available that enabled identification of specific Asian and Pacific Islander subpopulations in an investigation of the effects of immigrant status (nativity and duration) on health.

Descriptive tabulations (which included the white majority) support the view that Asians are a relatively healthy group, but evidence also exists that such a generalization should be qualified. Although the health of most Asian and Pacific Islander groups appears to be as good as or superior to that of whites in terms of most indicators, the respondent-evaluated health of Pacific Islanders and Vietnamese was worse, and a higher proportion of Pacific Islanders was bedridden for a week or more because of illness or disability.

Regression estimates that emerged after adjustment for a wide range of factors demonstrated that the health of Asian and Pacific Islander immigrants is superior to that of their native-born counterparts. Immigrants not only perceived they were healthier but also reported fewer activity limitations and bed days, and nearly all coefficients linking immigrant status to health status were highly statistically significant. Moreover, there was an almost perfectly consistent pattern of deterioration in health as length of residence in the United States increased.

Even after control for the powerful effect of immigrant status (along with other factors), health status varied substantially across Asian and Pacific Islander subpopulations. All other Asian and Pacific Islander groups seemed to be either less healthy or not significantly different in health status from the Japanese reference group. In particular, Vietnamese (with the recent and dramatic history of conflict in their nation of origin), Other Asians (who include a substantial number of refugees), and Pacific Islanders (whose health is apparently compromised by a greater tendency toward obesity and heavier cigarette smoking[35]) are two to three and a half times more likely to report poor or fair health and, except for Other Asians, are much more likely to encounter activity limitations. In addition, use by Asian and Pacific Islander immigrants of formal medical care increased with duration of immigration. In this instance at least, the strong tendency for the foreign born to become more similar to the native born the longer the former resided in the United States may be regarded as an advantage rather than a disadvantage.

Our study is subject to a number of limitations. One is the familiar problem of lack of information on attributes and conditions that would further advance our understanding of the outcomes of interest. A comparison of Chinese with Koreans—interesting in and of itself because of the confluence of similarities and differences that characterizes these two groups—would provide specific illustrations for what might otherwise legitimately be viewed as simply a conventional and substantively empty admission of imperfection. The adjusted model showed that both groups were at low risk of illness severe enough to require bed rest. However, the odds for Koreans' reporting health that was only fair or poor were *much* higher than the odds for Chinese, yet Koreans were most unlikely to have visited a physician in the past year or to have access to health care.

The explanation for the relatively good health of Chinese may lie in the fact that they, like the Japanese, have a long history of settlement in the United States (note that the explanation suggested here is in terms of a contextual variable [the length of time an immigrant *group* has been established at destination], not the length of time an *individual* immigrant has resided in the United States). That is, some quality of life and health advantages may accrue for groups that have had a longer period in which to develop positive social, economic, and political adaptations to a host society. Koreans, who are, in a historical context, a newer immigrant group, might well be expected to evidence poorer health. The observation that they are also the group least likely to visit a physician or to have a regular source of health care may be explicable partially in terms of their cultural preferences for traditional practitioners of "ethnomedicine"[36] and partially in terms of the large numbers of Koreans lacking health insurance.[33] Thus, it may be that variation in the health of minority groups, especially those comprising a large number of immigrants, can be fully understood only by taking into account additional factors, such as immigration history and diversity of cultural norms and values, for which data suitable for inclusion in statistical models are scant or absent.[36,37]

It might also be useful to conduct period-specific analyses. For example, the composition of pre- and post-1965 immigrant streams appears to differ substantially,[17] and the same may well be true of other temporal cut points when U.S. immigration law shifted course. Furthermore, a person's health status and whether he or she has systematic access to health care must depend on not only that person's financial circumstances and living arrangements (for which we controlled) but also on whether he or she has medical insurance. In addition, it might be more informative if finer distinctions were made with respect to health status. Finally, although the NHIS provides a large number of cases by typical standards, if a separate investigation of specific Asian and Pacific Islander populations is attempted, cell sizes become too small to permit stable estimates to be derived from multivariate models of the sort estimated here.

Despite these and other limitations, the present research makes it clear that immigration status exercises a powerful influence on the health of Asians and Pacific Islanders. Moreover, there is considerable support for the proposition that immigrant status is crucial to health in general and to the validity and complementarity of the positive immigration selectivity and acculturation hypotheses in particular.

Notes

1. Kitano, H., & Daniels, R. (1995). *Asian Americans: Emerging minorities.* Englewood Cliffs, NJ: Prentice Hall.

2. DaVita, C. J. (1996). The United States at mid-decade. *Popul Bull, 50,* 1–47.

3. Kuo, J., & Porter, K. (1998). *Health status of Asian Americans: United States, 1992–1994. Advance data, no. 298.* Washington, DC: U.S. Department of Health and Human Services.

4. O'Hare, W. J. (1992). A new look at poverty in America. *Popul Bull, 51,* 1–47.

5. Bradshaw, B. S., & Frisbie, W. P. (1992). Mortality of Mexican Americans and Mexican immigrants: Comparisons with Mexico. In J. R. Weeks & R. Ham-Chande (Eds.), *Demographic dynamics of the U.S.-Mexico border* (pp. 125–150). El Paso, TX: Texas Western Press.

6. Cabral, H., Fried, L. E., Levenson, S., et al. (1990). Foreign-born and U.S.-born black women: Differences in health behaviors and birth outcomes. *Am J Public Health, 80,* 70–72.

7. Hummer, R. A., Biegler, M., De Turk, P. B., et al. (1999). Race/ethnicity, nativity, and infant mortality in the United States. *Soc Forces, 77,* 1083–1117.

8. Hummer, R. A., Rogers, R. G., Nam, C. B., et al. (1999). Race/ethnicity, nativity and U.S. adult mortality. *Soc Sci Q, 80,* 136–153.

9. Marmot, M. G., Adelstein, A. M., & Bulusu, L. (1984). Lessons from the study of immigrant mortality. *Lancet, 112,* 1455–1457.

10. Rosenwaike, I., & Bradshaw, B. S. (1989). Mortality of the Spanish surname population of the Southwest: 1980. *Soc Sci Q, 70,* 631–649.

11. Singh, G. K., & Yu, S. M. (1996). Adverse pregnancy outcomes: Difference between U.S.- and foreign-born women in major U.S. racial and ethnic groups. *Am J Public Health, 86,* 837–843.

12. Lin-Fu, J. S. (1988). Population characteristics and health care needs of Asian Pacific Americans. *Public Health Rep, 103,* 18–27.

13. Singh, G., & Yu, S. M. (1993). Pregnancy outcomes among Asian Americans. *Asian Am Pacific Islander J Health, 1,* 63–68.

14. Blane, D. (1990). Social determinants of health—socioeconomic status, social class, and ethnicity. *Am J Public Health, 85,* 903–905.

15. Yu, E.S.H. (1991). The health risks of Asian Americans. *Am J Public Health, 81,* 1391–1393.

16. McGee, D. L., Liao, Y., Cao, G., et al. (1999). Self-reported health status and mortality in a multiethnic U.S. cohort. *Am J Epidemiol, 149,* 41–46.

17. Yang, P. Q. (1999). Quality of post-1965 Asian immigrants. *Popul Environ, 20,* 527–544.

18. Rosenwaike, I. (1991). Mortality of Hispanic populations. In I. Rosenwaike (Ed.), *Mortality of Hispanic populations.* New York: Greenwood Press, 3–11.

19. Scribner, R. (1996). Paradox as paradigm: The health outcomes of Mexican Americans. *Am J Public Health, 86,* 303–305.

20. Scribner, R., & Dwyer, J. H. (1989). Acculturation and low birthweight among Latinos in the Hispanic HANES. *Am J Public Health, 79,* 1263–1267.

21. Guendelman, S., & English, P. B. (1995). Effect of United States residence on birth outcomes among Mexican immigrants: An exploratory study. *Am J Epidemiol, 142*(Suppl.), 30–38.

22. Adams, P. F., & Benson, V. (1990). Current estimates from the National Health Interview Survey, 1989. *Vital Health Stat, 10,* 1–221.

23. Rogers, R. G., Hummer, R. A., & Nam, C. B. (2000). *Living and dying in the USA.* San Diego, CA: Academic Press,

24. Massey, J. T., Moore, T. F., Parsons, V. L., et al. (1989). Design and estimation from the National Health Interview Survey, 1985–94. *Vital Health Stat, 29,* 1–33.

25. Frisbie, W. P., Forbes, D., & Hummer, R. A. (1998). Hispanic pregnancy outcomes: Additional evidence. *Soc Sci Q, 79,* 149–169.

26. Shah, B. V., Barnwell, B. G., & Bieler, G. S. (1995). *SUDAAN user's manual, release 6.40.* Research Triangle Park, NC: Research Triangle Institute.

27. Thamer, M., Richard, C., Casebeer, A. W., et al. (1997). Health insurance coverage among foreign-born U.S. residents: The impact of race, ethnicity, and length of residence. *Am J Public Health, 87,* 96–102.

28. LeClere, F. B., Jensen, L., & Biddlecom, A. E. (1994). Health care utilization, family context, and adaptation among immigrants to the United States. *J Health Soc Behav, 35,* 370–384.

29. Idler, E., & Benyamini, Y. (1997). Self-rated health and mortality: A review of twenty-seven community studies. *J Health Soc Behav, 38,* 21–37.

30. Mossey, J. M., & Shapiro, E. (1982). Self-rated health: A predictor of mortality among the elderly. *Am J Public Health, 72,* 800–808.

31. Shetterly, S. M., Baxter, J., Mason, L. D., et al. (1996). Self-rated health among Hispanics vs. non-Hispanic white adults: The San Luis Valley Health and Aging Study. *Am J Public Health, 86,* 1798–1801.

32. vander Zanden, J. W. (1972). American minority relations (3rd ed.). New York: Ronald Press.

33. Huang, F. V. (1997). Health insurance coverage of the children of immigrants in the United States. *Matern Child Health J, 1,* 69–80.

34. Chen, M. S., Jr., & Hawks, B. L. (1995). A debunking of the myth of healthy Asian Americans and Pacific Islanders. *Sci Health Promot, 9,* 261–268.

35. Cundy, T., Gamble, G., Manuel, A., et al. (1993). Determinants of birthweight in women with established and gestational diabetes. *Aust N Z J Obstet Gynaecol, 33,* 249–254.

36. Kraut, A. M. (1990). Healers and strangers: Immigrant attitudes toward the physician in America: A relationship in historical perspective. *JAMA, 263,* 1807–1811.

37. Yamashiro, G., & Matsuoka, J. K. (1997). Help-seeking among Asian and Pacific Americans: A multiperspective analysis. *Soc Work, 42,* 176–186.

CHAPTER FOURTEEN

Differing Birthweight Among Infants of U.S.-Born Blacks, African-Born Blacks, and U.S.-Born Whites

Richard J. David
James W. Collins Jr.

During the past forty years, epidemiologic research has elucidated many important associations between the sociodemographic characteristics of mothers and the birthweight of infants.[1-4] For example, the extremes of childbearing age,[1] cigarette smoking,[2] inadequate prenatal care,[3] urban poverty,[4] and black race[5] are well-documented risk factors for low birthweight. Other obstetrical risk factors account for part of the racial disparity in birthweights, but differences persist.[6-9]

Although the incidence of low birthweight decreases in both blacks and whites as the number of risk factors declines, the improvement is faster among whites, resulting in a wider birthweight gap between blacks and whites among infants of low-risk women.[1,4] This has led some investigators to believe that genetic factors associated with race influence birthweight.[10-15] In the 1967 National Collaborative Perinatal Project, only 1 percent of the total variance in birthweight among 18,000 infants was accounted for by socioeconomic variables, leading the authors to conclude that "race behaves as a real biological variable in its effect on birth weight. This effect of race [is] presumably genetic."[10] The assumption

We are indebted to Steven Perry and the staff of the Illinois Department of Health for providing vital-records data; to James Bash and Barbara Sullivan for technical assistance; to Drs. Ugonna Chike-Obi, Richard Cooper, Helen Kusi, and Adeyemi Sobowali for useful comments; and to Susan Seidler for help in the preparation of the manuscript.

252

that black women differ genetically from white women in their ability to bear normal or large infants persists in more recent studies of fetal growth,[13,16] one of which, for example, refers to "genetic factors affecting growth, such as neonatal sex and race."[16]

Few data have been published on the birthweights of infants born to African-born women in the United States. Most African Americans trace their origins to western Africa, where the slave trade flourished in the seventeenth and eighteenth centuries.[17,18] It is estimated that U.S. blacks derive about three-quarters of their genetic heritage from West African ancestors and the remainder from Europeans.[18-21] To the extent that population differences in allele frequency underlie the observed differences in birthweight between blacks and whites in the United States, one would expect women of "pure" West African origin to bear smaller infants than comparable African Americans, considering the European genetic admixture in the latter. However, to our knowledge, no population of West African women delivering infants in the United States has been studied. We therefore undertook an analysis of racial differences in birthweight based on U.S.-born and African-born women giving birth in Illinois.

METHODS

Study Population

We obtained data on the birthweights of singleton black and white infants born in Illinois and the birthplaces of their mothers, using birth-certificate tapes for 1980 through 1995 from the Illinois Department of Public Health. All the white infants studied had U.S.-born mothers and were not of Latino origin. The mothers of the black infants fell into two groups: women born in sub-Saharan Africa and those born in the United States. We selected random samples of the white and black U.S.-born women in order to have groups convenient for analysis; these groups included 2.5 percent of white births and 7.5 percent of black births.

Black women born in the Western Hemisphere but not in the United States (that is, born in Canada, the Caribbean, or South America) were excluded from the study. Such designations of maternal origin were available for the period 1980 through 1988. During that period, birth records were coded with three separate fields: the mother's race, the mother's place of birth, and the mother's origin or descent. Women whose race was coded as "black," whose place of birth was coded as "not in Western Hemisphere," and whose origin or descent was coded as "Africa, excluding northern Africa" were considered to have immigrated from sub-Saharan Africa. According to the 1990 Census, 66 percent of African-born blacks living in Illinois for whom a sub-Saharan country of birth was recorded came from either Nigeria or Ghana.[22] From 1989 on, the variable indicating origin or descent was replaced by a variable specifically pertaining to Hispanic origin, but a new, detailed set of birthplace codes allowed us to identify births on the basis of the mother's country of birth. We therefore selected births from 1989 through 1995 in which the mother's birthplace was one of seventeen present-day countries corresponding to the area from which African slaves originated in the seventeenth and eighteenth centuries.[18,20]

Analysis of Birthweights

As a first step toward exploring the possible contribution of genetic factors to the racial disparity in outcomes of pregnancy, we compared the curves for the distribution of birthweight, the mean birthweights, and the rates of low birthweight (defined as the number of births of infants weighing less than 2,500 g per 100 live births) among infants born to U.S.-born blacks, African-born blacks, and U.S.-born whites. In addition, we computed rates of moderately low (1,500 to 2,500 g) and very low (<1,500 g) birthweight. Next, we determined the distribution of sociodemographic risk factors (the mother's age, education, and marital status; the trimester of first prenatal care, and the father's education) and reproductive risk factors (the overall number of pregnancies and whether there was a history of fetal loss or infant death) in the three groups of women. For the risk factors and outcomes, we calculated relative risks and 95 percent confidence intervals, using the infants of U.S.-born white women as the reference group.[23]

Because the three populations differed, we repeated the birthweight comparisons after adjustment for differences in risk profiles. We did so in three ways. First, we compared each African-born mother with two similar U.S.-born women, one white and one black, who were matched for age, education, marital status, prenatal care, parity, and history of fetal loss. Second, we used the REG procedure (SAS, release 6.07, Cary, N.C.) to create a model showing birthweight as a function of all the risk factors for which data were available, except paternal education (data on that variable were missing for 20 percent of births) and prior loss of an infant (prevalence, <5 percent). We then estimated mean differences in birthweight among the three subgroups, both by subtracting intercept terms estimated in three subgroup-specific models and by modeling the subgroups two at a time, with ethnic status entered as a dichotomous dummy variable.[24] Third, we repeated the birthweight analysis but limited it to subgroups of low-risk women defined according to social, demographic, and reproductive risk factors.

Our analysis used birth-certificate tapes from which the identifying information on the individual women and their infants had been removed. These data were provided by the Illinois Department of Health, which provides such "sterilized" birth tapes to researchers conducting epidemiologic studies.

RESULTS

The mean birthweight of the white infants was 3,446 g, as compared with 3,333 g for the infants of the African-born black women and 3,089 g for the infants of the U.S.-born black women (Table 14.1). The proportion of very low birthweight infants was similar for African-born blacks and U.S.-born blacks. Even though the infants born to African-born blacks had a slightly lower mean birthweight than the white infants, the overall distribution of birthweights was similar in the two groups and was different from that among the infants of U.S.-born blacks (Figure 14.1).

Table 14.2 shows the distribution of selected risk factors in the three groups of women. The African-born black women delivered the highest proportion of infants who were their mothers' fourth or subsequent children and had the highest proportion of previous fetal and infant deaths. The U.S.-born black women were the youngest, the least likely to be married, the least well educated, and the most likely to have received prenatal care late or not at all. The white women surpassed both groups of black women with regard to only one risk factor—primigravidity.

When the infants of African-born black women were compared with those of U.S.-born women matched for the mother's age, marital status, education,

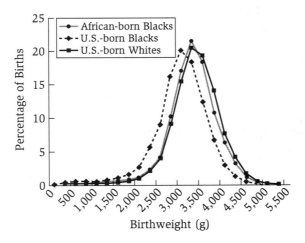

Figure 14.1 Distribution of Birthweights Among Infants of U.S.-Born White and Black Women and African-Born Black Women in Illinois, 1980–1995.

Note: The calculation of frequencies was based on all singleton births in Illinois. The study population included the infants of 3,135 black women born in sub-Saharan Africa, 43,322 black women born in the United States (a sample that included 7.5 percent of the total number of black women giving birth in Illinois), and 44,046 U.S.-born white women (2.5 percent of the total number of white women giving birth in Illinois).

Table 14.1. Birthweight Data in Illinois, 1980-1995, According to the Mother's Race and Place of Birth

Variable	Subgroup of Mothers			Relative Risk (95% CI) in Black Mothers*	
	U.S.-Born Whites	African-Born Blacks	U.S.-Born Blacks	African-Born	U.S.-Born
Raw data					
No. of births	44,046	3,135	43,322		
Mean birthweight (g)	3,446	3,333	3,089		
Low birthweight (% of infants)	4.3	7.1	13.2	1.6 (1.4–1.9)	3.1 (2.9–3.2)
Moderately low	3.6	4.8	10.6	1.3 (1.1–1.6)	3.0 (2.8–3.1)
Very low	0.7	2.3	2.6	3.2 (2.5–4.1)	3.5 (3.1–4.0)
Matched cases†					
No. of births	2,950	2,950	2,950		
Mean birthweight (g)	3,475	3,341	3,195		
Low birthweight (% of infants)	3.6	6.9	8.5	1.9 (1.5–2.4)	2.4 (1.9–2.9)
Moderately low	3.1	4.7	6.1	1.5 (1.2–2.0)	2.0 (1.5–2.5)
Very low	0.5	2.2	2.4	4.1 (2.4–7.0)	4.5 (2.6–7.7)

Note: Data on birthweight were missing for 19 infants (0.02 percent of the total). Low birthweight was defined as a weight of less than 2,500 g, moderately low birthweight as a weight of 1,500 to 2,499 g, and very low birthweight as a weight of less than 1,500 g.

*Relative risks shown are for the risk of low birthweight in the infants of women in the group shown as compared with the infants of U.S.-born white women. CI = confidence interval.

†In this analysis, each African-born black woman was matched with one U.S.-born white woman and one U.S.-born black woman for age, marital status, education and spouse's education, prenatal care, parity, and the presence or absence of previous fetal loss.

Table 14.2. Distribution of Selected Risk Factors in the Study Population, According to the Mother's Race and Place of Birth

Variable	Subgroup of Mothers			Relative Risk (95% CI) in Black Mothers*	
	U.S.-Born Whites	African-Born Blacks	U.S.-Born Blacks	African-Born	U.S.-Born
	Rate per 100				
Maternal age <20 years	8.8	1.5	28	0.2 (0.1–0.2)	3.1 (3.0–3.2)
Education <12 years					
Mother	13	8	36	0.6 (0.5–0.7)	2.9 (2.8–3.0)
Father	11	6	34	0.5 (0.4–0.6)	2.9 (2.9–3.0)
Mother unmarried	14	24	76	1.7 (1.6–1.8)	5.3 (5.2–5.4)
Late prenatal care or none	15	26	36	1.7 (1.6–1.8)	2.3 (2.3–2.4)
Gravidity					
1	34	22	29	0.6 (0.6–0.7)	0.9 (0.8–0.9)
>3	15	31	26	2.0 (1.9–2.1)	1.7 (1.6–1.7)
Prior death					
Fetus[†]	24	39	28	1.6 (1.5–1.7)	1.1 (1.1–1.2)
Infant	1.7	3.0	2.9	1.8 (1.5–2.2)	1.7 (1.6–1.9)

Note: Data on the number of previous pregnancies were obtained for 44,053 U.S.-born white women, 3,135 African-born black women, and 43,334 U.S.-born black women. For the other variables shown, there were missing data, as follows: maternal age, 0.01 percent; maternal education, 0.26 percent; paternal education, 16.4 percent; marital status, 0.05 percent; start of prenatal care, 1.38 percent; previous fetal death, 0.07 percent; and previous death of an infant, 0.36 percent.

*Relative risks shown are for the risk of low birthweight in the infants of women in the group shown as compared with the infants of U.S.-born white women. CI = confidence interval.

[†]This category includes spontaneous and induced abortions, miscarriages, and stillbirths, regardless of the period of gestation.

prenatal care, parity, and prior fetal loss and the father's education, the differences between the groups narrowed somewhat, but their relation did not change (Table 14.1). With white infants as the reference group, the relative risks for low and moderately low birthweight were both significantly higher among infants of U.S.-born blacks than among infants of African-born blacks. However, the relative risk of very low birthweight was similar in the two groups of infants born to blacks.

To gain more insight into the relative importance of the risk factors in the three groups, we used multiple regression analysis to study the changes in birthweight predicted by each factor. The models we constructed (Table 14.3) all showed a positive effect of being married (an increase of 60 to 124 g in predicted birthweight), having had one or two previous pregnancies (an increase of 29 to 50 g), and having no previous fetal loss (an increase of 19 to 55 g). Of the risk factors, only marital status had a statistically significant effect among the infants of African-born blacks.

On the basis of the multivariable models in Table 14.3, the birthweight of the infants of African-born blacks was 14 g less than that of the infants of U.S.-born whites after we controlled for risk factors. In another model, we looked at only the U.S.-born white women and the African-born black women, with race

Table 14.3. Regression Models Showing the Predicted Effects of Low-Risk Sociodemographic and Reproductive Variables in the Mother on the Birthweight of Infants in Each Subgroup, Defined According to the Mother's Race and Place of Birth

Variable	Subgroup of Mothers		
	U.S.-Born Whites (N = 44,046)	African-Born Blacks (N = 3135)	U.S.-Born Blacks (N = 43,322)
Birthweight (grams) with no protective factors present	3,144*	3,130*	2,942*
Maternal age >19 years	0	+146*	−25*
Maternal education >11 years	+128*	−26	+82*
Mother married	+118*	+60**	+124*
Prenatal care in 1st 3 months	+60*	−4	+47*
Gravida 2 or 3	+50*	+41	+29*
No prior fetal loss	+19***	+36	+55*

Note: The values show the increase or decrease in the predicted birthweight in each group, as estimated by arithmetically combining the predicted birthweight with no protective factors present with the sum of the protective factors, each multiplied by 1 if the factor was present or by 0 if it was absent. The p values indicate the stability of these point estimates; the greater the standard error of the coefficient, the less the statistical significance.

*$p < .001$; **$p < .05$; ***$p < .01$.

included as a dichotomous variable. In that analysis, the infants of the U.S.-born whites weighed 98 g more than the infants of the African-born blacks after adjustment for age, education, marital status, gravidity, prenatal care, and history of fetal loss. In a similar model that included only women born in the United States, the white infants weighed 248 g more than the black infants after adjustment for the same six variables.

Table 14.4 shows the mean birthweights and rates of low birthweight among infants born to the women at lowest risk—those twenty to thirty-nine years of age who began their prenatal care in the first trimester, had at least twelve years of education, and were married to men who also had at least twelve years of education. Sixty-six percent of the white women fit this profile, as compared with 50 percent of the African-born black women and 14 percent of the U.S.-born black women. The mean birthweight and rates of low birthweight of the infants born to African-born blacks were intermediate between the values for U.S.-born whites and those for U.S.-born blacks. However, when reproductive risk factors were included in the selection of low-risk women, the differences between the infants of U.S.-born whites and the infants of African-born blacks in mean birthweight and rates of both low and very low birthweight were narrowed, whereas the differences between the infants of U.S.-born whites and U.S.-born blacks were unchanged. The greatest change was in very low birthweight; the exclusion of women with a history of fetal loss resulted in nearly identical rates among infants of African-born blacks and those of U.S.-born whites, eliminating the significant excess of infants with very low birthweight born to African-born blacks.

DISCUSSION

The distribution of birthweights among infants of African-born black women approximated that among infants of U.S.-born white women. The rate of low birthweight births for African-born black women was between the rate for U.S.-born white women and that for U.S.-born black women. Adjusting for maternal risk factors in three ways shifted the magnitude of the differences in birthweight but did not alter the basic pattern. Among infants of African-born black women and those of U.S.-born black women, very low birthweight occurred at a similar frequency. Nevertheless, these data provide some evidence against the theory that there is a genetic basis for the disparity between white and black women born in the United States in the mean birthweights of their infants.

According to most studies, racial differences in birthweight persist independently of numerous social and economic risk factors.[8,9] This has led some investigators to suggest that the differences have a genetic basis.[11–14] Our findings

Table 14.4. Mean Birthweights and Rates of Low Birthweight Among Infants with Mothers at Low Risk, According to the Mother's Race and Place of Birth

Low-Risk Variables Studied	Subgroup of Mothers			Relative Risk (95% CI) in Black Mothers*	
	U.S.-Born Whites	African-Born Blacks	U.S.-Born Blacks	African-Born	U.S.-Born
Sociodemographic variables only†					
No. of births	29,012	1,577	6,181		
Mean birthweight (g)	3,497	3,344	3,243		
Low birthweight (rate per 100)	3.3	7.0	9.0	2.2 (1.8–2.6)	2.8 (2.5–3.1)
Very low birthweight (rate per 100)	0.6	2.4	1.8	4.3 (3.4–6.2)	3.3 (2.6–4.2)
Reproductive variables added‡					
No. of births	12,361	608	2,670		
Mean birthweight (g)	3,551	3,454	3,299		
Low birthweight (rate per 100)	2.4	3.6	7.5	1.5 (1.0–2.4)	3.0 (2.5–3.5)
Very low birthweight (rate per 100)	0.4	0.5	1.3	1.3 (0.4–4.2)	3.3 (2.2–5.2)

*Relative risks shown are for the risk of low birthweight in the infants of women in the group shown as compared with the infants of U.S.-born white women. CI = confidence interval.

†This analysis was limited to women twenty to thirty-nine years of age who began their prenatal care in the first trimester of pregnancy, had at least twelve years of education, and were married to men who also had at least twelve years of education.

‡This analysis was limited as described in the preceding note and also excluded primigravidas and mothers with a history of fetal or infant loss.

challenge the genetic concept of race as it relates to birthweight. The African-born women in our study were new immigrants from the same region from which the ancestors of most U.S. blacks came, but without the estimated 20 to 30 percent admixture of European genetic material that has occurred since the mid–seventeenth century.[18-21] If genetics played a prominent part in determining black–white differences in birthweight, the infants of the African-born black women should have had lower birthweights than those of the U.S.-born black women. We found the opposite: regardless of socioeconomic status, the infants of black women born in Africa weighed more than the infants of comparable black women born in the United States.

The birthweight distribution of the infants of African-born black women who delivered in Illinois is consistent with previous reports of the birthweights of infants of foreign-born black women of largely Caribbean origin.[25-28] Studies of groups of women from New York, Boston, and multiple states have had concordant results: black women born outside the United States have heavier infants than do those born inside the United States, even after adjustment for cigarette smoking, alcohol intake, and illicit drug use.

As data inconsistent with the genetic hypothesis of racial differences accumulate, social and psychophysiological hypotheses are advanced.[5,29-33] A woman's exposure as a young child to the effects of poverty or racial discrimination could adversely affect birthweight in the next generation.[28,34] The high educational level of African-born black women in Illinois indicates that rigorous selection occurs among African immigrants and suggests an overrepresentation of women born into affluent families, an elite subgroup in any developing nation.

Wilcox and Russell, in their extensive work on birthweight distributions, developed a model that can be applied to the birthweight curve of any group, partitioning it into an underlying Gaussian curve and a "residual" distribution of very low birthweight infants.[35] They proposed that the definition of normal birthweight differs for different groups, on the basis of the underlying distribution in the group under consideration. They attribute the residual births of very low birthweight infants to "disorganized, perhaps pathologic, processes"[35,36] that are presumably environmental in origin.

In our study, the proportions of very low birthweight infants born to African-born black women and to U.S.-born black women were similar. The factors that account for this finding are unclear. As in most published studies, the majority of the risk factors we examined were related to the course of pregnancy. In such a conceptualization, pregnancy is a relatively short-term condition, minimally related to past life experiences. In an attempt to broaden this concept, we studied how the outcome of prior pregnancy affected the disparity between blacks and whites in rates of very low birthweight. When we controlled for the outcome of prior pregnancy, we found that the rate of very low birthweight among infants of African-born black women more closely resembled that among infants of U.S.-born white women. This observation deserves further investigation.

Our study has important limitations. Vital records contain minimal clinical information. Data on cigarette smoking, weight before pregnancy, and weight gain during pregnancy might, if available, have explained some of our findings. In addition, the group of African-born black women studied, although more than ten times larger than the group studied previously,[37] was too small to permit stable estimates of very low birthweight in subgroups.

In summary, African-born black women have infants with a greater mean birthweight and a different birthweight distribution than do black women born in the United States.

Notes

1. Kleinman, J. C., & Kessel, S. S. (1987). Racial differences in low birth weight: Trends and risk factors. *N Engl J Med, 317,* 749–753.

2. Fox, S. H., Koepsell, T. D., & Daling, J. R. (1994). Birth weight and smoking during pregnancy: Effect modification by maternal age. *Am J Epidemiol, 139,* 1008–1015.

3. Murray, J. L., & Bernfield, M. (1988). The differential effect of prenatal care on the incidence of low birth weight among blacks and whites in a prepaid health care plan. *N Engl J Med, 319,* 1385–1391.

4. Collins, J. W., Jr., & David, R. J. (1990). The differential effect of traditional risk factors on infant birthweight among blacks and whites in Chicago. *Am J Public Health, 80,* 679–681.

5. David, R. J., & Collins, J. W., Jr. (1991). Bad outcomes in black babies: Race or racism? *Ethn Dis, 1,* 236–244.

6. Lieberman, E., Ryan, K. J., Monson, R. R., & Schoenbaum, S. C. (1987). Risk factors accounting for racial differences in the rate of premature birth. *N Engl J Med, 317,* 743–748.

7. Rawlings, J. S., Rawlings, V. B., & Read, J. A. (1995). Prevalence of low birth weight and preterm delivery in relation to the interval between pregnancies among white and black women. *N Engl J Med, 332,* 69–74.

8. Klebanoff, M. A., Shino, P. H., Berendes, H. W., & Rhoads, G. G. (1989). Facts and artifacts about anemia and preterm delivery. *JAMA, 262,* 511–515.

9. Sheehan, T. J., & Gregorio, D. I. (1995). Low birth weight in relation to the interval between pregnancies. *N Engl J Med, 333,* 386–387.

10. Naylor, A. F., & Myrianthopoulos, N. C. (1967). The relation of ethnic and selected socio-economic factors to human birth-weight. *Ann Hum Genet, 31,* 71–83.

11. Little, R. E., & Sing, C. F. (1987). Genetic and environmental influences on human birth weight. *Am J Hum Genet, 40,* 512–526.

12. Magnus, P. (1984). Further evidence for a significant effect of fetal genes on variation in birth weight. *Clin Genet, 26,* 289–296.

13. Hulsey, T. C., Levkoff, A. H., & Alexander, G. R. (1991). Birth weights of infants of black and white mothers without pregnancy complications. *Am J Obstet Gynecol, 164,* 1299–1302.

14. Goldenberg, R. L., Cliver, S. P., Cutter, G. R., et al. (1991). Black-white differences in newborn anthropometric measurements. *Obstet Gynecol, 78,* 782–788.

15. Wildschutt, H. I., Lumey, L. H., & Lunt, P. W. (1991). Is preterm delivery genetically determined? *Paediatr Perinat Epidemiol, 5,* 363–372.

16. Amini, S. B., Catalano, P. M., Hirsch, V., & Mann, L. I. (1994). An analysis of birthweight by gestational age using a computerized perinatal data base, 1975–1992. *Obstet Gynecol, 83,* 342–352.

17. Oliver, R., & Fage, J. D. (1988). *A short history of Africa* (6th ed.). New York: Facts on File.

18. Reed, T. E. (1969). Caucasian genes in American Negroes. *Science, 165,* 762–768.

19. Chakraborty, R., Kamboh, M. I., & Ferrell, R. E. (1991). "Unique" alleles in admixed populations: A strategy for determining "hereditary" population differences of disease frequencies. *Ethn Dis, 1,* 245–256.

20. Adams, J., & Ward, R. H. (1973). Admixture studies and the detection of selection. *Science, 180,* 1137–1143.

21. Glass, B., & Li, C. C. (1953). The dynamics of racial intermixture: An analysis based on the American Negro. *Am J Hum Genet, 5,* 1–20.

22. U.S. Bureau of the Census. (1993). *1990 Census of population: Social and economic characteristics: Illinois* (Section 1 of 2, CP-2-15). Washington, DC: U.S. Government Printing Office.

23. Schlesselman, J. J. (1982). *Case control studies: Design, conduct, analysis.* New York: Oxford University Press.

24. Kleinbaum, D. G., & Kupper, L. L. (1978). *Applied regression analysis and other multivariable methods.* North Scituate, MA: Duxbury Press.

25. Cabral, H., Fried, L. E., Levenson, S., Amaro, H., & Zuckerman, B. (1990). Foreign-born and U.S.-born black women: Differences in health behaviors and birth outcomes. *Am J Public Health, 80,* 70–72.

26. Kleinman, J. C., Fingerhut, L. A., & Prager, K. (1991). Differences in infant mortality by race, nativity status, and other maternal characteristics. *Am J Dis Child, 145,* 194–199.

27. Friedman, D. J., Cohen, B. B., Mahan, C. M., Lederman, R. I., Vezina, R. J., & Dunn, V. H. (1993). Maternal ethnicity and birthweight among blacks. *Ethn Dis, 3,* 255–269.

28. Valanis, B. M., & Rush, D. (1979). A partial explanation of superior birth weights among foreign-born women. *Soc Biol, 26,* 189–210.

29. Cooper, R. (1984). A note on the biologic concept of race and its application in epidemiologic research. *Am Heart J, 108,* 715–722.

30. Witzig, R. (1996). The medicalization of race: Scientific legitimization of a flawed social construct. *Ann Intern Med, 125,* 675–679.

31. Rowley, D. L., Hogue, C. J., Blackmore, C. A., et al. (1993). Preterm delivery among African-American women: A research strategy. *Am J Prev Med, 9*(Suppl.), 1–6.

32. Krieger, N., Rowley, D. L., Herman, A. A., Avery, B., & Phillips, M. T. (1993). Racism, sexism, and social class: Implications for studies of health, disease, and well-being. *Am J Prev Med, 9*(Suppl.), 82–122.

33. Geronimus, A. T. (1992). The weathering hypothesis and the health of African-American women and infants: Evidence and speculations. *Ethn Dis, 2,* 207–221.

34. Emanuel, I., Filakti, H., Alberman, E., & Evans, S.J.W. (1992). Intergenerational studies of human birthweight from the 1958 birth cohort: 1. Evidence for a multi-generational effect. *Br J Obstet Gynaecol, 99,* 67–74.

35. Wilcox, A. J., & Russell, I. T. (1983). Birthweight and perinatal mortality: I. On the frequency distribution of birthweight. *Int J Epidemiol, 12,* 314–318.

36. Wilcox, A. J., & Russell, I. T. (1990). Why small black infants have a lower mortality rate than small white infants: The case for population-specific standards for birth weight. *J Pediatr, 116,* 7–10.

37. Wasse, H., Holt, V. L., & Daling, J. R. (1994). Pregnancy risk factors and birth outcomes in Washington State: A comparison of Ethiopian-born and U.S.-born women. *Am J Public Health, 84,* 1505–1507.

CHAPTER FIFTEEN

Adverse Pregnancy Outcomes

Differences Between U.S.- and Foreign-Born Women in Major U.S. Racial and Ethnic Groups

Gopal K. Singh
Stella M. Yu

The nativity composition of the U.S. population has changed substantially in the past three decades, largely as a result of increased immigration from Asia and Latin America following the adoption of the Immigration Act of 1965.[1] The proportion of the foreign-born U.S. population rose by 70 percent from 1970 to 1990 (from 4.7 percent to about 8 percent). Indeed, the foreign-born population in 1990—19.8 million—was the largest in U.S. history.[1-3] In spite of this impressive growth of the foreign-born population, nativity status (that is, whether an individual is U.S. born or foreign born), as a primary factor of interest, has received relatively little attention in the analysis of health outcomes in general and pregnancy outcomes in particular.[4]

Foreign-born mothers have generally been shown to have significantly better pregnancy outcomes than their U.S.-born counterparts, even after a number of sociodemographic risk factors have been controlled for.[4-11] However, the studies that have examined the role of maternal nativity status have mostly focused on a few ethnic groups, particularly those of Hispanic origin.[5-8] Moreover, some of these studies have been based on localized samples or data sets and are therefore limited in their generalizability to the entire nation.[8-11] National-level

An earlier version of this chapter was presented at the 122nd annual meeting of the American Public Health Association, November 1994, Washington, D.C. We are grateful to Joyce Martin of the National Center for Health Statistics and to three anonymous reviewers for their helpful comments.

data have not been used to examine the impact of maternal nativity status on pregnancy outcomes for various racial and ethnic groups in the United States.

The main purpose of this study was to examine (1) whether there are significant differentials between U.S.-born and foreign-born mothers in risks for three adverse pregnancy outcomes—infant mortality, low birthweight, and preterm birth—even after a number of sociodemographic risk factors have been controlled and (2) whether these differentials, if they exist, vary across different racial and ethnic groups.

For our analysis, we considered the following major racial and ethnic groups: non-Hispanic whites, blacks, Chinese, Japanese, Filipinos, other Asians and Pacific Islanders, Mexicans, Puerto Ricans, Cubans, and Central and South Americans. Hawaiians and American Indians were excluded from the analysis because they are by definition native born. The other Asians and Pacific Islanders category, henceforth referred to as "other Asians," was largely made up of Asian Indians, Koreans, and Vietnamese.[12]

METHODS

Data

The data used in this study were derived primarily from the national Linked Birth and Infant Death Data Sets for the 1985, 1986, and 1987 birth cohorts.[13–15] The analysis of the linked files was supplemented by analyses of the 1988 National Maternal and Infant Health Survey and 1992 birth certificate data tapes. Detailed descriptions of the latter data sets have been provided elsewhere.[16–19]

Three years of data from linked birth and infant death records were pooled in order to provide stable and robust estimates of pregnancy outcome measures for U.S.- and foreign-born Asian and Hispanic subgroups. The study sample for most of the analysis consisted of 2,112,607 live births for non-Hispanic whites, 1,782,007 for blacks, 312,030 for Asian Americans, and 1,016,558 for Hispanics. Numbers of live births for the specific Asian American and Hispanic subgroups were as follows: Chinese, 50,572; Japanese, 23,919; Filipinos, 63,060; other Asians, 174,479; Mexicans, 740,382; Puerto Ricans, 109,874; Cubans, 29,935; and Central and South Americans, 136,367. It is important to note that all infant deaths and live births were classified according to maternal race and ethnicity.

Linked data on Hispanic origin were available only for twenty-three states and the District of Columbia. Therefore, we decided to exclude Hispanic origin from the pooled national-level analyses shown in Table 15.2, which were based on 100 percent data for Asian Americans during 1985 through 1987 and 2 percent and 5 percent random subsamples, respectively, of all white and black live births in 1986 from all fifty states and the District of Columbia. The smaller samples for the two latter groups yielded sufficiently large numbers of live births and infant deaths. This precluded us from having to perform the costly and impractical task of conducting a multivariate analysis of all white and black births, which totaled nearly 3.6 million in 1986 alone.

Variables

The dependent variables in this study were risk of infant mortality, low birthweight, and preterm birth. Infant mortality was defined as risk of death at less than one year of age. Infants weighing less than 2,500 g at birth were considered low birthweight, and those with less than thirty-seven weeks of gestation were considered preterm. Infant mortality and low birthweight were modeled as functions of the main covariates of interest (that is, nativity status and race/ethnicity) and such control variables as maternal age, marital status, education, birth order, place of residence, and timing of prenatal care. The preterm birth model included all of the covariates except prenatal care. The covariates just described have been identified in several studies as important risk factors for the three pregnancy outcomes;[20-24] they were measured here as categorical variables (as shown in Table 15.2).

Statistical Analysis

Multivariate logistic regression was used to analyze overall as well as ethnicity-specific nativity differentials in the pregnancy outcome measures just described. The parameters of the logistic models, which represented the effects of covariates (including those of nativity and ethnicity), were estimated by the maximum likelihood method; the LOGISTIC procedure of SAS, version 6,[25] was used in these estimations.

RESULTS

Figure 15.1 shows the nativity composition of mothers by ethnicity during 1985 through 1987. U.S.-born mothers in this study consisted of women born in the fifty states and the District of Columbia. Foreign-born or immigrant mothers consisted of women born outside the fifty states and the District of Columbia. For Puerto Rican mothers, the differentials are shown between women born in the fifty states and the District of Columbia and those born in Puerto Rico or abroad. With the exception of Japanese and Mexican mothers, Asian and Hispanic mothers were predominantly immigrants. About 46 percent of Japanese and 55 percent of Mexican mothers were foreign born. Over 47 percent of Puerto Rican mothers were born outside the fifty states and the District of Columbia. The Central and South American group included the highest proportion (98 percent) of foreign-born mothers; non-Hispanic whites and blacks evidenced the lowest proportions (5 percent and 7 percent, respectively).

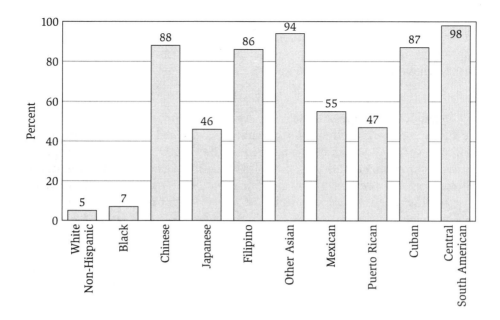

Figure 15.1 Percentage of Births to Mothers Born Outside the 50 States and the District of Columbia, by Maternal Race/Ethnicity: United States, 1985–1987.
Source: Data derived from the Linked Birth and Infant Death Data Sets, 1985, 1986, and 1987 birth cohorts.

Table 15.1 provides descriptive data on pregnancy outcomes and selected sociodemographic characteristics by nativity status and race/ethnicity. As can be seen in this table, foreign-born women had lower infant mortality rates than U.S.-born women for all racial/ethnic groups except Central and South Americans. Of all ethnicity and nativity groups, Chinese and Japanese immigrants had the lowest infant mortality rates, while U.S.-born blacks, Cubans, and Puerto Ricans had the highest rates. The largest nativity differentials in infant mortality were found for Cubans, other Asians, and blacks.

Ethnic and nativity differences in rates of low birthweight and preterm birth revealed a somewhat similar pattern. Except for other Asians, immigrants generally had lower rates of low birthweight than individuals born in the United States, with blacks, Chinese, and Mexicans showing the largest nativity differentials. Chinese and Mexican immigrants had the lowest rates of low birthweight, while U.S.-born blacks and Puerto Ricans had the highest rates. Except for other Asians and non-Hispanic whites, immigrants had lower proportions of preterm birth than individuals born in the United States. Other Asian immigrants evidenced a higher proportion of preterm birth than their U.S.-born counterparts. Blacks and Mexicans showed the largest nativity differentials in the rates of preterm birth.

Table 15.1. Pregnancy Outcomes and Selected Sociodemographic Characteristics, by Maternal Nativity Status and Race/Ethnicity: United States, 1985–1987

Characteristics	Non-Hispanic Whites*	Blacks	Chinese	Japanese	Filipinos	Other Asians	Mexicans*	Puerto Ricans*	Cubans*	Central and South Americans*
				U.S.-born mothers‡						
Infant mortality rate†	8.3	18.5	7.0	7.1	8.9	11.2	8.8	11.4	11.6	7.5
Low birthweight, %	5.5	13.1	6.5	6.5	8.0	6.3	6.6	9.4	7.0	6.8
Preterm birth, %	8.0	18.5	7.9	8.5	11.5	9.8	11.8	12.8	10.3	10.6
Maternal age <20 years, %	9.6	24.4	2.3	3.8	15.9	9.8	22.7	26.4	19.1	25.3
Maternal education <12 years, %	14.9	32.3	3.2	2.9	13.8	12.3	42.3	43.8	22.4	29.9
Maternal education ≥16 years, %	19.2	6.5	54.3	41.4	8.5	37.1	3.8	4.5	14.3	13.6
Mean education, years	13.0	11.9	14.8	14.4	12.6	13.7	11.4	11.4	12.6	12.3
Unmarried, %	14.0	64.0	8.9	10.2	29.0	18.9	29.6	54.2	23.2	65.1
Nonmetropolitan county, %	40.0	33.3	10.4	19.3	21.7	20.4	29.8	6.0	9.1	9.5
Live birth order ≥4, %	8.1	13.9	3.9	3.7	9.4	7.2	15.0	8.0	3.5	5.1
Prenatal care in 1st trimester, %	81.2	61.2	89.8	88.0	74.2	76.1	62.7	57.1	66.6	65.8
No prenatal care, %	1.1	3.8	0.4	0.5	1.0	1.5	3.7	9.4	4.4	2.8
No. live births	2,013,179	1,657,672	6,281	13,011	8,849	9,805	333,073	58,066	3,968	3,454
			Foreign- or Puerto Rican-born mothers							
Infant mortality rate†	7.6	13.7	5.8	6.1	6.9	7.9	7.6	10.4	7.1	7.8
Low birthweight, %	5.2	8.8	4.7	5.9	7.1	6.4	5.0	8.7	5.6	5.7
Preterm birth, %	8.0	13.1	7.1	7.2	10.8	10.9	10.0	12.3	9.0	10.1
Maternal age <20 years, %	4.1	6.7	0.6	1.4	3.4	5.3	13.1	14.5	4.8	7.7
Maternal education <12 years, %	11.2	28.1	15.2	5.5	12.7	23.7	74.6	46.7	19.5	35.8
Maternal education ≥16 years, %	26.6	13.9	33.8	39.0	42.2	30.9	2.6	5.5	16.2	8.3
Mean education, years	13.3	11.8	13.2	14.0	13.8	12.3	8.2	11.1	12.6	11.3
Unmarried, %	9.2	40.4	2.8	5.2	9.2	8.6	25.9	50.0	14.9	36.8
Nonmetropolitan county, %	21.4	6.6	9.1	16.7	14.8	20.1	15.7	6.5	3.5	3.0
Live birth order ≥4, %	8.7	13.7	4.3	4.3	7.1	16.5	20.9	16.1	5.9	11.5
Prenatal care in 1st trimester, %	82.5	60.8	80.8	82.8	78.2	70.2	57.1	58.3	83.5	59.2
No prenatal care, %	1.1	5.6	1.0	0.9	0.9	1.8	5.7	9.2	1.4	5.8
No. live births	99,428	124,335	44,291	10,908	54,211	164,674	407,309	51,808	25,967	132,913

Source: Data derived from the Linked Birth and Infant Death Data Sets, 1985, 1986, and 1987 birth cohorts.

*Based on data from 23 reporting states and the District of Columbia.

†Per 1,000 live births.

‡Born in the 50 states and the District of Columbia.

Table 15.1 also shows considerable ethnic and nativity difference in sociodemographic characteristics known to influence pregnancy outcomes. In general, the ethnic–nativity groups with the most favorable pregnancy outcomes appeared to have a lower prevalence of several risk factors. For instance, regardless of ethnicity, immigrants reported substantially lower rates of teenage birth than did individuals born in the United States; Chinese and Japanese immigrants had the lowest rates (0.6 percent and 1.4 percent, respectively). Immigrants were also considerably less likely to have out-of-wedlock births; the proportion of births to unmarried mothers was lowest among Chinese and Japanese immigrants and highest among U.S.-born blacks and Puerto Ricans. In addition, of all ethnic and nativity groups, U.S.-born Chinese mothers (54 percent) were most likely to have completed four or more years of college, followed by Filipino immigrants (42 percent) and U.S.- and foreign-born Japanese (41 percent and 39 percent); Mexican and Puerto Rican mothers, irrespective of their nativity status, were least likely to have completed four or more years of college. Because of higher immigrant fertility, the foreign-born women were generally more likely to have fourth- and higher order births than the U.S.-born women; however, the proportion of these high-parity births was lowest among the U.S.- and foreign-born Chinese and Japanese. Furthermore, not surprisingly, immigrants in most ethnic groups (except Cubans and non-Hispanic whites) were somewhat less likely to receive prenatal care in the first trimester than were individuals born in the United States.

Table 15.2 presents the results from the multivariate logistic analyses for the total population, showing the adjusted effect of each of the covariates on infant mortality, low birthweight, and preterm birth. Overall, regardless of ethnicity and other sociodemographic characteristics, U.S.-born women had 24 percent and 8 percent higher risks of infant mortality and low birthweight, respectively, than their immigrant counterparts. No significant differential in the risk of preterm birth was found between those born in the United States and those born elsewhere. In terms of ethnic differentials in infant mortality, only the black and other Asian groups were found to have significantly higher risks than whites—81 percent and 19 percent, respectively—after nativity and other covariates were controlled. However, relatively larger ethnic differentials existed in the risks of low-weight and preterm births. In comparison with whites, blacks, Filipinos, other Asians, and Japanese, respectively, had 113 percent, 59 percent, 38 percent, and 26 percent higher relative risks of low birthweight. The corresponding figures for the excess relative risk of preterm birth were 93 percent, 45 percent, 43 percent, and 9 percent.

The pregnancy outcome effects of the remaining covariates in Table 15.2 were consistent with those reported in previous studies.[4,12,20,22,24] Specifically, births to mothers nineteen years of age or younger and thirty-five years of age or older, out-of-wedlock and high-parity births, twin and multiple births, lower maternal

Table 15.2. Multivariate Logistic Regressions Showing Net Differentials in Pregnancy Outcomes, by Maternal Nativity Status and Other Sociodemographic Characteristics: United States, 1985–1987

	Odds Ratio (95% Confidence Interval)		
Covariate	Infant Mortality	Low Birthweight	Preterm Birth
Maternal nativity status			
Foreign born	1.00 —	1.00 —	1.00 —
U.S. born	1.24 (1.10, 1.39)	1.08 (1.04, 1.13)	0.99 (0.95, 1.03)
Race/ethnicity			
White	1.00 —	1.00 —	1.00 —
Black	1.81 (1.58, 2.07)	2.13 (2.01, 2.25)	1.93 (1.84, 2.02)
Chinese	0.92 (0.77, 1.10)	1.03 (0.97, 1.10)	0.98 (0.92, 1.03)
Japanese	0.90 (0.74, 1.09)	1.26 (1.18, 1.35)	1.09 (1.03, 1.16)
Filipino	1.06 (0.90, 1.24)	1.59 (1.50, 1.69)	1.45 (1.38, 1.52)
Other Asian	1.19 (1.03, 1.37)	1.38 (1.31, 1.46)	1.43 (1.37, 1.50)
Maternal age, years			
20–34	1.00 —	1.00 —	1.00 —
≤19	1.30 (1.14, 1.48)	1.10 (1.04, 1.16)	1.39 (1.33, 1.45)
≥35	1.18 (1.06, 1.32)	1.25 (1.20, 1.30)	1.24 (1.20, 1.28)
Marital status			
Married	1.00 —	1.00 —	1.00 —
Unmarried	1.36 (1.22, 1.50)	1.33 (1.28, 1.39)	1.45 (1.40, 1.50)
Birth order			
2–3	1.00 —	1.00 —	1.00 —
1	0.92 (0.85, 0.99)	1.32 (1.28, 1.36)	0.97 (0.95, 0.99)
≥4	1.09 (0.97, 1.21)	0.94 (0.89, 0.98)	1.21 (1.16, 1.25)
County of residence			
Nonmetropolitan	1.00 —	1.00 —	1.00 —
Metropolitan	0.93 (0.85, 1.01)	1.02 (0.98, 1.02)	0.94 (0.92, 0.97)
Plurality			
Single	1.00 —	1.00 —	1.00 —
Twin/multiple	6.02 (5.31, 6.82)	21.80 (20.68, 22.97)	6.67 (6.33, 7.03)
Maternal education, years			
<12	1.00 —	1.00 —	1.00 —
12	0.93 (0.82, 1.05)	0.85 (0.81, 0.90)	0.83 (0.80, 0.87)
≥13	0.78 (0.69, 0.89)	0.77 (0.73, 0.80)	0.72 (0.69, 0.75)
Unknown	0.99 (0.88, 1.11)	0.80 (0.76, 0.84)	0.87 (0.84, 0.90)
Trimester in which prenatal care began			
1st	1.00 —	1.00 —	— —
2nd	0.99 (0.90, 1.08)	1.00 (0.97, 1.04)	— —
3rd	0.74 (0.61, 0.89)	0.99 (0.93, 1.06)	— —
No care	2.95 (2.52, 3.46)	2.56 (2.38, 2.76)	— —
Model chi-square	1,208.47*	14,226.12*	8,935.09*
df	19	19	16
Number	387,083	386,718	378,723

Source: Data derived from the Linked Birth and Infant Death Data Sets, 1985, 1986, and 1987 birth cohorts. Adjustments made for race/ethnicity, maternal age, marital status, education, nativity status, county of residence, birth order, plurality, and prenatal care; the adjustment for preterm birth excluded prenatal care.

*p < .001.

education, and lack of prenatal care were all associated with increased risks of infant mortality, low birthweight, and preterm birth.

Table 15.3 shows how U.S.- and foreign-born differentials in risks of pregnancy outcomes differed according to race and ethnicity before and after adjustments for various sociodemographic characteristics through logistic regression. For the total population, the unadjusted (crude) nativity differentials were all significant, with U.S.-born mothers showing 51 percent, 22 percent, and 8 percent higher risks of infant mortality, low birthweight, and preterm birth, respectively, than foreign-born mothers. The adjusted nativity differentials for risk of pregnancy outcomes for the total population (also shown in Table 15.2) were much narrower, suggesting that the more favorable maternal risk profile for immigrants compared to U.S.-born women may partially account for the observed nativity differentials.

The conventional sociodemographic characteristics considered here do little to account for the observed nativity differentials in the three pregnancy outcomes for most of the ethnic groups. Because crude and adjusted nativity differentials were generally similar (see Table 15.3), only adjusted differentials were interpreted. The racial/ethnic immigrant groups that had significantly lower risks of infant mortality than individuals born in the United States included blacks, other Asians, Mexicans, Puerto Ricans, and Cubans. However, the reduced infant mortality risk was most pronounced for Cuban, other Asian, and black immigrants, who exhibited 39 percent, 27 percent, and 25 percent lower risks, respectively, than their U.S.-born counterparts of equivalent sociodemographic backgrounds.

Not only was the immigrants' risk of low birthweight significantly lower than that of the U.S.-born women, but the beneficial effects of immigrant status tended to vary according to race and ethnicity. For example, while U.S.-born Mexicans, Chinese, and blacks had 38 percent to 61 percent higher risks of low birthweight than their immigrant counterparts, U.S.-born Puerto Ricans, Central and South Americans, and Cubans showed only 10 percent to 24 percent higher risks than their immigrant or Puerto Rican–born counterparts. Moreover, other Asian immigrants showed an 11 percent higher risk of low birthweight than did their U.S.-born counterparts. A fairly similar pattern held for ethnicity-specific nativity effects on preterm births. While U.S.-born blacks showed a 31 percent higher risk of preterm birth than their immigrant counterparts, the U.S.- and foreign- or Puerto Rican–born differential was between 6 percent and 17 percent, respectively, for Puerto Ricans, Japanese, and Mexicans. Once again, other Asian immigrants showed a 16 percent higher risk of preterm birth than their U.S.-born counterparts.

While the beneficial effects of immigrant status may partly reflect positive selectivity (that is, the "healthy immigrant effect"), it may also serve as a proxy for a host of protective behavioral, cultural, and psychosocial factors such as

Table 15.3. Crude and Adjusted Differentials in Risks of Infant Mortality, Low Birthweight, and Preterm Birth Between U.S.- and Foreign-Born Mothers, by Race and Ethnicity: United States, 1985–1987

| Race/Ethnicity | Odds Ratio (95% Confidence Interval) | | No. Live Births |
	Crude*	Adjusted[†]	
	Infant Mortality		
White (non-Hispanic)[‡]	1.04 (0.93, 1.17)	0.98 (0.87, 1.10)	824,780[§]
Black	1.33 (1.22, 1.45)	1.33 (1.21, 1.45)	592,297**
Chinese	1.19 (0.85, 1.66)	1.18 (0.84, 1.66)	48,652
Japanese	1.11 (0.80, 1.55)	1.12 (0.80, 1.57)	23,416
Filipino	1.25 (0.97, 1.60)	1.03 (0.78, 1.35)	61,895
Other Asian	1.42 (1.16, 1.74)	1.37 (1.11, 1.68)	165,997
Mexican[‡]	1.14 (1.09, 1.20)	1.16 (1.09, 1.22)	718,558
Puerto Rican[‡,††]	1.17 (1.03, 1.31)	1.18 (1.04, 1.33)	104,975
Cuban[‡]	1.69 (1.22, 2.35)	1.63 (1.15, 2.30)	29,629
Central and South American[‡]	0.86 (0.56, 1.32)	0.80 (0.52, 1.23)	132,240
Total	1.51 (1.41, 1.62)	1.24 (1.10, 1.39)	387,083
	Low Birthweight		
White (non-Hispanic)[‡]	1.08 (1.03, 1.13)	1.04 (0.99, 1.09)	823,818[§]
Black	1.60 (1.54, 1.65)	1.61 (1.55, 1.67)	602,178**
Chinese	1.43 (1.28, 1.59)	1.45 (1.29, 1.64)	48,607
Japanese	1.09 (0.98, 1.22)	1.09 (0.97, 1.22)	23,390
Filipino	1.12 (1.02, 1.22)	1.04 (0.95, 1.14)	61,854
Other Asian	0.99 (0.91, 1.08)	0.90 (0.82, 0.98)	165,824
Mexican[‡]	1.36 (1.33, 1.39)	1.38 (1.35, 1.41)	717,884
Puerto Rican[‡,††]	1.10 (1.05, 1.14)	1.10 (1.05, 1.15)	104,857
Cuban[‡]	1.28 (1.12, 1.47)	1.24 (1.07, 1.43)	29,611
Central and South American[‡]	1.22 (1.06, 1.40)	1.18 (1.02, 1.36)	132,097
Total	1.22 (1.19, 1.25)	1.08 (1.04, 1.13)	386,718
	Preterm Birth		
White (non-Hispanic)[‡]	1.00 (0.96, 1.04)	0.96 (0.92, 1.00)	806,694[§]
Black	1.48 (1.44, 1.53)	1.31 (1.27, 1.35)	594,557**
Chinese	1.12 (1.02, 1.24)	1.08 (0.98, 1.20)	48,170
Japanese	1.19 (1.08, 1.31)	1.16 (1.05, 1.28)	23,072
Filipino	1.08 (1.01, 1.16)	0.97 (0.90, 1.05)	61,014
Other Asian	0.90 (0.84, 0.96)	0.86 (0.80, 0.93)	160,874
Mexican[‡]	1.20 (1.18, 1.22)	1.17 (1.15, 1.19)	701,750
Puerto Rican[‡,††]	1.04 (1.01, 1.08)	1.06 (1.02, 1.10)	107,168
Cuban[‡]	1.17 (1.04, 1.30)	1.11 (0.98, 1.25)	29,338
Central and South American[‡]	1.01 (0.90, 1.13)	0.99 (0.88, 1.12)	132,098
Total	1.08 (1.05, 1.10)	0.99 (0.95, 1.03)	378,723

Source: Data derived from the Linked Birth and Infant Death Data Sets, 1985, 1986, and 1987 birth cohorts. Differentials based on logistic regression models. The reference group was foreign- or Puerto Rican–born mothers.

*Unadjusted for the effects of other covariates.

[†]Adjusted for the effects of maternal age, marital status, education, birth order, place of residence, plurality, and prenatal care; the adjustment for preterm birth excluded prenatal care.

[‡]Based on data from 23 reporting states and the District of Columbia.

[§]40 percent sample of live births.

**35 percent sample of live births.

[††]Differentials between Puerto Rican women born in the 50 states and the District of Columbia and Puerto Rican women born in Puerto Rico or abroad.

low rates of tobacco, alcohol, and other substance use during pregnancy; social origin influences, including childhood socioeconomic status; better nutritional practices (for example, higher levels of breast-feeding, better/more balanced diets, lower levels of obesity); positive cultural attitudes toward maternity; and strong social and familial support.[4-11,20,26]

Although many of the cultural and psychosocial factors are difficult to operationalize and could not be addressed with vital statistics data, we can nonetheless present nativity-specific data on some of the behavioral and social factors, such as prenatal substance use, exposure to environmental tobacco smoke, household structure, breast-feeding, and whether the pregnancy was wanted. For instance, our analysis of the most recent birth certificate data indicates a considerably greater rate of cigarette smoking during pregnancy among U.S.-born mothers than among foreign-born mothers.[18] Figure 15.2 displays such information by race and ethnicity. As can be seen from this figure, U.S.-born

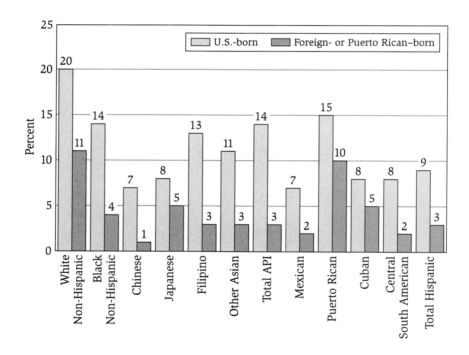

Figure 15.2 Percentage of Mothers Smoking During Pregnancy, by Maternal Race/Ethnicity and Nativity: United States, 1992.

Note: Smoking data exclude California, New York, Indiana, and South Dakota. Hispanic origin was not reported for New Hampshire. API = Asians and Pacific Islanders, including Hawaiians.

Source: Data derived from the 1992 natality data file, National Center for Health Statistics.

Hispanics, blacks, and Asians were, on average, three to five times more likely to smoke cigarettes than their immigrant counterparts. Even among non-Hispanic whites, U.S.-born mothers were almost twice as likely to smoke as their foreign-born counterparts. The rate of cigarette smoking was lowest among Chinese and Mexican immigrants and highest among U.S.-born non-Hispanic whites, Hawaiians, and Puerto Ricans.[18] Furthermore, based on the analysis of the 1988 National Maternal and Infant Health Survey data, mothers born in the United States were 2.3 and 3.9 times more likely to use alcohol and marijuana/cocaine during pregnancy, respectively, than their foreign-born counterparts.[16] In addition, U.S.-born non-Hispanic white, black, Asian, and Hispanic mothers were 1.3 to 1.9 times more likely than their immigrant counterparts to be exposed to environmental tobacco smoke during pregnancy.[16]

Household composition can be used to measure roughly the degree to which familial and social support may be available to mothers during their pregnancy.[27] Based on the 1988 National Maternal and Infant Health Survey data, black and Asian immigrant mothers were 6 percent to 9 percent more likely than their U.S.-born counterparts to live in households with their partners or extended family members,[16] environments generally regarded as more conducive to positive birth outcomes. Contrary to our expectation, Hispanic immigrants were somewhat more likely than U.S.-born Hispanics to live alone during pregnancy (10.0 percent versus 6.6 percent).[16] Breast-feeding, the optimal form of infant nutrition, has been linked to a reduced risk of infant mortality.[28] Our analysis of the 1988 National Maternal and Infant Health Survey data showed that foreign-born mothers were substantially more likely to breast-feed than U.S.-born mothers; this was especially true among black mothers, of whom immigrants were almost three times more likely to breast-feed than their U.S.-born counterparts.[16] Whether or not a pregnancy is wanted can influence birth outcome by encouraging positive maternal health behavior during pregnancy.[29,30] As the 1988 National Maternal and Infant Health Survey data indicate, Asian, Hispanic, and black immigrant mothers were, respectively, 43.2 percent, 21.8 percent, and 19.5 percent less likely than their U.S.-born counterparts to report that their babies were unwanted or mistimed.[16]

DISCUSSION

The results of this study strongly indicate that foreign-born/immigrant status is associated with a substantially reduced risk of infant mortality and low birthweight for the total population in general and for blacks, Cubans, Mexicans, and Chinese in particular. No appreciable difference in the risk of preterm birth existed between the U.S.-born and foreign-born women for the total population, although infants born to Japanese, Mexican, and black immigrant mothers exhibited about a 15 percent to 25 percent lower risk than their U.S.-born counterparts.

How does one address the observed ethnicity-specific nativity differentials in the risks of the pregnancy outcomes discussed here? The extent to which differences involving prenatal substance use, exposure to environmental tobacco smoke, household structure, breast-feeding, and whether the pregnancy is wanted vary by ethnicity may help account for a substantial portion of these differentials. However, to explain more fully the considerable differentials between U.S.- and foreign-born blacks, it may be necessary to look at not only the current life circumstances and socially disadvantaged position of U.S.-born blacks vis-à-vis foreign-born blacks but also their unique sociocultural and political historical background. Very few groups, if any, have experienced for so long the kind and degree of discrimination that U.S.-born blacks have faced.[31] Foreign-born blacks, on the other hand, have not had similar long-term exposure to socioeconomic and structural discrimination.

To understand further the nativity differentials, especially among such groups as Cubans, Mexicans, Chinese, and other Asians, it may be pertinent also to consider the varied circumstances under which members of different ethnic immigrant groups entered the United States. These circumstances, which broadly define the immigration process, include country-of-origin conditions, period of immigration, push and pull factors prompting the migration, criterion under which the individual immigrated (skill, refugee, or family reunification), place of destination within the United States, and U.S. immigration laws or restrictions in effect at the time of immigration.[1,32]

A word of caution is also in order. While data on infant mortality and low birthweight from linked records are considered to be very reliable, the accuracy of birth certificate data on gestational age has sometimes been questioned.[33-35] Gestational age data for this study, based primarily on last menstrual period, were missing for about 4 percent of the births.[13-15] Moreover, approximately 14 percent of the birth records were imputed for gestational age when the month of the last menstrual period was known but the day was not. The percentage of missing and imputed records tended to be higher for blacks, Mexicans, and other Asians than for other groups. Immigrants generally had a higher percentage of missing records but a somewhat lower percentage of imputed records.[36] Imputed and missing records may have introduced into our analysis two potentially different biases: while the effect of imputation may have been to slightly increase the proportion of preterm births,[37] the effect of missing records was likely to introduce a downward bias in the estimates of preterm birth.[33,34] These biases could mean a somewhat larger differential in preterm births between the U.S.- and foreign-born mothers in our ethnicity-specific analyses than may have actually been the case.

Finally, although we have emphasized only the substantial but varying effects of nativity status on pregnancy outcomes by ethnicity, it is also important to mention that several other critical factors, such as maternal age, education, marital status, and prenatal care, affected pregnancy outcomes differentially for immigrants and those born in the United States. As the findings of the study suggest, nativity status, in conjunction with ethnicity, may serve as an important axis of differentiation and stratification in analyses of pregnancy outcomes among the current U.S. population. Nativity differences should be considered in designing and carrying out ethnicity-specific interventions to prevent adverse pregnancy outcomes.

Notes

1. Jasso, G., & Rosenzweig, M. (1990). *The new chosen people: Immigrants in the United States.* New York: Russell Sage Foundation.

2. U.S. Bureau of the Census. (1993). *Statistical Abstract of the United States, 1993.* Washington, DC: Author.

3. U.S. Bureau of the Census. (1993). *Asians and Pacific Islanders in the United States.* Washington, DC: Author.

4. Kleinman, J. C., Fingerhut, L. A., & Prager, K. (1991). Differences in infant mortality by race, nativity status, and other maternal characteristics. *Am J Dis Child, 145,* 194–199.

5. Becerra, J., Hogue, C., Atrash, H., & Perez, N. (1991). Infant mortality among Hispanics: A portrait of heterogeneity. *JAMA, 265,* 217–221.

6. Guendelman, S., Gould, J., Hudes, M., et al. (1990). Generational differences in perinatal health among the Mexican American population: Findings from the HHANES 1982–1984. *Am J Public Health, 80*(Suppl.), 61–65.

7. Ventura, S., & Taffel, S. (1985). Childbearing characteristics of U.S.-born and foreign-born Hispanic mothers. *Public Health Rep, 100,* 647–652.

8. Collins, J. W., & Shay, D. K. (1994). Prevalence of low birthweight among Hispanic infants with United States–born and foreign-born mothers: The effect of urban poverty. *Am J Epidemiol, 139,* 184–192.

9. Cabral, H., Fried, L., Levenson, S., et al. (1990). Foreign-born and U.S.-born black women: Differences in health behaviors and birth outcomes. *Am J Public Health, 80,* 70–72.

10. Valanis, B., & Rush, D. (1979). A partial explanation of superior birth weights among foreign-born women. *Soc Biol, 26,* 198–210.

11. Valanis, B. (1979). Relative contributions of maternal social and biological characteristics to birth weight and gestation among mothers of different childhood socioeconomic status. *Soc Biol, 26,* 211–225.

12. Singh, G. K., & Yu, S. M. (1993). Pregnancy outcomes among Asian Americans. *Asian Am Pacific Islander J Health, 1,* 63–78.

13. U.S. Public Health Service. (1990). *Linked Birth/Infant Death Data Set: 1985 birth cohort, public use data tape documentation.* Hyattsville, MD: Author.

14. U.S. Public Health Service. (1991). *Linked Birth/Infant Death Data Set: 1986 birth cohort, public use data tape documentation.* Hyattsville, MD: Author.

15. U.S. Public Health Service. (1992). *Linked Birth/Infant Death Data Set: 1987 birth cohort, public use data tape documentation.* Hyattsville, MD: Author.

16. U.S. Public Health Service. (1991). *1988 National Maternal and Infant Health Survey: Public use data tape documentation.* Hyattsville, MD: Author.

17. Sanderson, M., Placek, P. J., & Keppel, K. G. (1991). The 1988 National Maternal and Infant Health Survey: Design, content, and data availability. *Birth, 18,* 26–32.

18. U.S. Public Health Service. (1994). *1992 Detail Natality File: Public use data tape documentation.* Hyattsville, MD: Author.

19. Ventura, S. J., Martin, J. A., Taffel, S. M., Mathews, T. J., & Clarke, S. C. (1994). Advance report of final natality statistics, 1992. *Mon Vital Stat Rep, 43*(5, Suppl.).

20. Institute of Medicine. (1985). *Preventing low birthweight.* Washington, DC: National Academy Press.

21. Eberstein, I. W. (1989). Demographic research on infant mortality. *Sociol Forum, 4,* 409–422.

22. Cramer, J. C. (1987). Social factors and infant mortality: Identifying high risk groups and proximate causes. *Demography, 24,* 299–322.

23. Nersesian, W. S. (1988). Infant mortality in socially vulnerable populations. *Annu Rev Public Health, 9,* 361–377.

24. Singh, G. K., & Kposowa, A. J. (1994). A comparative analysis of infant mortality in major Ohio cities: Significance of socio-biological factors. *Appl Behav Sci Rev, 2,* 77–94.

25. SAS Institute Inc. (1989). *SAS/STAT User's Guide: The LOGISTIC Procedure, Version 6*(4th ed.). Cary, NC: Author.

26. Brooks-Gun, J. (1991). Stress and support during pregnancy: What do they tell us about low birthweight? In H. Berendes, S. Kessel, & S. Yaffe (Eds.), *Advances in the Prevention of Low Birth Weight: An international symposium* (pp. 39–57). Washington, DC: National Center for Education in Maternal and Child Health.

27. Moss, N., & Carver, K. (1992, May). Explaining racial and ethnic differences in birth outcomes: The effect of household structure and resources. Paper presented at the annual meeting of the Population Association of America, Denver, CO.

28. Mosley, W. H., & Chen, L. C. (1984). An analytical framework for the study of child survival in developing countries? In W. H. Mosley & L. C. Chen (Eds.), Child survival: Strategies for research. *Popul Dev Rev, 10*(Suppl.), 15–45.

29. Weller, R. H., Eberstein, I. W., & Bailey, M. (1987). Pregnancy wantedness and maternal behavior during pregnancy. *Demography, 24,* 407–412.

30. Marsiglio, W., & Mott, F. (1988). Does wanting to become pregnant with a first child affect subsequent maternal behaviors and infant birth weight? *J Marriage Fam, 50,* 1023–1036.

31. James, S. A. (1993). Racial and ethnic differences in infant mortality and low birth weight: A psychosocial critique. *Ann Epidemiol, 3,* 130–136.

32. Lamberty, G., & Coll, C. G. (1994). Conclusion: Expanding on what is known about the health and development of Puerto Rican mothers and children. In G. Lamberty & C. G. Coll (Eds.), *Puerto Rican women and children: Issues in health, growth, and development* (pp. 255–276). New York: Plenum.

33. Berkowitz, G. S., & Papiernik, E. (1993). Epidemiology of preterm birth. *Epidemiol Rev, 15,* 415–443.

34. David, R. J. (1980). The quality and completeness of birth weight and gestational age data in computerized birth files. *Am J Public Health, 70,* 964–973.

35. Adams, M. M. (1995). The continuing challenge of preterm delivery. *JAMA, 273,* 739–740.

36. U.S. Public Health Service. (1989). *1987 Detail Natality File: Public use data tape documentation.* Hyattsville, MD: Author.

37. Taffel, S., Johnson, D., & Heuser, R. (1982). A method of imputing length of gestation on birth certificates. *Vital Health Stat, 2*(93).

CHAPTER SIXTEEN

Understanding the Hispanic Paradox

Luisa Franzini
John C. Ribble
Arlene M. Keddie

The purpose of this article is to review the literature on the health of Hispanics in the United States and to observe how it is influenced by socioeconomic variables. We were prompted to consider the health of this ethnic group because of our interest in the well-documented correlation in the general U.S. population between adverse social characteristics and mortality rates, as well as several other indicators of poor health. On the other hand, Hispanics, as a group, have mortality (but not morbidity) outcomes equal or surprisingly better than non-Hispanics in the United States, even though they rank low in most socioeconomic indicators.[1] The investigation of this "paradox" may provide additional insights into the ways that social factors affect the health of the population at large.

What follows is a review of the published evidence regarding the "Hispanic paradox," including documentation of this phenomenon with recent national vital statistics. We will also examine the hypotheses that have been put forth to explain it, and will suggest possibilities for further study of this interesting dilemma.

Our study was supported by funds from the Center for Society and Population Health, University of Texas School of Public Health. We thank Richard Wilkinson for discussions on the "Hispanic paradox" and comments on earlier drafts.

METHODS

We conducted computerized bibliographic searches of databases, including Medline (1966 through 1999) and Sociological Abstracts (1963 through 1999). Two types of computerized bibliographic searches were employed: a general search and eight focused searches.

The indexing term employed for the general search was "Hispanic-American mortality." The search yielded more than 300 articles, 76 of which were selected because their titles and abstracts pertained to some aspect of the Hispanic paradox.

Eight focused searches on specific diseases or factors believed to influence Hispanic health were carried out. The indexing terms and yields for the focused searches were diabetes in Hispanics (39 articles), HIV/AIDS in Hispanics (337 articles), migration (45 articles), risk factors in Hispanics (44 articles), acculturation in Hispanics (168 articles). Focused searches were also carried out for the following three studies: San Antonio Heart Study (118 articles), San Luis Valley Diabetes Study (40 articles), and Corpus Christi Heart Project (13 articles). We identified 98 articles relevant to the topics in the review by going through the titles and abstracts of the 804 articles generated by the focused searches.

There was some overlap in the 76 relevant articles located through the general search and the 98 relevant articles located through the focused searches. We identified additional relevant articles from the reference lists in the articles. Altogether, 183 articles relevant to this review were identified and read. We chose 89 of them, based on importance, originality, and avoidance of redundancy, to be reviewed in this chapter.

Data from the National Center for Health Statistics were taken directly from printed or Internet versions of U.S. government reports. Unless otherwise stated, the most recent data available in April 1999 were used.

The term *Hispanic* is used ambiguously throughout the literature. In this study, we use the term broadly to mean persons whose origins are the Spanish-speaking countries of the Americas (Mexico and the countries of Central and South America and the Caribbean). More specific definitions are given in the text as needed. In reviewing the specific articles, we use the term as it is defined in the original paper (Tables 16.1 and 16.2).

DOCUMENTATION OF THE HISPANIC PARADOX

Hispanic Socioeconomic Status

Hispanics as a group rank low in various measures of socioeconomic status. The average income of this group is much closer to that of blacks than of non-Hispanic whites (NHW), as is the proportion living in poverty. In 1998, the

Table 16.1. Selected Studies on Hispanic Health Outcomes

Authors	Definition of Hispanic	Data Source	Study Population	Outcomes
		Mortality		
Bradshaw & Fonner[9]	Spanish surname	Vital statistics	Texas, 1969–71	Mortality: males: SS similar to NHW; females: SS higher than NHW.
Schoen & Nelson[11]	Spanish surname	Vital statistics	California, 1969–71	Life expectancy: similar in SS and NHW.
Shai & Rosenwaike[12]	Nativity	Vital statistics	Mexican born and Puerto Rican born Cook County, 1979–81	Mortality: Mexican and Puerto Rican lower than NHW.
Rosenwaike[13]	Nativity	Vital statistics	Mexican born, Puerto Rican born, Cuban born Cook County, 1979–81	Mortality: Mexican, Cuban, and Puerto Rican lower in older groups, higher in younger groups.
Desenclos & Hahn[14]	Death certificate	Vital statistics	U.S., 1986–88	Years of life lost <65: higher in H than NHW.
Liao, Cooper, et al.[15]	Self-report	National Health Interview Survey	378,431 respondents (27,239 Hispanics) 1986–90	Mortality: younger age group: higher in H than NHW; older age group: lower in H than NHW.
Sorlie et al.[16]	Self-report	Current Population Survey and National Death Index (National Longitudinal Mortality Study)	700,000 respondents (40,000 Hispanics), 1979–87	Mortality: younger age group: similar in H and NHW; older age group: lower in H than NHW.

Infant Mortality

Study	Hispanic identifier	Data source	Population	Findings
Bradshaw & Frisbie[18]	Spanish surname	Vital statistics	San Antonio, Texas	Infant mortality: higher in SS than NHW in 1935; similar in 1985.
Williams et al.[19]	Spanish surname	Vital statistics	California	Neonatal and postneonatal mortality: similar in SS and NHW; birth-weight specific mortality rates: higher in SS than NHW.
Kleinman[20]	Mother's race/ethnicity as on birth certificate	Vital statistics	23 U.S. states	Infant mortality: equal or lower for most H subgroups and NHW.
Becerra et al.[21]	Mother's race/ethnicity as on birth certificate and nativity	Vital statistics	23 U.S. states	Neonatal and postneonatal mortality vary by H subgroups.
Engel et al.[22]	Mother's race/ethnicity as on birth certificate and nativity	Vital statistics	U.S. Puerto Rican women	Birthweight and postneonatal mortality: lower in PR born than U.S. born; neonatal mortality: higher in PR born than U.S. born.
Albrecht et al.[23]	Mother's race/ethnicity as on birth certificate	Vital statistics	U.S. Puerto Rican women	Birthweight, neonatal and post-neonatal mortality: vary by H subgroups.
Guendelman et al.[24]	Self-report	California Perinatal Reporting System	80,431 patients in prenatal care clinics, California, 1984–89	Fetal deaths: similar in H and NHW; lower than in African Americans.

(Continued)

Table 16.1. Selected Studies on Hispanic Health Outcomes (Continued)

Authors	Definition of Hispanic	Data Source	Study Population	Outcomes
Violence				
Rogers[25]	Self-report	National Health Interview Survey, Supplement on Aging	Sample of U.S. population, 1984	Health outcomes and mortality.
Rodriguez & Brindis[26]	Of Latin American origin or descendent	Literature review	Latino population	Homicide and nonfatal intentional injuries: higher in H than NHW; vary by H subgroups.
Shai & Rosenwaike[27]	Nativity	Vital statistics	Mexican, Puerto Rican and Cuban-born migrants	Homicide, suicide, accidents: vary by H subgroups.
AIDS				
Chiasson et al.[29]	Death certificate	Vital statistics	AIDS deaths in New York, 1983–98	Similar declines in HIV/AIDS mortality in H and NHW.
Lehner & Chiasson[30]	Self-report	Survey	Clinic in New York City	HIV seroprevalence and sex behavior.
Díaz & Klevens, et al.[32]	Self-report	Survey	Persons with AIDS reported to 12 local and state health departments	Exposure to HIV through drug use higher in Puerto Ricans than other H.
Montoya et al.[33]	Self-report	Survey	National sample	HIV risk highest in Puerto Ricans.
Davis et al.[34]	Self-report	Survey	National sample	HIV seroprevalence: higher in H than NHW.
Obiri et al.[36]	Death certificate	Vital statistics	New York City, 1983–94	Contribution of AIDS to years of potential life lost: higher in H than any other group.

CHD

Study	Ascertainment	Study design	Population	Findings
Goff et al.[37]	Spanish surname	Vital statistics	Deaths in Texas, 1980–89	Acute MI and chronic CHD mortality: lower in H men than NHW men; no difference among women.
Wild et al.[38]	Death certificate	Vital statistics	Deaths in California, 1985–90	Mortality from CHD and stroke: lower in H.
Mitchell et al.[39]	Self-report	Population-based survey (San Antonio Heart Study)	5,149 Mexican Americans and NHW, 25-64 years old	Relation between diabetes and prevalence of MI: similar in H and NHW.
Wei et al.[40]	Algorithm (self-report, SS, nativity)	Population-based survey (San Antonio Heart Study)	2,629 Mexican Americans and 1,136 NHW	All cause and cardiovascular disease mortality: similar in H and NHW; effect of risk factors similar.
Goff, Varas, et al.[41]	Self-report	Population-based surveillance (Corpus Christi Heart Project)	334 Mexican Americans and 348 NHW hospitalized for MI	MI survival disadvantage in H compared to NHW.
Goff, Ramsey, et al.[42]	Self-report	Population-based surveillance (Corpus Christi Heart Project)	1,228 men hospitalized for MI	MI 28-day case-fatality: higher in H than NHW.
Rewers, Shetterly, Hoag, et al.[43]	Self-report	Surveillance and survey (San Luis Valley Diabetes Study)	Residents of Alamosa and Conejos Counties, Colorado	Risk of CHD: lower in H diabetic than NHW diabetic; similar in nondiabetics.
Rewers, Shetterly, Baxter, et al.[44]	Self-report	Surveillance and survey (San Luis Valley Diabetes Study)	Residents of Alamosa and Conejos Counties, Colorado	Prevalence of CHD: lower in H diabetics than NHW diabetics.

(Continued)

Table 16.1. Selected Studies on Hispanic Health Outcomes (Continued)

Authors	Definition of Hispanic	Data Source	Study Population	Outcomes
Stroke				
Gillum[45]	Death certificate	Vital statistics	Hispanics and NHW in U.S., 1989–91	Stroke death rates similar in young H and NHW; lower in older H than NHW.
Sacco, Boden-Albala, et al.[46]	Self-report	Surveillance and survey (Northern Manhattan Stroke Study)	New York City, 1993–96	Stroke incidence for H intermediate between rates for NHW and AA.
Sacco, Hauser, et al.[47]	Skin pigmentation and surname	Medical records	Patients with stroke admitted to Columbia-Presbyterian Medical Center, NY, 1983–86	Better outcome one year after stroke for H than NHW and AA.
Cancer				
Rosenwaike[48]	Mexican born	Vital statistics	Deaths of Mexican born and whites, 1979–81	Cancer mortality from common cancers: lower in H; from rare cancers: higher in H.
Davis et al.[49]	Spanish surname and maiden name	Illinois State Cancer Registry	Hispanics and NHW Cook County, IL, 1986–87	Cancer incidence: lower for common cancers in H.
Gilliland et al.[50]	Self-report and Spanish surname	New Mexico Tumor Registry	New Mexico residents and American Indians in Arizona, 1969–94	Survival after cancer diagnosis: lower in H than NHW.
Rogers & Crank[51]	Mexican American; self-report	National Health Interview Survey	National sample, 1979–80	Smoking rates lower in H.
Balcazar et al.[52]	Mexican American	Literature review	571 Mexican American women	Cancer risk factors.

Diabetes,

Gardner et al.[55]	Self-report	Population-based survey (San Antonio Heart Study)	Three neighborhoods in San Antonio, Texas	Neighborhoods with higher % native American admixture as estimated from skin color had higher rates of NIDDM.
Hanis, Ferrell, et al.[57]	Self-report	Random sample of Starr County residents	Starr County, Texas	Prevalence and morbidity of diabetes: higher in Starr County.
Hamman et al.[58]	Self-report	Surveillance and survey (San Luis Valley Diabetes Study)	Residents of Alamosa and Conejos Counties, Colorado, 1983	Prevalence of NIDDM: higher in H than NHW.
Marshall, Hamman, Baxter, et al.[59]	Self-report	Case control study (San Luis Valley Diabetes Study)	767 residents of Alamosa and Conejos Counties, Colorado, 1984–86	Prevalence of NIDDM: higher in H than NHW after controlling for risk factors associated with NIDDM.
Baxter, Hamman, Lopez, et al.[60]	Self-report	Surveillance and survey (San Luis Valley Diabetes Study)	Residents of Alamosa and Conejos Counties, Colorado, 1983–88	Incidence of NIDDM: higher in H than NHW.
Perez-Stable et al.[61]	Self-report	HHANES and NHANES II	Sample of Mexican origin population, 1982–84	Self-reported diabetes: higher in H than U.S. population.

Note: H = Hispanic; NHW = non-Hispanic white; SS = Spanish surname; PR = Puerto Rican; AA = African American; NIDDM = non-insulin-dependent diabetes mellitus; CVD = cardiovascular disease; CHD = coronary heart disease; MI = myocardial infarction.

Table 16.2. Selected Studies on Possible Explanations for the Hispanic Paradox

Authors	Definition of Hispanic	Data Source	Study Population	Outcomes
		Data Reliability		
Rosenwaike & Bradshaw[64]	Spanish origin on death certificate and Spanish surname	Census and vital statistics	Arizona, California, Colorado, New Mexico, and Texas, 1980	Comparison of mortality for SS and from death certificate information.
Polednak[65]	Spanish origin on death certificate and Spanish surname	Vital statistics	Deaths in Connecticut, 1990–91	Comparison of mortality for SS and from death certificate information.
Sorlie, Rogot & Johnson[66]	Self-report	Current Population Survey and National Death Index (National Longitudinal Mortality Study)	43,000 deaths, 1979–85	Comparison of mortality from death certificate information and survey.
Polednak[67]	Spanish surname	Connecticut Tumor Registry	Connecticut residents, 1980–88	Lung cancer mortality lower in H men than NHW men. For women SS not good indicator of ethnicity.
Powell-Griner & Streck[68]	Spanish surname	Vital statistics	Texas residents, 1979	Underreporting of SS neonatal mortality.
		Salmon Bias/Healthy Migrant		
Abraido-Lanza et al.[72]	Self-report	Current Population Survey and National Death Index (National Longitudinal Mortality Study)	17,375 Hispanics and 301,718 NHW	Cuban and PR lower mortality than NHW. U.S.-born H lower mortality than U.S.-born NHW.
Fang et al.[75]	Nativity	Vital statistics	New York City residents, 1988–92	Higher mortality for U.S.-born H than foreign-born H.
Wei et al.[76]	Self-report	Population-based survey (San Antonio Heart Study)	3,735 residents of San Antonio, Texas	Higher mortality for U.S.-born Mexicans than foreign-born Mexicans.

Risk Factors

Jones, Gonzalez, Pillow, et al.[77]	Self-report	Local survey	22 Houston, Texas area women	Intake of dietary fiber higher in H.
Schaffer, Velie, et al.[78]	Self-report	Population-based sample	462 new mothers in California, 1989–91	Energy and nutrient intakes and health practices in the 3 months before pregnancy better in H.
Elder et al.[79]	Self-report	Population-based sample	358 Latino and 113 Anglo	Cancer risk related behaviors better in H.
Thompson, Demark-Wahnefried, et al.[80]	Self-report	Sample	15,060 participants to 7 study centers	Frequency of fruit and vegetables consumed lower in H.

Acculturation

Hazuda et al.[82]	Self-report	Population-based survey (San Antonio Heart Study)	1,288 Mexican American and 929 NHW in San Antonio, TX, 1979–82	Obesity and diabetes decrease with acculturation.
Angel & Cleary[84]	Self-report	National Opinion Research Center of the University of Chicago	Sample of 4,025 of U.S. population, 1980	Self-reported health and other health measures better in less-acculturated H.
Elder et al.[86]	Self-report	Survey	332 ESL students in San Diego, California	SES inversely related to CVD risk factors.
Scribner & Dwyer[91]	Self-report	HHANES, 1982–84	1,645 mothers of Mexican descent in HHANES	Less acculturated had lower risk of low birthweight.

Note: H = Hispanic; NHW = non-Hispanic white; SS = Spanish surname; PR = Puerto Rican; AA = African American; NIDDM = non-insulin-dependent diabetes mellitus; CVD = cardiovascular disease; CHD = coronary heart disease; MI = myocardial infarction.

median household income of Hispanics ($28,330) was substantially lower than that of NHW ($42,439), and only slightly higher than that of blacks ($25,351). Similar proportions of Hispanics (29 percent) and blacks (28 percent) were living below or near the poverty level. Over one-third of Hispanic children under eighteen years of age lived in or near poverty (33.6 percent), much closer to the proportion of black children (39.9 percent) than NHW children (10.4 percent) living in similar circumstances.[2] Not only was the income of Hispanics lower than that of NHW, it was also distributed somewhat less equally. In 1998, the Gini coefficient was higher in Hispanics (0.460) and blacks (0.466) than in whites (0.450).[3] The Gini coefficient is a measure of income inequality, with higher values representing higher inequality.[4]

Hispanics also rank low in education and job classification compared to both blacks and NHW. In 1996, more than 40 percent of Hispanics aged twenty-five to sixty-four years had completed fewer than twelve years of schooling compared to about 10 percent of NHW and 20 percent of blacks.[5] A smaller percentage of Hispanic workers (26 percent) have white-collar jobs compared to 52.6 percent of NHW and 33.5 percent of black workers.[5]

More Hispanics than any other racial/ethnic group are without health insurance. This is true for both men and women at each level of family income. In 1997, approximately 37 percent of Hispanics were uninsured, compared to 14 percent of NHW and 23 percent of blacks.[6] Hispanics were also less likely to use medical care. In 1995–1996, more Hispanics with health problems reported no physician contact within the past year than members of any other racial or ethnic group.[6]

Hispanic All-Cause Mortality

The Hispanic paradox appears to be a recent phenomenon. In Houston and San Antonio, Texas, in 1949–1951, mortality rates for individuals with Spanish surnames (SS) were slightly greater than those for other whites.[7,8] Studies in Texas conducted between 1969 and 1980 found that the all-cause mortality rates for SS males were similar to those for other white males, even though the rates for SS males under the age of forty-five were higher than those for other white males. In all age groups, the mortality rates for SS females were higher than those for other white females.[9,10] In California during the years 1969–1971, life expectancy at birth, fifteen, forty, and sixty-five years of age was very similar for individuals with Spanish surnames and other whites.[11]

The 1980 U.S. Census data permitted estimates of the mortality rates of persons residing in the United States who were born outside the country. All-cause mortality rates were consistently found to be lower for Hispanics compared to NHW in older, but not younger, age categories. In Chicago during the period 1979–1981, Cuban- and Mexican-born males and females had higher mortality rates than NHW in the younger age groups, but had lower mortality rates at older ages. Puerto Ricans had higher mortality rates than NHW in most age groups.[12,13]

Beginning in 1985, the National Center for Health Statistics provided information on ethnicity for many of the U.S. states that could be used to determine mortality rates of people of Hispanic origin. The data showed that the age-adjusted, all-cause mortality rate (per 100,000) for Hispanic males was 800.3 compared to 1,053.8 for NHW males. Mortality rates for females were 518.0 for Hispanics and 676.3 for NHW.[14]

Using data from the National Health Interview Survey for the years 1986–1990, Liao et al.[15] found that all-cause, age-adjusted mortality rates were lower for Hispanics (the ratio of Hispanic mortality rate to NHW mortality rate was 0.82 for men and 0.79 for women), but higher for ages under forty-five years, and lower for the older ages. Similarly, Sorlie et al.,[16] using the National Longitudinal Mortality Study matched to the National Death Index, reported that Hispanics have lower all-cause mortality rates than do NHW (0.74 for men and 0.82 for women). While significantly lower death rates were reported for both Hispanic men and women aged forty-five and older, there were no statistical differences in death rates between Hispanics and NHW aged twenty-five to forty-four. While in both Hispanics and NHW, lower income was associated with higher mortality rates; when mortality data were adjusted for income, there were significantly lower mortality rates for Hispanic men and women in each of the age groups, compared to the rates for NHW.

Age-adjusted mortality rates for 1998 from the National Center for Health Statistics (NCHS) indicate that all-cause death rates (per 100,000) for all ages combined were still lower for Hispanics (342.7) than for NHW (452.7).[2] Though all Hispanic subgroups have similar or lower mortality rates compared to the NHW rate, there was variation in mortality rates among the subgroups. Puerto Ricans had the highest mortality rates per 100,000 (419.7), Cubans the lowest (302.6), and Mexican Americans and other Hispanics fell into the middle range (365.2 and 320.8, respectively).[17]

Hispanic mortality rates were lower than those for NHW in all NCHS geographic regions of the United States for the years 1996–1998. On the state level, the results were mixed. Of the forty-four states for which there were adequate data, the rate ratios ranged from a low of 0.33 in Mississippi to a high of 1.14 in Minnesota.[17]

Figure 16.1 presents all-cause mortality by age groups and gender. It is clear that the Hispanic advantage in mortality is mainly among the middle and older age groups. Figure 16.2 presents variation by causes of death for Hispanics and NHW. The next section details differences in mortality between Hispanics and NHW at different stages of life, and links these differences to differences in causes of deaths.

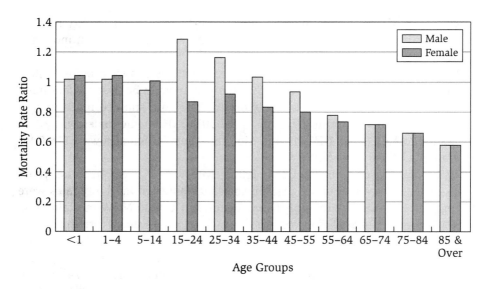

Figure 16.1 Hispanic/Non-Hispanic White All-Cause Mortality Rate Ratios, 1996–1998.

Note: A ratio of 1.0 indicates no difference between Hispanic and NHW mortality rates.

Source: Data from National Center for Health Statistics, *Health, United States, 2000.*

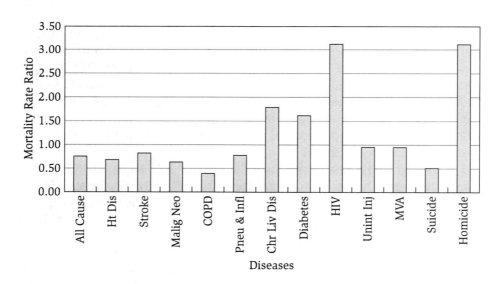

Figure 16.2 Hispanic/Non-Hispanic White Disease Specific Mortality Rate Ratios, 1998.

Note: A ratio of 1.0 indicates no difference between Hispanic and NHW mortality rates.

Source: Data from National Center for Health Statistics, *Health, United States, 2000.*

THE HISPANIC PARADOX FROM A LIFE CYCLE PERSPECTIVE

Infant Mortality: Lower Than Expected

In 1935, SS infants in San Antonio had higher mortality rates than did other white infants (197 per 1,000 live births for SS infants compared to 61 per 1,000 live births for other white infants).[18] Rates for both groups fell over the ensuing years, with a faster rate of decline among the SS infants. By 1980, the mortality rates for the two groups were about the same and remained so, at about 10 per 1,000 live births, through 1985.[18]

Williams et al.,[19] using a 1981 birth cohort in California, suggested that SS infants experienced low infant mortality rates largely due to a favorable birthweight distribution. Though SS and NHW infants had similar overall neonatal and postneonatal mortality rates, SS infants had higher birthweight-specific mortality rates for fetal and neonatal deaths, which may have resulted from inadequate medical care.

Infant mortality rates varied among Hispanic subgroups in data from the National Center for Health Statistics (1983–1984) from twenty-three states. Mexicans, Cubans, and Central and South Americans had neonatal, postneonatal, and infant mortality rates equal to or lower than the NHW rates. Puerto Rican rates were higher.[20] However, in contrast to Williams et al.,[19] there were no statistically significant differences in birthweight-specific mortality rates between NHW and Hispanics, or between NHW and any of the Hispanic subgroups.

Among Hispanics, infant mortality differed by maternal country of birth. The infants of U.S.-born Hispanic mothers were subject to slightly higher mortality rates compared to the infants of mothers born in Mexico, Puerto Rico, Cuba, and other Latin American countries.[21] However, according to NCHS data for the period 1983–1986, infants of Puerto Rican–born mothers had a lower risk of low birthweight and postneonatal mortality, but a statistically higher risk of neonatal mortality than the infants of U.S.-born Puerto Rican women.[22] Following up birth outcomes among Hispanics with the same data set for 1986 and 1987, Cubans had the lowest rates of adverse outcomes and Puerto Ricans the highest.[23]

Comparing fetal deaths among low-income women in California, Hispanic fetal death rates (7.8 per 1,000) were not significantly different from NHW rates (8.4 per 1,000), but both groups had significantly lower fetal death rates than did blacks (20.5 per 1,000).[24]

In the period 1995–1997, according to NCHS data, the Hispanic infant mortality rate of 6.1 per 1,000 live births was the same as that of NHW, and less than half the rate for blacks.[2] When infant mortality rates among mothers twenty years of age and older were stratified by maternal education, a clear gradient could be seen for NHW, with the lowest infant mortality rate found among the most highly educated. This relationship between infant mortality and maternal education was not so marked in the Hispanic population. At twelve years or less of maternal education, the Hispanic infant mortality rate of 5.8 per 1,000 live births was lower than the NHW rate of 9.1 per 1,000 live births.[2] Hispanic and NHW women have about the same frequency of infants weighing less than 2,500 grams (6.4 percent and 6.6 percent, respectively), and the same proportion of infants weighing less than 1,500 grams, 1.2 percent. Similar to the findings on infant mortality, the lack of a gradient by maternal education was also evident among Hispanics in relation to the proportion of infants with low birthweight.[2]

Youth: Higher Risk

For ages fifteen through forty-four, Hispanic males had higher mortality rates than did NHW. The reverse was true for young females (Figure 16.1). The higher death rates for Hispanic males reflected causes of death that are more prevalent among younger people, such as infectious diseases, including HIV/AIDS, and social pathologies, such as homicides, suicides, and drug abuse.[14,15,25] Hispanic mortality rates for males in this age group, excluding AIDS and homicide, were lower than corresponding NHW rates (87.5 versus 95.9, respectively, for ages fifteen to twenty-four; 95.0 versus 118.4 for ages twenty-five to thirty-four; and 201.6 versus 212.5 for ages thirty-five to forty-four).

Violence. Despite the unreliability of the recording of Hispanic origin on death certificates and in police reports, it is clear that mortality rates due to violent causes are consistently higher among Hispanics than among NHW.[26,27] The Hispanic population of the United States is younger and growing faster than the non-Hispanic population. Since crime is more common at a younger age, a greater percentage of the Hispanic population is potentially at risk of violence and violent death compared with non-Hispanics. The disproportionate number of Hispanics living in urban areas with a high incidence of poverty combined with the low educational achievement of many Hispanics, further places them at higher risk of violence.[26]

For blacks and Hispanics, homicide contributed more to premature mortality than did either heart disease or neoplasms; while among whites, mortality due to homicide was less than half that due to either of these physical conditions. For Hispanic males aged fifteen to twenty-four, the homicide rate was four times the rate for Anglo youth. There were variations in homicide rates by Hispanic subgroups, with Mexicans having the lowest rates, Cubans having the next lowest, and Puerto Ricans having the highest rates. Hispanic males and females also had higher rates of nonfatal intentional injuries than did NHW.[26]

Shai and Rosenwaike[27] considered homicide, suicide, and accidents (mainly attributed to motor vehicles) among Hispanics by nativity. Mortality profiles varied by nativity, with Mexican-born individuals having the highest death rates from accidents, Puerto Rican–born individuals having the highest homicide rates, and Cuban-born individuals having the highest suicide rates.

HIV/AIDS. In 1998, two-thirds of newly diagnosed AIDS cases in the United States were among minorities, 9,566 of whom were Hispanics.[28] Although the residents of New York City comprise only 3 percent of the U.S. population, they represent 16 percent of the country's AIDS cases, 71 percent of which occurred among blacks and Hispanics.[29] A cross-sectional study in New York City found that 87 percent of black and Hispanic men who have sex with men also have sex with women.[30] This could account for the tripling of the number of heterosexually acquired cases among blacks and Hispanics between 1991 and 1996.[31] Puerto Rican–born individuals, who had the highest rates of AIDS among Hispanics, were more likely to have been exposed to HIV through drug use than were other Hispanics.[32,33]

In 1998, 60 percent of persons living with AIDS were members of minority populations; 32,000 of these individuals were Mexican Americans.[28] Among five states with adequate data, seroprevalence rates among Hispanic women of childbearing age were higher than for NHW women, though not as high as for black women. Rates among Hispanic women were similar to rates among white women in two states (Texas and California).[34] In general, prevalence rates for AIDS in Texas were high among Hispanics and, between 1985 and 1996, were increasing in this population at a faster rate than for NHW.[35] Over the same time period, the percentage of female patients increased considerably in all races, particularly among Hispanics (from 2 percent in 1985 to 13 percent in 1996).[35]

Hispanics were also found to be at greater risk than whites of dying of HIV/AIDS.[28] While there has been a steep decline in mortality from AIDS in New York City between 1995 and 1998, mainly due to better treatment, the decline varied somewhat, but not substantially, by race/ethnicity and gender.[29]

Deaths from HIV/AIDS, being higher among younger individuals, contribute more to premature mortality than to total mortality. In New York City from 1983 to 1994, premature mortality decreased among NHW, but increased by 20 percent among blacks, and by 48 percent among Hispanics. The contribution of HIV/AIDS to total years of potential life lost (YPLL) before age sixty-five was greater among Hispanics than any other racial/ethnic group, accounting for 36.7 percent of YPLL in 1994, compared to 29.4 percent for NHW.[36]

Middle and Old Age: Chronic Diseases

From age fifty-five for males and age fifteen for females, Hispanic mortality rates were lower than for NHW (Figure 16.1). These lower mortality rates in the middle and old age groups reflect lower mortality from most of the chronic diseases that generally affect these age groups (Figure 16.2).

Cardiovascular Disease. While it can be said with a reasonable degree of certainty that total mortality from cardiovascular disease is not higher among Hispanics than among NHW, results from studies of cardiovascular disease among Hispanics are not consistent, especially for men. The evidence seems stronger that there is no appreciable difference in the prevalence, incidence, or case-fatality of cardiovascular disease between the two ethnic groups of women.

Studies based on vital statistics[37,38] show a clear Hispanic cardiovascular disease mortality advantage; however, these studies are subject to misclassification bias of both ethnicity and the underlying cause of death.

National cohort studies based on data linkage have shown lower or not statistically different cardiovascular mortality rates for Hispanics relative to NHW.[15,16] Sorlie et al.[16] found significantly lower mortality rates due to cardiovascular disease for Hispanics compared to NHW, after adjusting for age and income, among all age groups of men and women over forty-five. Liao et al.[15] found that mortality rates for cardiovascular disease were not significantly different between Hispanics and NHW for any age or gender group.

Three local cohort studies, likely to suffer less from biases but more limited in terms of generalizability, have shown inconsistent results. In the San Antonio Heart Study,[39] the age-adjusted prevalence of myocardial infarction at baseline was significantly lower for Mexican American men than for NHW men but similar for both groups of women. After 3,765 of these subjects had been followed for seven to eight years, there were no statistically significant differences in cardiovascular disease mortality rates.[40] The Corpus Christi Heart Project,[41,42] a population-based surveillance study of cardiac events in Nueces County, Texas, reported that Mexican Americans had a poorer twenty-eight-day and twenty-five-month prognosis after suffering a myocardial infarction than did NHW, controlling for a variety of risk factors. The San Luis Valley Diabetes Study,[43,44] a population-based cohort study of diabetic and nondiabetic Hispanic and NHW residents of Alamosa and Conejos counties in Colorado, reported a significant ethnic difference in prevalence and incidence of coronary heart disease, favoring Hispanics only among diabetic males.

Stroke. The age-adjusted stroke mortality rates were lower for Hispanics than for NHW (Figure 16.2). Sorlie et al.[16] found significantly lower cerebrovascular disease mortality rates in Hispanic men as compared to their NHW counterparts, and lower rates, of borderline significance, in Hispanic women. However, differences in total cerebrovascular mortality between the two ethnic groups varied with age. Below age sixty-five, death rates were not significantly different; however, at older ages, the Hispanic rates dropped below those of NHW, a trend that increased with age.[45]

Few incidence or case-fatality rates exist on stroke by Hispanic ethnicity. The Northern Manhattan Stroke Study[46] found age-adjusted incidence rates for Hispanics intermediate between those of non-Hispanic blacks and whites. However, 78 percent of these Hispanics were either Puerto Rican or Dominican and do not represent the ethnic mix found in other parts of the United States. In a two-year follow-up study of patients admitted for stroke to the Neurological Institute of Columbia-Presbyterian Medical Center, Hispanics had the lowest risk of stroke recurrence or death throughout the first year of follow-up, compared to blacks and NHW.[47]

Analyses of data from the 1989–1991 National Health Interview Surveys indicated a pattern of lower total stroke mortality among Hispanics, especially after age sixty-five. These data also indicate equal or higher incidence, but lower case-fatality, among Hispanics compared to NHW.[47] Other studies are needed to confirm these results because of the small number of Hispanics with stroke for this time period.

Cancer. Hispanics had much lower age-adjusted mortality rates for all malignant neoplasms combined than did NHW (Figure 16.2). While Hispanics had lower mortality rates from types of cancer that are more prevalent among the U.S. population at large, they suffered higher mortality from forms of cancer that are more rare in this country. In 1997, the mortality rate ratio (Hispanic mortality rate/NHW mortality rate) for all neoplasms was 0.61.[2] For respiratory cancer, it was 0.38; breast cancer, 0.66; colorectal cancer, 0.64; and prostate cancer, 0.68.[2] Lower death rates from these common cancers accounted for lower Hispanic mortality from all cancers combined.

Hispanics suffered higher mortality from cancers in specific sites. The rate ratios, with NHW as the referent, were 1.73 for stomach cancer, 2.44 for liver cancer, 1.13 for pancreatic cancer, and 2.14 for cervical cancer.[48] Although Hispanics often experienced higher case-fatality rates, possibly due to late diagnosis, incidence rates among Hispanics compared to other groups reflected their mortality rates, indicating that their lower overall mortality due to cancer was a consequence of lower incidence of this disease.[48–50] This was possibly due to different risk factor profiles, which put Hispanics at lower risk for certain common cancers, while increasing their risk for others.[51,52]

Diabetes Mellitus. There were several reports indicating that diabetes, particularly non-insulin-dependent diabetes mellitus (NIDDM), disproportionately affects Hispanics in Texas and Colorado.[53–56] For example, in Starr County, Texas (which is 98 percent Mexican American), the reported prevalence of NIDDM was two to five times that of the general U.S. population.[57] In two Colorado counties, the age-adjusted prevalence (per 1,000) of confirmed NIDDM was 21 in NHW males, 44 in Hispanic males, 13 in NHW females, and 62 in Hispanic females.[58] Hispanics were 3.5 (95% CI, 2.4–4.9) times more likely than NHW to have NIDDM. The risk reduced to 1.9 (95% CI, 1.2–2.9) after taking into account age, sex, family history of NIDDM, income, skinfold measurements, and waist-hip ratios.[59]

The increased prevalence of NIDDM in Hispanics was related to increased incidence.[60] The rate ratio comparing incidence rates for Hispanics to those for NHW was 3.1 (95% CI, 2.3–4.2). Self-reported diabetes mellitus (which included insulin-dependent as well as NIDDM) in the Hispanic Health and Nutrition Examination Survey (1982–1984) was 6.8 percent and 7.6 percent among Mexican American men and women, respectively, compared to the U.S. population rates of 2.9 percent for men and 3.8 percent for women.[61] In the Behavioral Risk Factor Surveillance Survey (1994–1997), the age-adjusted percentage of self-reported diabetes was 8.0 (95% CI, 7.4–8.5) for Hispanics and 4.0 (95% CI, 3.9–4.1) for NHW.[62]

Gardner et al.[55] suggested that the epidemic of NIDDM in Mexican Americans is confined to that part of the population with a substantial Native American heritage. They inferred from skin tone the prevalence of Native American genes among individuals in various neighborhoods of San Antonio, Texas, and found that neighborhoods with the highest percentage of "Native American admixture" had the highest rates of NIDDM. However, neighborhoods with a high proportion of Mexican Americans of dark skin color also tended to be the least acculturated and the poorest.

The susceptibility of Hispanics to diabetes is also reflected in disease-related mortality figures. The age-adjusted mortality rate (per 100,000) from diabetes in 1998 for Hispanics was 18.4; for NHW, 11.5; for blacks, 28.8; and for Native Americans, 29.6.[2]

The foregoing data strongly suggest that Hispanics are more susceptible to diabetes mellitus than are NHW. Chakraborty et al.,[63] however, question whether or not Hispanic ethnicity is, in itself, a risk factor for NIDDM. They point out that Hispanics in the United States are both genetically and culturally heterogeneous. They speculate that the actual risk factor(s) for NIDDM may co-vary with Hispanic ethnicity.

POSSIBLE EXPLANATIONS FOR THE HISPANIC PARADOX

Data Reliability

Before further investigating the Hispanic paradox, it is important to consider artifactual explanations. The question of data reliability in the numerator and denominator used in calculating mortality rates has been raised in the literature. The problem arises when census data are used in the denominator and death certificate information is used in the numerator. Possible underreporting of Hispanic deaths on death certificates would bias mortality rates downward and give an inaccurate picture of mortality differences among racial/ethnic groups. However, this is not believed to be a serious problem as lower Hispanic mortality is reported from studies that do not use death certificate information to assess ethnicity (as discussed later).

In 1978, a question on Hispanic origin was added to the death certificates in several states, but only in 1989 did the National Center for Health Statistics add an item on Hispanic origin to the U.S. Standard Certificate of Death.[64] The use of the Hispanic origin item in calculating Hispanic mortality has been criticized because of its possible inaccuracy. When introduced, it was not recorded on a significant portion of death certificates, though the occurrence of missing Hispanic origin has been decreasing over time.[65] The reliability of the Hispanic-origin item is further in question because demographic information on the death certificate is recorded by a hospital, funeral director, or coroner in an unstructured and unstandardized manner.[66] Corresponding questions in the census are answered by a knowledgeable household member, implying a lack of homogeneity in reporting Hispanic origin on the death certificate and the census. Despite these problems, a study by Sorlie et al.[66] comparing demographic characteristics on the death certificate with those reported in the baseline interview of the National Longitudinal Mortality Study found that the agreement for the Hispanic yes/no item was 98.7 percent for all known values. However, this high level of agreement could be verified for only approximately one-quarter of the sample because 72.8 percent of the death certificates did not indicate Hispanic origin. Since the deaths in this study occurred before the introduction of the Hispanic-origin item on the U.S. Standard Certificate of Death, the low response rate is not surprising.

Before the introduction of the Hispanic-origin item on death certificates, Hispanic mortality was calculated using Spanish surname lists that have been developed by the U.S. Bureau of the Census since 1950 (1953, 1963, and 1973). The advantages of using this method to determine Hispanic ethnicity are that Spanish surnames can be assessed without any query about the origin of the descendents, and names are rarely missing on death certificates. The use of Spanish surnames has several limitations, however. Some Hispanics do not have Spanish surnames. Some persons coded as having Spanish surnames are not Hispanic; for example, Italians have similar last names, and non-Hispanic women may be married to men with Spanish surnames. Hispanic women married to men without Spanish surnames, and their offspring, are not included.[64] The complication of women taking their husband's surname can be addressed by considering the father's surname (that is, the maiden name) for married women.[65,67] The father's surname is reported on death certificates and, in one study, was found to be missing in only approximately 6 percent of female death certificates.[65] Despite these limitations, some studies have suggested the use of

Spanish surnames is preferable to answers to the Hispanic-origin item on the death certificate in identifying Hispanic deaths because use of Spanish surnames gives consistent mortality estimates since the same Spanish surname list is used to identify Hispanics in the numerator (death certificates) and the denominator (census data).[64,67] Studies using Spanish surnames and comparing mortality rates among Hispanics and NHW tend to find lower Hispanic mortality.[11,64,65] Studies of infant mortality have found only small discrepancies between the Hispanic origin item on the death certificate and the use of Spanish surnames.[68]

Other studies have circumvented the problem of numerator-denominator inconsistencies by considering nativity rather than ethnic origin.[12,13] Place of birth is an item that has been on both the census and the death certificate for many decades. The limitation of this approach is that it excludes U.S.-born Hispanics, and cannot estimate overall Hispanic mortality. Also, it cannot differentiate between the health effects of being an immigrant and being Hispanic.

Longitudinal cohort studies, where ethnicity is determined at baseline and individuals are followed over a period of time, provide the strongest support for the substantive nature of the Hispanic paradox, since these studies avoid numerator-denominator bias and can examine Hispanic ethnicity among the U.S. born as well as the foreign born. Two such studies confirm the substantive nature of the Hispanic paradox by finding lower age-adjusted mortality for Hispanics compared to NHW.[15,16] These two studies provide evidence for the genuine existence of lower-than-expected Hispanic mortality rates, because they avoid the possibility of substantial numerator-denominator bias in their design. They lend support to the existence of a Hispanic paradox that is not an artifact of the data.

Salmon Bias Hypothesis

The salmon bias hypothesis suggests that Hispanics tend to return to their birth country after they retire or became seriously ill. If Hispanics return to their birth country to die, their deaths are not recorded in the U.S. vital statistics and they became "statistically immortal."[69] The artificially lower numerator biases Hispanic mortality downward. Though not substantiated, the hypothesis has been mentioned as possibly biasing estimates of Hispanic mortality.[12,66,67] Studies of return migration suggest that the salmon bias hypothesis is plausible, as a large percentage of foreign-born Hispanics return to their home country (though it is not clear if the return is permanent).[70,71]

Only recently, Abraido-Lanza et al.[72] attempted to study systematically the salmon bias hypothesis. Since the salmon bias hypothesis is based on the notion that foreign-born Hispanics desire to return to their home country in order to die among their families, we would expect U.S.-born Hispanics to similarly desire to die among their families and remain in the United States. Therefore, the salmon bias should not be present in mortality rates among U.S.-born Hispanics. Similarly, we would not expect a salmon bias in the mortality rates for Cubans, who cannot return to Cuba for political reasons, and for Puerto Ricans, since the deaths of Puerto Ricans, whether they die on the island or on the mainland, are recorded in the U.S. vital statistics. Since all of these groups were found to have lower mortality rates than NHW, this study provided evidence against the salmon bias hypothesis.

Healthy Migrant Hypothesis

The healthy migrant hypothesis is based on the notion that the healthiest and strongest members of a population migrate. These migrants bring with them their superior health and other advantages. There is evidence to support this notion. In international data, the mortality rate of immigrants is lower than that of the residents of their country of origin.[73] In the United States, foreign-born persons have lower mortality rates than U.S.-born citizens.[74] Among immigrants to the United States, those who have been residing in the United States for longer periods of time have worse health than do recent arrivals.[74]

Among Hispanics, several studies have compared Hispanic mortality for U.S. born and foreign born by country of origin.[12,72,75,76] Fang et al.[75] found that in New York, Puerto Rican– and U.S.-born Hispanics have less favorable mortality than Hispanics born in Central America, South America, and the Caribbean. Finally, the San Antonio Heart Study[76] found age- and sex-adjusted all-cause mortality rates per 1,000 person years of 3.8 for NHW, 5.7 for U.S.-born Mexican Americans, and 3.6 for foreign-born Mexican Americans, supporting the healthy migrant hypothesis. However, because of the low number of deaths (eighty-five for U.S.-born Mexican Americans, eleven for foreign-born Mexican Americans, and forty for NHW) these results should be interpreted with caution. While these studies do not contradict the healthy migrant hypothesis, factors other than the healthy migrant effect could well account for differences in mortality between foreign-born Hispanics and NHW.

Recently, Abraido-Lanza et al.[72] specifically tested the healthy migrant hypothesis. They reasoned that U.S.-born Hispanics "are not subject to the migratory selective processes" and therefore, if U.S.-born Hispanics have lower mortality rates than U.S.-born NHW, something other than migratory selective processes must be involved. Some have argued that healthier migrants pass on their genetic and lifestyle advantages to the next generation, so that lower mortality among the second and later generations could still be due to a healthy migrant effect. If true, this argument weakens the Abraido-Lanza test. A further test of the healthy migrant hypothesis is based on differences in mortality between Hispanic immigrants and other white immigrants. If the healthy migrant effect explains the lower mortality rates among Hispanics, there should be no differences in mortality between migrants from Latin America and other regions of the world, particularly Europe, since they are also affected by selective migration. As European migrants did not appear to have the same mortality advantages relative to U.S.-born whites that Hispanic migrants had relative to U.S.-born Hispanics, the study suggests that the healthy migrant hypothesis is not a major explanation for the Hispanic paradox.[72]

Risk Factors

Hispanics differ from the non-Hispanic population with regard to several risk factors for disease. Furthermore, many of these risk factors differ by Hispanic ethnicity and are not universal across the entire group. Compared to NHW, Hispanics tend to have lower rates of childhood immunizations; have nearly equal mean serum levels of cholesterol, but a higher prevalence of hypertension; have much higher rates of diabetes; have about an equal proportion of overweight men, but a higher proportion of overweight women and children; engage in less recreational exercise; have a higher proportion of mothers receiving prenatal care; and are less likely to live in areas with high air quality.[2] However, Hispanics also have a lower prevalence of cigarette smoking,[51] smoke fewer cigarettes when they smoke,[51] consume diets high in fiber[77-79] but possibly lower in fruits and vegetables,[80] and are likely to become pregnant at an earlier age.[81] Their risk factor profiles are, therefore, mixed compared to those of non-Hispanics. Lower prevalences of some risk factors, such as cigarette smoking, may protect them against some diseases, while equal or higher prevalences of others, such as obesity, appears to put them more at risk. It is not clear what role all of these factors play in the Hispanic paradox, since Hispanics' health behaviors are not, in all respects, superior to those of non-Hispanics; however, differences in risk factors profiles could contribute to lower incidence rates among Hispanics for some diseases.

Acculturation and Culture

Acculturation can be conceptually defined as the process by which an individual raised in one culture enters the social structure and institutions of another, and internalizes the prevailing attitudes and beliefs of the new culture.[82] It can result in complete assimilation or the creation of a new composite culture, combining aspects of both the original and adopted cultures.[83] As such, it is a complex phenomenon. This concept is measured in a variety of ways across studies, from primary spoken language only[84] to multidimensional scales with several components.[52,76,82,85] Acculturation could influence health through a direct effect on health behaviors and access to the health care system.[52,82,84,86] It could also influence health through the degree of social support and the extent of social networks available,[87] through values specific to a culture that may affect psychological well-being,[88] through changes in an individual's reference group and acceptance by that group,[87,89] and through changes in socioeconomic status.[90]

Acculturation has been shown to have a beneficial effect on some health behaviors and outcomes and a detrimental effect on others. Specifically, a higher degree of assimilation to mainstream U.S. culture has been associated with a higher proportion of low birthweight infants,[87,91] lower childhood immunization levels,[85] lower consumption of fiber,[52] higher blood pressure (men),[86] and higher prevalence of cigarette smoking (women).[52] However, it has also been associated with lower prevalence of obesity and diabetes,[82] lower levels of fat consumption,[52] lower total cholesterol (women),[86] higher HDL cholesterol (men),[86] and lower alcohol use (men).[86]

In general, a lower level of acculturation seems supportive of mothers, which is then reflected in better birth outcomes.[89,91] In Alameda County, California, Hispanic mothers living in enclaves which were at least 30 percent Hispanic gave birth to a lower proportion of low birthweight infants than did NHW women living in the same enclaves. The enclave created an environment supportive of motherhood, including the promotion of healthy pregnancies and good nutrition, while providing prohibitions against smoking, alcohol, and drug abuse.[87]

Less acculturated Hispanics, by definition, identify more strongly with the prevailing values of their culture. One such intrinsic value is the concept of *respeto,* indicating respect for elders or those with experience. Although this could raise the status of the elderly within traditional Hispanic enclaves, bolstering their sense of purpose and self-esteem, it is also possible that younger generations of more acculturated family members may not share these values. No empirical studies could be found that test any possible association between *respeto* and the health of the elderly.[88]

Another well-documented Hispanic value is *familismo,* the centrality of the family and pseudo-family.[88,92-94] However, it is not known if *familismo* actually increases the social support available to Hispanics relative to NHW, or simply provides a different but qualitatively similar type of social support.[92] A growing literature of sociological studies on *familismo* and Hispanic family structure exists,[94] but the possible connections between this kind of social support and health have not been established.

The mixed effects of acculturation on health outcomes and behavioral risk factors may be due partly to a high degree of confounding by socioeconomic status (SES). Education, which is one indicator of socioeconomic status, is a vehicle by which the acculturation process often takes place. No study has systematically compared health outcomes among those with low levels of education and low levels of acculturation (the majority of first-generation immigrants), and those with low SES but high acculturation (mainly U.S.-born Hispanics).

James[89] put forth the hypothesis that a strong ethnic identity is protective of health. Identification with positive subcultural images and values is thought to be a crucial buffer against either racial or economic marginalization by the dominant society. For this reason, he believes Mexican Americans to be at an advantage relative to African Americans, who have had to reconstruct a positive ethnic identity after a history of slavery and forced segregation. Although protective of racial minorities and the economically disadvantaged, low levels of acculturation would offer no additional benefits to those higher in the social hierarchy.[89] This seems true in the case of birth outcomes among Hispanics,[91] but too few studies have been done to allow us to form conclusions about the effect of either the acculturation process or Hispanic culture on other aspects of health.

CONCLUSIONS AND SUGGESTIONS FOR FUTURE RESEARCH

For the past twenty years, there has been widespread evidence of a Hispanic paradox in the United States, in which most Hispanic groups are characterized by low income, low levels of education, and high proportions of workers in blue-collar or unskilled occupations, but have low all-cause and infant mortality rates. This paradox is mainly apparent for mortality and less so, if at all, for morbidity. A closer look reveals that this paradox is a complex picture, with variations by age, gender, type of Hispanic group, acculturation, country of birth, and specific disease or cause of death. The lower all-cause mortality rates seem mainly attributable to lower mortality among the older groups for the diseases that kill the majority of Americans.

The causes of this paradox are largely unknown. Despite suggestions of bias in vital statistics, we can be reasonably certain that the paradox is real for the following subgroups of Hispanics: infants, older Hispanics, Mexican Americans, the foreign born, and the unacculturated. The explanations put forward to explain the Hispanic paradox, such as the salmon bias and healthy migrant effects and different risk behaviors, may contribute to, but do not completely explain, the unexpected favorable health outcomes of Hispanics. The reasons for the Hispanic paradox are likely to be social in origin and multifactorial. There may be some aspect of Hispanic, particularly Mexican culture, itself, that is protective. If the reasons are largely cultural, the paradox will exist only for as long as a large percentage of Hispanics remains culturally distinct from the rest of the U.S. population and does not adopt Anglo norms. A rare window of opportunity now exists to learn more about how cultural factors influence an individual's health and well-being, which could ultimately be beneficial to all. Well-designed empirical studies need to be conducted to determine the protective effects of immigrant status, positive identification with a subculture, and the influence of acculturation on health behaviors, and to ascertain which aspects of Hispanic culture may be contributing to the mortality advantage that some members of this population enjoy.

Notes

1. Markides, K. S., & Coreil, J. (1986). The health of Hispanics in the Southwestern United States: An epidemiologic paradox. *Public Health Rep, 101,* 253–265.

2. National Center for Health Statistics. (2000). *Health, United States, 2000, with adolescent health chartbook.* Washington, DC: U.S. Government Printing Office.

3. U.S. Census Bureau. (1999). *Historical income tables.* Washington, DC: Author.

4. Sen, A. K. (1973). *On economic inequality.* Oxford, UK: Clarendon Press.

5. Pamuk, E., Makuc, D., Heck, K., Reuben, C., & Lochner, K. (1998). Socioeconomic status and health chartbook. In National Center for Health Statistics, *Health, United States, 1998.* Hyattsville, MD: National Center for Health Statistics.

6. Kaiser Family Foundation. (2000). *Racial and ethnic disparities in access to health insurance and health care.* Washington, DC: Author.

7. Ellis, J. M. (1959). Mortality differences for a Spanish-surname population group. *Southwestern Soc Sci Q, 39,* 314–321.

8. Ellis, J. M. (1962). Spanish-surname mortality differences in San Antonio, Texas. *J Health Hum Behav, 3,* 125–217.

9. Bradshaw, B. S., & Fonner, E. (1978). The mortality of Spanish-surnamed persons in Texas: 1969–1971. In F. D. Bean & W. P. Frisbie (Eds.), *Demography of racial and ethnic groups* (pp. 261–281). San Diego, CA: Academic Press.

10. Bradshaw, B. S., Frisbie, W. P., & Eifler, C. W. (1985). Excess and deficit mortality due to selected causes of death and their contribution to differences in life expectancy of Spanish-surnamed and other white males, 1970 and 1980. In U.S. Department of Health and Human Services, *Report of the Secretary's Task Force on Black and Minority Health: Vol. 1. Executive summary* (pp. 43–65). Washington, DC: U.S. Government Printing Office.

11. Schoen, R., & Nelson, V. E. (1981). Mortality by cause among Spanish-surnamed Californians, 1969–71. *Soc Sci Q, 62,* 259–274.

12. Shai, D., & Rosenwaike, I. (1987). Mortality among Hispanics in metropolitan Chicago: An examination based on vital statistics data. *J Chronic Dis, 40,* 445–451.

13. Rosenwaike, I. (1987). Mortality differentials among persons born in Cuba, Mexico, and Puerto Rico residing in the United States, 1979–81. *Am J Public Health, 77,* 603–606.

14. Desenclos, J. A., & Hahn, R. A. (1992). Years of potential life lost before age 65, by race, Hispanic origin, and sex: United States, 1986–1988. *Morbid Mortal Wkly Rep, 41,* 13–23.

15. Liao, Y., Cooper, R. S., Cao, G., et al. (1998). Mortality patterns among adult Hispanics: Findings from the NHIS, 1986 to 1990. *Am J Public Health, 88,* 227–232.

16. Sorlie, P. D., Backlund, E., Johnson, N. J., & Rogot, E. (1993). Mortality by Hispanic status in the United States. *JAMA, 270,* 2464–2468.

17. Hoyert, D. L., Kochanek, K. D., & Murphy, S. L. (1999). Deaths: Final data for 1997. *Natl Vital Stat Rep, 47,* 1–2.

18. Bradshaw, B. S., & Frisbie, W. P. (1992). Mortality of Mexican Americans and Mexican immigrants: Comparisons with Mexico. In J. R. Weeks & R. H. Chande (Eds.), *Demographic dynamics of the U.S.-Mexico border* (pp. 125–150). El Paso, TX: Texas Western Press.

19. Williams, R. L., Binkin, N. J., & Clingman, E. J. (1986). Pregnancy outcomes among Spanish-surname women in California. *Am J Public Health, 76,* 387–391.

20. Kleinman, J. C. (1990). Infant mortality among racial/ethnic minority groups, 1983–1984. *Morbid Mortal Wkly Rep, 39,* 31–39.

21. Becerra, J. E., Hogue, C.J.R., Atrash, H. K., & Perez, N. (1991). Infant mortality among Hispanics: A portrait of heterogeneity. *JAMA, 265,* 217–221.

22. Engel, T., Alexander, G. R., & Leland, N. L. (1995). Pregnancy outcomes of U.S.-born Puerto Ricans: The role of maternal nativity status. *Am J Prev Med, 11,* 34–39.

23. Albrecht, S. L., Clarke, L. L., Miller, M. K., & Farmer, F. L. (1996). Predictors of differential birth outcomes among Hispanic subgroups in the United States: The role of maternal risk characteristics and medical care. *Soc Sci Q, 77,* 407–433.

24. Guendelman, S., Chavez, G., & Christianson, R. (1994). Fetal deaths in Mexican-American, black and white non-Hispanic women seeking government-funded prenatal care. *J Community Health, 19,* 319–330.

25. Rogers, R. (1995). Sociodemographic characteristics of long-lived and healthy individuals. *Popul Dev Rev, 21,* 33–58.

26. Rodriguez, M. A., & Brindis, C. D. (1995). Violence and Latino youth: Prevention and methodological issues. *Public Health Rep, 110,* 260–267.

27. Shai, D., & Rosenwaike, I. (1988). Violent deaths among Mexican-, Puerto Rican- and Cuban-born migrants in the United States. *Soc Sci Med, 26,* 269–276.

28. Carter-Pokras, O., & Woo, V. (1999). Health profile of racial and ethnic minorities in the United States. *Ethn Health, 4,* 117–120.

29. Chiasson, M. A., Berenson, L., Li, W., et al. (1999). Declining HIV/AIDS mortality in New York City. *J Acquir Immune Defic Syndr, 21,* 59–64.

30. Lehner, T., & Chiasson, M. A. (1998). Seroprevalence of human immunodeficiency virus type I and sexual behaviors in bisexual African-American and Hispanic men visiting a sexually transmitted disease clinic in New York City. *Am J Epidemiol, 147,* 269–272.

31. Lehner, T., Muthambi, B., & Chiasson, M. A. (1997). *HIV/AIDS in New York City.* New York: HIV Prevention Planning Group of New York City, New York City Department of Health.

32. Diaz, T., Klevens, M., & the Group TSthaASP. (1997). Differences by ancestry in sociodemographics and risk behaviors among Latinos with AIDS. *Ethn Dis, 7,* 200–206.

33. Montoya, I. D., Bell, D. C., Richard, A. J., Carlson, J. W., & Trevino, R. A. (1999). Estimated HIV risk among Hispanics in a national sample of drug users. *J Acquir Immune Defic Syndr, 21,* 42–50.

34. Davis, S. F., Rosen, D. H., Steinberg, S., Wortley, P. M., Karon, J. M., & Gwinn M. (1998). Trends in HIV prevalence among childbearing women in the United States, 1989–1994. *J Acquir Immune Defic Syndr, 19,* 158–164.

35. VitalStats. (1997). The changing demographics of AIDS in Texas. *Tex Med, 93,* 19.

36. Obiri, G. U., Fordyce, E. J., Singh, T. P., & Forlenza, S. (1998). Effects of HIV/AIDS versus other causes of death on premature mortality in New York City, 1983–1994. *Am J Epidemiol, 147,* 840–845.

37. Goff, D. C., Ramsey, D. J., Labarthe, D. R., & Nichaman, M. Z. (1993). Acute myocardial infarction and coronary heart disease mortality among Mexican Americans and non-Hispanic whites in Texas, 1980 through 1989. *Ethn Dis, 3,* 64–69.

38. Wild, S. H., Laws, A., Fortmann, S. P., Varady, A. N., & Byrne, C. D. (1995). Mortality from coronary heart disease and stroke for six ethnic groups in California, 1985 to 1990. *Ann Epidemiol, 5,* 432–439.

39. Mitchell, B. D., Haffner, S. M., Hazuda, H. P., Patterson, J. K., & Stern, M. P. (1992). Diabetes and coronary heart disease risk in Mexican Americans. *Ann Epidemiol, 2,* 101–106.

40. Wei, M., Mitchell, B. D., Haffner, S. M., & Stern, M. P. (1996). Effects of cigarette smoking, diabetes, high cholesterol, and hypertension on all-cause mortality and cardiovascular disease mortality in Mexican Americans. *Am J Epidemiol, 144,* 1058–1065.

41. Goff, D. C., Varas, C., Ramsey, D. J., Wear, M.L., Labarthe, D. R., & Nichaman, M. Z. (1993). Mortality after hospitalization for myocardial infarction among Mexican Americans and non-Hispanic whites: The Corpus Christi Heart Project. *Ethn Dis, 3,* 55–63.

42. Goff, D. C., Ramsey, D. J., Labarthe, D. R., & Nichaman, M. Z. (1994). Greater case-fatality after myocardial infarction among Mexican Americans and women than among non-Hispanic whites and men. *Am J Epidemiol, 139,* 474–483.

43. Rewers, M., Shetterly, S. M., Hoag, S., Baxter, J., Marshall, J., & Hamman, R. F. (1993). Is the risk of coronary heart disease lower in Hispanics than in non-Hispanic whites? The San Luis Valley Diabetes Study. *Ethn Dis, 3,* 44–54.

44. Rewers, M., Shetterly, S. M., Baxter, J., Marshall, J., & Hamman, R. F. (1992). Prevalence of coronary heart disease in subjects with normal and impaired glucose tolerance and non-insulin-dependent diabetes mellitus in a biethnic Colorado population. *Am J Epidemiol, 135,* 1321–1330.

45. Gillum, R. F. (1995). Epidemiology of stroke in Hispanic Americans. *Stroke, 26,* 1707–1712.

46. Sacco, R. L., Boden-Albala, B., Gan, R., et al. (1998). Stroke incidence among white, black, and Hispanic residents of an urban community: The Northern Manhattan Stroke Study. *Am J Epidemiol, 147,* 259–268.

47. Sacco, R. L., Hauser, W. A., Mohr, J. P., & Foulkes, M. A. (1991). One-year outcome after cerebral infarction in whites, blacks, and Hispanics. *Stroke, 22,* 305–311.

48. Rosenwaike, I. M. (1988). Cancer mortality among Mexican immigrants in the United States. *Public Health Rep, 103,* 195–201.

49. Davis, F. G., Persky, V. W., Ferre, C. D., Howe, H. L., Barrett, R. E., & Haenszel, W. M. (1995). Cancer incidence of Hispanics and non-Hispanic whites in Cook County, Illinois. *Cancer, 75,* 2939–2945.

50. Gilliland, F. D., Hunt, W. C., & Key, C. R. (1998). Trends in the survival of American Indian, Hispanic and non-Hispanic white cancer patients in New Mexico and Arizona, 1969–1994. *Cancer, 82,* 1763–1783.

51. Rogers, R. G., & Crank, J. (1988). Ethnic differences in smoking patterns: Findings from NHIS. *Public Health Rep, 103,* 387–393.

52. Balcazar, H., Castro, F. G., & Krull, J. L. (1995). Cancer risk reduction in Mexican-American women: The role of acculturation, education, and health risk factors. *Health Educ Q, 22,* 61–84.

53. Stern, M. P., Gaskill, S. P., Allen, C. R., Garza, V., Gonzalez, J. L., & Waldrop, R. H. (1981). Cardiovascular risk factors in Mexican Americans in Laredo, Texas. *Am J Epidemiol, 113,* 546–555.

54. Stern, M. P., Gaskill, S. P., Hazuda, H. P., Gardner, L. I., & Haffner, S. M. (1983). Does obesity explain excess prevalence of diabetes among Mexican Americans? Results of the San Antonio Heart Study. *Diabetologia, 24,* 272–277.

55. Gardner, L. I., Stern, M. P., Haffner, S. M., et al. (1984). Prevalence of diabetes in Mexican Americans: Relationship to percent of gene pool derived from Native American sources. *Diabetes, 33,* 86–92.

56. Stern, M. P., Rosenthal, M., Haffner, S. M., Hazuda, H. P., & Franco, L. J. (1984). Sex differences in the effects of sociocultural status on diabetes and cardiovascular risk factors in Mexican Americans: The San Antonio Heart Study. *Am J Epidemiol, 120.*

57. Hanis, C. L., Ferrell, R. E., Barton, S. A., et al. (1983). Diabetes among Mexican Americans in Starr County, Texas. *Am J Epidemiol, 118,* 659–672.

58. Hamman, R. F., Marshall, J. A., Baxter, J., et al. (1989). Methods and prevalence of non-insulin-dependent diabetes mellitus in a biethnic Colorado population: The San Luis Valley Diabetes Study. *Am J Epidemiol, 129,* 295–311.

59. Marshall, J., Hamman, R. F., & Baxter, J., et al. (1993). Ethnic differences in risk factors associated with the prevalence of non-insulin-dependent diabetes mellitus: The San Luis Valley Diabetes Study. *Am J Epidemiol, 137,* 706–718.

60. Baxter, J., Hamman, R. F., Lopez, T. K., Marshall, J., Hoag, S., & Swenson, C. J. (1993). Excess incidence of known non-insulin-dependent diabetes mellitus (NIDDM) in Hispanics compared with non-Hispanic whites in the San Luis Valley, Colorado. *Ethn Dis, 3,* 11–21.

61. Perez-Stable, E. J., McMillen, M. M., Harris, M. I., et al. (1989). Self-reported diabetes in Mexican Americans: HHANES 1982–84. *Am J Public Health, 79,* 770–772.

62. Centers for Disease Control and Prevention. (1999). Self-reported prevalence of diabetes among Hispanics—United States, 1994–1997. *Morbid Mortal Wkly Rep, 48*, 8–12.

63. Chakraborty, B. M., Fernandez-Esquer, M. E., & Chakraborty, R. (1999). Is being Hispanic a risk factor for non-insulin-dependent diabetes mellitus (NIDDM)? *Ethn Dis, 9*, 278–283.

64. Rosenwaike, I., & Bradshaw, B. S. (1988). The status of death statistics for the Hispanic population of the Southwest. *Soc Sci Q, 69*, 722–736.

65. Polednak, A. P. (1995). Estimating mortality in the Hispanic population of Connecticut, 1990 to 1991. *Am J Public Health, 85*, 998–1001.

66. Sorlie, P. D., Rogot, E., & Johnson, N. J. (1992). Validity of demographic characteristics on the death certificate. *Epidemiology, 3*, 181–184.

67. Polednak, A. P. (1993). Lung cancer rates in the Hispanic population of Connecticut, 1980–88. *Public Health Rep, 108*, 471–476.

68. Powell-Griner, E., & Streck, D. (1982). A closer examination of neonatal mortality rates among the Texas Spanish surname population. *Am J Public Health, 72*, 993–999.

69. Pablos-Mendez, A. (1994). Letter to the editor. *JAMA, 271*, 1237–1238.

70. Gasso, G., & Rosenzweig, M. (1982). Estimating the emigration rates of legal immigrants using administrative and survey data. *Demography, 19*, 279–290.

71. Reichert, J., & Massey, D. S. (1979). Patterns of U.S. migration from a Mexican sending community: A comparison of legal and illegal migrants. *Int Migration Rev, 13*, 599–623.

72. Abraido-Lanza, A. F., Dohrenwend, B. P., Ng-Mak, D. S., & Turner, J. B. (1999). The Latino mortality paradox: A test of the "salmon bias" and healthy migrant hypotheses. *Am J Public Health, 89*, 1543–1548.

73. Marmot, M. G., Adelstein, A. M., & Bulusu, L. (1984). Lessons from the study of immigrant mortality. *Lancet, 2*, 1455–1457.

74. Stephen, E. H., Foote, K., Hendershot, G. E., & Schoenborn, C. A. (1994). *Health of the foreign-born population: United States, 1989–90* (Advance Data, No. 241). Atlanta, GA: Centers for Disease Control and Prevention.

75. Fang, J., Madhavan, S., & Alderman, M. H. (1997). The influence of birthplace on mortality among Hispanic residents of New York City. *Ethn Dis, 7*, 55–64.

76. Wei, M., Valdez, R. A., Mitchell, B. D., Haffner, S. M., Stern, M. P., & Hazuda, H. P. (1996). Migration status, socioeconomic status, and mortality rates in Mexican Americans and non-Hispanic whites: The San Antonio Heart Study. *Ann Epidemiol, 6*, 307–313.

77. Jones, L. A., Gonzalez, R., Pillow, P. C., et al. (1997). Dietary fiber, Hispanics, and breast cancer risk. *Ann N Y Acad Sci, 837*, 524–536.

78. Schaffer, D. M., Velie, E. M., Shaw, G. M., & Todoroff, K. P. (1998). Energy and nutrient intakes and health practices of Latinas and white non-Latinas in the 3 months before pregnancy. *J Am Diet Assoc, 98*, 876–884.

79. Elder, J. P., Castro, F. G., de Moor, C., et al. (1991). Differences in cancer-risk-related behaviors in Latino and Anglo adults. *Prev Med, 20,* 751–763.

80. Thompson, B., Demark-Wahnefried, W., Taylor, G., et al. (1999). Baseline fruit and vegetable intake among adults in seven 5-a-day study centers located in diverse geographic areas. *J Am Diet Assoc, 99,* 1241–1248.

81. Poston, D.L.J., & Dan, H. (1996). Fertility trends in the United States. In D. L. Peck & J. S. Hollingsworth (Eds.), *Demographic and structural change: The effects of the 1980s on American society* (pp. 85–100). Westport, CT: Greenwood.

82. Hazuda, H. P., Haffner, S. M., Stern, M. P., & Eifler, C. W. (1988). Effects of acculturation and socioeconomic status on obesity and diabetes in Mexican Americans. *Am J Epidemiol, 128,* 1289–1301.

83. Keefe, S., & Padilla, A. (1987). *Chicano ethnicity.* Albuquerque: University of New Mexico Press.

84. Angel, R., & Cleary, P. D. (1984). The effects of social structure and culture on reported health. *Soc Sci Q, 65,* 814–828.

85. Anderson, L. M., Wood, D. L., & Sherbourne, C. D. (1997). Maternal acculturation and childhood immunization levels among children in Latino families in Los Angeles. *Am J Public Health, 87,* 2018–2021.

86. Elder, J. P., Woodruff, S. L., Candelaria, J. G., et al. (1998). Socioeconomic indicators related to cardiovascular disease risk factors in Hispanics. *Am J Health Behav, 22,* 172–185.

87. Peete, C. T. (1999). The importance of place of residence in health outcomes research: How does living in an ethnic enclave affect low birth weight deliveries for Hispanic mothers? *Dissertation Abstracts Int, 60,* 1777-A.

88. Bassford, T. L. (1995). Health status of Hispanic elders. *Clin Geriatr Med, 11,* 25–38.

89. James, S. A. (1993). Racial and ethnic differences in infant mortality and low birth weight: A psychosocial critique. *Ann Epidemiol, 3,* 130–136.

90. Hazuda, H. P. (1985). Differences in socioeconomic status and acculturation among Mexican Americans and risk of cardiovascular disease. In U.S. Department of Health and Human Services, *Report of the Secretary's Task Force on Black and Minority Health: Vol. 1. Executive summary* (pp. 367–390). Washington, DC: U.S. Government Printing Office.

91. Scribner, R., & Dwyer, J. H. (1989). Acculturation and low birth weight among Latinos in the Hispanic HANES. *Am J Public Health, 79,* 1263–1267.

92. Keefe, S. E., Padilla, A. M., & Carlos, M. L. (1979). The Mexican-American extended family as an emotional support system. *Hum Organ, 38,* 144–152.

93. Mirowsky, J., & Ross, C. (1984). Mexican culture and its emotional contradictions. *J Health Soc Behav, 25,* 2–13.

94. Vega, W. A. Hispanic families in the 1980s: A decade of research. (1990). *J Marriage Fam, 52,* 1015–1024.

CHAPTER SEVENTEEN

Levels of Racism

A Theoretic Framework and a Gardener's Tale

Camara Phyllis Jones

Race-associated differences in health outcomes are routinely documented in this country, yet for the most part they remain poorly explained. Indeed, rather than vigorously exploring the basis of the differences, many scientists either adjust for race or restrict their studies to one racial group.[1] Ignoring the etiological clues embedded in group differences impedes the advance of scientific knowledge, limits efforts at primary prevention, and perpetuates ideas of biologically determined differences between the races.

The variable *race* is only a rough proxy for socioeconomic status, culture, and genes, but it precisely captures the social classification of people in a race-conscious society such as the United States. The race noted on a health form is the same race noted by a salesclerk, a police officer, or a judge, and this racial classification has a profound impact on daily life experience in this country. That is, the variable race is not a biological construct that reflects innate differences[2-4] but a social construct that precisely captures the impacts of racism.

For this reason, some investigators now hypothesize that race-associated differences in health outcomes are in fact due to the effects of racism.[5,6] In light of the Department of Health and Human Services' Initiative to Eliminate Racial and Ethnic Disparities in Health by the Year 2010,[7,8] it is important to examine the potential effects of racism in causing race-associated differences in health outcomes.

LEVELS OF RACISM: A FRAMEWORK

I have developed a framework for understanding racism on three levels: institutionalized, personally mediated, and internalized. This framework is useful for raising new hypotheses about the basis of race-associated differences in health outcomes, as well as for designing effective interventions to eliminate those differences. In this framework, "institutionalized racism" is defined as differential access to the goods, services, and opportunities of society by race. Institutionalized racism is normative, sometimes legalized, and often manifests as inherited disadvantage. It is structural, having been codified in our institutions of custom, practice, and law, so there need not be an identifiable perpetrator. Indeed, institutionalized racism is often evident as inaction in the face of need.

Institutionalized racism manifests itself both in material conditions and in access to power. With regard to material conditions, examples include differential access to quality education, sound housing, gainful employment, appropriate medical facilities, and a clean environment. With regard to access to power, examples include differential access to information (including one's own history), resources (including wealth and organizational infrastructure), and voice (including voting rights, representation in government, and control of the media). It is important to note that the association between socioeconomic status and race in the United States has its origins in discrete historical events but persists because of contemporary structural factors that perpetuate those historical injustices. In other words, it is because of institutionalized racism that there is an association between socioeconomic status and race in this country.

"Personally mediated racism" is defined as prejudice and discrimination, where prejudice means differential assumptions about the abilities, motives, and intentions of others according to their race, and discrimination means differential actions toward others according to their race. This is what most people think of when they hear the word "racism." Personally mediated racism can be intentional as well as unintentional, and it includes acts of commission as well as acts of omission. It manifests as lack of respect (poor or no service, failure to communicate options), suspicion (shopkeepers' vigilance; everyday avoidance by others, including street crossing, purse clutching, and standing when there are empty seats on public transportation), devaluation (surprise at competence, stifling of aspirations), scapegoating (the Rosewood incident,[9,10] the Charles Stuart case,[11-14] the Susan Smith case[15-18]), and dehumanization (police brutality, sterilization abuse, hate crimes).

"Internalized racism" is defined as acceptance by members of the stigmatized races of negative messages about their own abilities and intrinsic worth. It is characterized by their not believing in others who look like them, and not believing in themselves. It involves accepting limitations to one's own full humanity, including one's spectrum of dreams, one's right to self-determination, and one's range of allowable self-expression. It manifests as an embracing of "whiteness" (use of hair straighteners and bleaching creams, stratification by skin tone within communities of color, and "the white man's ice is colder" syndrome); self-devaluation (racial slurs as nicknames, rejection of ancestral culture, and fratricide); and resignation, helplessness, and hopelessness (dropping out of school, failing to vote, and engaging in risky health practices).

The following allegory is useful for illustrating the relationship between the three levels of racism (institutionalized, personally mediated, and internalized) and for guiding our thinking about how to intervene. I use this story in my teaching on race and racism at the Harvard School of Public Health as well as in my public lectures.

LEVELS OF RACISM: A GARDENER'S TALE

When my husband and I bought a house in Baltimore, there were two large flower boxes on the front porch. When spring came we decided to grow flowers in them. One of the boxes was empty, so we bought potting soil to fill it. We did nothing to the soil in the other box, assuming that it was fine. Then we planted seeds from a single seed packet in the two boxes. The seeds that were sown in the new potting soil quickly sprang up and flourished. All of the seeds sprouted, the most vital towering strong and tall, and even the weak seeds made it to a middling height. However, the seeds planted in the old soil did not fare so well. Far fewer seeds sprouted, with the strong among them only making it to a middling height, while the weak among them died. It turns out that the old soil was poor and rocky, in contrast to the new potting soil, which was rich and fertile. The difference in yield and appearance in the two flower boxes was a vivid, real-life illustration of the importance of environment. Those readers who are gardeners will probably have witnessed this phenomenon with their own eyes.

Now I will use this image of the two flower boxes to illustrate the three levels of racism. Let's imagine a gardener who has two flower boxes, one that she knows to be filled with rich, fertile soil and another that she knows to be filled with poor, rocky soil. This gardener has two packets of seeds for the same type of flower. However, the plants grown from one packet of seeds will bear pink blossoms, while the plants grown from the other packet of seeds will bear red blossoms. The gardener prefers red over pink, so she plants the red seed in the rich fertile soil and the pink seed in the poor rocky soil. And sure enough, what I witnessed in my own garden comes to pass in this garden too. All of the red flowers grow up and flourish, with the fittest growing tall and strong and even the weakest making it to a middling height. But in the box with the poor rocky soil, things look different. The weak among the pink seeds don't even make it, and the strongest among them grow only to a middling height (Figure 17.1).

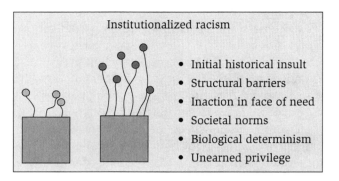

Figure 17.1 Institutionalized Racism.

In time the flowers in these two boxes go to seed, dropping their progeny into the same soil in which they were growing. The next year the same thing happens, with the red flowers in the rich soil growing full and vigorous and strong, while the pink flowers in the poor soil struggle to survive. And these flowers go to seed. Year after year, the same thing happens. Ten years later the gardener comes to survey her garden. Gazing at the two boxes, she says, "I was right to prefer red over pink! Look how vibrant and beautiful the red flowers look, and see how pitiful and scrawny the pink ones are" (Figure 17.2).

This part of the story illustrates some important aspects of institutionalized racism. There is the initial historical insult of separating the seed into the two different types of soil; the contemporary structural factors of the flower boxes, which keep the soils separate; and the acts of omission in not addressing the differences between the soils over the years. The normative aspects of institu-

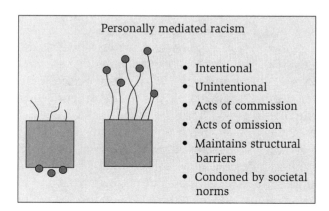

Figure 17.2 Personally Mediated Racism.

tionalized racism are illustrated by the initial preference of the gardener for red over pink. Indeed, her assumption that red is intrinsically better than pink may contribute to a blindness about the difference between the soils.

Where is personally mediated racism in this gardener's tale? That occurs when the gardener, disdaining the pink flowers because they look so poor and scraggly, plucks the pink blossoms off before they can even go to seed. Or when a seed from a pink flower has been blown into the rich soil, and she plucks it out before it can establish itself.

And where is the internalized racism in this tale? That occurs when a bee comes along to pollinate the pink flowers and the pink flowers say, "Stop! Don't bring me any of that pink pollen—I prefer the red!" The pink flowers have internalized the belief that red is better than pink, because they look across at the other flower box and see the red flowers strong and flourishing (Figure 17.3).

What are we to do if we want to put things right in this garden? Well, we could start by addressing the internalized racism and telling the pink flowers, "Pink is beautiful!" That might make them feel a bit better, but it will do little to change the conditions in which they live. Or we could address the personally mediated racism by conducting workshops with the gardener to convince her to stop plucking the pink flowers before they have had a chance to go to seed. Maybe she'll stop, or maybe she won't. Yet, even if she is convinced to stop plucking the pink flowers, we have still done nothing to address the poor, rocky condition of the soil in which they live.

What we really have to do to set things right in this garden is address the institutionalized racism. We have to break down the boxes and mix up the soil, or we can leave the two boxes separate but fertilize the poor soil until it is as rich as the fertile soil. When we do that, the pink flowers will grow at least as strong and vibrant as the red (and perhaps stronger, for they have been selected for survival). And when they do, the pink flowers will no longer think that

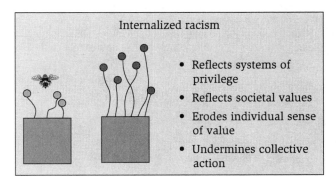

Figure 17.3 Internalized Racism.

red pollen is better than pink, because they will look over at the red flowers and see that they are equally strong and beautiful. And although the original gardener may have to go to her grave preferring red over pink, the gardener's children who grow up seeing that pink and red are equally beautiful will be unlikely to develop the same preferences.

This story illustrates the relationship between the three levels of racism. It also highlights the fact that institutionalized racism is the most fundamental of the three levels and must be addressed for important change to occur. Finally, it provides the insight that once institutionalized racism is addressed, the other levels of racism may cure themselves over time. Perhaps the most important question raised by this story is *Who is the gardener?* After all, the gardener is the one with the power to decide, the power to act, and the control over the resources.

In the United States, the gardener is our government (Figure 17.4). As the story illustrates, there is particular danger when this gardener is not concerned with equity. The current Initiative to Eliminate Racial and Ethnic Disparities in Health by the Year 2010 is to be lauded as the first explicit commitment by the government to achieve equity in health outcomes.

Many other questions arise from this simple story. What is the role of public health researchers in vigorously exploring the basis of pink-red disparities, including the differences in the soil and the structural factors and acts of omission that maintain those differences? How can we get the gardener to own the whole garden and not be satisfied when only the red flowers thrive? If the gardener will not invest in the whole garden, how can the pink flowers recruit or grow their own gardener?

The reader is invited to share this story with family members, neighbors, colleagues, and communities. The questions we raise and the discussions we generate may be the start of a much needed national conversation on racism.

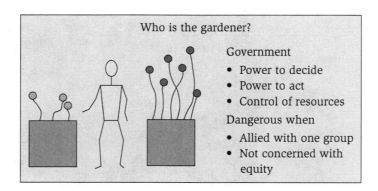

Figure 17.4 Who Is the Gardener?

Notes

1. Jones, C. P., LaVeist, T. A., & Lillie-Blanton, M. (1991). "Race" in the epidemiologic literature: An examination of the *American Journal of Epidemiology, 1921–1990. Am J Epidemiol, 134,* 1079–1084.

2. Cooper, R., & David, R. (1986). The biological concept of race and its application to public health and epidemiology. *J Health Polit Policy Law, 11,* 97–116.

3. Cavalli-Sforza, L. L., Menozzi, P., & Piazza, A. (1994). *The history and geography of human genes.* Princeton, NJ: Princeton University Press.

4. Williams, D. R. (1997). Race and health: Basic questions, emerging directions. *Ann Epidemiol, 7,* 322–333.

5. Krieger, N., Rowley, D. L., Herman, A. A., Avery, B., & Phillips, M. T. (1993). Racism, sexism, and social class: Implications for studies of health, disease, and well-being. *Am J Prev Med, 9*(6, Suppl.), 82–122.

6. Jones, C. P. (1994). *Methods for comparing distributions: Development and application exploring "race"-associated differences in systolic blood pressure.* Unpublished dissertation, Johns Hopkins School of Hygiene and Public Health, Baltimore, MD.

7. *President Clinton announces new racial and ethnic health disparities initiative* (White House Fact Sheet). (1998, February 21). Washington, DC: U.S. Department of Health and Human Services Press Office.

8. U.S. Department of Health and Human Services. *The initiative to eliminate racial and ethnic disparities in health.* Retrieved May 29, 2000, from http://raceand-health.hhs.gov/

9. Jones, M. D., Rivers, L. E., Colburn, D. R., Dye, R. T., & Rogers, W. W. *A documented history of the incident which occurred at Rosewood, Florida, in January 1923.* Retrieved May 29, 2000, from http://members.aol.com/klove01/ rosehist.txt

10. Love, K. *Materials on the destruction of Rosewood Florida.* Retrieved May 29, 2000, from http://members.aol.com/klove01/rosedest.htm

11. Canellos, P. S., & Sege, I. (1989, October 24). Couple shot after leaving hospital: Baby delivered. *Boston Globe,* p. 1, Metro/Region sec.

12. Jacobs, S. (1989, December 29). Stuart is said to pick out suspect. *Boston Globe,* p. 1, Metro/Region sec.

13. Cullen, K., Murphy, S., Barnicle, M., et al. (1990, January 5). Stuart dies in jump off Tobin Bridge after police are told he killed his wife: The Stuart murder case. *Boston Globe,* p. 1, Metro/Region sec.

14. Graham, R. (1990, January 11). Hoax seen playing on fear, racism: The Stuart murder case. *Boston Globe,* p. 1, Metro/Region sec.

15. Davis, R. (1994, October 27). Prayers lifted up for abducted boys: Tots whisked off in S.C. carjacking Tuesday. *USA Today,* p. 10A.

16. Terry, D. (1994, November 6). A woman's false accusation pains many blacks. *New York Times,* p. 32, sec. 1.

17. Harrison, E. (1994, November 9). Accused child killer's family apologizes to blacks. Race relations: Susan Smith's brother says that his sister's false claim that an African American man kidnapped her sons was a "terrible misfortune." *Los Angeles Times,* p. A9.

18. Lewis, C. (1994, November 16). The game is to blame the blacks. *Philadelphia Inquirer,* p. A15.

CHAPTER EIGHTEEN

Racism as a Stressor
for African Americans

A Biopsychosocial Model

Rodney Clark
Norman B. Anderson
Vernessa R. Clark
David R. Williams

Given the historical and contemporary existence of racism in American society, one might suspect there would be an equally substantial literature examining the effects of racism on African Americans. Yet research exploring the biological, psychological, and social effects of racism among African Americans is virtually nonexistent. The purpose of this chapter is threefold: (1) to provide a brief overview of how the concept of racism has been addressed in the scientific literature, (2) to review studies exploring the existence of intergroup and intragroup racism, and (3) to present a conceptual model for systematic studies of the biopsychosocial effects of perceived racism among African Americans. This chapter represents perhaps the first attempt to synthesize research examining perceptions of intergroup and intragroup racism and their biopsychosocial effects among African Americans.

CONCEPTUALIZATIONS OF RACISM

Despite its ubiquity in everyday language, no consensus on the definition of racism has emerged from the scientific literature.[1] In this chapter, *racism* is

We are grateful to James Blumenthal, Karen Gil, and William Jenkins for their helpful comments on earlier versions of this chapter.

operationally defined as beliefs, attitudes, institutional arrangements, and acts that tend to denigrate individuals or groups because of phenotypic characteristics or ethnic group affiliation. Unlike other conceptualizations that describe racism as a relationship between members of oppressed and nonoppressed groups, this more comprehensive definition of racism encompasses beliefs, attitudes, arrangements, and acts either held by or perpetuated by members of a different ethnic group (intergroup racism) and by members of the same ethnic group (intragroup racism).

Although numerous conceptualizations of racism have been used in the scientific literature, they can be placed into two broad categories: attitudinal or behavioral.[2] Attitudinal racism and ethnic prejudice have both been used to represent attitudes and beliefs that denigrate individuals or groups because of phenotypic characteristics or ethnic group affiliation.[3] According to Yetman,[3] behavioral racism (ethnic discrimination), in contrast, is any act of an individual or institution that denies equitable treatment to an individual or a group because of phenotypic characteristics or ethnic group affiliation.

EVIDENCE OF RACISM

Reviews of the survey literature suggest that despite improvements in ethnic group attitudes among Caucasians over the last three decades,[4] there remain "important signs of continued resistance to full equality of black Americans."[5] Examples include more objective findings of intergroup racism in higher education,[6] the restaurant industry,[7] housing rentals and sales,[8] automotive sales,[9] and hiring practices,[10] as well as more subjective experiences of intergroup racism reported by African Americans.[2,11-15]

Although research exploring intergroup racism abounds in the literature, relatively few studies have assessed the impact of intragroup racism among African Americans. Of the studies that have assessed the impact of intragroup racism among African Americans, the majority have focused on skin tone variations. For example, many African Americans once endorsed the idea that darker-skinned African Americans were inherently inferior to lighter-skinned African Americans.[16,17] Additionally, African American fraternities, sororities, business and social organizations, churches, preparatory schools, and historically black colleges and universities routinely excluded African Americans on the basis of skin tone and hair texture.[17,18] In summary, the available research evidence suggests that perceptions of both intergroup and intragroup racism have persisted and continue to exert a significant effect on the well-being of many African Americans.[2,5,8-10,14,18-24]

BIOPSYCHOSOCIAL EFFECTS OF PERCEIVED RACISM IN AFRICAN AMERICANS: A CONTEXTUAL MODEL

Examining the effects of intergroup racism and intragroup racism in African Americans is warranted for at least three important reasons. First, if exposure to racism is perceived as stressful, it may have negative biopsychosocial sequelae[25-30] that might help explain intergroup differences in health outcomes.[31-33] Second, differential exposure to and coping responses following perceptions of racism may help account for the wide within-group variability in health outcomes among African Americans. Third, if exposure to racism is among the factors related to negative health outcomes in African Americans, specific intervention and prevention strategies could be developed and implemented to lessen its deleterious impact. These strategies would provide a needed supplement to efforts aimed at reducing health disparities in American society.

Despite hypothesized links between perceptions of racism and health outcomes,[15,21,32,34-40] few studies have examined the effects of perceived racism within a comprehensive and empirically testable biopsychosocial model (see Figure 18.1). This proposed model is consistent with the conceptualizations of other researchers[25,41,42] who have proposed relationships between biopsychosocial factors and specific health outcomes. Although unique in that it is tailored to apply to perceptions of racism, the model builds on the more general stress-coping model proposed by Lazarus and Folkman.[29]

The principal tenet of this proposed model is that the perception of an environmental stimulus as racist results in exaggerated psychological and physiological stress responses that are influenced by constitutional factors, sociodemographic factors, psychological and behavioral factors, and coping responses. Over time, these stress responses are posited to influence health outcomes. Furthermore, the perception of environmental stimuli as racist and the ensuing coping responses are postulated to be a function of a complex interplay between an array of psychological, behavioral, constitutional, and sociodemographic factors. Although it is possible for psychological, behavioral, constitutional, and sociodemographic factors to influence coping responses directly, for simplicity of illustration these connections are not included in Figure 18.1. The remainder of this section is devoted to explicating each component of the model and highlighting its relevance to research on health outcomes in African Americans. Following the discussion of "environmental stimuli," the section is divided into subsections delineating the moderator and mediator variables in the proposed model. Consistent with the work of Baron and Kenny,[43] moderator variables are defined herein as factors that influence the direction or magnitude of

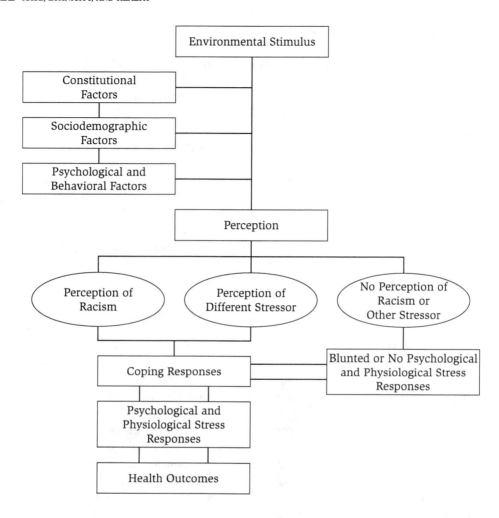

Figure 18.1 A Contextual Model to Examine the Biopsychosocial Effects
of Perceived Racism.

the relationship between predictor and criterion variables. Mediator variables,
on the other hand, are operationalized herein as factors that may account, at
least in part, for the relationship between predictor and criterion variables.

Environmental Stimuli

African Americans are disproportionately exposed to environmental stimuli that
may be sources of chronic and acute stress.[14,24,28,44] The historical basis for
many of these exposures has been experienced by few, if any, other ethnic
groups to the extent it has by African Americans.[21,28] A myriad of these stimuli

(especially interpersonal) could be perceived as involving racism. For example, more than 50 percent of African Americans attribute substandard housing, lack of skilled labor and managerial jobs, and lower wages for African Americans to ethnic discrimination.[2] Moreover, given that psychological and physiological stress responses are more sensitive to an individual's perception of stressfulness than to objective demands,[26,45] there is no a priori way of determining if an environmental stimulus will be perceived as racist by an individual.[46]

Distinguishing between chronic and acute sources of perceived racism may be particularly instructive, given that these two sources of stress may differentially predict self-reported health status.[15] Moreover, the combined effects of chronic and acute perceptions have the potential to contribute to psychological and physiological sequelae that may be particularly toxic in African Americans.[2,11,35] Therefore, perceived racism as a potential source of stress should be viewed as having both chronic and acute dimensions.

Moderator Variables

Constitutional Factors. Numerous constitutional factors are hypothesized to influence the relationship between exposure to environmental stimuli and health outcomes. For example, among many African Americans, skin tone has been associated with perceptions of ethnic discrimination,[22,47] occupational status,[20,22] and personal income.[22] In addition to skin tone, family history of hypertension has been the focus of studies examining intergroup and intragroup differences in cardiovascular reactivity, resting blood pressure, and the prevalence of essential hypertension. Findings from studies examining the predictive utility of these markers to independently differentiate groups at varying levels of hypertension risk have been mixed.[32,40,48–51] A growing body of research suggests, however, that family history of hypertension and skin tone influence the development of hypertension indirectly. That is, these constitutional factors may interact with sociodemographic variables to increase the risk of negative health outcomes like hypertension.[32,52–55]

Sociodemographic Factors. One sociodemographic factor that is particularly relevant to the proposed model is socioeconomic status (SES). SES is associated with perceptions of racism,[56] ethnicity,[5,57] and biopsychosocial functioning.[15,52] Research has suggested that the relationship between SES and the other components of this model is complex.[56] That is, some research has found a positive relationship between SES and discrimination, whereas other studies suggest that SES is inversely related to experiences of discrimination among African Americans.[2] It is plausible that the pattern of association between SES and racism among African Americans depends, in part, on what dimension of racism is assessed. For example, with measures that tap subtler expressions of racism, it is probable that higher SES African Americans report perceiving their environments as more discriminatory because of their tendency to negotiate environments where racism is less overt. Conversely, lower SES African Americans may be more sensitive to overt racism and as a result report more racism on measures that assess more overt expressions of racism and those that assess institutionally mediated dimensions of racism (for example, access to good jobs).

Moreover, SES has been found to interact with ethnicity in that lower SES African Americans appear to be more vulnerable to some negative health outcomes than are higher SES African Americans and many other ethnicity-SES groups. At least two explanations can be forwarded to help explain findings that African Americans at comparable educational levels have a higher prevalence of hypertension and all-cause mortality than do Caucasians.[58] First, within SES groups, the distribution of wealth among African Americans and Caucasians is not comparable.[52,57] Second, relative to Caucasians, African Americans report exposure to more stressors like racism and other unfair treatment.[15,59] As a consequence, African Americans may have to utilize coping responses more frequently to deal with these added stressors than do Caucasians, thereby increasing the likelihood of both resource strain-behavioral exhaustion and psychological and physiological distress. It is probable therefore that lower SES African Americans are not only exposed to more chronic stressors than higher SES African Americans but may also have fewer resources with which to cope with these stressors, leading to more deleterious health outcomes.[11]

Relative to other components of this model, there has been less research exploring associations between perceived racism, other sociodemographic factors, and health outcomes. For example, age and gender may influence health outcomes through their association with the amount and frequency of potential stress exposure, the cognitive appraisal process, coping responses, and stress responses.[18,22,27,52] Adams and Dressler[46] reported that age was inversely related to perceptions of racism and injustice in a community sample of African Americans. Although this finding seemed paradoxical, these authors reasoned that older African Americans may have come to accept discriminatory treatment and not to label it as such. This subsample may be similar to those in Krieger[59] and Krieger and Sidney,[38] who did not report being recipients of unfair treatment yet showed elevated resting blood pressure levels. Krieger and Sidney[38] suggested that denial may be one important coping response members of ethnic minority groups may use in dealing with racism that may have health consequences.

Psychological and Behavioral Factors. Depending on individual factors, any event may be perceived as stressful[60] and involving racism.[46] Various psychological and behavioral factors may influence how individuals perceive and respond to environmental stimuli.[46,60–62] Additionally, these factors may "play a potential role in the presentation or treatment of almost every general medical condition" (p. 676).[63] Type A behavior, cynical hostility, neuroticism, self-esteem, obsessive-compulsive disorder, hardiness, perceived control, and anger expression-suppression are among the psychological and behavioral factors that are postulated to influence the stress process, cardiovascular outcomes, and immune functioning.[46,60,62,64–67] For example, research has suggested that of the usual ways by which African Americans cope with anger, the affective state most commonly reported to follow perceptions of racism,[68] is related to cardiovascular reactivity and resting blood pressure.[69,70] It remains to be determined if and how these psychological and behavioral factors influence the relationship between perceived racism and health status.

Mediator Variables

Racism as a Perceived Stressor. *Perceived racism* refers to the subjective experience of prejudice or discrimination. Therefore, perceived racism is not limited to those experiences that may "objectively" be viewed as representing racism. For example, subtler forms of racism include belief systems and symbolic behaviors that promulgate the ideology of "free will."[24,71] Although the ideology of free will may not be inherently racist, Yetman remarked, "when applied to black Americans, the belief system of free will is racist in that it refuses to recognize or acknowledge the existence of external impingements and disabilities (such as prejudice and discrimination) and instead imputes the primary responsibility for black disadvantages to blacks themselves" (p. 15).[3] Although many Caucasians who are proponents of free will may not view their beliefs or actions as racist, such beliefs and actions may be perceived as serious or threatening (for example, involving racism) by some African Americans.

During the past twenty years, several self-report measures have been developed to assess perceived racism. These include scales by Allan-Claiborne and Taylor,[72] Barbarin,[73] Harrell,[74] Landrine and Klonoff,[39] McNeilly, Anderson, Armstead, et al.,[75] Thompson, Neville, Weathers, Poston, and Atkinson,[76] and Utsey and Ponterotto.[77] Although these scales vary in their multidimensionality, each one has the potential to facilitate empirical investigations that disentangle the complex relationship between ethnically relevant stressors and health outcomes.

Whereas other self-report measures of stress have been accepted widely (for example, those assessing job strain, life events, and daily hassles), there may be a tendency to discount reports of racism simply because they involve a subjective component. Such a tendency to discount perceptions of racism as stressful is inconsistent with the stress literature, which highlights the importance of the appraisal process. For example, Lazarus and Folkman[29] noted that it is both the individual's evaluation of the seriousness of an event and his or her coping responses that determine whether a psychological stress response will ensue. That is, the perception of demands as stressful is more important in initiating stress responses than objective demands that may or may not be perceived as stressful.[45,78] With this in mind, the initiation of psychological stress responses as a result of perceiving environmental stimuli as involving racism would qualify these stimuli as stressors.

Coping Responses. Even among African Americans who perceive certain stimuli as stressful, whether ethnically based or not, there are likely to be wide individual differences in psychological and physiological stress responses. The magnitude and duration of these stress responses will depend on the availability and use of coping responses. Coping responses that do not attenuate stress responses are considered maladaptive and may negatively affect health.[61,78] That is, when maladaptive coping responses are used, the perception of an environmental event as racist will trigger psychological and physiological stress responses. If an individual fails to replace these maladaptive coping responses with more adaptive ones, this model further predicts a continued state of heightened psychological and physiological activity.[79] A similar stress response pattern would be expected in African Americans who perceive the stimulus as a stressor without racist content.

Adaptive coping responses, on the other hand, are postulated to mitigate enduring psychological and physiological stress responses, thereby reducing the potentially untoward effects of racism on health. As such, it may be possible to identify coping responses that influence the relationship between perceived racism and stress responses. Both adaptive and maladaptive coping responses would be expected to influence the duration and intensity of psychological and physiological stress responses.[26] A potential limitation of this model is that some individuals may not report perceiving any stressor or may inhibit the expression of psychological responses (for example, anger) yet show exaggerated physiological responses to stimuli.[42,80–82] To partially address this potential limitation, social desirability and repression measurements could be used to help identify individuals who exhibit this response pattern.

Coping responses to ethnically relevant stimuli have been conceptualized as general[61,69,83] or specific.[38,59,61,68,69,84] *General coping responses* refer to strategies that are usually used to deal with stressful stimuli—irrespective of their nature. In the only published study to investigate the efficacy of general coping strategies as moderators of the perceived racism-cardiovascular reactivity relationship, Armstead et al.[69] found that as Anger Out scores on the Framingham and Anger Expression scales increased, blood pressure levels decreased after viewing racist video scenes. Research has suggested that the effects of more general coping responses, such as "John Henryism,"[85] social support,[86] and religious participation,[21] may be particularly relevant for African Americans and may interact with sociodemographic factors to modify risk for negative health outcomes like elevated blood pressure.[25,85,87]

Racism-specific coping responses refer to cognitions and behaviors used to mitigate the effects (for example, psychological and physiological) of perceived racism. Although numerous investigators have examined the relationship between general coping responses and health outcomes, few have sought to identify specific coping responses African Americans use in response to perceptions of racism. Two notable exceptions include recent studies by McNeilly, Anderson, Armstead, et al.[75] and Harrell[74] that outlined a broad range of emotional and coping responses to racism and a method for measuring them. Given their recent addition to the literature, published research examining the efficacy of these coping measures as predictors of health outcomes does not yet exist. To date, only six published studies[15,38,59,61,69,84] have examined the relationship between racism-specific coping responses and physiological responses and health status.

The observed association between racism-specific coping responses and health outcomes varies depending on the outcome under consideration. For example, after adjusting for sociodemographic and psychological factors, Williams, Yu, Jackson, and Anderson[15] found that passive and active coping responses to discrimination (including ethnic-group discrimination) were related to increased psychological distress, poorer well-being, and more chronic conditions among African Americans. In two of the laboratory studies, racism-specific coping responses were not related to cardiovascular responses to ethnically relevant stressors.[69,84] Conversely, Clark and Harrell[61] found that scores on the "cognitive flexibility" dimension of a coping scale were positively associated with initial resting systolic blood pressure and time to recovery for diastolic blood pressure. Their findings suggest that individuals who use the cognitive flexibility style to cope with perceived racism may process the racist content of the stimulus longer than do individuals using more active coping responses.

Over time, chronic perceptions of racism coupled with more passive coping responses may lead to frequent increases in and prolonged activation of sympathetic functioning resulting in higher resting systolic blood pressure levels. Many authors have proposed that such chronic stress-induced sympathetic activation may be among the factors that lead to hypertension (for a review see Manuck, Kasprowicz, and Muldoon[88]). For instance, Krieger[59] found that African American women (forty-five years old and older) who responded to unfair treatment (for example, racism and gender discrimination) with passive coping responses (for example, keeping quiet and accepting treatment) were 4.4 times more likely to have self-reported hypertension than were African American women whose coping techniques were more active. Similarly, Krieger and Sidney[38] found that among African American working-class men and women, passive coping responses were associated with markedly higher resting blood pressure levels.

Additionally, the efficacy of various coping strategies in reducing the chronic and acute psychological and physiological effects of ethnically relevant stimuli may depend, in part, on the frequency of the perceived stressor and the context or setting in which racism is perceived. For example, although coping responses like projection and denial may be adaptive with acute stressors, they may be maladaptive when used to negotiate chronic stressors.[26,38,80,82] Similarly, whereas expressing emotional reactions to peers may be adaptive in some contexts, this approach may be maladaptive in others.

Psychological and Physiological Stress Responses. Numerous psychological stress responses may follow perceptions of racism. These responses include anger, paranoia, anxiety, helplessness-hopelessness, frustration, resentment, and fear.[68,69] Psychological stress responses may, in turn, influence the use of subsequent coping responses.[26,28,29,60] For example, perceptions of racism that engender anger may lead to coping responses that include anger suppression, hostility, aggression, verbal expression of the anger, or the use of alcohol or other substances to blunt angry feelings.[35,69,89–92] These psychological responses are not necessarily independently occurring phenomena, given that responses to primary stressors may elicit prolonged psychological responsiveness and sociocultural adjustment.[60,93] For example, chronic feelings of helplessness-hopelessness may evoke feelings of frustration, depression, resentment, distrust, or paranoia[94–96] that lead to passivity, overeating, avoidance, or efforts to gain control.[68]

Physiological responses following exposure to psychologically stressful stimuli most notably involve immune, neuroendocrine, and cardiovascular functioning.[27,41,97,98] In the immune system, for example, two immune reactions (humoral and cellular) may be affected. In response to chronic stress, the adrenal gland produces hormones that suppress the activity of B and T lymphocytes, thereby preventing the body from destroying or neutralizing foreign substances (for example, bacteria and viruses) and increasing vulnerability to disease.[98] In one meta-analysis of the stress-immune literature, Herbert and Cohen[99] found that chronic and interpersonal stressors are related to lower natural killer cell activity. Research suggests that immune responses to these chronic and acute stressors are not transient.[100] For example, in studies examining the chronic stress associated with caregiving and immune functioning, researchers have found that spouses who are caring for partners with Alzheimer's dementia show decreased cellular immunity and prolonged respiratory infections[101] and decreased expression of the growth hormone mRNA.[102] Results from immune function tests on blood samples have also shown that laboratory-induced conflict among married couples is associated with lowered immune functioning that persists well after the experimental session.[103] Additionally, it has recently been demonstrated that stress-induced immune changes may slow the healing process.[104] Although tentative, these studies suggest that perceived stress is related to decreases in immune functioning (for example, lower helper T cells, lower natural killer cell cytotoxic activity, and higher antibody titers to the Epstein-Barr virus) that may increase susceptibility for an array of health outcomes.[98,105–107]

Stress-induced neuroendocrine responses include activation of the pituitary-adrenocortical and hypothalamic-sympathetic-adrenal medullary systems.[26,27] Findings from human and animal studies have suggested that the activation of these systems results in numerous physiological changes. For example, in response to acute stressors, these changes include the release of antidiuretic hormone, prolactin, growth hormone, glucocorticoids, epinephrine, norepinephrine, adrenocorticotropic hormone (which influences the production of cortisol via the adrenal gland), cortisol, and β-endorphin.[27,108,109] Concurrent with these neuroendocrine changes, there is an increase in cardiovascular activity. According to Herd, the cardiovascular responses include "increased rate and force of cardiac contraction, skeletal muscle vasodilation, venoconstriction, splanchnic vasoconstriction, renal vasoconstriction, and decreased renal excretion of sodium" (p. 326).[27] Upon repeated exposure to acute stressors, the magnitude and duration of these neuroendocrine and cardiovascular responses would depend, in part, on an individual's ability to successfully cope with the stressor.[26,110–113]

Health Outcomes. Psychological and physiological responses to perceptions of racism may, over time, be related to numerous health outcomes. For example, Fernando[94] postulated that as a potential added stressor for many African Americans, perceived racism may influence the genesis of depression by (1) posing transient threats to self-esteem, (2) making the group's failure to receive normative returns more salient, and (3) contributing to a sense of helplessness. Although some research has suggested that reports and expectations of discrimination are associated with depressive symptomatology among African Americans[75] and adolescent immigrants,[114] other reports have questioned the validity of these discriminatory reports and expectations. For example, Taylor, Wright, and Ruggiero[115] concluded that mental health problems like depression could affect perceptions of life experiences and lead individuals to perceive discriminatory practices that do not exist.

Although studies explicating the long-term health effects of perceived racism remain limited, there is a growing body of research in the more general stress literature that documents the relationship between stress and health. For example, stress has been linked to low birthweight and infant mortality,[28] depression,[116] the healing process,[104] breast cancer survival,[117] heart disease,[118–120] mean arterial blood pressure changes,[121] and chronic obstructive pulmonary disease.[122] Additionally, research suggests that exposure to stress is related to upper respiratory infections and the development of clinical colds.[106] There is some suggestion, however, that the duration of stress exposure moderates the relationship between stress exposure and cold susceptibility. For example, Cohen et al.[105] found that exposure to chronic psychological stressors (lasting one month or longer)—not acute stressors—is related to cold susceptibility.

Although not all studies have found support for the hypothesized perceived racism-health status association,[34] significant relationships between perceptions of racism and resting blood pressure[38] and subjective well-being[14,123] have been documented. In one multistage area probability sample of 1,106 African American and Caucasian adults in the Detroit metropolitan area, Williams, Yu, Jackson, and Anderson[15] found that unfair treatment attributed to racial or ethnic discrimination and racial or ethnic discrimination over the lifetime predicted psychological distress, well-being, number of bed days, and chronic conditions for African Americans. Among Caucasians, racial or ethnic discrimination over the lifetime predicted psychological distress and well-being.

The focus of this chapter has been on the role of racism as a perceived stressor and its implications for health. It is also possible, however, that racism may affect health even when it is not perceived as a stressor. For example, institutional racism[21,124] may reduce access to goods, services, and opportunities for African Americans in ways that have important health consequences. In a recent study, for example, it was found that ethnicity is a strong determinant of physicians' recommendations for critical cardiac assessments for patients experiencing chest pain, even among patients with similar risk factors, clinical features, and economic resources.[125] In this instance, institutional racism in health care may have dire consequences for the health of African Americans—even when no individual racism may be perceived. Therefore, perceived racism may be one of several possible pathways by which racism may affect health.

Summary

Despite the different sampling schemes and data quantification methodologies and the paucity of studies, the results of the research reviewed in this section were generally consistent. The perception of racism usually resulted in psychological and physiological stress responses. To deal with the effects of perceived racism, African Americans were found to use various coping strategies. These strategies were associated with physiological reactivity and health status. The research reviewed in this section does provide a basis for a stress and coping approach to the study of the effects of perceived racism.

CONCLUSIONS AND RECOMMENDATIONS

The purpose of this chapter was to provide a discussion of the potential usefulness of studying the biopsychosocial effects of perceived racism within a stress and coping model. Research examining the psychological, physiological, and social effects of perceived racism was presented. Overall, research in this area is lacking, and the research that has been conducted is without conceptual and methodological cohesion. As a step toward advancing this field of study, a contextual model was presented that may serve as a guide for systematic investigations of perceived racism and its biopsychosocial concomitants and sequelae. On the basis of the proposed model, research examining the effects of ethnically relevant stressors like racism may contribute to a better understanding of interethnic and intraethnic group health disparities. Given that available research also suggests that non-African Americans not only perceive racism but that such perceptions also adversely affect their psychological well-being,[15,126] this stress and coping analysis could be expanded to include other populations. Interdisciplinary investigations, examining the following questions, are encouraged to broaden the knowledge base in this area.

1. What Is the Relationship Between Perceived Racism and Health Outcomes for African Americans?

Epidemiologic investigations are needed to elucidate the relationship between perceived racism and the risk of maladies like hypertension, cardiovascular disease, infant mortality, low birthweight, cancer, depression, anxiety disorders, disruptive behavior disorders, and substance abuse and dependence.

2. What Are the Psychological and Physiological Concomitants of Perceived Racism?

Laboratory and ambulatory monitoring studies would be instrumental in identifying the sympathetic, immune, adrenocortical, and psychological responses that are associated with ethnically relevant stressors.

3. What Are Some of the General and Racism-Specific Responses Used in Response to Perceived Racism?

Psychophysiological, psychoneuroimmunological, and epidemiologic studies are also needed to determine whether general and racism-specific coping responses are differentially effective in mitigating the effects of perceived racism.

4. Does the Context in Which Racism Is Perceived Modify Its Psychological and Physiological Effects?

Psychological and sociological investigations are needed to determine whether the magnitude and duration of psychological stress responses such as anger, avoidance, denial, passivity, aggression, hostility, helplessness, and assertiveness vary as a function of the setting in which racism is perceived and the subtlety of the racist stimuli. Psychophysiological and psychoneuroimmunological studies examining sympathetic, immune, and adrenocortical responses to stressors that involve blatant versus subtle racist stimuli are also needed.

5. What Other Factors Influence the Relationship Between Perceived Racism and Health Outcomes?

Further research is needed to determine whether there are other factors that moderate or mediate the effects of perceived racism.

Notes

1. Farley, J. E. (1988). Orientation: Basic terms and concepts. In *Majority-minority relations* (2nd ed., pp. 1–11). Englewood Cliffs, NJ: Prentice Hall.

2. Sigelman, L., & Welch, S. (1991). *Black Americans' views of racial inequality: The dream deferred.* New York: Cambridge University Press.

3. Yetman, N. (1985). Introduction: Definitions and perspectives. In N. Yetman (Ed.), *Majority and minority: The dynamics of race and ethnicity in American life* (4th ed., pp. 1–20). Boston: Allyn & Bacon.

4. Schuman, H., Steeh, C., & Bobo, L. (1985). *Racial attitudes in America.* Cambridge, MA: Harvard University Press.

5. Jaynes, G. D., & Williams, R. M., Jr. (1989). *A common destiny: Blacks and American society.* Washington, DC: National Academy Press.

6. Farrell, W. C., Jr., & Jones, C. K. (1988). Recent racial incidents in higher education: A preliminary perspective. *Urban Rev, 20,* 211–226.

7. Schuman, H., Singer, E., Donovan, R., & Sellitz, C. (1983). Discriminatory behavior in New York restaurants, 1950 and 1981. *Soc Indicators Res, 13,* 69–83.

8. Yinger, J. (1995). *Closed doors, opportunities lost: The continuing costs of housing discrimination.* New York: Sage.

9. Ayres, I. (1991). Fair driving: Gender and race discrimination in bargaining for a new car. *Am Econ Rev, 85,* 304–321.

10. Kirschenman, J., & Neckerman, K. M. (1991). We'd love to hire them, but . . . : The meaning of race for employers. In C. Jenkins & P. E. Peterson (Eds.), *The urban underclass* (pp. 203–232). Washington, DC: Brookings Institution.

11. Feagin, J. R. (1991). The continuing significance of race: Antiblack discrimination in public places. *Am Sociol Rev, 56,* 101–116.

12. Mays, V. M., Coleman, L. M., & Jackson, J. S. (1996). Perceived race-based discrimination, employment status, and job stress in a national sample of black women: Implications for health outcomes. *J Occupat Health Psychol, 1,* 319–329.

13. Phillip, S. F. (1998). African-American perceptions of leisure, racial discrimination, and life satisfaction. *Percept Mot Skills, 87,* 1418.

14. Thompson, V.L.S. (1996). Perceived experiences of racism as stressful life events. *Community Ment Health J, 32,* 223–233.

15. Williams, D. R., Yu, Y., Jackson, J., & Anderson, N. (1997). Racial differences in physical and mental health: Socioeconomic status, stress, and discrimination. *J Health Psychol, 2,* 335–351.

16. Gatewood, W. B., Jr. (1988). Aristocrats of color: South and North, the black elite, 1880–1920. *J South Hist, 54,* 3–20.

17. Okazawa-Rey, M., Robinson, T., & Ward, J. V. (1986). Black women and the politics of skin color and hair. *Women's Studies Q, 14,* 13–14.

18. Neal, S. M., & Wilson, M. L. (1989). The role of skin color and features in the black community: Implications for black women and therapy. *Clin Psychol Rev, 9*, 323–333.

19. Essed, P. (1991). *Everyday racism.* Claremont, CA: Hunter House.

20. Hughes, M., & Hertel, B. R. (1990). The significance of color remains: A study of life chances, mate selection, and ethnic consciousness among black Americans. *Soc Forces, 68*, 1105–1120.

21. Jones, J. M. (1997). *Prejudice and racism* (2nd ed.). New York: McGraw-Hill.

22. Keith, V. M., & Herring, C. (1991). Skin tone and stratification in the black community. *Am J Sociol, 97*, 760–778.

23. Kinder, D. R., & Mendelberg, T. (1995). Cracks in American apartheid: The political impact of prejudice among desegregated whites. *J Politics, 57*, 402–424.

24. Sears, D. O. (1991). Symbolic racism. In P. A. Katz & D. A. Taylor (Eds.), *Eliminating racism: Profiles in controversy* (pp. 53–84). New York: Plenum.

25. Anderson, N. B., McNeilly, M., & Myers, H. (1991). Autonomic reactivity and hypertension in blacks: A review and proposed model. *Ethn Dis, 1*, 154–170.

26. Burchfield, S. R. (1979). The stress response: A new perspective. *Psychosom Med, 41*, 661–672.

27. Herd, J. A. (1991). Cardiovascular responses to stress. *Physiol Rev, 71*, 305–330.

28. James, S. A. (1993). Racial and ethnic differences in infant mortality and low birth weight: A psychosocial critique. *Ann Epidemiol, 3*, 130–136.

29. Lazarus, R. S., & Folkman, S. (1984). *Stress, appraisal, and coping.* New York: Springer.

30. Selye, H. (1983). The stress concept: Past, present, and future. In C. L. Cooper (Ed.), *Stress research* (pp. 1–20). New York: Wiley.

31. Dressler, W. W. (1991). Social class, skin color, and arterial blood pressure in two societies. *Ethn Dis, 1*, 60–77.

32. Klag, M. J., Whelton, P. K., Coresh, J., Grim, C. E., & Kuller, L. H. (1991). The association of skin color with blood pressure in U.S. blacks with low socioeconomic status. *JAMA, 265*, 599–602.

33. U.S. Department of Health and Human Services. (1985). *Report of the Secretary's task force on black and minority health.* Washington, DC: U.S. Government Printing Office.

34. Browman, C. L. (1996). The health consequences of racial discrimination: A study of African Americans. *Ethn Dis, 6*, 148–153.

35. Cooper, R. S. (1993). Health and the social status of blacks in the United States. *Ann Epidemiol, 3*, 137–144.

36. King, G., & Williams, D. R. (1995). Race and health: A multi-dimensional approach to African American health. In B. C. Amick, S. Levine, D. C. Walsh, & A. Tarlov (Eds.), *Society and health* (pp. 93–130). New York: Oxford University Press.

37. Krieger, N., Rowley, D. L., Herman, A. A., Avery, B., & Phillips, M. T. (1993). Racism, sexism, and social class: Implications for studies of health, disease, and well-being. *Am J Prev Med, 9*, 82–122.

38. Krieger, N., & Sidney, S. (1996). Racial discrimination and blood pressure: The CARDIA study of young black and white adults. *Am J Public Health, 86*, 1370–1378.

39. Landrine, H., & Klonoff, E. A. (1996). The Schedule of Racist Events: A measure of racial discrimination and a study of its negative physical and mental health consequences. *J Black Psychol, 22*, 144–168.

40. Tyroler, H. A., & James, S. A. (1978). Blood pressure and skin color. *Am J Public Health, 68*, 1170–1172.

41. Andersen, B. L., Kiecolt-Glaser, J. K., & Glaser, R. (1994). A biobehavioral model of cancer stress and disease course. *Am Psychol, 49*, 389–404.

42. Jorgensen, R. S., Johnson, B. T., Kolodziej, M. E., & Schreer, G. E. (1996). Elevated blood pressure and personality: A meta-analytic review. *Psychol Bull, 120*, 293–320.

43. Baron, R. M., & Kenny, D. A. (1986). The moderator-mediator variable distinction in social psychological research: Conceptual, strategic, and statistical considerations. *J Pers Soc Psychol, 51*, 1173–1182.

44. Outlaw, F. H. (1993). Stress and coping: The influence of racism on the cognitive appraisal processing of African Americans. *Issues Ment Health Nurs, 14*, 399–409.

45. Matheny, K. B., Aycock, D. W., Pugh, J. L., Curlette, W. L., & Cannella, K.A.S. (1986). Stress coping: A qualitative and quantitative synthesis with implications for treatment. *Couns Psychol, 14*, 499–549.

46. Adams, J. P., & Dressler, W. W. (1988). Perceptions of injustice in a black community: Dimensions and variations. *Human Relations, 41*, 753–767.

47. Udry, J. R., Bauman, K. E., & Chase, C. (1971). Skin color, status, and mate selection. *Am J Sociol, 76*, 722–733.

48. Anderson, N. B., Lane, J. D., Taguchi, F., & Williams, R. B., Jr. (1989). Patterns of cardiovascular responses to stress as a function of race and parental hypertension in men. *Health Psychol, 8*, 525–540.

49. Hohn, A. R., Riopel, D. A., Keil, J. E., Loadholt, C. B., Margolius, H. S., Halushka, P. V., Privitera, P. J., Webb, J. G., Medley, E. S., Schuman, S. H., Rubin, M. I., Pantell, R. H., & Braunstein, M. L. (1983). Childhood familial and racial differences in physiologic and biochemical factors related to hypertension. *Hypertension, 5*, 56–70.

50. Korol, B., Bergfeld, G. R., & McLaughlin, L. J. (1975). Skin color and autonomic nervous system measures. *Physiol Behav, 14*, 575–578.

51. Lawler, K. A., & Allen, M. T. (1981). Risk factors for hypertension in children: Their relationship to psychophysiological responses. *J Psychosom Res, 23*, 199–204.

52. Anderson, N. B., & Armstead, C. A. (1995). Toward understanding the association of socioeconomic status and health: A new challenge for the biopsychosocial approach. *Psychosom Med, 57,* 213–225.

53. Ernst, F. A., Jackson, I., Robertson, R. M., Nevels, H., & Watts, E. (1997). Skin tone, hostility, and blood pressure in young normotensive African Americans. *Ethn Dis, 7,* 34–40.

54. Harburg, E., Gleiberman, L., Russell, M., & Cooper, M. L. (1991). Anger-coping styles and blood pressure in black and white males: Buffalo, New York. *Psychosom Med, 53,* 153–164.

55. Harburg, E., Gleiberman, L., Roeper, P., Schork, M. A., & Schull, W. J. (1978). Skin color, ethnicity, and blood pressure in Detroit blacks. *Am J Public Health, 68,* 1177–1183.

56. Forman, T. A., Williams, D. R., & Jackson, J. S. (1997). Race, place, and discrimination. *Perspect Soc Problems, 9,* 231–261.

57. Williams, D. R., & Collins, C. (1995). Socioeconomic and racial differences in health. *Annu Rev Sociol, 21,* 349–386.

58. Pappas, G., Queen, S., Hadden, W., & Fisher, G. (1993). The increasing disparity and mortality between socioeconomic groups in the United States, 1960 and 1986. *N Engl J Med, 329,* 103–109.

59. Krieger, N. (1990). Racial and gender discrimination: Risk factors for high blood pressure? *Soc Sci Med, 12,* 1273–1281.

60. Pearlin, L. I. (1989). The sociological study of stress. *J Health Soc Behav, 30,* 241–256.

61. Clark, V. R., & Harrell, J. P. (1982). The relationship among Type A behavior, styles used in coping with racism, and blood pressure. *J Black Psychol, 8,* 89–99.

62. Wiebe, D. J., & Williams, P. G. (1992). Hardiness and health: A social psychophysiological perspective on stress and adaptation. *J Soc Clin Psychol, 11,* 238–262.

63. American Psychiatric Association. (1994). *Diagnostic and statistical manual of mental disorders* (4th ed.). Washington, DC: Author.

64. Bandura, A., Taylor, C. B., & Williams, S. L. (1985). Catecholamine secretion as a function of perceived coping self-efficacy. *J Consult Clin Psychol, 53,* 406–414.

65. Everson, S. A., Goldberg, D. E., Kaplan, G. A., Julkunen, J., & Solonen, J. T. (1998). Anger expression and incident hypertension. *Psychosom Med, 60,* 730–735.

66. Larkin, K. T., Semenchuk, E. M., Frazer, N. L., Suchday, S., & Taylor, R. L. (1998). Cardiovascular and behavioral response to social confrontation: Measuring real-life stress in the laboratory. *Ann Behav Med, 20,* 294–301.

67. Miller, G. E., Dopp, J. M., Myers, H. F., Stevens, S. Y., & Fahey, J. L. (1999). Psychosocial predictors of natural killer cell mobilization during marital conflict. *Health Psychol, 18,* 262–271.

68. Bullock, S. C., & Houston, E. (1987). Perceptions of racism by black medical students attending white medical schools. *J Natl Med Assoc, 79,* 601–608.

69. Armstead, C. A., Lawler, K. A., Gorden, G., Cross, J., & Gibbons, J. (1989). Relationship of racial stressors to blood pressure responses and anger expression in black college students. *Health Psychol, 8,* 541–556.

70. Johnson, E. H., & Browman, C. L. (1987). The relationship of anger expression to health problems among black Americans in a national survey. *J Behav Med, 10,* 103–116.

71. McConahay, J. B., & Hough, J. C. (1976). Symbolic racism. *Journal of Social Issues, 32,* 23–45.

72. Allan-Claiborne, J. G., & Taylor, J. (1981). The racialistic incidents inventory: Measuring awareness of racialism. In O. A. Barbarin, P. R. Good, O. M. Pharr, & J. A. Siskind (Eds.), *Institutional racism and community competence* (pp. 172–178). Rockville, MD: U.S. Department of Health and Human Services.

73. Barbarin, O. A. (1996). The IRS: Multidimensional measurement of institutional racism. In R. L. Jones (Ed.), *Handbook of tests and measurements for black populations* (Vol. 2, pp. 375–398). Hampton, VA: Cobb and Henry.

74. Harrell, S. P. (1997). *The Racism and Life Experiences Scales (RaLES).* Unpublished manuscript, California School of Professional Psychology, Los Angeles.

75. McNeilly, M. D., Anderson, N. B., Armstead, C. A., Clark, R., Corbett, M. O., Robinson, E. L., Pieper, C. F., & Lipisto, M. (1996). The Perceived Racism Scale: A multidimensional assessment of the perception of white racism among African Americans. *Ethn Dis, 6,* 154–166.

76. Thompson, C. E., Neville, H., Weathers, P. L., Poston, W. C., & Atkinson, D. R. (1990). Cultural mistrust and racism reaction among African-American students. *J College Student Develop, 31,* 162–168.

77. Utsey, S. O., & Ponterotto, J. G. (1996). Development and validation of the Index of Race-Related Stress (IRRS). *J Couns Psychol, 43,* 490–501.

78. Burchfield, S. R. (1985). Stress: An integrative framework. In S. R. Burchfield (Ed.), *Stress: Psychological and physiological interactions* (pp. 381–394). New York: Hemisphere.

79. Selye, H. (1976). *The stress of life.* New York: McGraw-Hill.

80. Jorgensen, R. S., Gelling, P. D., & Kliner, L. (1992). Patterns of social desirability and anger in young men with a parental history of hypertension: Association with cardiovascular activity. *Health Psychol, 11,* 403–412.

81. Ruggiero, K. M., & Taylor, D. M. (1997). Why minority group members perceive or do not perceive the discrimination that confronts them: The role of self-esteem and perceived control. *J Pers Soc Psychol, 72,* 373–389.

82. Sommers-Flanagan, J., & Greenberg, R. P. (1989). Psychosocial variables and hypertension: A new look at an old controversy. *J Nerv Ment Dis, 177,* 15–24.

83. Sutherland, M. E., & Harrell, J. P. (1986–1987). Individual differences in physiological responses to fearful, racially noxious, and neutral imagery. *Imagination, Cognition and Personality, 6,* 133–150.

84. Myers, L. J., Stokes, D. R., & Speight, S. L. (1989). Physiological responses to anxiety and stress: Reactions to oppression, galvanic skin potential, and heart rate. *J Black Studies, 20,* 80–96.

85. James, S. A., Hartnett, S. A., & Kalsbeek, W. D. (1983). John Henryism and blood pressure differences among black men. *J Behav Med, 6,* 259–278.

86. McNeilly, M., Anderson, N. B., Robinson, E. F., McManus, C. F., Armstead, C. A., Clark, R., Pieper, C. F., Simons, C., & Saulter, T. D. (1996). The convergent, discriminant, and concurrent criterion validity of the perceived racism scale: A multidimensional assessment of white racism among African Americans. In R. L. Jones (Ed.), *Handbook of tests and measurements for black populations* (Vol. 2, pp. 359–374). Hampton, VA: Cobb and Henry.

87. James, S. A., Strogatz, D. S., Wing, S. B., & Ramsey, D. L. (1987). Socioeconomic status, John Henryism, and hypertension in blacks and whites. *Am J Epidemiol, 126,* 664–673.

88. Manuck, S., Kasprowicz, A., & Muldoon, M. (1990). Behaviorally-evoked cardiovascular reactivity and hypertension: Conceptual issues and potential associations. *Ann Behav Med, 12,* 17–29.

89. Cornell, D. G., Peterson, C. S., & Richards, H. (1999). Anger as a predictor of aggression among incarcerated adolescents. *J Consult Clin Psychol, 67,* 108–115.

90. Grier, W. H., & Cobbs, P. M. (1968). *Black rage.* New York: Basic Books.

91. Harris, M. B. (1992). Beliefs about how to reduce anger. *Psychol Rep, 70,* 203–210.

92. Novaco, R. W. (1985). Anger and its therapeutic regulation. In M. A. Chesney & R. Rosenman (Eds.), *Anger and hostility in cardiovascular and behavioral disorders* (pp. 203–226). New York: Hemisphere/McGraw-Hill.

93. Anderson, L. P. (1991). Acculturative stress: A theory of relevance to black Americans. *Clin Psychol Rev, 11,* 685–702.

94. Fernando, S. (1984). Racism as a cause of depression. *Int J Soc Psychiatry, 30,* 41–49.

95. Peterson, C., Maier, S. F., & Seligman, M.E.P. (1993). *Learned helplessness: A theory for the age of personal control.* New York: Oxford University Press.

96. Seligman, M.E.P. (1975). *Helplessness: On depression, development, and death.* San Francisco: W. H. Freeman.

97. Cacioppo, J. (1994). Social neuroscience: Autonomic, neuroendocrine, and immune responses to stress. *Psychophysiology, 31,* 113–128.

98. Cohen, S., & Herbert, T. B. (1996). Health psychology: Psychological factors and physical disease from the perspective of human psychoneuroimmunology. *Annu Rev Psychol, 47,* 113–142.

99. Herbert, T. B., & Cohen, S. (1993). Stress and immunity in humans: A meta-analytic review. *Psychosom Med, 55,* 364–379.

100. Stone, A. A., Valdimarsdottir, H. B., Katkin, E. S., Burns, J., & Cox, D. S. (1993). Effects of mental stressors on mitogen-induced lymphocyte responses in the laboratory. *Psychol Health, 8,* 269–284.

101. Kiecolt-Glaser, J. K., Dura, J. R., Speicher, C. E., Trask, O. J., & Glaser, R. (1991). Spousal caregivers of dementia victims: Longitudinal changes in immunity and health. *Psychosom Med, 53,* 345–362.

102. Wu, H., Wang, J., Cacioppo, J. T., Glaser, R., Kiecolt-Glaser, J. K., & Malarkey, W. B. (1999). Chronic stress associated with spousal caregiving of patients with Alzheimer's dementia is associated with down regulation of B-lymphocyte GH mRNA. *J Gerontol: Series A, Biological Sciences and Medical Sciences, 54,* 212–215.

103. Kiecolt-Glaser, J. K., Malarkey, W. B., Chee, M., Newton, T., Cacioppo, J. T., Mao, H., & Glaser, R. (1993). Negative behavior during marital conflict is associated with immunological down-regulation. *Psychosom Med, 55,* 395–409.

104. Kiecolt-Glaser, J. K., Marucha, P. T., Malarkey, W. B., Mercado, A. M., & Glaser, R. (1995, November 4). Slowing of wound healing by psychological stress. *Lancet, 346,* 1194–1196.

105. Cohen, S., Frank, E., Doyle, W. J., Skoner, D. P., Rabin, B. S., & Gwaltney, J. M., Jr. (1998). Types of stressors that increase susceptibility to the common cold in healthy adults. *Health Psychol, 17,* 214–223.

106. Cohen, S., Tyrrell, D.A.J., & Smith, A. P. (1991). Psychological stress and susceptibility to the common cold. *N Engl J Med, 325,* 606–612.

107. Kiecolt-Glaser, J. K., & Glaser, R. (1995). Psychoneuroimmunology and health consequences: Data and shared mechanisms. *Psychosom Med, 57,* 269–274.

108. Anisman, H., Kokkinidis, L., & Sklar, L. S. (1985). Neurochemical consequences of stress: Contributions of adaptive processes. In S. R. Burchfield (Ed.), *Stress: Psychological and physiological interactions* (pp. 67–98). New York: Hemisphere.

109. McCance, K. L. (1990). Stress and disease. In K. L. McCance & S. E. Huether (Eds.), *Pathophysiology: The biologic basis for disease in adults and children* (pp. 279–293). St. Louis, MO: Mosby.

110. Brandenberger, G., Follenius, M., Wittersheim, G., & Salame, P. (1980). Plasma catecholamines and pituitary adrenal hormones related to mental task demand under quiet and noise conditions. *Biol Psychol, 10,* 239–252.

111. Cohen, F., & Lazarus, R. S. (1979). Coping with the stresses of illness. In G. S. Stone, F. Cohen, & N. E. Adler (Eds.), *Health psychology: A handbook* (pp. 77–112). San Francisco: Jossey-Bass.

112. Light, K. C., & Obrist, P. A. (1980). Cardiovascular response to stress: Effects of opportunity to avoid shock, shock experience, and performance feedback. *Psychophysiology, 17,* 243–252.

113. Ursin, H., Baade, E., & Levine, S. (Eds.). (1978). *Psychobiology of stress: A study of coping men.* New York: Academic Press.

114. Rumbaut, R. G. (1994). The crucible within: Ethnic identity, self-esteem, and segmented assimilation among children of immigrants. *Int Migration Rev, 28,* 748–794.

115. Taylor, D. M., Wright, S. C., & Ruggiero, K. (1991). The personal/group discrimination discrepancy: Responses to experimentally induced personal and group discrimination. *J Soc Psychol, 131,* 847–858.

116. Kendler, K. S., Kessler, R. C., Walters, E. E., MacLean, C., Neale, M. C., Heath, A. C., & Eaves, L. J. (1995). Stressful life events, genetic liability, and onset of an episode of major depression in women. *Am J Psychiatry, 152,* 833–842.

117. Spiegel, D., Bloom, H. C., Kraemer, J. R., & Gottheil, E. (1989, October 14). Effect of psychosocial treatment on survival of patients with metastatic cancer. *Lancet, 2,* 888–901.

118. Jiang, W., Babyak, M., Krantz, D. S., Waugh, R. A., Coleman, R. E., Hanson, M. M., Frid, D. J., McNulty, S., Morris, J. J., O'Connor, C. M., & Blumenthal, J. A. (1996). Mental stress-induced myocardial ischemia and cardiac events. *JAMA, 275,* 1651–1656.

119. Kamarck, T., & Jennings, J. R. (1991). Biobehavioral factors in sudden cardiac death. *Psychol Bull, 109,* 42–75.

120. Rozanski, A., Blumenthal, J. A., & Kaplan, J. (1999). Impact of psychological factors on the pathogenesis of cardiovascular disease and implications for therapy. *Circulation, 99,* 2192–2217.

121. Clark, R., & Armstead, C. A. (in press). Family conflict predicts blood pressure changes in African American adolescents. *J Adolesc.*

122. Narsavage, G. L., & Weaver, T. E. (1994). Physiologic status, coping, and hardiness as predictors of outcomes in chronic obstructive pulmonary disease. *Nurs Res, 43,* 90–94.

123. Jackson, J. S., Brown, T. N., Williams, D. R., Torres, M., Sellers, S. L., & Brown, K. (1996). Racism and the physical and mental health status of African Americans: A thirteen-year national panel study. *Ethn Dis, 6,* 132–147.

124. Williams, D. R., Yu, Y., & Jackson, J. (1997, July). *The costs of racism: Discrimination, race, and health.* Paper presented at the joint meeting of the Public Health Conference on Records and Statistics and Data User's Conference, Washington, DC.

125. Schulman, K. A., Berlin, J. A., Harless, W., Kerner, J. F., Sistrunk, S., Gersh, B. J., Dube, R., Taleghani, C. K., Burke, J. E., Williams, S., Eisenberg, J. M., & Escarce, J. J. (1999). The effects of race and sex on physicians' recommendations for cardiac catheterization. *N Engl J Med, 340,* 618–626.

126. Serafica, F. C., Schwebel, A. I., Russell, R. K., Isaac, P. D., & Myers, L. B. (Eds.). (1990). *Mental health of ethnic minorities.* New York: Praeger.

CHAPTER NINETEEN

Is Skin Color a Marker for Racial Discrimination?

Explaining the Skin Color–Hypertension Relationship

Elizabeth A. Klonoff
Hope Landrine

Numerous studies have revealed that dark-skinned blacks have significantly higher rates of hypertension than their lighter-skinned cohorts and have noted that the high rates for dark-skinned blacks may account for racial differences in hypertension prevalence.[1-9] Although this relationship between skin color and hypertension among blacks is clear, the meaning of it is not. Two major explanations for it have been advanced. The *genetic explanation* argues that hypertension is in part linked to genetic blackness; dark-skinned blacks have higher rates of hypertension because they are more genetically black than their lighter-skinned counterparts (who have greater "genetic admixture"; genetic whiteness). Alternatively, the *social explanation* argues that hypertension is in part linked to stress: dark-skinned blacks have higher rates of hypertension because they experience higher levels of (stressful) racial discrimination than their lighter-skinned cohorts (for a discussion see Krieger, Sidney, and Coakley[10]). These two explanations have been widely accepted despite the absence of empirical evidence for them: those who interpret the skin color–hypertension relationship as a function of genetic admixture have never assessed genetic differences (but instead have assumed skin color to be a proxy for those). Likewise, those who interpret the skin color–hypertension relationship as a function of racial

This work was supported by funds provided by University of California Tobacco-Related Disease Research Program Grant 8RT-0013 and by California Department of Health Services Tobacco Control Section Grant 94-20962.

discrimination have not assessed discrimination (but instead have assumed skin color to be a marker for it).[10] Both arguments are clearly circular.

Hence, to understand the skin color–hypertension relationship, the assumption that skin color is a marker for racial admixture must be tested empirically, and the assumption that skin color is a proxy for racial discrimination similarly must be tested empirically. To date, only one study has directly tested the assumption that skin color among blacks is related to differential exposure to racial discrimination. Using a brief measure of exposure (ever) to racial discrimination in seven situations, Krieger and her colleagues[10] found that skin color *was not* associated with self-reported discrimination in five of the seven situations and was only weakly associated with discrimination in the remaining two situations (that is, discrimination by the police/courts and discrimination at school). Strong associations between skin color and gender were found, in which black women had significantly lighter skin than black men, as measured with a Photovolt 577 reflectance meter.

Unfortunately, Krieger et al.[10] measured the extent to which blacks have *ever* experienced discrimination. However, racial discrimination is so common that 80 to 95 percent of blacks in health studies report experiencing discrimination of some type,[8–10] leaving little variance to be associated with skin color. Thus, to test the widely held assumption that skin color is associated with differential exposure to racial discrimination, a comprehensive, reliable, valid measure of the frequency of discrimination (as opposed to discrimination ever) is needed.[10] This study used such a measure to assess the skin color–discrimination relationship.

METHOD

Subjects

Three hundred black adults (195 women, 105 men) participated. Their ages ranged from 15 to 79 years (mean = 38.72 years, σ = \$21,422). Their education levels were as follows: 15.5 percent were high school dropouts, 22.2 percent were high school graduates, 38.7 percent had taken some college courses, and 21.5 percent had college degrees.

Procedure

Black health educators asked blacks in public settings (for example, beauty parlors, community centers) in south-central Los Angeles to complete a survey.

Materials

The anonymous survey contained the Schedule of Racist Events,[11,12] demographic questions, a question on skin color, and Krieger's racism scale;[8] the latter was included to establish further the validity of the Schedule of Racist

Events and was not entered into any analyses, given the lack of a relationship between scores on that scale and skin color.[10]

The Schedule of Racist Events (SRE) measures the frequency of a variety of types of racial discrimination (for example, in salaries, by store clerks) in blacks' lives (Table 19.1). Types of racial discrimination are conceptualized as culturally specific, stressful events (that is, racist events) that are analogous to the generic (can happen to anyone) stressful life events (for example, getting fired) that are measured by popular stress inventories such as the PERI-LES.[13] The SRE also measures people's appraisals of the stressfulness of the racist events, in a manner similar to the Perceived Stress Scale[14,15] and the Hassles Scale.[16] The logic behind the appraisal (versus the events) approach to measuring stress is that two people may experience the same stressful event (getting fired, being

Table 19.1. Sample Items from the Schedule of Racist Events

Circle **1** = if the event has NEVER happened to you
Circle **2** = if the event happened ONCE IN A WHILE (less than 10% of the time)
Circle **3** = if the event happened SOMETIMES (10–25% of the time)
Circle **4** = if the event happened A LOT (26–49% of the time)
Circle **5** = if the event happened MOST OF THE TIME (50–70% of the time)
Circle **6** = if the event happened ALMOST ALL OF THE TIME (more than 70% of the time)

1. How many times have you been treated unfairly by *teachers and professors* because you are Black?

   How many times IN YOUR ENTIRE LIFE?   1   2   3   4   5   6
   How many times IN THE PAST YEAR?   1   2   3   4   5   6

                                        Not at all stressful   Very stressful
   How stressful was this for you?   1   2   3   4   5   6

2. How many times have you been treated unfairly by *your employers, bosses, and supervisors* because you are Black?

4. How many times have you been treated unfairly by *people in service jobs* (by store clerks, waiters, bartenders, bank tellers, and others) because you are Black?

10. How many times have you been *accused or suspected of doing something wrong* (such as stealing, cheating, not doing your share of the work, or breaking the law) because you are Black?

17. How many times have you been *made fun of, picked on, pushed, shoved, hit, or threatened with harm* because you are Black?

15. How many times have you been *called a racist name* like nigger, coon, jungle bunny, or other names?

16. How many times have you *gotten into an argument or a fight about something racist that was done to you or done to somebody else?*

called a nigger) with equal frequency, but one may find it very stressful while the other dismisses it. Theoretically, the event should have a greater negative impact on the individual who appraised it as stressful.[14] Hence some stress researchers take the frequency-of-events and others the appraisal-of-events approach to measuring stress. The SRE uses both: it is an eighteen-item scale on which blacks estimate the frequency with which they have experienced specific racist events and then give their appraisals of those experiences. Each item is answered on a scale that ranges from 1 (the event never happened to me) to 6 (the event happens almost all of the time). Items are completed once for the frequency of the racist events in the past year, again for the frequency of the events in one's entire lifetime, and again for the appraisal of the stressfulness of each event, as shown by the examples in Table 19.1. These are treated as the subscales Recent Racist Events (range, 18–108), Lifetime Racist Events (range, 18–108), and Appraisal Racist Events (range, 17–102).

As shown in Table 19.2, the SRE has an exceptionally high reliability. The SRE also has strong validity as a measure of stressful events and as a measure

Table 19.2. Reliability of the Schedule of Racist Events

Racist Events	No. of Items	Mean	σ	Internal Consistency Reliability, Cronbach's α	Split-Half Reliability, r	1-Month Test-Retest Reliability, r
		Reliability for the standardization sample*				
Recent	18	40.99	19.82	.949	.928	.956
Lifetime	18	53.93	21.99	.953	.907	.946
Appraisal	17	51.47	21.61	.936	.919	.963
		Reliability for the cross-validation sample†				
						SE
Recent	18	38.75	17.18	.947	.839	0.753
Lifetime	18	45.86	18.41	.940	.827	0.808
Appraisal	17	44.23	20.34	.943	.822	0.892
		Reliability for the current sample				
Recent	18	53.04	11.71	.956	.938	1.34
Lifetime	18	63.78	13.09	.966	.947	1.52
Appraisal	17	65.53	25.39	.966	.933	1.52

*Adapted from Landrine, H., & Klonoff, E. A. (1996). The Schedule of Racist Events: A measure of racial discrimination and a study of its negative physical and mental health consequences. *J Black Psychol, 22*(2), 144–168.

†Adapted from Klonoff, E. A., & Landrine, H. (1999). Cross-validation of the Schedule of Racist Events. *J Black Psychol, 25,* 231–254.

of racism: the SRE has stronger relationships with the PERI-LES and the Hassles (stress scales) than those scales do with each other (Table 19.3, top) and has strong relationships to Krieger's brief measure of racism as well[8] (Table 19.3, bottom). All items in each SRE subscale load on a single factor.[12] The construct validity of the SRE was established through structural equation modeling.[17]

To assess skin color, blacks rated their skin as follows: 1 = very light-skinned, 2 = light-skinned, 3 = medium-skinned, 4 = dark-skinned, 5 = very dark-skinned. Those rating themselves 1 or 2 were categorized as light, those rating themselves 3 were categorized as medium, and those who rated themselves 4 or 5 were categorized as dark.

Table 19.3. Validity of the Schedule of Racist Events

Convergent Validity as a Means of Stress (Standardization Sample)*			
	Hassles Frequency	PERI-LES	Hassles Intensity (Appraisal)
PERI-LES	.19 n.s.		
Hassles intensity	−.28 n.s.	.16 n.s.	
SRE Recent	.54 (.0005)	.27 (.001)	.22 n.s.
SRE Lifetime	.54 (.0005)	.32 (.0005)	.31 (.05)
SRE Appraisal	.37 (.016)	.24 (.005)	.46 (.003)

Convergent Validity as a Measure of Racism (Current Sample)†			
Krieger (1990) Discrimination Items: "Have you ever been treated unfairly because of your race?" (yes = 1, no = 0)	Recent Racist Events	Lifetime Racist Events	Appraised Racist Events
At school	.36	.39	.35
Getting a job	.35	.46	.40
At work	.38	.48	.49
Getting housing	.45	.55	.49
In medical care	.44	.45	.45
By the police	.42	.45	.38
Total score on Krieger items	.64	.71	.67

*n.s. = not significant. The data on the standardization sample have not been reported elsewhere.

†All correlations are point biserial except that for total score, which is a normal, bivariate correlation. All r's in the bottom of the table are significant at .005.

RESULTS

Analysis of Skin Color Groups

To assess the relationship between skin color and experiencing racial discrimination, a MANOVA was conducted using the three skin color groups (light, medium, dark) as the grouping factor and the three SRE subscales and income as the dependent variables. The MANOVA was significant (Wilks's $\lambda = .799$; $F[8,352] = 5.209$; $p = .00005$); follow-up ANOVAs, post hoc comparisons, and chi-square analyses are listed in Table 19.4. As shown in Table 19.4 (top), dark-skinned blacks reported significantly more frequent racial discrimination in the past year (recent racism) and in the course of their lifetimes (lifetime racism) and also found that racism to be more subjectively stressful (appraised racism) than did other blacks. Skin color was also associated with income, gender, and education (Table 19.4, bottom). Light-skinned blacks tended to be women and were more likely than dark-skinned blacks to be college educated and less likely to be high school dropouts.

Analysis of Racial Discrimination Groups

An alternative way to assess the relationship between skin color and discrimination is to group subjects into high versus low racial discrimination groups and

Table 19.4. Analysis of Skin Color Groups

Dependent Variable	Group 1 Light (n = 56)	Group 2 Medium (n = 106)	Group 3 Dark (n = 132)	$F^{\dagger}$	Tukey HSD
Recent racism	41.59	43.69	56.25	10.09**	$1 = 2 < 3$
Lifetime racism	50.85	55.18	72.50	16.13**	$1 = 2 < 3$
Appraised racism	55.25	54.18	72.99	13.20**	$1 = 2 < 3$
Income	$22,443	$32,923	$30,841	3.20*	$1 < 2$
Gender					
Men	14.8%	32.0%	39.1%	$\chi^2_{(df\,2)} = 10.28, p = .006$	
Women	85.2%	68.0%	60.9%		
Education					
<H.S.	9.8%	8.9%	22.4%	$\chi^2_{(df\,6)} = 16.39, p = .012$	
H.S. grad	21.6%	17.8%	24.8%		
Some college	41.2%	44.6%	39.2%		
≥College grad	27.5%	28.7%	13.6%		

$^{\dagger}df = 2,182$ for each F.

$*p = .043$; $**p = .0005$.

then examine the association of these groups with skin color. Cluster analysis of cases (CAC) was used to define discrimination groups empirically. In CAC, the program, rather than the researcher, creates groups that differ on the dependent variables, thereby avoiding groups defined by arbitrary cut-points that are prone to experimenter bias. The program was instructed to create two groups that differ maximally on the three SRE scales. K-means cluster analysis with centroid sorting was used because of the relatively large number of cases; cluster centers were iteratively estimated from the data.[18] As shown in Table 19.5 (top), the ensuing low and high discrimination clusters differed significantly on all SRE scales, with the high-discrimination cluster scoring twice as high on each scale. Chi-square analyses, t tests (Table 19.5, bottom), and logistic regression (Table 19.6) were then used to examine relationships.

As shown in Table 19.5 (bottom), high racial discrimination subjects were significantly older than low discrimination subjects, no doubt because lifetime racism scores increase with age (length of lifetime). The high and low racial discrimination groups did not differ in their incomes but did differ in education,

Table 19.5. Analysis of Racial Discrimination Groups

Dependent Variable	Cluster 1: Low Discrimination Group ($n = 147$)	Cluster 2: High Discrimination Group ($n = 110$)	Cluster Analysis ANOVA F*
SRE Recent	36.60	69.55	318.54
SRE Lifetime	45.35	87.36	606.69
SRE Appraisal	44.71	86.01	451.84
Age	36.26 ($\sigma = 13.7$)	40.75 ($\sigma = 14.1$)	$t_{(df\,233)} = -2.45$, $p = .02$
Income	$30,212 ($\sigma = 22,234$)	$29,593 ($\sigma = 20,122$)	$t_{(df\,182)} = 0.193$, $p = .85$ (ns)
Education			
H.S. dropout	10.9%	21.5%	$\chi^2_{(df\,3)} = 12.59$,
H.S. grad	15.9%	27.1%	$p = .006$
Some college	48.6%	32.7%	
≥College grad	24.6%	18.7%	
Skin color			
Light	26.9%	8.5%	$\chi^2_{(df\,2)} = 38.37$,
Medium	44.8%	24.5%	$p = .0005$
Dark	28.3%	67.0%	
Gender			
Women	74.5%	57.0%	$\chi^2_{(df\,1)} = 8.51$,
Men	25.5%	43.0%	$p = .004$

*$df = 1,255$ and $p < .0005$ for each F.

Table 19.6. Stepwise Logistic Regression Predicting Membership in the High Discrimination Cluster from Income, Age, Gender, Education, and Skin Color

Variable Selected	β	SE	Coef./SE	OR	95% CI
Reference Group: Light-Skinned					
1. Skin color					
Medium	0.654	0.6243	1.048	1.92	0.566, 6.539
Dark	2.39	0.6057	3.948	10.93	3.334, 35.821
Reference Group: Women					
2. Gender					
Men	1.097	0.373	2.939	2.995	1.441, 6.226

gender, and skin color. The high discrimination group had significantly more high school dropouts and significantly fewer college graduates than the low racial discrimination group. The high discrimination group also had significantly fewer light-skinned blacks and significantly more dark-skinned blacks than the low discrimination group: 67 percent of high discrimination subjects were dark-skinned and only 8.5 percent were light-skinned. The low discrimination group also was predominantly women (74.5 percent). As shown in Table 19.6, a stepwise logistic regression predicted membership in the high discrimination group from these variables: income, age, education group, gender, and skin color group (light, medium, dark). Only skin color and gender predicted membership in the high discrimination group. Dark-skinned blacks were 10.9 times more likely than light-skinned blacks to be in the high discrimination group, and men were 3 times more likely than women to be in that group.

DISCUSSION

When divided into skin color groups, analyses revealed that dark-skinned blacks reported significantly more frequent and more stressful experiences with racial discrimination than the lighter-skinned cohorts. Similarly, when clustered into groups that differ maximally in discrimination, analyses revealed that 67 percent of subjects who experience frequent discrimination were dark-skinned and only 8.5 percent were light-skinned. Dark-skinned blacks were eleven times more likely to be in the high discrimination group than were their light-skinned counterparts. Likewise, gender was the only status variable consistently associated with skin color and discrimination in all analyses: 74.5 percent of light-skinned blacks were women and hence women tended to be in the low discrimination group.

These results suggest that there is a strong relationship between skin color and exposure to racial discrimination among blacks and that this relationship may be strong enough for skin color to indeed be treated as a marker for racial discrimination. However, this study is limited by the use of self-reported (instead of measured) skin color. Nonetheless, a strong relationship between gender and skin color was found here despite using self-reported skin color, and it matches Krieger et al.'s finding using measured skin color;[10] this implies that these self-reports of skin color, albeit inferior to direct measurement, nonetheless may be a valid procedure for assessing skin color among blacks. The gender–skin color relationship found here and in the Krieger et al. study[10] is consistent with evidence that black women have greater concerns about skin color than black men and (unlike black men) use skin-bleaching creams;[19] hence, black women self-reported lighter skin than did black men in this study and, when their skin was measured by Krieger et al.,[10] they did indeed have lighter skin than black men.

In addition to being limited by the use of self-reported skin color, this study is limited by its modest, nonrandom sample, and hence the findings must be regarded as preliminary. However preliminary they may be, these findings nonetheless provide the first empirical evidence for the view that skin color among blacks is a marker for racial discrimination, and so provide the first tentative empirical support for the social explanation of the skin color–hypertension relationship. Clearly, studies with large samples are now needed in which skin color, hypertension, and discrimination are all measured; then the hypothesis that discrimination is the moderator variable explaining the skin color–hypertension relationship can finally be empirically tested. Such studies would benefit from using the SRE as the measure of racial discrimination, because it is comprehensible enough to be sensitive to differences among blacks by skin color and has clear psychometric integrity.

Notes

1. Coresh, J., Klag, M. J., Whelton, P. K., & Kuller, L. H. (1991). Left ventricular hypertrophy and skin color among American blacks. *Am J Epidemiol, 134,* 129–136.

2. Gleiberman, L., Harburg, E., Frone, M. R., Russel, M., & Cooper, M. L. (1995). Skin color, measures of socioeconomic status, and blood pressure among blacks in Erie County, New York. *Ann Hum Biol, 22,* 69–73.

3. Harburg, E., Erfrut, J. C., Hauenstein, L. S., Chape, C., Schull, W. J., & Schork, M. A. (1973). Socioecological stress, suppressed hostility, skin color, and black-white male blood pressure. *Psychosom Med, 35,* 276–295.

4. Harburg, E., Gleiberman, L., Roeper, P., Schork, M. A., & Schull, E. J. (1978). Skin color, ethnicity, and blood pressure. *Am J Public Health, 68,* 1177–1183.

5. Klag, M. J., Whelton, P. K., Coresh, J., Grim, C. E., & Kuller, L. H. (1991). The association of skin color with blood pressure in U.S. blacks with low socioeconomic status. *JAMA, 265,* 599–602.

6. Keil, J. E., Tyroler, H. A., Sandifer, S. H., & Boyle, E., Jr. (1977). Hypertension: Effects of social class and racial admixture: The results of a cohort study of the black population of Charleston, South Carolina. *Am J Public Health, 67,* 634–639.

7. Keil, J. E., Sandifer, S. H., Loadholt, C. B., & Boyle, E., Jr. (1981). Skin color and education effects on blood pressure. *Am J Public Health, 71,* 532–534.

8. Krieger, N. (1990). Racial and gender discrimination: Risk factors for high blood pressure? *Soc Sci Med, 30,* 1273–1281.

9. Krieger, N., & Sidney, S. (1996). Racial discrimination and blood pressure: The CARDIA study. *Am J Public Health, 86,* 1370–1378.

10. Krieger, N., Sidney, S., & Coakley, E. (1998). Racial discrimination and skin color in the CARDIA study: Implications for public health research. *Am J Public Health, 88,* 1308–1313.

11. Landrine, H., & Klonoff, E. A. (1996). The Schedule of Racist Events: A measure of racial discrimination and a study of its negative physical and mental health consequences. *J Black Psychol, 22*(2), 144–168.

12. Klonoff, E. A., & Landrine, H. (1999). Cross-validation of the Schedule of Racist Events. *J Black Psychol, 25,* 231–254.

13. Dohrenwend, B. S., Krasnoff, L., Askenasy, A., & Dohrenwend, B. P. (1978). Exemplification of a method for scaling life events. *J Health Soc Behav, 19,* 205–229.

14. Cohen, S. (1986). Contrasting the Hassles scale and the Perceived Stress Scale: Who's really measuring appraised stress? *Am Psychol, 41,* 716–718.

15. Cohen, S., Kamarck, T., & Mermelstein, R. (1983). A global measure of perceived stress. *J Health Soc Behav, 24,* 385–396.

16. Kanner, A. D., Coyne, J. C., Schaeffer, C., & Lazarus, R. S. (1981). Comparison of two modes of stress measurement. *J Behav Med, 4,* 1–39.

17. Klonoff, E. A., Landrine, H., & Ullman, J. B. (1999). Racial discrimination and psychiatric symptoms among blacks. *Cult Divers Ethnic Minor Psychol, 5*(4), 329–339.

18. Anderberg, M. R. (1973). *Cluster analysis for applications.* New York: Academic Press.

19. Russel, K., Wilson, M., & Hall, R. (1992). *The color complex: The politics of skin color among African Americans.* New York: Harcourt Brace Jovanovich.

CHAPTER TWENTY

John Henryism and the Health
of African Americans

Sherman A. James

In this presentation, I will discuss how "John Henryism"—a strong behavioral predisposition to cope actively with psychosocial environmental stressors—interacts with low socioeconomic status to influence the health of African Americans. Hypertension, a leading cause of disability and premature death among African Americans, will be the focal health problem, although much of what I will say has implications for understanding other "stress-related" health problems that affect African Americans disproportionately. Early on, I will describe the scientific and folkloric background of the John Henryism hypothesis, after which I will summarize the empirical data produced thus far by our group testing the validity of the hypothesis. In the concluding section, I will explore the deeper *cultural* meaning of John Henryism for African Americans (both men and women), arguing that the concept of John Henryism may have something important to tell us about the relationship between African Americans and selected core values of American culture. I shall begin with a word about the magnitude of the problem of hypertension in black Americans,

This chapter was originally presented as the Roger Allan Moore Lecture on Values and Medicine: Ethical, Religious and Cultural Perspectives, Harvard University School of Medicine, March 25, 1993. The empirical research on the relationship between John Henryism and blood pressure described in this paper was made possible by grants (IIL33211) to the author from the National Heart, Lung, and Blood Institute of the National Institutes of Health. The author thanks Jay Kaufman and Christine Wenner for their valuable assistance in preparing this manuscript.

then move quickly into a discussion of the circumstances that gave rise to the John Henryism hypothesis. (The terms "black American" and "African American" are used interchangeably in this discussion.)

HYPERTENSION IN BLACK AMERICANS: THE MAGNITUDE OF THE PROBLEM

Hypertension remains one of the most important health problems affecting African Americans, in both rural and urban settings. Depending on the clinical cut-points used to define the disorder, blacks in the United States are two to four times more likely than whites to develop hypertension by age fifty.[1] Largely because of their greater risk for hypertension, blacks are three to four times more likely than whites to suffer a stroke[2] and two to five times more likely to develop end-stage kidney disease.[3] The reasons for the excess risk and greater clinical severity of hypertension in African Americans are not known. Hypotheses abound, however, and in the main, focus on (unspecified) *genetic* factors presumed to be linked in some way to African ancestry, and on *environmental* factors such as diet, high levels of psychosocial stress, and poor access to medical care.[4]

While the relative contribution of genetic and environmental factors to the well-documented excess risk for hypertension in African Americans is still a matter of debate,[5] one fact is clear and universally accepted: socioeconomic status (whether measured by education, occupation, or income) and hypertension tend to be *inversely* associated, for both blacks and whites;[4] that is, as the education, income, or occupation of an individual *increases*, his or her overall risk for hypertension *decreases*.

Using education to indicate socioeconomic status, Figure 20.1 provides a good illustration of both the magnitude of the black-white differences in hypertension typically observed in (community-based) studies and the aforementioned inverse association between hypertension and socioeconomic status. The data are from the Hypertension Detection and Follow-Up Program (HDFP),[6] a large multicommunity study conducted in the United States in the 1970s to assess the effectiveness of "stepped-care" antihypertensive drug therapy in preventing heart attacks and strokes among women and men with established hypertension. Figure 20.1 shows the relationship between years of education completed (less than ten to college graduates) and the prevalence of hypertension (mean diastolic blood pressure ≥ 95 mmHg, or treated) among the 159,000 middle-aged blacks and whites who underwent eligibility screening in their homes. Approximately 45 percent of African Americans with less than ten years of formal schooling were hypertensive, compared to 22 percent of whites. This excess prevalence of hypertension among blacks varied between $1\frac{1}{2}$- to 2-fold

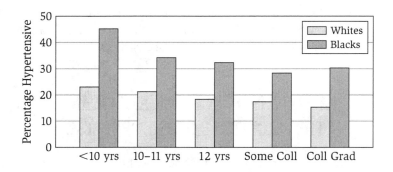

Figure 20.1 Prevalence of Hypertension by Level of Education, Whites, and Blacks: The HDFP Study, 1977.

Note: Hypertension defined as DBP ≥ 95 mmHg, or currently taking antihypertensive drugs.
HDFP = Hypertension Detection and Follow-up Program, First Screening.

Source: Reprinted with permission from the *American Journal of Epidemiology.*

for each of the remaining education categories. Equally apparent for both blacks and whites, however, was a stepwise decrease in the prevalence of hypertension with increasing levels of education. This pattern of a strong *differential* risk for hypertension by socioeconomic status and by race remained even after taking into account the age and body weight of study participants.[6]

While the nearly twofold excess risk for hypertension among African Americans across *all* educational categories is compatible with the hypothesis that hypertension in blacks has a genetic basis, these data are equally compatible with the hypothesis that unrelieved psychosocial stress—generated by environments in which African Americans live and work—is primarily responsible for their heightened susceptibility to this disorder. In addition, proponents of the psychosocial perspective[7] argue that a similar level of education for blacks and whites—whether at the high or low end of the scale—does not mean that the day-to-day psychosocial stressors (or the problem-solving resources to combat such stressors) are equal for the two groups. Thus, taken alone, education may be a seriously misleading indicator of the comparability of socioeconomic status for blacks and whites.

JOHN HENRYISM: THE SCIENTIFIC AND FOLKLORIC BACKGROUND

In the early and mid-1970s, several provocative papers were published which demonstrated that "high-effort" coping (that is, sustained cognitive and emotional engagement) with difficult psychosocial stressors produces substantial increases in heart rate and systolic blood pressure, increases which persist as long as individuals *actively* work at trying to eliminate the stressor. Some of these studies were controlled laboratory experiments[8] and some were field-based studies of "real-life" stressors.[9-11] In the laboratory, a prototypical stressor—one which rarely failed to induce large increases in heart rate and systolic blood pressure—was the threat of electric shock. To avoid receiving the shock, individuals (typically healthy male undergraduates) had to perform some specified behavior very quickly following the unpredictable appearance of a light. While the field-based studies were less well controlled than the laboratory studies, they were also less artificial. In one study,[9] for example, researchers monitored changes in the blood pressure of male, blue-collar factory workers whose plant was about to be closed permanently. Blood pressures of the men increased as the plant closing date approached, and remained elevated over baseline values until the men found new employment or, alternatively, gave up their *active* search for new jobs.

In another study, by Harburg et al.,[11] conducted in Detroit, the blood pressures of blacks and whites were measured to determine if individuals residing in "high-stress" neighborhoods—that is, neighborhoods characterized by high unemployment, high crime, high residential mobility, and so forth—had higher blood pressure on average than individuals residing in "low-stress" neighborhoods. No differences in mean blood pressure by residential area were observed for whites, but average blood pressures as well as the prevalence of hypertension were higher for blacks who resided in high-stress neighborhoods than they were for those in low-stress neighborhoods. Interestingly, these effects were greater for men than for women. Moreover, subsequent analyses revealed that these effects were limited to men under forty years of age. This latter finding led the investigators to speculate that the younger black men—in contrast to their older counterparts—may still have been trying to deal in a very *active* manner with the difficult psychosocial stressors they confronted daily. Such high-effort coping, the investigators reasoned, could be accompanied by sharp elevations in heart rate and blood pressure throughout each day, forming a pattern of sympathetic arousal which, over the course of years, could dysregulate basic blood pressure control mechanisms and lead to established hypertension.[11]

In a perceptive commentary on this body of research, Syme[12] observed that persons of lower socioeconomic status (especially blacks in these positions) by definition face more difficult psychosocial environmental stressors than more economically privileged individuals. He then advanced the intriguing hypothesis that *prolonged, high-effort coping* with difficult psychosocial stressors could be the most parsimonious explanation of both the inverse association between socioeconomic status and hypertension typically observed in U.S. communities and the increased risk for this disorder in black Americans.

It was my good fortune to come across this literature, and Syme's commentary,[12] shortly after I had met a fascinating, retired black farmer named *John Henry* Martin. His name could hardly have been more appropriate, since his life story[13] contained a number of features that evoked the legend of John Henry, the "steel-driving man." The legend is familiar to most Americans of a "certain" age; but in brief, John Henry, the steel-driving man, was known far and wide among late-nineteenth-century railroad and tunnel workers[14] for the remarkable physical strength and endurance he displayed in his work. It was at the mouth of the Big Bend tunnel in West Virginia, in the early 1870s, so the story goes,[14,15] that John Henry beat a mechanical steam drill in a famous steel-driving contest pitting "man against machine." The race was extremely close throughout, but, with a series of powerful blows from his 9 lb. hammer in the closing seconds of the race, John Henry emerged the victor. Moments after the contest ended, however, John Henry dropped dead from complete physical and mental exhaustion.

John Henry Martin, the retired black farmer, also won an epic battle against "the machine." In his case, however, the "machine" was the ruthlessly exploitative sharecropping system of the rural South. Martin was born into an extremely poor, sharecropping family in 1907, in the Upper Piedmont region of the state of North Carolina. As a child, he was not able to attend school beyond the second grade; but as an adult, he somehow taught himself to read and write. Even more impressively, however, through unrelenting hard work and determination (that is, *effortful active coping*), John Henry Martin—against tremendous odds—freed himself and his offspring from the debt bondage of the sharecropper system. Specifically, by the time he was forty years of age, he owned seventy-five acres of fertile North Carolina farmland. Like the legendary steel driver, however, John Henry Martin also paid a price for his victory. By his late fifties, he suffered from hypertension, arthritis, and a case of peptic ulcer disease so severe that 40 percent of his stomach had to be removed.[13]

The connection between the life story of John Henry Martin and the scientific literature (especially Syme's commentary) on how prolonged, high-effort coping with psychosocial stressors over many years might increase risk for hypertension was, for me, instantaneous. Not only was John Henry Martin's life an example par excellence of such coping, it was emblematic, I believed, of the larger protracted struggle of African American men and women (especially those in the working classes) to free themselves from pervasive and deeply entrenched systems of social and economic oppression. Intrigued by the connections that the scientific works by Obrist, Harburg, Syme and others had helped me to see, I resolved to pursue the "active coping–hypertension" hypothesis, with special emphasis on African Americans. Furthermore, in tribute to John Henry Martin, and the larger historical drama that I believe his life story represents, I decided to provide a context—cultural as well as historical—for the active coping hypothesis by referring to it in my own work as the "John Henryism hypothesis." Thus, "John Henryism" is a synonym for prolonged, high-effort coping with difficult psychosocial environmental stressors.

THE JOHN HENRYISM HYPOTHESIS

The John Henryism hypothesis assumes that lower socioeconomic status individuals in general, and African Americans in particular, are routinely exposed to psychosocial stressors (for example, chronic financial strain, job insecurity, and subtle or perhaps not so subtle social insults linked to race or social class) that require them to use considerable energy each day to manage the psychological stress generated by these conditions. However, the hypothesis also assumes that not all individuals so exposed will respond to these noxious conditions with high-effort coping. Some will, while others will not; or perhaps more accurately, some will respond with effortful active coping for a time, and then give up, while others—encouraged by their success—will persist. The John Henryism hypothesis predicts that it is the latter group—those lower socioeconomic status individuals who persist with effortful active coping *under difficult conditions* who drive up the overall prevalence of hypertension in lower socioeconomic groups. By this logic, if we were to categorize individuals into two broad groups—those strongly predisposed to cope actively with psychosocial stressors (that is, a "high" John Henryism group) and those less predisposed to do so (that is, a "low" John Henryism group)—we would expect to see the highest mean blood pressure level in those individuals who are simultaneously characterized by low socioeconomic status and high John Henryism. Figure 20.2 summarizes these expectations: among low socioeconomic status individuals

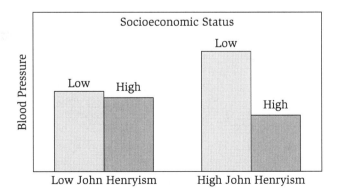

Figure 20.2 Theoretical Expectations.

with high levels of John Henryism, the strong sympathetic nervous system arousal induced by frequent high-effort coping is expected to result, over time, in the highest mean blood pressure levels of any group. For individuals categorized as low in John Henryism, and for whom strong sympathetic nervous system arousal is presumed to occur less frequently, mean blood pressure levels are expected to differ little by socioeconomic status. In formal terms, the John Henryism hypothesis is summarized as follows:

> **The inverse association between socioeconomic status and blood pressure will be much more pronounced (that is, more striking) for individuals who score high on John Henryism than for those who score low.**

THE MEASUREMENT OF JOHN HENRYISM

John Henryism is measured by a twelve-item scale called The John Henryism Scale for Active Coping, or the JHAC12.* Questions for the JHAC12 were developed by this author following a close reading of scholarly works on the legend of John Henry.[14-16] Three mutually reinforcing themes emerged as important to capture in any empirical measure of John Henryism: (1) efficacious mental and physical vigor, (2) a strong commitment to hard work, and (3) a single-minded determination to succeed. Each of the twelve questions, in varying degrees,[†] reflects these three themes. Here are three sample items from the JHAC12:

1. I've always felt that I could make of my life pretty much what I wanted to make of it.

2. Once I make up my mind to do something, I stay with it until the job is completely done.

3. When things don't go the way I want them to, that just makes me work even harder.

A "completely true" response to any question results in a score of 5 for that question; a "completely false" response results in a score of 1. Thus, for the scale as a whole, John Henryism scores can range from a low of 12 to a high of 60. For hypothesis testing, individuals are classified as "high" in John Henryism if they score above the sample median and "low" in John Henryism if they score at or below the median.

---

*Copies of the JHAC12 are available upon request from the author.

†Cronbach's alpha, a measure of internal consistency for unidimensional scales, varies between 0.70 and 0.80 for the JHAC12.

THE RESEARCH SETTING

To date, three independent, cross-sectional investigations of the John Henryism hypothesis have been conducted by our group.[17-19] Each study was conducted in North Carolina, specifically in the coastal plains region of that state, where death rates due to stroke and heart disease are among the highest in the country.[20] The first two studies[17,18] were conducted in Edgecombe County and the third[19] in Pitt County. Both communities are predominantly rural; however, Pitt County has experienced more rapid urbanization and economic diversification than Edgecombe County in recent decades. Because of the more diversified economy in Pitt County (where our work continues), we were able to include a reasonably large number of professional, middle-class blacks in our sample.

For simplicity, the following summary of research findings from these three studies presents data for diastolic blood pressure and/or the prevalence of hypertension only. The findings for systolic blood pressure were uniformly similar to those for diastolic pressure.

SUMMARY OF RESEARCH FINDINGS

The first study[17] was a pilot, designed in part to field test the original version of the John Henryism Scale. A random, household sample of 132 working-class black men, ages seventeen to sixty, were interviewed and their blood pressures measured. A 91 percent response rate was achieved. As in the HDFP study,[6] socioeconomic status in this pilot investigation was measured by years of formal education: men who had completed high school were assigned to the "high" socioeconomic status category, and those who had not to the "low" category.

Consistent with findings in most other published studies, non–high school graduates in the pilot study had higher ($p \leq .05$) adjusted diastolic blood pressures than high school graduates: 81.1 mmHg versus 77.1 mmHg (see Figure 20.3). However, in keeping with our theoretical expectations, when the men were divided into high and low John Henryism groups, the difference in mean blood pressure for high school graduates versus nongraduates in the low John Henryism group was very small—1.7 mmHg; whereas in the high John Henryism group the observed difference was considerably larger—6.3 mmHg (see Figure 20.4).

Our second study[18] provided an opportunity to test the John Henryism hypothesis for the first time in whites (n men = 195, and n women = 203) and in a larger sample of blacks that included both men ($n = 190$) and women ($n = 232$). Study participants were again selected at random (90 percent response rate) from households in the community. The sample of whites consisted largely of skilled blue-collar and lower midlevel white-collar workers,

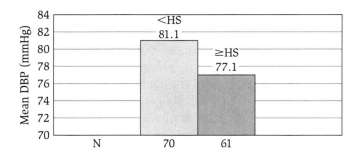

Figure 20.3 Mean Diastolic Blood Pressure (mmHg) by Level of Education: The Pilot Study, 1983.

Note: Mean DBP adjusted for age, body mass index (BMI), time of day, and smoking; $p = .05$ for the <HS versus ≥HS comparison of mean DBP.

Source: Reprinted with permission from the *Journal of Behavioral Medicine.*

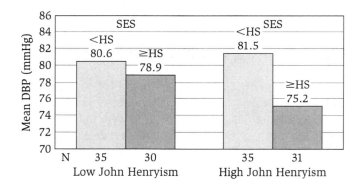

Figure 20.4 Mean Diastolic Blood Pressures (mmHg) for the Four Education–John Henryism Groups: The Pilot Study, 1983.

Note: Mean DBP adjusted for age, BMI, time of day, and smoking. Adjusted $p = .10$ for <HS versus ≥HS for the high John Henryism stratum.

Source: Reprinted with permission from the *Journal of Behavioral Medicine.*

while the sample of blacks consisted primarily of unskilled and semiskilled workers. To test the John Henryism hypothesis, participants were restricted to persons between twenty-one and fifty years of age. All analyses were initially race and sex specific; however, since the sex-specific analyses produced similar results for men and women, data for the two sexes were pooled within race, in order to increase statistical power. The findings were thus reported for whites and blacks separately but without regard to gender.

Contrary to the findings of most published studies, education—as an indicator of socioeconomic status—was not inversely associated with blood pressure in this second study. This was true for both whites and blacks. While an alternative measure for blacks of socioeconomic status,[‡] which combined respondent information on education and occupation, was inversely associated with blood pressure, a similarly constructed composite indicator for whites[§] did not alter the original null findings for whites. Subdividing whites into high and low John Henryism subgroups also produced null findings (that is, findings which did not conform to our theoretical expectations as depicted in Figure 20.2).

Blacks with better occupations (for example, higher level, blue-collar jobs) and at least some high school—the high socioeconomic status group in Figure 20.5—had a lower ($p \le .06$) mean diastolic blood pressure than did blacks with low-level occupations and similarly low levels of education (80.4 mmHg versus 78.1 mmHg). When the respondents were subsequently divided into high and low John Henryism subgroups (Figure 20.6), however, the difference in blood pressure by level of socioeconomic status was much larger for persons scoring high on John Henryism (3.8 mmHg) than for those scoring low on John Henryism (1 mmHg).

The results were even more striking when prevalence of hypertension (Figure 20.7) was the outcome. Differences in hypertension prevalence by socioeconomic status were very small for blacks scoring low on John Henryism (25 percent versus 23.4 percent); but for those scoring high on John Henryism, hypertension prevalence was almost *three* times greater for persons in the lower socioeconomic status group (31.4 percent) versus those in the higher group (11.5 percent). Indeed, the 11.5 percent prevalence of hypertension in the high socioeconomic status–high John Henryism subgroup is usually low for any group of adult blacks. This suggests that the combination of high socioeconomic status and high John Henryism could be *protective* against hypertension for black adults, a possibility that deserves further study.

Because of the apparent greater sensitivity of our theoretical model for blacks, as well as the greater magnitude and severity of the problem of hypertension in blacks, we decided to focus on African Americans exclusively in our third study (1992). In Pitt County, we interviewed 1,784 individuals (80 percent response rate), all of whom were between twenty-five and fifty years of age in 1988.**

[‡]For blacks, the composite measure of socioeconomic status was constructed as follows: high = nine years or more of formal schooling plus at least a semiskilled (for example, truck driver, painter) or skilled job (for example, carpenter, electrician, secretary); low = less than nine years of schooling or an unskilled job (for example, farm laborer, domestic worker).

[§]For whites, the composite measure of socioeconomic status was constructed as follows: high = high school graduate or more, plus a white-collar job (for example, businessman, nurse, teacher, plant manager); low = non–high school graduate or a blue-collar job (for example, electrician, mechanic, assembly-line worker).

**The Pitt County study was designed to be longitudinal; that is, we will track changes in blood pressure as study participants age and then relate these changes to their baseline (1988) dietary practices, physical activity levels, body weight and body fat distribution, psychological stress, socioeconomic status, and John Henryism scores. Data collection for the 1988–1993 follow-up period was conducted from February 1 through July 31, 1993.

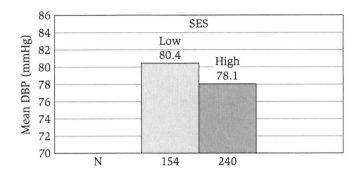

Figure 20.5 Mean Diastolic Blood Pressure (mmHg) by Socioeconomic Status: Edgecombe County, NC, 1987.

Note: Mean DBP adjusted for age, sex, age × sex interaction, and BMI; $p = .06$ for the association between SES and mean DBP.

Source: Reprinted with permission from the *American Journal of Epidemiology.*

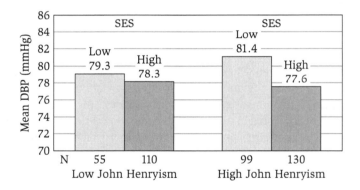

Figure 20.6 Mean Diastolic Blood Pressures (mmHg) for the Four SES–John Henryism Groups: Edgecombe County, NC, 1987.

Note: Mean DBP adjusted for age, sex, age × sex interaction, and BMI; $p =$ n.s. for the test of the SES × John Henryism regression interaction term.

Source: Reprinted with permission from the *American Journal of Epidemiology.*

Socioeconomic status was again measured by a combination of education and occupation; however, the larger sample size, along with a deliberate oversampling of blacks in middle-class neighborhoods, made it possible to create three as opposed to two socioeconomic status groups. The lowest socioeconomic category consisted of non–high school graduates who were also unskilled workers; the medium category consisted of semiskilled and skilled blue-collar workers, most of whom had finished high school; and the highest category was composed of skilled blue-collar and white-collar workers, all of whom had either post–high

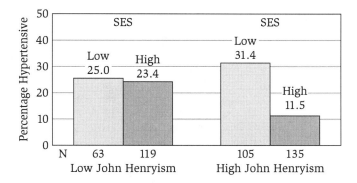

Figure 20.7 Adjusted Prevalence of Hypertension in Blacks for the Four SES–John Henryism Groups: Edgecombe County, NC, 1987.

Note: Mean DBP adjusted for age, sex, age × sex interaction, and BMI. Hypertension defined as DBP ≥ 90 mmHg, or currently taking antihypertensive medication; $p = .02$ for the test of the SES × John Henryism logistic regression interaction term.

Source: Reprinted with permission from the *American Journal of Epidemiology.*

school technical training or college degrees. In the following summary, only the findings for hypertension prevalence will be discussed; the conclusions reached also apply to systolic and diastolic blood pressure.

Figure 20.8 summarizes the prevalence of hypertension for the three socio-economic categories just described. Data for men and women were again combined. A very modest and nonstatistically significant ($p ≥ .05$) inverse association between socioeconomic status and hypertension prevalence was observed: 25.5 percent, 24.6 percent, and 23.6 percent for the low, medium, and high socioeconomic groups, respectively. Division of the sample into high and low John Henryism subgroups produced similarly unimpressive gradients (data not shown). Thus, despite the greater socioeconomic heterogeneity of the study population in Pitt County and our efforts to capture this heterogeneity in a sensitive manner, the findings failed to support our a priori predictions. In an attempt to understand why this occurred, we decided to concentrate our attention on the high socioeconomic status group whose surprisingly high 23.6 percent hypertension prevalence was, at least to us, an anomaly.

The exploratory analyses which followed revealed that self-reported psychological stress (measured by the Perceived Stress Scale developed by Sheldon Cohen and colleagues at Carnegie Mellon University) was quite high among managerial level, white-collar workers, especially men. Since psychological stress scores were positively and significantly ($p ≤ .05$) associated with mean blood pressures for both men and women in the Pitt County study population, these elevated stress scores for male white-collar workers raised the prevalence of hypertension to a surprisingly high level for the high socioeconomic status group as a whole.

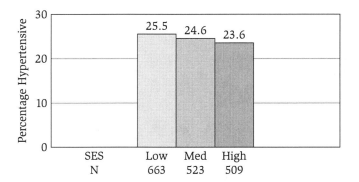

Figure 20.8 Adjusted Prevalence of Hypertension in Black Adults Aged 25 to 50 Years, by Socioeconomic Status: Pitt County, NC, 1992.

Note: Mean DBP adjusted for age, sex, age × sex, BMI, waist-hip ratio, and physical activity. Hypertension defined as DBP ≥ 90 mmHg, or currently taking antihypertensive medication; p = n.s. for the test of the association between socioeconomic status (SES) and hypertension prevalence.

Source: Reprinted with permission from the *American Journal of Epidemiology.*

Interestingly, this insight strengthens the argument that chronic psychological stress plays a significant role in creating and maintaining the well-known inverse association between socioeconomic status and hypertension. The argument can be summarized as follows: when chronic psychological stress is *higher* among lower socioeconomic status groups than among groups of higher socioeconomic status (and this is the usual case), the inverse association between socioeconomic status and blood pressure will be strong. However, when this is not the case—when chronic psychological stress does not vary in expected ways with socioeconomic status—the anticipated inverse association between socioeconomic status and blood pressure will be weak or perhaps nonexistent. We reasoned that the latter circumstance occurred in the Pitt County study.

To test the merits of this alternative explanation, we conducted a special post hoc test of the John Henryism hypothesis, with full appreciation, of course, of the scientific limitations of this post hoc analysis. First, we excluded all high socioeconomic status persons (n = 234) whose psychological stress scores were above the sample median. We then excluded all low socioeconomic status persons (n = 322) whose stress scores were below the sample median. These exclusions resulted in a strong (but theoretically expected) inverse association between socioeconomic status and psychological stress for the remaining members (n = 1,131) of the study sample.

How did the study findings change as a result of excluding individuals who were "discordant" on socioeconomic status and perceived stress? As shown in Figure 20.9, the inverse association between socioeconomic status and hypertension prevalence was considerably stronger: 24.7 percent, 23.4 percent, and

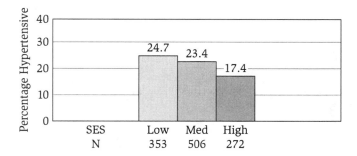

Figure 20.9 Adjusted Prevalence of Hypertension in Black Adults Aged 25 to 50 Years, by Socioeconomic Status: Pitt County, NC, 1992.

Note: Adjusted for age, sex, age × sex, BMI, waist-hip ratio, alcohol consumption, and physical activity. Respondents ($n = 556$) discordant on SES and perceived stress are excluded.

Source: Reprinted with permission from the *American Journal of Epidemiology.*

17.4 percent for the low, medium and high socioeconomic categories, respectively. Moreover, Figure 20.10 shows what occurred when these same respondents were subdivided into high and low John Henryism groups. Note that hypertension prevalence varied little by socioeconomic status in the low John Henryism group, but a strong (and theoretically expected) *inverse* association was observed in the high John Henryism group. In relative terms, the 35 percent hypertension prevalence in the low socioeconomic status–high John Henryism group is quite striking. We can be fairly certain, however, that it is not high psychological stress, per se, that so dramatically increased risk for hypertension in this group.[††] Rather, the *combination* of high stress (now significantly correlated with low socioeconomic status) and prolonged, high-effort coping with such stress is probably responsible for this strong elevation in risk and for the resulting strong, inverse *social* gradient in risk observed for persons scoring high on John Henryism.

No cross-sectional study, regardless of how intriguing the findings might be, can provide definitive evidence for cause-and-effect relationships. Our three cross-sectional studies,[17–19] as summarized previously, are no exception. To provide a more convincing case for the validity of the John Henryism hypothesis, we must demonstrate that the combination of low socioeconomic status and

---

[††]Recall that the exclusions forced all low socioeconomic status individuals in these analyses to have psychological stress scores *above* the sample median. Hence, if high stress scores alone dramatically increased risk for hypertension, both low socioeconomic status groups shown in Figure 20.10—those persons who scored low on John Henryism ($n = 215$) as well as those who scored high ($n = 138$)—would show dramatic elevations of hypertension prevalence. This was clearly not the case.

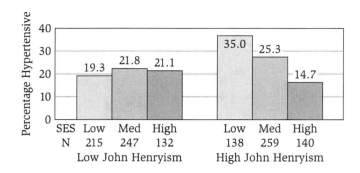

Figure 20.10 Adjusted Prevalence of Hypertension in Black Adults Aged 25 to 50 Years, by Socioeconomic Status and Level of John Henryism: Pitt County, NC, 1992.

Note: Respondents (n = 556) discordant on SES and perceived stress are excluded.

Source: Reprinted with permission from the *American Journal of Epidemiology.*

high John Henryism at one point in time contributes to an accelerated increase in blood pressure by some well-defined, second point in time. As noted elsewhere,[6] this is a major research objective of our ongoing work in Pitt County. If average increases in blood pressure (for example, from 1988 to 1993) follow the same pattern shown in Figure 20.10, this would provide much more persuasive scientific evidence that prolonged high-effort coping with chronic psychological stress that is structurally linked to low socioeconomic status is causally related to increased risk for hypertension in African Americans. Such findings, if observed, would have major societal, public health, and clinical importance.

I wish now to offer some speculations on the possible deeper cultural meaning of John Henryism for African Americans. This discussion is motivated by a long-standing interest of mine in the origins of John Henryism in black Americans, an interest which was deepened and challenged by the opportunity this discussion has afforded to link John Henryism to certain core values of American culture.

JOHN HENRYISM, AFRICAN AMERICANS, AND AMERICAN CULTURE

Perhaps the first issue to be addressed when considering the meaning of John Henryism for African Americans is the role of gender. The masculine imagery in the legend of John Henry is indeed quite strong.[15,16] Hence, it is understandable that many individuals automatically assume that the John Henryism hypothesis and its larger implications apply exclusively to black men. This is not the case. The scientific findings produced thus far apply equally to black men and black women. Moreover, black men and black women—unlike their white counterparts—score virtually identically on the JHAC12. In the Edgecombe County study,[18] for example, blacks—both men and women—had significantly higher ($p \leq .01$) age-adjusted John Henryism scores than whites. (This racial difference persisted even after we controlled, statistically, for education, marital status, and life satisfaction.) The rank order of mean John Henryism scores by race-sex was black men (53.3), black women (53.1), white men (51.5), and white women (50.1). Race-sex–specific information on John Henryism scores from settings outside the rural South are still quite limited, but at least two other studies,[21,22] both conducted in urban settings, reported the same rank order of scores by race-sex that we observed in Edgecombe County.

Collectively, these findings suggest that John Henryism in African Americans has a cultural as well as an economic basis. The economic basis is fairly easy to discern. African Americans clearly face more economic hardships than do whites; and, unlike whites, most blacks in the United States are routinely exposed to a most pernicious psychosocial stressor—racial discrimination—which further erodes their economic security and psychological well-being. Because black men and black women are more or less equally exposed to economic hardship linked to racial discrimination, the necessity that both groups might feel to cope in an effortful, active manner with these conditions undoubtedly contributes to the similarity in their John Henryism scores.[‡‡]

Having said this, we must now try to go beyond a purely economic perspective if we are to achieve a deeper, richer understanding of the "origins" and meaning of John Henryism for African Americans. Let me now propose the idea that John Henryism emerged as a widespread behavioral phenomenon among black Americans in the years and decades immediately following the Civil War; that it was in effect a strategy, a cultural adaptation, if you will, on the part of a newly freed people faced with the daunting task of creating for themselves an *American* identity. To be authentic that identity had to, first of all, acknowledge and find meaning in African Americans' past enslavement. Second, it had to make possible a culturally coherent (for blacks themselves) expression of core American values such as "hard work," "self-reliance," and "freedom." And, finally, it had to provide a pragmatic (that is, peaceful and effective) means to resist the new forms of oppression to which blacks, even as "freed" people, were

---

‡‡Though black men and black women score similarly on John Henryism, it is possible that their scores are significantly influenced by environmental factors (for example, racial discrimination and economic hardship) to which both groups are exposed as well as by environmental factors (for example, gender discrimination) to which only one group is exposed. This topic clearly deserves further study.

being increasingly subjected. With its strong, explicit emphasis on hard work and self-reliance, and its equally strong but more implicit emphasis on resistance to environmental forces that arbitrarily constrain personal freedom, the concept of John Henryism embodies, albeit imperfectly, all of the above.

I believe that two powerful currents of socialization converged in the lives of the Freedmen during this critical period to form a cultural crucible within which a viable African American identity could be forged. The first, as suggested in the important scholarship by Blassingame,[23] Gutman,[24] and Berlin et al.,[25] among others, was the heroic work of slave families over generations to maintain the self-esteem and optimism of a people in bondage so that when freedom came, they would be psychologically prepared for it.

The second current of socialization addressed the need of the Freedmen to become a literate people and thus develop a deeper understanding of the political and social implications of their hard-won freedom. This latter work, as is well-known, was carried out by the black churches and by missionary societies, many of which were based in New England.[26,27] Work by these groups gave a much needed focus to (but could not have succeeded without) the strong psychological and cultural resources that the Freedmen brought with them out of slavery. Here Litwack's description of the cultural and religious values that the New England missionaries and black church leaders attempted to impart to the Freedmen is particularly relevant to the thesis that these values may have found coherent *secular* expression in the behavioral predisposition I call John Henryism:

> Teachers and missionaries alike, whatever their race or affiliation, could agree on the critical need to provide the recently freed slaves with prerequisites of civilization and citizenship, and these would be nothing less than the virtues esteemed by mid-nineteenth-century Americans and taught in nearly every school and from every pulpit—*industry, frugality, honesty, sobriety, marital fidelity, self-reliance, self-control, godliness, and love of country* [p. 452, emphasis added].[26]

While it is highly unlikely that the Freedmen accepted these teachings uncritically, it is reasonable to conclude that many, perhaps the majority, recognized the utility of these values as the best available strategy for individual and group advancement in a society that would remain hostile to their presence for generations to come.

Was it pure coincidence, then, that this same crucial period, roughly the early 1870s, gave birth to the legend of John Henry? This tale of the folk (that is, the black folk) objectified the anxiety and the determination of a newly freed people about to embark upon a quest for economic security and a new cultural identity; but in the face of such formidable odds, could their quest possibly succeed? Given that this epic drama is still unfolding, none of us knows with certainty the answer to this question. However, if I read the legend of John Henry correctly, and if I understand its strong echo in the exemplary life of John Henry Martin,[§§] the black North Carolina farmer, the answer would seem to be "yes—but not without struggle, and not without a price."

Notes

1. Roberts, J., & Rowland, M. (1981). *Hypertension in adults 25–74 years of age, United States, 1971–1975* (Vital and Health Statistics, Series II: Data from the National Health Survey, no. 221, DHHS Publication No. [PHS] 81-1671). Hyattsville, MD: National Center for Health Statistics.

2. Hildreth, C., & Saunders, E. (1991). Hypertension in blacks: Clinical overview. In E. Saunders (Ed.), *Cardiovascular diseases in blacks* (pp. 85–96). Philadelphia: F. A. Davis.

3. Lopes, A. A., Port, F. K., James, S. A., & Agodoa, L. (1993). The excess risk of treated end-stage renal disease in blacks in the United States. *J Am Soc Nephrol, 3,* 1961–1971.

4. Tyroler, H. A. (1986). Hypertension. In J. M. Last (Ed.), *Public health and preventive medicine* (12th ed., pp. 1195–1214). Norwalk, CT: Appleton-Century-Crofts.

5. Saunders, E. (Ed.). (1991). *Cardiovascular diseases in blacks.* Philadelphia: F. A. Davis.

6. Hypertension Detection and Follow-up Program Cooperative Group. (1977). Race, education, and prevalence of hypertension. *Am J Epidemiol, 106,* 351–361.

7. Williams, D. R. (1992). Black-white differences in blood pressure: The role of social factors. *Ethn Dis, 2,* 126–141.

8. Obrist, P. A., Gaebelein, C. J., Teller, E. S., Langer, A. W., Grignoto, A., Light, K. C., & McCubbin, J. A. (1978). The relationship among heart rates, carotid dp/dt, and blood pressure in humans as a function of the type of stress. *Psychophysiology, 15,* 102–115.

9. Kasl, S. V., & Cobb, S. (1970). Blood pressure changes in men undergoing job loss: A preliminary report. *Psychosom Med, 32,* 19–38.

10. Cobb, S., & Rose, R. M. (1973). Hypertension, peptic ulcer and diabetes in air traffic controllers. *JAMA, 224,* 489–492.

11. Harburg, E. H., Erfurt, J. C., Hauenstein, L. S., Chape, C., Schull, W. I., & Schork, M. A. (1973). Socioecological stressor areas and black-white blood pressure. *J Chronic Dis, 26,* 595–611.

12. Syme, S. L. (1979). Psychosocial determinants of hypertension. In E. Oresti & C. Klint (Eds.), *Hypertension determinants, complications and intervention* (pp. 95–98). New York: Grune and Stratton.

[§§]John Henry Martin died in 1989, at eighty-one years of age.

13. James, S. A. (1993). The narrative of John Henry Martin. *Southern Cultures,* (Inaugural issue), 83–106.

14. Williams, B. (1983). *John Henry: A bio-bibliography.* Westport, CT: Greenwood Press.

15. Johnson, G. B. (1927). *John Henry: Tracking down a Negro legend.* Chapel Hill: University of North Carolina Press.

16. Levine, L. (1977). *Black culture and black consciousness: Afro-American folk thought from slavery to freedom.* Oxford, UK: Oxford University Press.

17. James, S. A., Hartnett, S., & Kalsbeck, W. D. (1983). John Henryism and blood differences among black men. *J Behav Med, 6,* 259–278.

18. James, S. A., Strogatz, D. S., Wing, S. B., & Ramsey, D. (1987). Socioeconomic status, John Henryism and hypertension in blacks and whites. *Am J Epidemiol, 126,* 664–673.

19. James, S. A., Keenan, N. L., Strogatz, D. S., Browning, S. R., & Garrett, J. M. (1992). Socioeconomic status, John Henryism, and blood pressure in black adults: The Pitt County study. *Am J Epidemiol, 135,* 59–67.

20. Mason, T. J., Fraumeni, J. R., & Hoover, R. (1981). *An atlas of mortality from selected diseases* (NIH Publication No. 81-2397). Washington, DC: U.S. Government Printing Office.

21. Weinrich, S. P., Weinrich, M. C., & Keil, J. E. (1988). The John Henryism and Framingham Type A Scales: Measurement properties in elderly black and whites. *Am J Epidemiol, 128,* 165–178.

22. McKetney, E. (1991). *John Henryism, education and blood pressure in young adults: The CARDIA study.* Unpublished doctoral dissertation, University of California, Berkeley, CA.

23. Blassingame, J. W. (1979). *The slave community: Plantation life in the antebellum South.* New York: Oxford University Press.

24. Gutman, H. G. (1976). *The black family in slavery and freedom, 1750–1925.* New York: Vintage Books.

25. Berlin, I., Fields, B. J., Miller, S. F., Reidy, J. P., & Rowland, L. S. (Eds.). (1992). *Free at last: A documentary history of slavery, freedom, and the Civil War.* New York: New Press.

26. Litwak, L. F. (1979). *Been in the storm so long: The aftermath of slavery.* New York: Vintage Books.

27. Anderson, J. D. (1988). *The education of blacks in the South, 1860–1935.* Chapel Hill: University of North Carolina Press.

CHAPTER TWENTY-ONE

Racial Residential Segregation

A Fundamental Cause of Racial Disparities in Health

David R. Williams
Chiquita Collins

Racial disparities are large and pervasive across multiple indicators of health status. Mortality data for the United States reveal that compared to the white population, African Americans (or blacks) have an elevated death rate for eight of the ten leading causes of death.[1] Especially disconcerting is evidence revealing that black-white disparities in health have not narrowed over time. For example, age-adjusted all-cause mortality for African Americans was one and a half times as high as that of whites in 1998, identical to what it was in 1950.[1] Moreover, the black:white ratios of mortality from coronary heart disease, cancer, diabetes, and cirrhosis of the liver were larger in the late 1990s than in 1950.[2] In the case of infant mortality, the black:white ratio increased from 1.6 in 1950 to 2.4 in 1998.[1] Such large and persistent racial disparities in health are inconsistent with widely supported American values of equality in society.

Healthy People 2010 is a major planning initiative of the United States government that seeks to eliminate racial and ethnic disparities in health in six target areas by the year 2010. The success of this initiative is contingent on identifying and addressing the fundamental causes of these disparities. Researchers have long emphasized the importance of distinguishing basic fundamental

Preparation of this paper was supported by grants MH59575 and MH57425 from the National Institute of Mental Health and the John D. and Catherine T. MacArthur Foundation Research Network on Socioeconomic Status and Health. We wish to thank Scott Wyatt for research assistance and Kathleen Boyle for preparing the manuscript.

causes from surface or proximate ones.[3-7] Basic causes are those responsible for generating a particular outcome. Changes in these factors produce corresponding change in outcomes. In contrast, although proximate factors (surface causes) are related to outcomes, changes in these factors do not lead to changes in the relevant outcomes. Accordingly, interventions to reduce or eliminate racial disparities in health that focus only on proximate causes will have only limited effectiveness.

In this chapter we argue that racial residential segregation is the cornerstone on which black-white disparities in health status have been built in the United States. Segregation is a fundamental cause of differences in health status between African Americans and whites because it shapes socioeconomic conditions for blacks not only at the individual and household levels but also at the neighborhood and community levels. We review evidence that suggests that segregation is a key determinant of racial differences in socioeconomic mobility and, additionally, can create social and physical risks in residential environments that adversely affect health.

NATURE AND ORIGINS OF RESIDENTIAL SEGREGATION

Although residential segregation is a neglected variable in contemporary discussions of racial disparities in health, it has long been identified as the central determinant of the creation and perpetuation of racial inequalities in America.[8-12] Segregation refers to the physical separation of the races in residential contexts. It was imposed by legislation, supported by major economic institutions, enshrined in the housing policies of the federal government, enforced by the judicial system, and legitimized by the ideology of white supremacy that was advocated by the church and other cultural institutions.[11-13] These institutional policies combined with the efforts of vigilant neighborhood organizations, discrimination on the part of real estate agents and home sellers, and restrictive covenants to limit the housing options of blacks to least desirable residential areas. In both Northern and Southern cities, levels of black-white segregation increased dramatically from 1860 to 1940 and have remained strikingly stable since then.[12]

The segregation of African Americans is distinctive. Although most immigrant groups have experienced some residential segregation in the United States, no immigrant group has ever lived under the high levels of segregation that currently exist for African American population.[12] In the early twentieth century, immigrant enclaves were never homogeneous to one immigrant group. In most immigrant ghettos, the ethnic immigrant group after which the enclave was named did not constitute a majority of the population of that area, and most members of European ethnic groups did not live in immigrant enclaves.[12,14]

The Civil Rights Act of 1968 made discrimination in the sale or rental of housing units illegal in the United States, but studies reveal that subtle and explicit discrimination in housing persists.[15] Thus, although African Americans express higher support than other racial/ethnic groups for residence in integrated neighborhoods,[16] analyses of the 2000 Census data document that the residential exclusion of blacks remains high and distinctive.[17] Nationally, the index of dissimilarity (a measure of segregation) for the United States declined from 0.70 in 1990 to 0.66 in 2000.[17] An index of 0.66 means that 66 percent of blacks would have to move to eliminate segregation.[18] Generally, a dissimilarity index value above 0.60 is thought to represent extremely high segregation.[19] In the 2000 Census, there were more than seventy-four Metropolitan Statistical Areas (MSAs) with dissimilarity scores greater than 0.60. Instructively, these metropolitan areas contain the majority of the black population. In the last decade, segregation has declined the most in smaller, growing cities, especially those of the Southwest and West, and has remained relatively stable in the large metropolitan areas of the Northeast and Midwest. The decline in segregation has been due to the reduction in the number of all-white census tracts and has had no impact on very high percentage African American census tracts, the residential isolation of most African Americans, or the concentration of urban poverty.[17]

SEGREGATION AND HEALTH STATUS: INDIVIDUAL AND HOUSEHOLD SES

Researchers have identified socioeconomic status (SES) as a fundamental cause of the observed social inequalities in health[4-6] and in particular of racial differences in health.[7] Yet health researchers and practitioners have given inadequate attention to the *causes* of racial disparities in SES. Racial differences in SES are the predictable results of the successful implementation of institutional policies and arrangements, with residential segregation being a prominent one in the U.S. context. By determining access to educational and employment opportunities for African Americans, residential segregation has truncated their socioeconomic mobility and been a central mechanism by which racial inequality has been created and reinforced in the United States.[12-13]

SEGREGATION AND EDUCATIONAL OPPORTUNITY

First, residential segregation has led to highly segregated elementary and high schools and is a fundamental cause of racial differences in the quality of education. For most Americans, residence determines which public school students can attend, and the funding of public education is under the control of local government. Thus, community resources importantly determine the quality of neighborhood schools. There is a very strong relationship between residential segregation and the concentration of poverty. Nationally, the correlation between the percentage of poor students in a school and the percentage of minority students (black and Hispanic) was 0.66 in 1991.[20] In metropolitan Chicago, the correlation between the percentages of poor and nonwhite students was 0.90 for elementary schools in 1989.[21] Although there are millions of poor whites in the U.S., poor white families tend to be dispersed throughout the community with many residing in desirable residential areas.[22] Accordingly, in 96 percent of predominantly white schools, the majority of students come from middle-class backgrounds.[21]

Levels of segregation for black and Latina and Latino students are currently on the increase.[23] One recent study found that as a growing number of minority families moved to the suburbs from 1987 to 1995, residential segregation there led to increased levels of segregation in suburban schools.[24]

The concentration of poverty, not racial composition per se, is the basic cause of the problems that plague segregated schools. Compared to schools in middle-class areas, segregated schools have lower average test scores, fewer students in advanced placement courses, more limited curricula, less qualified teachers, less access to serious academic counseling, fewer connections with colleges and employers, more deteriorated buildings, higher levels of teen pregnancy, and higher dropout rates.[21] These conditions often give rise to peer pressure against academic achievement and in support of crime and substance use. Black and Latina and Latino students are concentrated in urban schools that have different and inferior courses and lower levels of achievement than the schools attended by white students in adjacent suburban school districts. Thus, racial residential segregation leads to racial differences in high school dropout and graduation rates, competencies and knowledge of high school graduates, preparation for higher education, and the probability of enrollment in college.

SEGREGATION AND EMPLOYMENT OPPORTUNITIES

Second, *institutional* discrimination, based on residential segregation, severely restricts employment opportunities, and thus income levels, for African Americans. In the last several decades there has been a mass movement of low-skilled, high-paying jobs from many of the urban areas where blacks are concentrated.[22,25-26] This has created a "spatial mismatch" in which African Americans reside in areas that do not offer ready access to high paying entry-level jobs. It has also led to a "skills mismatch" in which the available jobs in the urban areas where African Americans live require levels of skill and training that many do not have. Some corporations explicitly use the racial composition of areas in their decision-making process regarding the placement of new plants and the relocation of existing ones.[27] Negative racial stereotypes of African Americans and the areas where they are concentrated play an important role in many of these decisions.[28-29] Thus, during routine "non-racial" restructuring, relocation, and downsizing, employment facilities are systematically moved to suburban and rural areas where the proportions of African Americans in the labor force are low. For example, a *Wall Street Journal* analysis of over 35,000 U.S. companies found that African Americans were the only racial group that experienced a net job loss during the economic downturn of 1990–1991.[30] African Americans had a net job loss of 59,000 jobs, while there was a net gain of 71,100 for whites, 55,100 for Asians, and 60,000 for Latinas and Latinos.

Residential segregation also affects employment opportunities by isolating blacks in segregated communities from both role models of stable employment and social networks that could provide leads about potential jobs.[22] The social isolation created by these structural conditions in segregated residential environments can then induce cultural responses that weaken the commitment to norms and values that may be critical for economic mobility. For example, long-term exposure to conditions of concentrated poverty can undermine a strong work ethic, devalue academic success, and remove the social stigma of imprisonment as well as of educational and economic failure.[31]

THE CONSEQUENCES OF SEGREGATION: RACIAL DIFFERENCES IN SES

After a thorough empirical analysis of the effects of segregation on young African Americans making the transition from school to work, Cutler et al. concluded that the elimination of residential segregation would lead to the disappearance of black-white differences in earnings, high school graduation rates, and idleness and would reduce racial differences in single motherhood by two-thirds.[32] Segregation is thus a central force in producing the large racial differences in socioeconomic circumstances evident in Table 21.1. In 1998, whites had higher levels of income and education attainment but lower levels of poverty and unemployment than African Americans. Other data reveal that large racial differences in unemployment persist even at equivalent levels of education.[33]

Many socioeconomic indicators are not equivalent across race.[34-35] For example, a given level of education may not reflect the same degree of educational preparation and skills. There are also racial differences in the income returns for a given level of education, with blacks, especially black males, earning less income than whites at comparable levels of education (Table 21.1). In addition, American women of all racial groups earn less than their similarly

Table 21.1. Selected Socioeconomic Indicators for Black and White Populations: United States, 1998

Indicator	Black	White
Median household income	$25,351	$40,912
Poverty indicators		
Population below poverty level (%)	26.1	10.5
Children <18 years old below poverty level (%)	36.4	14.4
People ≥65 years old below poverty level (%)	26.4	8.9
Educational attainment of those age 25 years and older		
High school graduate or higher (%)	76.0	83.7
College graduate or higher (%)	14.7	25.0
Population ≥16 years old unemployed (%)	8.9	3.9
Personal income by education, ages 25–64 years		
Median income, high school graduate, male	$22,099	$29,789
Median income, college graduate, male	$39,278	$53,158
Median income, high school graduate, female	$14,355	$15,733
Median income, college graduate, female	$33,865	$31,454
Household income by education of survey respondent ≥25 years old, 1996[40]		
Median income, high school graduate, male	$36,020	$41,200
Median income, college graduate, male	$54,500	$67,952
Median income, high school graduate, female	$23,556	$37,000
Median income, college graduate, female	$47,100	$64,007
Wealth (1995)[36]		
Median net worth	$ 7,073	$49,030
Median net worth, lowest income quintile	$ 1,500	$ 9,720
Median net worth, highest income quintile	$40,866	$123,781

Note: Data are for 1998, except as noted.

Source: Data drawn from U.S. Bureau of the Census. (2000). *Statistical abstract of the United States.* Washington, DC: U.S. Government Printing Office; except as noted.

educated male counterparts. This gender difference in earnings combined with racial differences in household structure (black households are more likely than white ones to be headed by a female) means that, especially for women, racial differences in individual earnings at equivalent levels of education understate racial differences in household income. National data,[112] as shown in Table 21.1, indicate that in 1996, black households with a college-educated male earned 80 cents for every dollar earned by a comparable white household. Such racial differences in the returns to education are evident at all levels of educational preparation but are more marked for women than for men. Households of black women who completed high school earned 64 cents for every dollar earned by comparable white households, and households of black women with a college degree earned 74 cents for every dollar earned by comparable white households.

The largest racial difference evident in Table 21.1 is for wealth. The median net worth of whites is almost six times that of blacks. This underscores the extent to which racial differences in income understate racial differences in economic status and resources. At every level of income, blacks have considerably less wealth than whites.[36] For example, the net worth at the lowest quintile of income is $9,720 for white households compared to $1,500 for African American households. At the highest quintile of income white households have a net worth of $123,781 compared to $40,866 for black households. Racial differences in wealth also link the current situation of blacks to historical processes of segregation. For most American families, housing equity is a major source of wealth. Thus, today's black-white differences in wealth are, to a considerable degree, a direct result of the institutional discrimination in housing practiced in the past that limited the home ownership opportunities of blacks.[37] However, racial differences in housing equity also reflect contemporary segregation because African Americans tend to receive smaller returns on their investment in a home than whites do. The growth in housing equity over time is smaller for black homeowners in highly segregated areas than for owners of comparable homes in other areas.[37]

RACE, SES, AND HEALTH

SES accounts for much of the racial differences in health, yet it is frequently found that SES differences, within each racial group, are substantially larger than overall racial differences.[2,38–39] Table 21.2 illustrates the key role that SES plays in racial/ethnic differences in health with national data on self-rated health and activity limitation.[1] The rate of activity limitation due to chronic conditions is higher for blacks than for whites, and blacks are more likely to report being in fair or poor health than whites. When stratified by economic status, the rates of activity limitation are almost identical for blacks and whites, suggesting that the higher prevalence of low income among African Americans completely accounts for the observed black-white difference on this outcome.

Table 21.2. Percentage of Individuals Reporting Fair or Poor Health and Activity Limitations, by Black and White Race and by Household Income: United States, 1997

Household Income	Percentage Reporting Activity Limitations		Percentage Reporting Fair or Poor Health	
	Black	White	Black	White
Poor	29.4	29.5	25.6	20.6
Near poor	20.0	20.7	19.5	14.1
Nonpoor	10.7	10.7	9.6	5.7
Total	17.0	13.2	15.8	8.0

Source: National Center for Health Statistics. (2000). *Health, United States, 2000, with adolescent health chartbook.* Hyattsville, MD: U.S. Department of Health and Human Services.

The black-white pattern for self-rated health reflects the more familiar pattern in which income predicts variation in health for both groups, but blacks report poorer health than whites at all levels of income. Such a pattern exists for other health outcomes, such as coronary heart disease mortality and life expectancy.[40] The residual effect of race, after SES is controlled for, could reflect the nonequivalence of individual indicators of SES across race, racial differences in community context, the long-term consequences of exposure to adversity in childhood, and the effect of other aspects of racism. Two studies have reported that perceptions of discrimination make an incremental contribution to explaining racial differences in self-rated health after SES is accounted for.[41–42]

In the United States, large and persistent black-white differences in health co-occur with large and persistent black-white differences in SES. The *Economic Report of the President* in 1998 documented that there was little change in the economic gap between blacks and whites in the last quarter of the twentieth century.[43] In 1978, black households earned 59 cents for every dollar earned by white households and had a poverty rate that was 3.5 times as high and an unemployment rate that was 1.9 times as high. In 1996, African American households earned 59 cents for every dollar earned by white households and had a poverty rate that was 2.5 times as high and an unemployment rate that was twice as high.

Analysis of economic and health data for the last fifty years reveals that the narrowing of the black-white gap in economic status was associated with a parallel narrowing of the black-white gap in health; similarly, a widening of the racial gap in SES was associated with a widening gap in health.[44] Specifically, between the late 1960s and the mid-1970s, as a result of the gains of the civil rights movement, there was some narrowing of the black-white gap in income.[43] There was a corresponding narrowing of the racial gap in health status. That is, between 1968 and 1978, across multiple causes of death, black men and women experienced a larger decline in mortality, both on a percentage and an absolute basis, than their white counterparts did.[45] Life expectancy data for this period show larger gains for blacks than whites on both a relative and an absolute basis. During the early 1980s, in the wake of substantial changes in social and economic policies at the national level, the health status of economically vulnerable populations worsened in several states.[46–47] Similarly, the black-white gap in health status widened between 1980 and 1991 for multiple health outcomes, including life expectancy, excess deaths, and infant mortality.[35,48]

SEGREGATION AND THE EFFECTS OF PLACE

Segregation can also adversely affect health by creating a broad range of pathogenic residential conditions that can induce adverse effects on health status. Measures of segregation appear to capture some of the effects of racism at the area level, and these community-level effects are one reason for the persistence of racial differences in health status even after controls are introduced for individual variations in SES.[49] The available evidence clearly indicates that racial segregation has created distinctive ecological environments for African Americans. For example, although numerically there are more poor whites than poor African Americans in the United States, most poor white people are residentially located next to nonpoor people, while most poor African Americans are concentrated in high-poverty neighborhoods.[22] An analysis of the 171 largest cities in the United States indicated that there was not even one city where whites lived in comparable ecological conditions to blacks in terms of poverty rates and single-parent households.[50] Sampson and Wilson concluded: "The worst urban context in which whites reside is considerably better than the average context of black communities."[50]

A growing number of studies using multilevel analyses indicate that social and economic characteristics of residential areas are associated with a broad range of health outcomes independent of individual indicators of SES.[51] For example, Diez Roux and colleagues found that even after adjustment for education, income, and occupational status and a broad range of biomedical and behavioral risk factors for coronary heart disease (smoking, exercise, hypertension, diabetes, obesity, and LDL and HDL cholesterol) people residing in disadvantaged neighborhoods had a higher incidence of heart disease than people who lived in more advantaged neighborhoods.[52] Several studies have specifically operationalized residential segregation and related the level of segregation to rates of morbidity and mortality. This body of research has found that residential segregation is related to elevated risks of cause-specific and overall adult mortality,[53-56] infant mortality,[57-60] and tuberculosis.[61] At the same time, one study found that the degree of residential segregation was unrelated to infant mortality rates.[62] There are multiple characteristics of low-SES environments, in general, and segregated environments, in particular, that are likely to be related to health. We now consider some of the ways in which residence in segregated areas can adversely affect health. Because of the paucity of work in this area, we include the related work of Sally Macintyre and colleagues from Scotland that illustrates area variations in risk factors for disease.

SEGREGATION AND NEIGHBORHOOD AND HOUSING QUALITY

Residential segregation can lead to large differences in neighborhood quality. Racial residential segregation has also let to unequal access for most blacks to a broad range of services provided by municipal authorities. Political leaders have been more likely to cut spending and services in poor neighborhoods, in general, and in African American neighborhoods, in particular, than in more affluent

areas.[31,63–64] Poor people and members of minority groups are less active politically than their more economically and socially advantaged peers, and elected
officials are less likely to encounter vigorous opposition when services are
reduced in the areas in which large numbers of poor people and people of color
live. This disinvestment of economic resources in these neighborhoods has led
to a decline in the urban infrastructure, physical environment, and quality of life
in those communities.[65–66] The selective out-migration of many whites and some
middle-class blacks from cities to the suburbs has also reduced the urban tax
base and the ability of some cities to provide a broad range of supportive social
services to economically deprived residential areas.

Racial differences in neighborhood quality persist at all levels of SES. Middle-
class suburban African Americans reside in neighborhoods that are less segregated than those of poor, central-city blacks.[67] However, compared to their white
counterparts, middle-class blacks are more likely to live in poorer quality neighborhoods, with white neighbors who are less affluent than they are. That is,
middle-class blacks are less able than their white counterparts to translate their
higher economic status into desirable residential conditions. One recent analysis of 1990 Census data revealed that suburban residence does not buy better
housing conditions for blacks.[68] The suburban locations where African
Americans reside tend to be equivalent or inferior to those of central cities.

Research by Macintyre and colleagues[69–70] of four neighborhoods in Glasgow,
Scotland, that varied in economic characteristics illustrate the ways in which
neighborhood areas can vary in the provision of resources that support health.
These researchers found that neighborhood areas differed in access to public
and private transportation, exposure to personal and property crime, amenities,
neighborliness, and problems such as litter, noxious odors, and discarded needles. U.S. research has also found that poor, segregated African American neighborhoods are also characterized by high mobility, low occupancy rates, high
levels of abandoned buildings and grounds, and more commercial and industrial facilities, and inadequate municipal services and amenities, including police
and fire protection.[71] Neighborhood problems are associated with ill health.
For example, Collins and colleagues[49] found a positive association between a
woman's negative rating of her neighborhood (in terms of police protection,
municipal services, cleanliness, quietness, and schools) and the likelihood of
having a low-birthweight infant.

The quality of housing is also likely to be poorer in highly segregated areas,
and poor housing conditions can also adversely affect health. Multiple housing
stressors (dampness or condensation, inadequate heat, problems with noise and
vibration from outside, the lack of space and the lack of private space, as well as
the presence of environmental hazards) varied by area in the four contrasting
neighborhoods in Glasgow, Scotland.[72] Similarly, U.S. data indicate that crowding, substandard housing, elevated noise levels, decreased ability to regulate

temperature and humidity, as well as elevated exposure to noxious pollutants and allergens (including lead, smog, particulates, and dust mites) are all common in poor, segregated communities.[66,71] These aspects of the physical environment have been shown to adversely affect health.[71,72]

SEGREGATION AND HEALTH BEHAVIORS

Research also reveals that the socioeconomic characteristics and segregation levels of particular areas can lead to dramatic variations in factors conducive to the practice of healthy or unhealthy behaviors. In Glasgow, there were more athletic tracks, playing fields, and swimming pools in economically advantaged neighborhoods than in economically disadvantaged ones.[69] U.S. research also reveals that a lack of recreational facilities and concerns about personal safety can also discourage leisure time physical exercise. For example, analysis of data from the 1996 Behavioral Risk Factor surveys for five states found a positive association between the perception of neighborhood safety and physical exercise.[73] Instructively, this association was somewhat larger among members of racial/ethnic minorities than among whites.

Segregation can also lead to racial differences in the purchasing power of a given level of income for a broad range of services, including those that are necessary to support good health. Many commercial enterprises avoid segregated urban areas: as a result, the available services are fewer in quantity, poorer in quality, and often higher in price than those available in less segregated urban and suburban areas. On average, blacks pay higher costs than whites for housing, food, insurance, and other services.[35] The consumption of nutritious food items is positively associated with their availability, and the availability of healthful products in grocery stores varies across different counties as well as zip codes.[74] Thus, the high cost and poor quality of grocery items in segregated neighborhoods can lead to poorer nutrition.

Researchers have long noted that both the tobacco and alcohol industry have heavily targeted poor minority communities with advertising for their products.[75–79] These marketing strategies include greater intensity of large highway billboard advertising in minority communities, the increasing use of smaller but more visible billboards, the concentration of alcohol and tobacco ads in print outlets with large minority readerships, and the increasing level of corporate sponsorship of athletic, cultural, civic, and entertainment events targeted to minority consumers.[79] Moreover, tobacco and alcohol use are coping strategies that are frequently employed to obtain escape and relief from the personal suffering and deprivation that characterizes many disadvantaged environments. Many segregated areas have high levels of multiple sources of stress, including violence, financial stress, family separation, chronic illness, death, and family turmoil.[71]

Research reveals that increased exposure to stress is positively associated with tobacco, alcohol, and drug use.[80-83] One recent study of African Americans in ten different census tracts in Southern California found a positive association between cigarette smoking and a measure of lifetime exposure to segregation.[84]

Data from Scotland have documented an area effect on the practice of a broad range of health behaviors, independent of individual characteristics.[85] That is, even after adjustment for age, gender, and individual indicators of SES, the data show that people living in more economically deprived neighborhoods were more likely to smoke, less likely to consume healthy foods (such as fruits, vegetables, and whole grain bread), more likely to consume unhealthy foods (such as sweets, cakes, processed meats, and french fries), and less likely to exercise than their counterparts in wealthier neighborhoods.[85] Not surprisingly, residents of more economically deprived neighborhoods were shorter, had higher body mass indexes, larger waist circumferences, and higher waist-hip ratios than their peers in more economically advantaged residential areas.[86]

MEDICAL CARE

Segregation is also likely to adversely affect access to high-quality medical care. The four Glasgow neighborhoods varied in the quality of primary health care services (health clinics, physician offices, dentists, opticians, and pharmacies).[69] African Americans face challenges in accessing medical care, and it is likely that these are more acute in segregated areas. Health care facilities are more likely to close in poor and minority communities than in other areas.[87-88] One recent study of New York City neighborhoods revealed that pharmacies in minority neighborhoods were less likely than pharmacies in other areas to have adequate medication in stock to treat persons with severe pain.[89] Other recent research documents that irrespective of residence, African Americans and members of other minority groups are less likely than whites to receive appropriate medical treatment after they gain access to medical care.[90] This pattern exists across a broad range of medical procedures and institutional contexts and is not accounted for by differences in SES, insurance, or disease severity. The causes of these disparities have not been identified, but it is likely that unconscious discrimination based on negative stereotypes of race and residence plays a role.[91-92]

SEGREGATION AND CRIME, HOMICIDE, AND SOCIAL CONTEXT

An investigation of segregation also sheds light on the racial differences in some health outcomes that have strong environmental components. African Americans are much more likely than whites to be victims of all types of crime, including homicide.[33] Of the fifteen leading causes of death in the United States, the black-white gap is largest for homicide. In 1996, the death rate from homicide for African Americans was 30.6 per 100,000 population—virtually identical to the rate of 30.5 in 1950.[1] Several studies have found that segregation is positively associated with the risk of being a victim of homicide for blacks,[31,93-96] although this finding is not uniform.[97] Table 21.3 presents the homicide rates for men and women for 1994–1995, stratified by race and education. Irrespective of racial status, the homicide rate was strongly patterned by SES. For both men and women, the racial gaps were large even at identical levels of education, with, for example, the homicide rate for black males in the highest education category exceeding that for white males in the lowest education group. These dramatic racial differences may reflect an important area effect.

Sampson's research on the causes of urban violence clearly suggests that the elevated homicide rate of African Americans is a consequence of residential segregation.[98] His research indicates that in black urban communities characterized by high rates of poverty, there are only very small pools of employable or stably employed males. Social science research has long documented that high male unemployment and low wage rates for males are associated with increased rates of female-headed households for both blacks and whites.[99] Lack of access to jobs produces high rates of male unemployment and underemployment, which in turn underlies the high rates of out-of-wedlock births, the large numbers of female-headed households, the "feminization of poverty," and the extreme concentration of poverty in many black communities.[100-101] In turn, single-parent households lead to lower levels of social control and supervision. Sampson documented a strong association between family structure and violent crime.[98] Importantly, the relationship between family structure and violent crime for whites was identical in size and magnitude to that for blacks. Thus, the elevated rates of violent crime and homicide for African Americans are determined by the structural conditions of their residential contexts. Relatedly, residential segregation also contributes to racial differences in drug use. A study

Table 21.3. Homicide Rate Among Adults 25–44 Years of Age, by Educational Attainment, Sex, and Black and White Race, 1994–1995

	Male		Female	
Education	Black	White	Black	White
<12 years	163.3	25.0	38.2	10.2
12 years	110.7	10.6	22.0	4.7
≥13	32.4	2.9	9.4	1.6
Total (1995)[1]	77.9	11.0	17.4	3.3

Source: Data drawn from National Center for Health Statistics. (1998). *Health, United States, 1998, with socioeconomic status and health chartbook.* Hyattsville, MD: U.S. Department of Health and Human Services; except as noted.

using national data revealed that elevated rates of cocaine use by blacks and Hispanics in individual-level data could be completely explained when individuals were grouped into neighborhood clusters based on census characteristics.[102]

RESEARCH DIRECTIONS

This chapter has focused heavily on the experience of African Americans. Research is needed to explore the extent to which segregation affects the health of other minority populations and to identify the fundamental causes of all racial/ethnic disparities in health. Similar to the pattern for African Americans, long-term data for American Indians served by the Indian Health Service indicate widening American Indian–white disparities for multiple causes of death.[103] For example, the American Indian mortality rate for diabetes was 1.3 times higher than that of whites in 1955, but 3.7 times higher in 1993. Similarly, the American Indian:white mortality ratio for liver cirrhosis increased from 2.9 in 1955 to 4.6 in 1993. Reservations are another prominent example of residential segregation that deserves careful examination in identifying the basic causes of the health challenges faced by many American Indians and Alaskan Natives.

Segregation is a factor that may also adversely affects Hispanics, although its impact on the Hispanic population is likely to be smaller than that for African Americans. Levels of segregation of Hispanics from whites are moderate compared to levels for African Americans.[104] Even under conditions of high immigration, there has not been the expected large increase in residential segregation for Hispanics in recent decades.[104] Mainland Puerto Ricans are the exception to this generalization. Because of their relatively higher level of African ancestry, Puerto Ricans are distinctive among Hispanic groups in having high levels of segregation.[104] More important than segregation as a determinant of the low SES levels of other Hispanic subgroups is the immigration of large numbers of relatively unskilled persons with low levels of educational attainment.[105] The lower levels of segregation for most Hispanic groups suggest that the long-term socioeconomic trajectory of Hispanics is likely to be somewhat better than that of African Americans.[106] However, the Hispanic population faces considerable difficulties with socioeconomic mobility due to substantial barriers to occupational mobility and persisting educational disadvantages.[105] The situation of Hispanics highlights the heterogeneity of minority populations and the importance of paying attention to the specific circumstances of each population group.

The consequence of segregation for whites is another issue worthy of careful empirical scrutiny. One recent study found that segregation was associated with elevated mortality for whites in cities high on two indices of segregation.[54] However, it is not clear whether this reflects an adverse effect of some of the structural characteristics of highly segregated cities or a selection effect in which more vulnerable whites (in terms of SES, age, and health) opted not to migrate out of highly segregated cities.

Finally, research is needed to catalogue and quantify the specific aspects of the social and physical environments of segregated neighborhoods that are plausibly linked to health. The assessment strategies that have been used in Chicago[107] and Glasgow[70] are good places to start. However, such approaches must be expanded to capture potentially health-enhancing aspects of residence in segregated areas. Mental health researchers have long documented that the mental health is enhanced when group members reside in enclaves with higher concentrations of their group.[108–110] The conditions under which segregation can positively and negatively affect health are not well understood. Additionally, theoretically driven multilevel analytic models are needed that will identify how characteristics of the physical and social environment relate to each other and combine with individual predispositions and characteristics in additive and interactive ways to influence health.

CONCLUSION

It is widely recognized that a pervasive and persistent pattern of racial disparities across a broad range of indicators of health status is determined by a complex, multifactorial web of causation. One effective way to eliminate these disparities is to identify and eliminate the "spiders" responsible for creating the web in the first place.[111] The evidence reviewed suggests that racial residential segregation, an institutional manifestation of racism, is one of the most important "spiders" responsible for persisting black-white inequalities in health. Inattention to eliminating residential segregation and the conditions created by it may limit the utility of well-intentioned efforts to reduce racial disparities in health. Thus, effective efforts to reduce racial disparities in health status should seriously grapple with reducing racial disparities in socioeconomic circumstances and with targeting interventions not only to individuals but also to the geographic contexts in which they live.

Notes

1. National Center for Health Statistics. (2000). *Health, United States, 2000, with adolescent health chartbook*. Hyattsville, MD: U.S. Department of Health and Human Services.

2. Williams, D. R. (1999). Race, SES, and health: The added effects of racism and discrimination. *Ann N Y Acad Sci, 896*, 173–188.

3. Lieberson, S. (1985). *Making it count: The improvement of social research and theory*. Berkeley: University of California Press.

4. House, J. S., Kessler, R. C., Herzog, A. R., Mero, R., Kinney, A., & Breslow, M. (1990). Age, socioeconomic status, and health. *Milbank Q, 68,* 383–411.

5. Link, B. G., & Phelan, J. (1995). Social conditions as fundamental causes of disease. *J Health Soc Behav* (extra issue), 80–94.

6. Williams, D. R. (1990). Socioeconomic differentials in health: A review and redirection. *Soc Psychol Q, 53*(2), 81–99.

7. Williams, D. R. (1997). Race and health: Basic questions, emerging directions. *Ann Epidemiol, 7*(5), 322–333.

8. Myrdal, G. (1944). *An American dilemma: The Negro problem and modern democracy.* New York: Harper & Brothers.

9. Clark, K. B. (1965). *Dark ghetto: Dilemmas of social power.* New York: Harper and Row.

10. National Advisory Commission on Civil Disorders. (1988). *Report of the National Advisory Commission on Civil Disorders* (The Kerner report). New York: Pantheon Books.

11. Cell, J. (1982). *The highest stage of white supremacy: The origin of segregation in South Africa and the American South.* New York: Cambridge University Press.

12. Massey, D. S., & Denton, N. A. (1993). *American apartheid: Segregation and the making of the underclass.* Cambridge, MA: Harvard University Press.

13. Jaynes, G. D., & Williams, R. M. (1989). *A common destiny: Blacks and American society.* Washington, DC: National Academy Press.

14. Lieberson, S. (1980). *A piece of the pie: Black and white immigrants since 1880.* Berkeley: University of California Press.

15. Fix, M., & Struyk, R. J. (1993). *Clear and convincing evidence: Measurement of discrimination in America.* Washington, DC: Urban Institute Press.

16. Bobo, L., & Zubrinsky, C. L. (1996). Attitudes on residential integration: Perceived status differences, mere in-group preference, or racial prejudice? *Soc Forces, 74*(3), 883–909.

17. Glaeser, E. L., & Vigdor, J. L. (2001). *Racial segregation in the 2000 Census: Promising news.* Washington, DC: Brookings Institution, Survey Series.

18. Massey, D. S., & Denton, N. (1988). The dimensions of residential segregation. *Soc Forces, 67,* 281–315.

19. Massey, D. S., & Denton, N. A. (1989). Hypersegregation in U.S. metropolitan areas: Black and Hispanic segregation along five dimensions. *Demography, 26,* 373–392.

20. Orfield, G. (1993, December). *The growth of segregation in American schools: Changing patterns of separation and poverty since 1968* (Report of the Harvard Project on School Desegregation to the National School Boards Association). New York: New Press.

21. Orfield, G., & Eaton, S. E. (1996). *Dismantling desegregation: The quiet reversal of Brown v. Board of Education.* New York: New Press.

22. Wilson, W. J. (1987). *The truly disadvantaged.* Chicago: University of Chicago Press.

23. Orfield, G. (2001, July). Schools more separate: Consequences of a decade of resegregation. Cambridge, MA: Harvard University, the Civil Rights Project.

24. Reardon, S. F., & Yun, J. T. (2001). Suburban racial change and suburban school segregation, 1987–95. *Sociol Educ, 74,* 79–101.

25. Wilson, W. J. (1996). *When work disappears: The world of the new urban poor.* New York: Knopf.

26. Kasarda, J. D. (1989). Urban industrial transition and the underclass. *Ann Am Acad Political Soc Sci, 501,* 26–47.

27. Cole, R. E., & Deskins, D. R., Jr. (1988). Racial factors in site location and employment patterns of Japanese auto firms in America. *Calif Manage Rev, 31*(1), 9–22.

28. Kirschenman, J., & Neckerman, K. M. (1991. "We'd love to hire them, but . . .": The meaning of race for employers. In C. Jencks & P. E. Peterson (Eds.), *The urban underclass* (pp. 203–232). Washington, DC: Brookings Institution.

29. Neckerman, K. M., & Kirschenman, J. (1991). Hiring strategies, racial bias, and inner-city workers. *Soc Problems, 38,* 433–447.

30. Sharpe, R. (1993, September 14). In latest recession, only blacks suffered net employment loss. *Wall Street Journal,* p. A1.

31. Shihadeh, E. S., & Flynn, N. (1996). Segregation and crime: The effect of black social isolation on the rates of black urban violence. *Soc Forces, 74*(4), 1325–1352.

32. Cutler, D. M., Glaeser, E. L., & Vigdor, J. L. (1997). Are ghettos good or bad? *Q J Econ, 112*(3), 827–872.

33. Council of Economic Advisers for the President's Initiative on Race. (1998). *Changing America: Indicators of social and economic well-being by race and Hispanic origin.* Washington, DC: U.S. Government Printing Office.

34. Kaufman, J. S., Cooper R. S., & McGee, D. L. (1997). Socioeconomic status and health in blacks and whites: The problem of residual confounding and the resiliency of race. *Epidemiology, 8,* 621–628.

35. Williams, D. R., & Collins, C. (1995). U.S. socioeconomic and racial differences in health. *Annu Rev Sociol, 21,* 349–386.

36. Davern, M. E., & Fisher, P. J. (2001). *Household net worth and asset ownership, 1995* (U.S. Bureau of the Census, Current Population Reports, Household Economic Studies Series P70-71). Washington, DC: U.S. Government Printing Office.

37. Oliver, M. L., & Shapiro, T. M. (1997). *Black wealth/white wealth: A new perspective on racial inequality.* New York: Routledge.

38. Sorlie, P., Rogor, E., Anderson, R., & Backlund, E. (1992). Black-white mortality differences by family income. *Lancet, 340,* 346–350.

39. Navarro, V. (1990). Race or class versus race and class: Mortality differentials in the United States. *Lancet, 336,* 1238–1240.

40. National Center for Health Statistics. (1998). *Health, United States, 1998, with socioeconomic status and health chartbook.* Hyattsville, MD: U.S. Department of Health and Human Services.

41. Williams, D. R., Yu, Y., Jackson, J., & Anderson, N. (1997). Racial differences in physical and mental health: Socioeconomic status, stress, and discrimination. *J Health Psychol, 2*(3), 335–351.

42. Ren, X. S., Amick, B., & Williams, D. R. (1999). Racial/ethnic disparities in health: The interplay between discrimination and socioeconomic status. *Ethn Dis, 9*(2), 151–165.

43. *Economic report of the president, with the annual report of the Council of Economic Advisers.* Washington, DC: U.S. Government Printing Office. (1998).

44. Williams, D. R. (2001). Race and health: Trends and policy implications. In J. A. Auerbach & B. K. Krimgold (Eds.), *Income, socioeconomic status, and health: Exploring the relationships* (pp. 67–85). Washington, DC: Academy for Health Services Research and Health Policy, National Policy Association.

45. Cooper, R. S., Steinhauer, M., Schatzkin, A., & Miller, W. (1981). Improved mortality among U.S. blacks, 1968–1978: The role of antiracist struggle. *Int J Health Serv, 11,* 511–522.

46. Mandinger, M. (1985). Health service funding cuts and the declining health of the poor. *N Engl J Med, 313,* 44–47.

47. Lurie, N., Ward, N. B., Shapiro, M. F., & Brook, R. H. (1984). Termination from Medi-Cal: Does it affect health? *N Engl J Med, 311,* 480–484.

48. National Center for Health Statistics. (1994). *Excess deaths and other mortality measures for the black population, 1979–81 and 1991.* Hyattsville, MD: U.S. Public Health Service.

49. Collins, J. W., David, R. J., Symons, R., Handler, A., Wall, S., & Andes, S. (1998). African-American mothers' perception of their residential environment, stressful life events, and very low birthweight. *Epidemiology, 9,* 286–289.

50. Sampson, R. J., & Wilson, W. J. (1995). Toward a theory of race, crime, and urban inequality. In J. Hagan & R. D. Peterson (Eds.), *Crime and inequality* (pp. 37–54). Stanford, CA: Stanford University Press.

51. Pickett, K. E., & Pearl, M. (2001). Multilevel analyses of neighbourhood socioeconomic context and health outcomes: A critical review. *J Epidemiol Community Health, 55,* 111–122.

52. Diez Roux, A. V., Merkin, S. S., Arnett, D., Chambless, L., Massing, M., Nieto, J., Sorlie, P., Szklo, M., Tyroler, H. A., & Watson, R. L. (2001). Neighborhood of residence and incidence of coronary heart disease. *N Engl J Med, 345*(2), 99–106.

53. Polednak, A. P. (1993). Poverty, residential segregation, and black/white mortality rates in urban areas. *J Health Care Poor Underserved, 4,* 363–373.

54. Collins, C. A., & Williams, D. R. (1999). Segregation and mortality: The deadly effects of racism? *Sociol Forum, 14*(3), 495–523.

55. Fang, J., Madhavan, S., Bosworth, W., & Alderman, M. H. (1998). Residential segregation and mortality in New York City. *Soc Sci Med, 47,* 469–476.

56. Guest, A. M., Almgren, G., & Hussey, J. M. (1998). The ecology and race and socioeconomic distress: Infant and working-age mortality in Chicago. *Demography, 35*(1), 25–34.

57. LaVeist, T. A. (1989). Linking residential segregation and infant mortality race disparity in U.S. cities. *Sociol Soc Res, 73,* 90–94.

58. LaVeist, T. A. (1992). The political empowerment and health status of African-Americans: Mapping a new territory. *Am J Sociol, 97*(4), 1080–1095.

59. LaVeist, T. A. (1993). Beyond dummy variables and sample selection: What health services researchers ought to know about race as a variable. *Health Serv Res, 29,* 1–16.

60. Polednak, A. P. (1991). Black-white differences in infant mortality in 38 standard metropolitan statistical areas. *Am J Public Health, 81,* 1480–1482.

61. Acevedo-Garcia, D. (2001). Zip code–level risk factors for tuberculosis: Neighborhood environment and residential segregation in New Jersey, 1985–1992. *Am J Public Health, 91*(5), 734–741.

62. Polednak, A. P. (1996). Trends in U.S. urban black infant mortality, by degree of residential segregation. *Am J Public Health, 86*(5), 723–726.

63. Wallace, R. (1990). Urban desertification, public health and public order: "Planned shrinkage," violent death, substance abuse, and AIDS in the Bronx. *Soc Sci Med, 31,* 801–813.

64. Wallace, R. (1991). Expanding coupled shock fronts of urban decay and criminal behavior: How U.S. cities are becoming "hollowed out." *J Quantitative Criminology, 7*(4), 333–356.

65. Alba, R. D., & Logan, J. R. (1993). Minority proximity to whites in suburbs: An individual-level analysis of segregation. *Am J Sociol, 98*(6), 1388–1427.

66. Bullard, R. D. (1994). Urban infrastructure: Social, environmental, and health risks to African Americans. I. L. Livingston (Ed.), *Handbook of black American health: The mosaic of conditions, issues, policies and prospects* (pp. 315–330). Westport, CT: Greenwood Press.

67. Alba, R. D., Logan, J. R., & Stults, B. J. (2000). How segregated are middle-class African Americans? *Soc Problems, 47*(4), 543–558.

68. Harris, D. R. (1999). *All suburbs are not created equal: A new look at racial differences in suburban locations* (Research Report No. 99-440). Ann Arbor: University of Michigan, Population Studies Center.

69. Macintyre, S., Maciver, S., & Sooman, A. (1993). Area, class and health: Should we be focusing on places or people? *J Soc Politics, 22*(2), 213–234.

70. Sooman, A., & Macintyre, S. (1995). Health and perceptions of the local environment in socially contrasting neighbourhoods in Glasgow. *Health & Place, 1*(1), 15–26.

71. Evans, G. W., & Saegert, S. (2000). Residential crowding in the context of inner city poverty. In S. Wapner, J. Demick, T. Yamamoto, et al. (Eds.), *Theoretical perspectives in environment-behavior research* (pp. 247–267). New York: Kluwer Academic/Plenum.

72. Ellaway, A., & Macintyre, S. (1998). Does housing tenure predict health in the UK because it exposes people to different levels of housing related hazards in the home or its surroundings? *Health & Place, 4*(2), 141–150.

73. Centers for Disease Control and Prevention. (1999). Neighborhood safety and the prevalence of physical inactivity—Selected states, 1996. *Morbid Mortal Wkly Rep, 48*(7), 143–146.

74. Cheadle, A., Psaty, B. M., Curry, S., Wagner, E., Diehr, P., Koepsell, T., & Kristal, A. (1991). Community-level comparisons between the grocery store environment and individual dietary practices. *Prev Med, 20,* 250–261.

75. Hacker, A. G., Collins, R., & Jacobson, M. (1987). *Marketing booze to blacks.* Washington, DC: Center for Science in the Public Interest.

76. Rabow, J., & Watt, R. (1982). Alcohol availability, alcohol beverage sales, and alcohol-related problems. *J Studies Alcohol, 43,* 767–801.

77. Maxwell, B., & Jacobson, M. (1989). *Marketing disease to Hispanics: The selling of alcohol, tobacco, and junk foods.* Washington, DC: Center for Science in the Public Interest.

78. Mayberry, R. M., & Price, P. A. (1993). Targeting blacks in cigarette billboard advertising: Results from down South. *Health Values: The Journal of Health Behavior, Education & Promotion, 17*(1), 28–35.

79. Moore, A. J., Williams, J. D., & Qualls, W. J. (1996). Target marketing of tobacco and alcohol-related products to ethnic minority groups in the United States. *Ethn Dis, 6*(1,2), 83–98.

80. Linsky, A. S., Straus, M. A., & Colby, J. P. (1985). Stressful events, stressful conditions and alcohol problems in the United States: A partial test of Bales's theory. *J Stud Alcohol, 46*(1), 72–80.

81. Singer, M. (1986). Toward a political economy of alcoholism. *Soc Sci Med, 23,* 113–130.

82. Conway, T., Ward, H., Vickers, R., & Rahe, R. (1981). Occupational stress, and variation in cigarette, coffee, and alcohol consumption. *J Health Soc Behav, 22,* 155–165.

83. Benfari, R., Ockene, J., & McIntyre, K. (1982). Control of cigarette smoking from a psychological perspective. *Annu Rev Public Health, 3,* 101–128.

84. Landrine, H., & Klonoff, E. A. (2000). Racial segregation and cigarette smoking among blacks: Findings at the individual level. *J Health Psychol, 5*(2), 211–219.

85. Ellaway, A., & Macintyre, S. (1996). Does where you live predict health related behaviours? A case study in Glasgow. *Health Bull, 56*(6), 443–446.

86. Ellaway, A., Anderson, A., & Macintyre, S. (1997). Does area of residence affect body size and shape? *Int J Obesity, 21,* 304–308.

87. Whiteis, D. G. (1992). Hospital and community characteristics in closures of urban hospitals, 1980–1987. *Public Health Rep, 107*(4), 409–416.

88. McLafferty, S. (1982). Neighborhood characteristics and hospital closures: A comparison of the public, private, and voluntary hospital systems. *Soc Sci Med, 16*(19), 1667–1674.

89. Morrison, R. S., Wallenstein, S., Natale, D. K., Senzel, R. S., & Huang, L.-L. (2000). "We don't carry that": Failure of pharmacies in predominantly nonwhite neighborhoods to stock opioid analgesics. *N Engl J Med, 342*(14), 1023–1026.

90. Mayberry, R. M., Mili, F., & Ofili, E. (2000). Racial and ethnic differences in access to medical care. *Med Care Res Rev, 57*(Suppl. 1), 108–145.

91. Williams, D. R., & Rucker, T. D. (2000). Understanding and addressing racial disparities in health care. *Health Care Financing Rev, 21*(4), 75–90.

92. van Ryn, M., & Burke, J. (2000). The effect of patient race and socio-economic status on physicians' perceptions of patents. *Soc Sci Med, 50*(6), 813–828.

93. Logan, J. R., & Messner, S. F. (1987). Racial residential segregation and suburban violent crime. *Soc Sci Q, 68,* 510–527.

94. Rosenfield, R. (1986). Urban crime rates: Effects of inequality, welfare dependency, region and race. In J. Byrne & R. Sampson (Ed.), *The social ecology of crime.* New York: Springer-Verlag.

95. Potter, L. (1991). Socioeconomic determinants of white and black life expectancy differentials. *Demography, 28,* 303–320.

96. Krivo, L. J., & Peterson, R. D. (1996). Extremely disadvantaged neighborhoods and urban crime, *Soc Forces, 75*(2), 619–650.

97. Sampson, R. J. (1985). Race and criminal violence: A demographically disaggregated analysis of urban homicide. *Crime and Delinquency, 31,* 47–82.

98. Sampson, R. J. (1987). Urban black violence: The effect of male joblessness and family disruption. *Am J Sociol, 93*(2), 348–382.

99. Bishop, J. H. (1980). Jobs, cash transfers, and marital instability: A review and synthesis of the evidence. *J Hum Resources, 15,* 301–334.

100. Testa, M., Astone, N. M., Krogh, M., et al. (1993). Employment and marriage among inner-city fathers. In W. J. Wilson (Ed.), *The ghetto underclass* (pp. 96–108). Newberry Park, CA: Sage.

101. Wilson, W., & Neckerman, K. M. (1986). Poverty and family structure: The widening gap between evidence and public policy issues. In S. H. Danziger & D. H. Weinberg (Eds.), *Fighting poverty* (pp. 232–259). Cambridge, MA: Harvard University Press.

102. Lillie-Blanton, M., Martinez, R. M., Taylor, A. K., & Robinson, B. G. (1993). Latina and African American women: Continuing disparities in health. *Int J Health Serv, 23*(3), 555–584.

103. Indian Health Service. (1997). *Trends in Indian Health.* Rockville, MD: U.S. Department of Health and Human Services.

104. Massey, D. S. (2001). Residential segregation and neighborhood conditions in U.S. metropolitan areas. In N. J. Smelser, W. J. Wilson, & F. Mitchell (Eds.), *America becoming: Racial trends and their consequences* (Vol. 1, pp. 391–434). Washington, DC: National Academy Press.

105. Camarillo, A. M., & Bonilla, F. (2001). Hispanic in a multicultural society: A new American dilemma? In N. J. Smelser, W. J. Wilson, & F. Mitchell (Eds.), *America becoming: Racial trends and their consequences* (Vol. 1, pp. 103–134). Washington, DC: National Academy Press.

106. Williams, D. R. (2001). Racial variations in adult health status: Patterns, paradoxes and prospects. In N. J. Smelser, W. J. Wilson, & F. Mitchell (Eds.), *America becoming: Racial trends and their consequences* (Vol. 2, pp. 371–410). Washington, DC: National Academy Press.

107. Raudenbush, S. W., & Sampson, R. J. (1999). Ecometrics: Toward a science of assessing ecological settings, with application to the systematic social observation of neighborhoods. *Sociol Methodology, 29,* 1–41.

108. Faris, R. E., & Dunham, W. H. (1965). *Mental disorders in urban areas: An ecological study of schizophrenia and other psychoses.* Chicago: University of Chicago Press.

109. Levy, L., & Rowitz, L. (1973). *The ecology of mental disorder.* New York: Behavioral Publications.

110. Halpern, D. (1993). Minorities and mental health. *Soc Sci Med, 36,* 597–607.

111. Krieger, N. (1994). Epidemiology and the web of causation: Has anyone seen the spider? *Soc Sci Med, 39*(7), 887–903.

112. U.S. Bureau of the Census. (2000). *Statistical abstract of the United States.* Washington, DC: U.S. Government Printing Office.

CHAPTER TWENTY-TWO

U.S. Socioeconomic and Racial Differences in Health

Patterns and Explanations

David R. Williams
Chiquita Collins

C lass is a very widely used concept in the social sciences in general, and sociology in particular. Although no consensus exists on exactly what it means and how it should be measured, class, however defined, has proven to be remarkably robust in elucidating the complexities of social and historical processes and in predicting variations within and between social groups in living conditions and life chances, skill levels and material resources, relative power and privilege. Health status is one arena where the effects of class are readily evident.

Similarly, race is one of the major bases of division in American life, and throughout U.S. history racial disparities in health have been pervasive. The vast majority of studies focus on the black-white contrast, but a rapidly growing literature describes variations in health status within and between America's increasingly diverse racial populations. The U.S. government requires all federal statistical reporting agencies to recognize four racial groups (American Indian or Alaskan Native, Asian or Pacific Islander, black, and white) and one ethnic category (Hispanic). Given that racial taxonomies are socially constructed and arbitrary, we treat all of these categories as racial groups. Moreover, since

Preparation of this paper was supported by Grant AG-07904 from the National Institute on Aging. We wish to thank Greg Duncan, James S. House, and Sherman James for helpful comments on an earlier version of this chapter.

group designations should reflect generally recognized definitions as well as individual dignity, and there are varying views within racial groups with regard to terminology, we treat the following paired categories as alternative labels: American Indian or Native American, Hispanic or Latino, and black or African American.

This chapter reviews the evidence for persisting inequalities in health by socioeconomic status (SES) and race. We focus on the magnitude of the differences, the trends over time, and the major explanatory factors invoked to account for these variations. Methodological issues are also discussed, and directions for future research are outlined. We begin with a consideration of SES differences in health.

SOCIOECONOMIC STATUS AND HEALTH

SES is widely used as a proxy for social class in studies that examine variations in the distribution of disease, and it continues to be a remarkably robust determinant of variations in the rates of illness and death. The terms SES and social class are used interchangeably in the literature, but we treat SES as the preferred term except when explicit theories of social class are invoked. SES is typically assessed more in line with Weberian notions of stratification (income, education, occupation, and ownership of property) than with the Marxist emphasis on relationship to the system of production.

Recent reviews reveal that SES remains a persistent and pervasive predictor of variations in health outcomes.[1-10] A robust inverse association between SES and health status dates back to our earliest records and exists in all countries where it has been examined. Some of the clearest recent evidence for the United States comes from studies of mortality rates. Descriptive data from the National Longitudinal Mortality Study (NLMS) reveal, for example, that higher levels of both income and education are associated with lower rates of mortality.[11] For blacks and whites, males and females, the mortality ratios for persons with a total family income of less than $5,000 (in 1980 dollars) per year were at least twice those of persons with incomes greater than $50,000 per year. Other recent studies have also found a strong inverse relationship between SES and mortality.[12-16]

Research interest in the association between SES and mental health status has been declining over time,[17] but recent findings continue to demonstrate a powerful role for SES. The Epidemiologic Catchment Area study (ECA), the largest study of psychiatric disorders ever conducted in the United States, found that low SES predicted elevated rates of a broad range of psychiatric conditions.[18,19] Moreover, this inverse association between SES and psychiatric disorders was evident for both blacks and whites.[20]

The direction of causality between SES and health has been debated in the literature. The positive association between SES and health could reflect selection or "drift" processes where poor health is the cause of low SES. The competing social causation hypothesis views the elevated rates of illness among low-SES populations as a consequence of their low socioeconomic circumstances. The direction of influence cannot be assessed in the typical study, but a growing number of cohort studies suggest that although health-driven downward social mobility occurs, it makes only a minor contribution to SES differences in health.[4,21,22]

Widening Inequality

The extent to which the association between SES and health has been widening in recent decades has emerged as a major issue in the SES literature. Three U.S. studies have compared SES differences in mortality in recent studies with those reported by Kitagawa and Hauser[23] from the 1960 Matched Records Study. Feldman et al. found that mortality differentials by education increased substantially for white men between 1960 and 1984.[13] Duleep noted that the observed mortality differentials by education and income in the late 1970s for men aged twenty-five to sixty-five years old were not smaller than those in 1960.[14] A comparison of 1960 mortality differentials with those from the 1986 National Mortality Follow-Back Survey found evidence for an increase in socioeconomic disparity.[15]

Much of the widening disparity in health status reflects more rapid gains in health status for high-SES than for low-SES groups, but for some health indicators, evidence suggests a worsening health status at the low end of the socioeconomic spectrum. A recent study by Wagener and Shatzkin,[24] for example, documents that although the SES differential in breast cancer narrowed between 1969 and 1989, breast cancer mortality has been declining for women in high-SES counties in the United States, but rising for women in low-SES counties.

Differences between SES groups in accessibility, utilization, and quality of care, or differences in the benefits derived from medical care, are contributing factors to the widening inequality. Mandinger shows that in the wake of the large budget cuts in health and social service spending early in the Reagan administration, an increase occurred in the number of pregnant women not receiving prenatal care, in the incidence of anemia in pregnant women, and in infant mortality rates among poverty populations in twenty states.[25] Similarly, Lurie et al. found evidence of significant deterioration in access to care, satisfaction with care, and health status in a population of medically indigent adults in California six months after their termination from Medicaid.[26] For example, their mean diastolic blood pressure increased by 10 points (mmHg).

However, an increase in economic inequality is apparently the major driving force behind widening health disparities. Since the mid-1970s in the United

States, there have been an increase in income inequality, a growing concentration of wealth among the highest income groups, and a worsening of the economic conditions of a substantial portion of the population.[27] The economic expansion of the 1980s was accompanied by a deterioration in the standard of living for a majority of households. Compared to the 1970s, in the 1980s more American adults fell from middle- to low-income status, and low-income families found it increasingly difficult to climb into the middle class.[28] This polarization of the income distribution may have resulted from changes in the economy that led to a decline in manufacturing jobs and simultaneous increases in both low-wage (service industry and low-skilled) and high-wage (high-technology industries) employment.

Income inequality has also increased in Western European countries,[27] and a pattern of widening socioeconomic differentials in mortality is also evident in England, France, Finland, Norway, and the Netherlands.[29,30] A study of mortality trends over time in England, Wales, and the Netherlands documents most clearly for England and Wales, although the pattern for the Netherlands is consistent, that a widening of mortality differences between SES groups is partly due to differences in the decline of mortality from conditions amenable to medical intervention. However, the contribution of medical care is limited. The higher SES groups also experienced larger improvements in mortality than did their lower SES counterparts from those causes of death where medical care does not play a major role.[31]

Nature of the Gradient

The nature of the SES gradient in health status has generated considerable interest. Some studies indicate a stepwise progression of risk in the relationship between SES and health status, with each higher level of SES associated with better health status. The most impressive evidence of this pattern comes from the Whitehall Study of civil servants in England.[32,33] This study population consists of adults mainly from one ethnic group, residing in one geographic area, stably employed in white-collar jobs, with limited exposure to industrial hazards. Workers in the lowest occupational grades had a rate of mortality three times higher than those in the highest occupational grades. However, each higher grade of employment had lower levels of mortality and better health status than the prior grade. Further, homeowners engaged in professional employment who own two cars have lower mortality than their counterparts who own only one car.[34] Thus, elevated rates of disease and death are not restricted to the low occupational grades but are evident even for privileged groups, when compared to those of highest SES.

Some recent reviews have noted a similar pattern in at least some studies conducted in the United States, and they have concluded that this finely graded pattern is characteristic of the association between SES and health status.[6,7]

Accordingly, there has been great interest in understanding the determinants of this finely stratified mortality difference that appears to run from top to bottom of the social hierarchy. Several studies document that the gradient is nonetheless characterized by a threshold that predicts a weakening of the association between SES and health. That is, beyond some level of SES, usually around the median for income, additional increases in SES have little or a greatly diminished effect in reducing mortality and morbidity rates. For example, both the Kitagawa and Hauser[23] and the Pappas et al.[15] studies of mortality document diminishing returns to increases in socioeconomic status after a certain level of income. House et al. also report a similar pattern for morbidity indicators.[35] The health gains due to income are small for households above $20,000 per year. Recent analyses of the association between income and mortality in the Panel Study of Income Dynamics (PSID) also find large reductions in the mortality rate associated with increases in income at low levels of SES, but smaller declines in mortality linked to additional income at higher levels of SES.[36] Wilkinson reports a similar pattern for income data in Great Britain.[4]

Evidence suggests that even in a single study, patterns of association vary for different indicators of SES. For example, Rogot[11] found in the NLMS a continuous linear gradient between income and mortality for African Americans and whites, males and females, aged twenty-five to sixty-four. In contrast, although an inverse association exists between education and mortality, a graded pattern of association was not evident for all of the four race-sex groups. Clearly needed now are more systematic efforts to identify the conditions under which particular indicators of SES manifest patterns of linear or nonlinear associations with health outcomes. We need to identify the thresholds after which weaker effects of SES are observed, and we also need to identify the social, psychological, material, and especially occupational resources and risks that characterize each level of SES.

Measuring Socioeconomic Position

Numerous variables are used to measure SES: income, education, and occupational status are the most common. Although SES tends to be related to health outcomes irrespective of the indicator used, each SES measure has its own set of advantages and limitations. Some researchers suggest that education is the most stable and robust indicator of SES[23,37] or the most practical and convenient in some contexts.[38]

However, the education measure suffers from several limitations.[9] First, in at least some national data, inequalities in health associated with income are larger than those associated with education, so that using education as a measure of SES may minimize estimates of social inequalities in health. Second, the lack of volatility in education levels for most adults precludes assessing how health status is affected by changes in SES. Third, many studies that use education as an indicator of SES take an individualistic approach and do not incorporate information about the education level of other members of the household. Fourth, as discussed in greater detail later, the return for a given level of education varies importantly by race and gender.

Numerous problems appear with the measure of income. Analyses using income are more likely than those of some other SES indicators to be open to reverse causation arguments. That is, poor health can lead to declines in income, so that the association between low income and health status can be a cause rather than a consequence. In addition, income information may be especially sensitive for some individuals, resulting in higher nonresponse rates for income questions than for other SES indicators. Measuring income well can also be costly and time consuming. Income is probably best measured by the Survey of Income and Program Participation, which uses fifty questions to assess annual income. Moreover, the poverty measure, a widely used indicator of income, is almost forty years old and of questionable current applicability.[39,40]

Income is also a more unstable measure of SES than is either education or occupation. Family incomes throughout the life cycle are characterized by considerable volatility, with many households experiencing sharp losses in income, and a substantial portion of the population is at risk of experiencing such losses. Duncan shows, for example, that between 1969 and 1979 in the United States, between 20 percent and 35 percent of women between the ages of twenty-five and seventy-five experienced poverty at least once.[41] The rates of poverty were higher among women than among men. Persistent poverty, defined as living in poverty for more than half of the eleven-year period, increased with age from 5 percent among women aged twenty-five to forty-five to 11 percent among those in the sixty-six- to seventy-five-year-old age group. Thus, volatility of income also was patterned by age. Measures of education miss this dynamic component of SES, and although highly educated persons are not completely shielded from the volatility of income, they tend to be protected from income drops to near-poverty levels.

Rather than using the volatility of income as a reason not to collect income information, the dynamic nature of income highlights the importance and potential contribution of indicators of long-term economic well-being. Three longitudinal studies have documented that measures of average income capturing long-term exposure to economic deprivation are more strongly related to childhood health outcomes than are single-year indicators of economic status.[42-44] These findings highlight the importance of having longitudinal data with multiyear or long-term measures of income. This larger effect for long-term economic deprivation may reflect the fact that families may use assets or credit to cushion the impact of short-term economic losses.

Permanent income or wealth may thus be better a measure of economic status than is annual household income. In addition, wealth may be more strongly linked to social class location than is earned income. In a study of 100,000 black, white, and Hispanic youth between 1973 and 1990, parental home ownership had a large effect on both school dropout and college entry independent of parental income, education, and occupational status.[45] More health studies should include indicators of assets or wealth. In the National Longitudinal Survey (NLS) of the Labor Market Experience of Mature Men, Mare[12] found that family assets were strongly related to mortality independent of the effects of education and first occupation. Studies in Britain also find that home and car ownership are predictive of decreased mortality risk.[34] The extent to which traditional measures of economic consumption such as the monthly cost of housing and food are predictors of health status is another important but neglected issue.

Occupational status is likely to be a better indicator of long-term income than is income at a single point in time. Nonetheless, there is some volatility to occupational status, and this may also have consequences for health. A national study of black and white male workers found that one-third of the sample changed occupational class over the seven to thirteen years of follow-up.[46] Compared to whites who remained in professional and technical jobs between the baseline and follow-up surveys, African American and white males who remained in the lower occupational classes or made certain transitions, especially into lower occupational classes, had significantly higher rates of new cases of hypertension.

Considering multiple measures of occupational status can also shed light on underlying processes. Mare studied the association of father's occupation, first occupation, and current occupation to mortality in the NLS.[12] Father's occupation was inversely related to mortality, but the effects of first occupation on mortality were stronger than those of father's occupation, and they appeared to be due to the ability of sons from higher SES origins to acquire more schooling. Current occupation and family assets were also linked to mortality. The association between multiple measures of occupation and mortality can be complex. Moore and Hayward found in the NLS data that the occupational category with the highest mortality risk for longest occupation was different from that for most recent occupation.[47]

A practical barrier to the use of occupation for analyses of national mortality data in the United States is that the numerator and denominator do not use the same units of measurement. Denominator data come from the census, which collects information about current occupation. The twenty-one states that record occupational information on death certificates collect information about usual, instead of current, occupation.[9] The collection of uniform data about both current and usual occupation could alleviate this problem.

Krieger and Fee[9] emphasize that social class should be measured at the level of the individual, the household, and the neighborhood. At the individual level, class-based (occupational) measures can capture exposure to occupational health risks, while household SES measures can provide information regarding standards of living and cultural patterns. Community-level measures of SES can provide information about neighborhood-related conditions such as exposure to environmental hazards and levels of neighborhood violence. Two California studies have found that measures of deprivation based on area characteristics were associated with mortality independent of individual socioeconomic status indicators.[16,48] Moreover, Krieger[48] found that a deprivation measure based on census block characteristics (a smaller unit of analysis) explained more variance than did the one based on the characteristics of the census tract. These studies document that area characteristics provide additional information about social inequalities in health that are not captured by individual-level data. Similarly, British studies have found a robust relationship between area-based measures of social deprivation and health status.[49,50] Future research needs to identify the specific characteristics of residential environments that are deleterious to health.

Greater attention also needs to be given to theoretically driven measures of social class. Krieger[48] found that a relational measure of social class (that emphasizes social class location based on relationship to others and to property through employment) was more strongly related to women's reproductive history outcomes than was a measure of household poverty. The three class categories utilized were working class, not working class, and other class. An alternative measure for assessing objective class location distinguishes social class based on the possession of productive assets, property assets, skill assets, and organizational assets.[51] There is growing awareness that SES, as well as social class, attempts to capture a dynamic multidimensional process, and greater attention needs to be given to modeling the joint effects of SES variables.

Other Emerging Issues

The age patterning of the association between SES and mortality has been addressed in recent studies. Early studies noted that SES differentials in health status tend to be largest during middle age but are relatively small at older ages.[52] Analyses of the NLMS data found that although the association between education and mortality exists for persons aged sixty-five or older, it is not as strong as at the younger ages.[11] Similarly, House et al.,[35] using two national probability samples, document that the association between SES and morbidity (chronic conditions, functional status, and activity limitation) is most marked between ages forty-five to sixty-four but narrows with increasing age. Replications and extensions of these cross-sectional findings with short-term longitudinal data provide further support for this pattern with both income and education.[53] However, the evidence is not uniform. Recent analyses by Wu and Ross found the opposite pattern.[54] Using two nationally representative telephone samples, they found that educational differences for three measures of health (physical functioning, self-reported health, and physical well-being) widen with increasing age. It is not clear if these findings reflect differences in the measurement of health status or the coverage of the population.

Women are overrepresented among the poor, but the nature of the association between SES and women's health status is not well understood. The measurement of occupation has been particularly problematic for women. Findings are inconsistent for the few studies that have assessed the association between occupation and women's health. Strong linear SES gradients have been found in some studies, while others report relatively weaker associations than those obtained for men.[55,56] In some studies occupation has been unrelated to mortality risk for women.[57–59]

It is likely that these inconsistencies reflect, at least in part, the limitations of the measurement of SES. Frequently, married women are assigned to the occupational class of their husband, while single women are given their own or their father's class position. The assignment of women to the occupational status of male relatives is increasingly problematic given the growing number of women who are employed outside of the home and the increasing number of female-headed households.[37] Most of the widely used classification systems are based on the occupational patterns of men. Gender-based differences in income and education within occupations and the gender segregation of employment suggest that the inclusion of women may require modifications in occupational classification schemes.[60,61]

Evidence from the United Kingdom reveals that for married women, social class based on the husband's occupation predicts mortality better than does social class based on the woman's own occupation.[62] For single women, own social class is a powerful predictor. A recent study of the relationship between objective class location and subjective class identification for men and women in the United Sates, Sweden, Norway, and Australia found that husband's class location is a major determinant of subjective class identity for women.[51] Thus, women's increasing independence from men appears not to undermine the conventional view of class analysis. These findings also suggest the importance of studying social class at the household level, as opposed to only the individual level, for women.

There is growing interest in understanding the contribution of biological factors to human behavior in general and processes of social stratification in particular. Ellis's review suggests that genetic and physiological factors account for a substantial portion of the variation in both adult education and earning levels.[63] For example, sex hormone levels, especially testosterone, are associated with individuals' career choices, and some twin studies suggest that as much as 40 to 50 percent of the variation in vocational interest can be attributed to genetic factors. However, cause and effect remain problematic because a person's experiences also affect hormone levels. In addition, the determinants of individual risks of disease are often different from those of population risks of disease.[64] It is likely that genetic factors play a larger role in the causes of individual variations in disease than they do in socioeconomic group differences in health status. While guarding against biological determinism is important, social scientists need to give greater attention to the biological mechanisms and processes through which social factors affect health and to the interrelationships between genetic factors and social variables. Much remains to be understood about the ways in which genetic susceptibilities combine additively or interactively with exposures in the social and physical environment to affect health at different stages of the life cycle and for persons living under varying environmental conditions.

RACIAL/ETHNIC DIFFERENCES IN HEALTH STATUS

The United States is relatively unusual among industrialized countries in that it reports the health status of its population based on race.[65] Most other countries focus on social class differences. For most of this century, the contrast between whites and nonwhites (a category that consisted almost exclusively of blacks) was the basis of differentiation. Since the late 1970s there has been a growing emphasis on collecting more data on the racial and ethnic minority populations that constitute an increasing proportion of the American population. Recent reviews reveal that race and ethnicity remain potent predictors of variations in health status.[66-69]

The most recent report card on the health of the U.S. population presents infant and adult mortality rates by race.[70] Infant mortality rates are reported for major subgroups of the Asian and Pacific Islander American (APIA) and the Hispanic population, but subgroup differences were not available for adult mortality. The infant mortality rate for blacks is twice that of whites, and American Indians also have elevated infant mortality rates compared to the white population. The APIA population and its four major subgroups have rates that are lower than those of whites, while the rate for Hispanics is equivalent to that of whites. However, variation occurs within the Hispanic category: Puerto Ricans have higher infant mortality rates than do the other Hispanic groups and the white population. The report also revealed that the age-adjusted death rate for the entire black population is dramatically higher than that of whites, but all of the other racial/ethnic populations have death rates lower than the white population, with the APIA population having the lowest death rates.

These overall data mask important patterns of variation for subgroups of these populations and for specific health conditions, a point readily evident in recent overviews of the health of the Hispanic population.[71,72] While Latinos have lower death rates for the two leading causes of death (heart disease and cancer) than do non-Hispanics, they also have higher mortality rates than do non-Hispanic whites for tuberculosis, septicemia, chronic liver disease and cirrhosis, diabetes, and homicide. Death rates of Hispanics also exceed those of whites in the fifteen to forty-four age group.[73] Moreover, Hispanics have elevated rates of infectious diseases such as measles, rubella, tetanus, tuberculosis, syphilis, and AIDS. The prevalence of obesity and glucose intolerance are also particularly high, especially among Mexican Americans. Similar to the findings for infant mortality, adult mortality rates for Puerto Ricans are higher than the rates of other Hispanic groups. However, even among Puerto Ricans, the mortality rate is lower than for white non-Hispanics and considerably lower than for African Americans.

Specific subgroups of the APIA population have elevated rates of morbidity and mortality across a number of health indicators. The Native Hawaiian population has the highest cancer rates of any APIA population in the United States[74] and the highest death rates due to heart disease of any racial group in the United States.[75] Rates of stomach cancer are high among Japanese Americans, and Chinese Americans have an incidence of liver cancer that is four times higher than that of the white population.[74] Very high rates of obesity are evident for Native Hawaiians and Samoans, and these populations, along with Asian Indians, Japanese Americans, and Korean Americans, have prevalence rates of diabetes that are more similar to those of the black population than those of the white population.[76] Death rates for Native Americans are high for the under-forty-five age group, and suicide rates for American Indian youth are two to four times higher than those of any other racial group.[73] Native American youth also have higher levels of alcohol and other drug use than does any other racial group.[77]

Worsening Health Status

As part of the increasing income inequality in the United States, the gains in economic status of blacks relative to that of whites have stagnated in recent years.[78] Moreover, on several economic indicators there has been an absolute decline in the economic status of African Americans. For example, unlike the pattern for white families, the pattern for low-income black and Hispanic families shows an absolute decline in family income since 1973, and weekly wage and salary income declined for all black and Hispanic males below the 90th percentile of income between 1979 and 1987. Similarly, the percentage of black children living in poverty increased from 41 percent to 44 percent between 1979 and 1988.[79] Similar to the findings noted earlier for SES, this decline in black economic well-being and increase in black-white inequality is associated with worsening black health across a number of health status indicators.

The gap in life expectancy between blacks and whites widened between 1980 and 1991 from 6.9 years to 8.3 years for males and from 5.6 years to 5.8 years for females.[80] Moreover, for every year between 1985 and 1989, the life expectancy for both African American men and women declined from the 1984 level, although an upturn has been reported in the most recent data.[70] A slower rate of decline among blacks than whites for heart disease is the chief contributor to the widening racial gap in life expectancy, while HIV infection, homicide, diabetes, and pneumonia are major causes of decreasing life expectancy for blacks.[81]

The age-adjusted death ratios for blacks and whites were greater in 1991 than in 1980, and the annual number of excess deaths for the African American population, compared to the white population, increased from 60,000 in 1980 to 66,000 in 1991.[80] During this period, the overall age-adjusted death rate decreased more rapidly for white males and females than for their black counterparts. Under the age of seventy, three causes of death—cardiovascular disease, cancer, and problems resulting in infant mortality—account for 50 percent of the excess deaths for black males and 63 percent of the excess deaths for black females. Homicide accounts for 19 percent of the excess deaths for black males and 6 percent for black females. An analysis of death rates between 1900 and the present reveals that black-white health inequality among men is currently at an all-time high for this century.[82] In some depressed urban environments there has been no improvement in the health status of the black population over time. For example, Freeman[83] shows that in contrast to a steady decline in national mortality rates for both blacks and whites between 1960 and 1980, there was no change in mortality for African Americans in Harlem over this twenty-year period. However, the potential contribution of selection processes via migration to this pattern was not assessed.

The gap in infant mortality rates for white and black babies widened for each sex between 1980 and 1991.[80] Rates of both preterm delivery[84] and low birth-weight[80] have remained stable for white women but have been increasing among African Americans. A widening differential between African Americans and whites is also evident for rates of sexually transmitted diseases.[85] Between 1986 and 1989, cases of gonorrhea and syphilis decreased by 50 percent and 11 percent, respectively, for whites. In contrast, gonorrhea declined by only 13 percent for blacks while syphilis increased by 100 percent. The increase in syphilis is thought to be associated with increases in the use of crack cocaine and related increases in prostitution.

Major Historical Events

This recent evidence of deterioration in the health of the African American population emphasizes the importance of considering the larger historical context in understanding the health status of population groups. Mullings has suggested that the civil rights movement, for example, has had important positive effects on black health.[86] By reducing occupational and educational segregation, it improved the SES position of at least a segment of the black population and also influenced public policy to make health care accessible to larger numbers of people. Consistent with this hypothesis, one study found that between 1968 and 1978, blacks experienced a larger decline in mortality rates (both on a percentage and absolute basis) than whites.[87]

More recently, the presidential campaign of Jesse Jackson may have had a positive short-term impact on the health of the African American population. Using four-wave data from the National Study of Black Americans that span the period 1979–80 to 1992, Jackson et al. found that during the third wave of data collection (1988), the reported levels of physical and mental well-being were at their highest.[88] In addition, the proportions of respondents reporting that they had experienced racial discrimination and that they perceived whites as wanting to keep blacks down were at their lowest levels. Contemporaneously, Jesse Jackson, a black male, was making the most successful run for the presidency of the United States that had ever been made by an African American in the history of the United States. These researchers suggest that this political event may have had spillover effects for black adults' perceptions of America's racial climate and their health status.

The massive internal migration of blacks in the United States earlier this century has been an important influence on the African American population. Although the initial economic and longer-term political gains linked to migration may have had positive health consequences, the black migration may have also had profound adverse effects on health.[89] First, the black migration disproportionately distributed the African American population to urban residential areas where living conditions are hostile to life and health. Unlike the white urban poor who are dispersed throughout the city, with many residing in relatively safe and comfortable neighborhoods, the black poor are concentrated in depressed central-city neighborhoods[90] where the stress of poor urban environments can lead to illness.[16,91] A recent study in Harlem, one of the poorest areas of New York City, documented that black males between the ages of twenty-five and forty-four in Harlem are six times more likely to die than are their white counterparts in the United States.[92] Moreover, the life expectancy of blacks in Harlem is lower than that of persons in Bangladesh, one of the poorest countries in the world.

Wilson suggests that the concentration of black poverty in the inner city is due to the out-migration of middle-class blacks to other areas.[90] In contrast, Massey and Gross found that three complementary mechanisms were responsible:[93] the wholesale abandonment of black and racially mixed areas by middle-class whites, the selective migration of poor people into black neighborhoods, and the net movement into poverty of blacks living in segregated areas. Living conditions in inner-city areas are also deteriorating over time. The economic status of central-city African Americans has declined relative to other urban blacks. In 1940, central-city blacks earned 10 percent more than did other black urban dwellers, but by 1980 they were receiving 10 percent less.[78] There is also growing concern about the health consequences of stress in residential environments, such as the high level of community violence in many depressed urban environments.[94]

The internal migration of the African American population also affected health by changing health behaviors in ways that lead to high risks of disease and death. With the great migration and urbanization of black Americans came a dramatic rise in their use of alcohol and tobacco, and a reversal in the racial distribution of alcohol and tobacco use.[95] During the first half of the twentieth century, the prevalence of cigarette smoking and alcohol abuse was higher for whites than for blacks. The great migration shifted a considerable portion of the black population from the relatively "dry" rural South, where social life revolved around churches and family associations, to the "wet" areas of the urban North, where taverns and associated alcohol use were an integral part of social life.[96] Moreover, by producing feelings of alienation, powerlessness, and helplessness, life in urban settings created the need for individuals to mask these feelings or obtain temporary relief from them by consuming tobacco and alcohol. African Americans have been special targets of the advertising of both the tobacco and the alcohol industries,[97,98] targeting that dates back to the 1950s.[99]

A recent provocative theory designed to account for the high rates of hypertension among African Americans also gives a central role to historical factors.[100] According to the "slavery hypothesis," the historic conditions of slavery, especially those linked to capture in Africa and the transatlantic slave voyage, resulted in the preferential survival of those Africans who had a genetic propensity to conserve sodium and water. Contemporary African Americans have inherited this trait, which is responsible for the elevated rates of high blood pressure. Despite its deceptive simplicity and intuitive appeal, like earlier biological explanations, this hypothesis locates racial disparities in health inside the individual and pays scant attention to current living conditions. Serious questions have been raised regarding the plausibility of a historic genetic "bottleneck" being a key determinant of current genetic characteristics,[101] and about the validity of the historic data that have been invoked to support this theory.[102] Moreover, there is abundant evidence that the current social circumstances of African Americans play a major role in accounting for their elevated rates of high blood pressure.[103]

Race and SES

Socioeconomic differences between racial groups are largely responsible for the observed patterns of racial disparities in health status. Race is strongly correlated with SES and is sometimes used as an indicator of SES. For example, while 11 percent of the white population is poor, poverty rates for the African American and Hispanic population are 33 percent and 29 percent, respectively. Not surprisingly, differentials in health status associated with race are smaller than those associated with SES. For example, in 1986, persons with an annual household income of $10,000 or less were 4.6 times more likely to be in poor health than those with income over $35,000, while blacks were 1.9 times more likely to be in poor health than whites.[65] Thus, race differentials were less than half of the SES differentials.

Researchers frequently find that adjusting racial disparities in health for SES substantially reduces these differences. In some cases the race disparity disappears altogether when adjusted for SES.[104,105] Two recent studies provide striking evidence of the contribution of SES to observed racial differences in violence and illegal drug use. Greenberg and Schneider[106] showed that rates of violent deaths in New Jersey were associated not with race per se, but with residence in urban areas with a high concentration of undesirable environmental characteristics such as waste incinerators, landfills, and deserted factories. Violent deaths from homicide, poisoning/drug use, falls, fires, and suicide in these marginal areas were ten times higher for males and six times higher for females than for their counterparts in the rest of New Jersey. Moreover, deaths in these marginal areas were high for whites and Hispanics as well as blacks, females as well as males, and middle-aged and elderly populations as well as youthful populations. Lillie-Blanton et al.[107] also found that a twofold higher prevalence of crack cocaine use for blacks and Hispanics compared to whites was reduced to nonsignificance when adjusted for census indicators of social environmental risk factors. Thus, failure to adjust racial differences for SES can reinforce racial prejudices and perpetuate racist stereotypes, diverting both public opinion and research dollars from the underlying social factors that are responsible for the pattern of risk distribution.

More frequently, it is found that adjustment for SES substantially reduces but does not eliminate racial disparities in health.[9,82,108] That is, within each level of SES, blacks generally have worse health status than whites. One recent study found higher infant mortality rates among college-educated black women than among their similarly situated white peers.[109] Moreover, some studies find that the black-white mortality ratio actually increases with rising SES. This is clearly the case for infant mortality, where the black-white gap is narrowest among women who have not completed high school, and highest among women with a college education.[10]

Kessler and Neighbors emphasize the importance of systematically testing for interactions between race and socioeconomic status.[110] They reanalyzed data from eight epidemiologic surveys and demonstrated that although controlling for SES reduced to nonsignificance the association between race and psychological distress, low-SES blacks had higher rates of distress than did low-SES whites. However, the findings have not been uniform. Analyses of data from the large ECA study found that low-SES white males had higher rates of psychiatric disorders than did their black peers.[20] Among women, low-SES black females had higher levels of substance abuse disorders than did their white peers. These findings suggest the importance of distinguishing distress from disorder, as well as the need to understand the interactions among race, gender, and class.

One reason for the persistence of racial differences despite adjustment for SES is that the commonly used SES indicators do not fully capture the economic status differences between households of different races. For example, racial differences in wealth are much larger than those for income. There are large racial differences in the inheritance of wealth and intergenerational transfers of wealth. Table 22.1 shows that while white households have a median net worth of $44,408, the net worth was $4,604 for black households and $5,345 for Hispanic households.[111] Compared to white households, black households had a significantly greater percentage of their net worth in durable goods such as housing and motor vehicles, and a significantly lower percentage of their net worth in financial assets. Moreover, at every income level, the net worth of black and Hispanic households is dramatically less than that of white households. Thus, in studies of racial comparisons, measures of assets are necessary for the identification of the economic status of the household.

In some cases where blacks are more exposed to particular risk factors, these risk factors appear to have weaker effects for the black population. In a national study in which black children constituted 75 percent of those in the category of lowest long-term income, persistent poverty was unrelated to either stunting or wasting for blacks, unlike the strong pattern evident for non-Hispanic whites and Hispanics.[42] Similarly, although black infants have twice the low birthweight

Table 22.1. Median Net Worth in 1991 by Monthly Household Income Quintiles for Whites, Blacks, and Hispanics

Household Income	White	Black	Hispanic
All	$44,408	$4,604	$5,345
Lowest quintile	$10,257	$1	$645
Second quintile	$25,602	$3,299	$3,182
Third quintile	$33,503	$7,987	$7,150
Fourth quintile	$52,767	$20,547	$19,413
Highest quintile	$129,394	$54,449	$67,435

Source: Eller, T. J. (1994). *Household wealth and asset ownership, 1991* (U.S. Bureau of the Census, Current Population Reports, P70–34). Washington DC: U.S. Government Printing Office.

risk of whites, low birthweight is more strongly linked to infant mortality in the neonatal period for blacks than for whites.[112]

Racism

Another reason for the failure of SES indicators to completely account for racial differences in health is the failure of most studies to consider the effects of racism on health. A growing body of theoretical and empirical work suggests that racism is a central determinant of the health status of oppressed racial and ethnic populations.[10,38,82,113,114] Racism is viewed as incorporating ideologies of superiority, negative attitudes and beliefs toward racial and ethnic outgroups, and differential treatment of members of those groups by both individuals and societal institutions. Racism can affect health in at least three ways.[38,82]

First, it can transform social status so that SES indicators are not equivalent across race. There are large differences related to race in the quality of elementary and high school education, so that blacks bring fewer basic skills to the labor market than whites do.[115] In addition, as Table 22.2 indicates, whites receive higher income returns from education than blacks and Hispanics.[116]

Table 22.2. Median Earnings in 1990 by Education (Years of School Completed) for White, Black, and Hispanic, Male and Female Full-Time Workers

Education Level	Males		
	White	Black	Hispanic
8 years or less	16,906	16,961	13,913
9–11 years	21,048	16,778	17,868
12 years	26,526	20,271	20,932
Some college	31,336	25,863	26,380
College degree	28,263	30,532	33,074
Graduate	47,787	36,851	42,315

Education Level	Females		
	White	Black	Hispanic
8 years or less	11,826	11,364	11,231
9–11 years	14,010	13,643	12,586
12 years	17,552	16,531	16,298
Some college	21,547	19,922	20,881
College degree	26,822	26,881	22,555
Graduate	31,991	31,119	30,133

Source: U.S. Bureau of the Census. (1991). *Money income of households, families, and persons in the United States* (Current Population Reports, P-60, No. 174). Washington, DC: U.S. Government Printing Office.

These racial differences are larger among males than among females, and the black-white income gap for males does not become narrower with increasing years of education. In addition, although Hispanic males do better than their black peers at the higher levels of education, the same is not true for Hispanic females. These data indicate that simply equalizing levels of education would still leave a large racial gap in earned income.

Dressler also indicates that the pattern of income production varies for black and white households.[117] Black households are more likely than white ones to rely on several wage earners to contribute to total household income. Middle-class blacks are also more likely than their white peers to be recent and tenuous in that class status.[118] College-educated blacks, for example, are almost four times more likely than their white peers to experience unemployment.[119] Researchers have also emphasized that the purchasing power of a given level of income varies by race,[113,120] with blacks paying higher prices than whites for a broad range of goods and services in society, including food and housing. African Americans also have higher rates of unemployment and underemployment than do whites. Moreover, employed blacks are more likely than their white peers to be exposed to occupational hazards and carcinogens, even after adjusting for job experience and education.[121]

Second, racism can restrict access to the quantity and quality of health-related desirable services such as public education, health care, housing, and recreational facilities. Recent studies have found a positive association between residential segregation and mortality rates for both adults[122] and infants.[123,124] The relationship between segregation and infant mortality exists for blacks but not for whites. A recent review of racial differences in medical care found that even after adjusting for severity of illness, SES, and/or insurance status, blacks were less likely to receive a wide range of medical services than were whites.[125]

Third, the experience of racial discrimination and other forms of racism may induce psychological distress that may adversely affect physical and mental health status as well as the likelihood of engaging in violence and addiction. Recent reviews reveal that a small but growing body of evidence indicates that the experience of racial discrimination is adversely related to a broad range of health outcomes.[10,38] In addition, the internalization of racist ideology is also adversely associated with morbidity.[38]

In color-conscious American society, skin color may be an important determinant of the degree of exposure to racial discrimination, access to valued resources, and the intensity of the effort necessary to obtain those resources.[117] Dressler[117] has employed darker skin color as an objective indicator of low social status within the black population and found that status inconsistency based on the relation of skin color to lifestyle (ownership of material goods and engaging in status-enhancing behaviors) is associated with elevated rates of hypertension. Independent of education level, persons with darker skin color and higher lifestyle had the highest levels of blood pressure. Klag et al. also found an interaction between skin color and SES in a sample of blacks.[126] Darker skin color was associated with elevated rates of hypertension for low- but not high-SES blacks. Consistent with the notion that darker-skinned African Americans may experience higher levels of discrimination, analyses of data from the National Study of Black Americans found that skin color was a stronger predictor of occupational status and income of blacks than was parental SES.[127]

Age may be a proxy for the cumulative exposure to racism and adverse living conditions. There is an intriguing age patterning of at least some of the racial disparities in health. For both obesity and high blood pressure, racial differences are absent in childhood but emerge in early adulthood.[103,128] Similarly, neonatal mortality rates increase with age of the mother from the teens through the twenties for blacks and Puerto Ricans, while an opposite pattern is evident for whites and Mexican Americans.[129] These patterns may reflect a lagging effect of environmental exposure or a marked change in health status, as young adults are forced to confront restricted socioeconomic opportunities and truncated options.[103] Geronimus has proposed a "weathering hypothesis" to account for this pattern: for disadvantaged populations,[129] age is a proxy for chronic exposure to adverse living conditions, with older age reflecting cumulative exposure to environmental assaults and the consequent increase in biological vulnerability.

Acculturation

The health profile of the Hispanic population in general and Mexican Americans in particular has seriously questioned the dominant paradigm that focuses heavily on SES and medical care as key explanatory factors for racial differences in health. Although Mexican Americans are low in SES and have low rates of health insurance, utilization of medical care, and preventive health care, they have rates of infant mortality, overall mortality, and many chronic illnesses that are lower than those of African Americans and comparable to those of Anglos.[67] Moreover, several recent studies have noted that unlike the pattern for other racial groups, SES is unrelated to health outcomes such as blood pressure and low birthweight for Mexican Americans or foreign-born Mexican Americans.[130,131] It is unclear whether this pattern reflects a healthy immigrant effect, protective effects of host cultures, or differences in the historical time period across societies in the secular distribution of disease. For example, SES has opposite effects in the earlier versus the later periods of the heart disease epidemic. A role for acculturation is suggested by the fact that foreign-born Hispanics have a better health profile than do their counterparts born in the United States. Rates of infant mortality, low birthweight, cancer, high blood pressure, adolescent pregnancy, and psychiatric disorders increase with length of stay in the United States.[72]

Migration studies of the Chinese and Japanese show that rates of some cancers such as prostate and colon increase when these populations migrate to the United States, while the rates of other cancers such as liver and cervix decline.[132]

It has been hypothesized that the cultural factors resident in traditional Mexican culture enhance the health of Mexican immigrants.[133] However, exactly what these protective cultural symbols, attitudes, or experiences are has not been clearly identified. As groups migrate from one culture to another, immigrants often adopt the diet and behavior patterns of the new culture. At the same time the transition to a new culture can also generate stress that may have adverse consequences for health. Several behaviors that adversely affect health status increase with acculturation. These include decreased fiber consumption, decreased breast feeding, increased use of cigarettes and alcohol especially in young women, driving under the influence of alcohol, and the use of illicit drugs.[72] Acculturation also brings declines in caloric intake and fat, and reduced rates of diabetes and obesity.

Earlier studies of acculturation and heart disease among the Japanese immigrants to the United States provide a useful model for identifying and studying the health consequences of different aspects of culture.[134] Rogler et al.[135] have also outlined directions for improvement in the conceptualization and measurement of acculturation and for assessing its relationship to health.

Conceptualization of Race

Researchers have recently emphasized that we need to give more attention to what race is and why it is related to health status. They emphasize that our fundamental assumptions about what race is will shape the research questions developed to understand racial disparities in health.[10,38,113,117] Historically, explanations for differences in health between the races focused on biological differences between racial groups. The biological approach views racial taxonomies as meaningful classifications of genetic differences between human population groups. The available scientific evidence shows that such a view of race is seriously flawed. Our current racial categories do not capture biological distinctiveness. Racial groups are more alike than different in terms of biological characteristics and genetics, and no specific scientific criteria distinguish different racial groups. Williams et al.[38] note that unlike the social sciences, medicine and epidemiology have been slower in rejecting the now scientifically discredited biological view of race. They argue that an emphasis on biological sources of racial variations in health are least threatening to the status quo. Biological explanations focus on factors that reside within the individual and develop solutions that target individuals. They can effectively divert attention from current societal arrangements and policies that shape the health status of population groups.

Diseases that have a clear genetic component account for only a tiny part of racial disparities in health. For example, sickle cell anemia in African Americans accounts for three-tenths of 1 percent of the total number of excess deaths in the black population.[120] Thus, racial differences in biology are not the primary cause of racial variations in health and disease. Although the genetic contribution to racial variations in health status is likely to be small, researchers should be attentive to interactions between biological variables and environmental ones.

Studies that have examined the ways in which race is used in health and medical research document that race and ethnicity are widely used in the health literature to stratify or adjust results and to describe the sample or population of the study.[136,137] However, the terms used for race are seldom defined, and race is frequently employed in a routine and uncritical manner to represent ill-defined social and cultural factors. Researchers seldom specify how race is measured. A more deliberate, purposeful, and theoretically informed explication of race is needed.[137] Race is a proxy for specific historical experiences and a powerful marker of current social and economic conditions that determine exposure to pathogenic factors. Advances in our understanding of the role of race in health are contingent on efforts to directly assess the critical aspects of race that are implicated in health outcomes.

Problems with Racial Data

There is growing awareness of serious reliability and validity problems with the measurement of race and ethnicity.[138] One study of a large national population found that fully one-third of the U.S. population reported a different racial or ethnic status one year after their initial interview.[139] There is also considerable discrepancy, especially for American Indians, Hispanics, and APIAs, between interviewer-observed race and respondent self-report. Massey[140] found, in a large national sample, that 6 percent of persons who reported themselves as black, 29 percent of self-identified APIAs, 62 percent of self-identified American Indians, and 80 percent of persons who self-identified with an "other" category (70 percent of whom were Hispanic) were classified by the interviewer as white. Given that racial status on death certificates is typically based on observer identification, the undercount problem in the numerator for mortality rates may be especially acute for some minority populations. Variations in the classification of race by different administrative systems can affect reported rates of health conditions, and this has also emerged as a major concern.[138]

The implications of census undercount for the quality of health data for racial and ethnic populations have also been receiving increasing attention.[38,141] Census data are routinely used to construct sampling frames for population-based epidemiologic studies, to adjust obtained samples for nonresponse, and to calculate denominators for mortality and selected morbidity rates. Any rate that uses an undercounted denominator is overestimated in exact proportion to the undercount in the denominator. For all five-year age groups of black men ages thirty to fifty-four, the estimated net undercount is almost 20 percent. Estimates of undercount based on demographic analysis are available only at the national level, and rates are probably even higher in selected geographic areas.

There is growing awareness that the Latino, APIA, and Native American populations are characterized by considerable heterogeneity in sociodemographic characteristics as well as the distribution of disease and risk factors for disease.[69,72] Failure to attend to the variations in health indicators within a racial category can prevent the identification of health needs for some specific groups. Increasing attention has also been given to the heterogeneity of the black population.[38] The major white ethnic groups are also characterized by distinctive histories and cultures, but little recent attention has been given to exploring ethnic variations in health for the non-Hispanic white population.

The classification of persons of mixed racial parentage is a significant issue facing data collection agencies, and American society more generally. The numbers of interracial couples and of children from these unions have been increasing steadily over time. The health risks associated with multiracial status have not been systematically studied. Morton et al. studied the birthweight of infants of mixed race in Hawaii and found that such infants had birthweights intermediate between those of their parents' racial groups.[142] A recent study suggests that the relationship between multiracial status and health may be complex: for example, infants born to black mothers and white fathers were more likely to be low in birthweight than those born to white mothers and black fathers.[143]

The noncoverage of selected racial/ethnic subgroups in population-based epidemiologic surveys is a matter of continuing concern. In addition to precluding our understanding of the distribution of disease in certain populations, the unavailability of data also has policy implications. For example, due to the lack of baseline data, there were fewer Healthy People 2000 objectives for the APIA population than for any other racial group.[75] Healthy People 2000 is a national health planning initiative that has defined a set of measurable health targets to improve the health status of the American population by the year 2000. Because it has increasingly become a basis for the allocation of funds to support public health programs, lack of objectives can importantly determine the distribution of economic resources.

MECHANISMS UNDERLYING SES AND RACIAL DIFFERENCES IN HEALTH

Research on the determinants of health has suggested that a broad range of factors, such as stress in family home and work environments, health practices, social ties, and attitudinal orientations, are important determinants of health.

Typically, inadequate attention is given to the ways in which the social distribution of risk factors and resources for health is constrained by societal norms and structures. A growing body of evidence suggests that risk factors for health outcomes are related to SES and race.[5,35,53,144] The distribution of risk factors and resources is shaped by the conditions under which people live and work. Researchers should also be attentive to interactions between social status and risk factors because evidence suggests that comparable stressful events, for example, have stronger negative effects on low-SES persons than on those of higher status.[145]

Medical Care

Inadequate use of medical care, especially preventive medical care, by the poor and members of racial/ethnic minority populations is generally viewed as an important determinant of their health status. There are racial and socioeconomic status differences in the quantity and quality of medical care.[146] A study of deaths of blacks and whites in Alameda County, California,[147] found that deaths due to causes amenable to medical intervention accounted for about one-third of the excess total death rate of blacks relative to whites. Recent reviews of the evidence on the contribution of medicine to health status indicate that the role of medicine is frequently overstated and that the removal of economic barriers alone will not eliminate social disparities in health care utilization.[5,6]

However, equitable access to medical care is important and crucial to preventing further deterioration of the health status of disadvantaged populations.[5] For many disease conditions, such as cancer, tuberculosis, and hypertension, the higher incidence rates among African Americans do not account for the higher mortality rates.[148] The higher mortality rate may result from later initial diagnosis of disease, comorbidity, delays in treatment, or other gaps in the quality of care. Thus, preventive medical care, appropriate early intervention in the course of an illness, and medical management of chronic disease can play important roles in enhancing the quantity and quality of life. Some evidence indicates that medical care has a greater impact on the health status of vulnerable racial and low-SES groups than on their more advantaged counterparts.[5] For disadvantaged groups faced with multiple deficits, medical care may be a critical health-protective resource, while the incremental contribution of medicine is more limited for groups that already enjoy many social advantages.

Health Behavior

Health behaviors are important determinants of health. A U.S. Surgeon General's report indicated that unhealthy behavior or lifestyle accounts for half of the annual number of deaths in the United States.[149] In comparison, 20 percent are due to environmental factors, 20 percent to genetics, and 10 percent to inadequate medical care. Health practices such as better nutrition and eating habits; diminished tobacco, alcohol, and drug abuse; and more exercise can dramatically improve health. The federal report on black and minority health also identified health behaviors as the major determinants of the excess levels of mortality in minority populations in the United States.[150]

Cigarette smoking is responsible for more than one in six deaths annually in the United States, for a total of 430,000 deaths.[151] A growing body of evidence suggests that smoking is increasingly concentrated among the lowest socioeconomic groups and minority populations. The prevalence of smoking is higher for black and Hispanic men than for whites. There is a paradox to black rates of smoking. Compared to whites, African American smokers start smoking later and smoke fewer cigarettes per day, but they are more adversely affected by smoking.[152] In particular, there has been a sharper rise in lung cancer incidence among blacks than whites. Part of this difference may reflect differences in occupational exposures.[152] A much greater proportion of blacks than whites work in occupations where they are exposed to occupational hazards such as toxic chemicals, dust, and fumes. Another factor accounting for this difference is the tendency for blacks to smoke cigarettes with higher tar content than those smoked by whites. More than 75 percent of black smokers use high-tar cigarettes compared to 56 percent of whites and 69 percent of other races. Blacks are also three times more likely than other groups to smoke menthol cigarettes.[151] In general, blue-collar and service workers are more likely to smoke nonfilter cigarettes than are professional managerial workers, and blacks are disproportionately represented in the former category.

Working Conditions

In one of the earliest sociological treatises on the association between social class and health, Engels noted that the average longevity of the upper classes in Liverpool in 1840 was thirty-five years, compared to twenty-two years for businessmen and better-placed craftsmen, and only fifteen years for operatives and day-laborers.[153] He identified conditions of work including machine-paced employment, long hours, exposure to dust, fumes, other bad atmospheric conditions, and having to maintain uncomfortable body positions as major mechanisms responsible for excess mortality. Most recent U.S. studies utilize income and education as indicators of SES and neglect the role of occupational conditions. Low-SES persons are more likely to be employed in occupational settings where there is an elevated risk of exposure to toxic substances and bad working conditions, but the role of occupational conditions tends to be neglected. Moore and Hayward's study is an exception to this pattern.[47] They used data from the NLS and found that the aspects of the occupational environment that accounted for the association between occupation and mortality varied with the occupational indicator utilized. For longest occupation, the substantive complexity of the job (routinization and autonomy) is the major factor, while social skills and physical and environmental demands are the major factors accounting for the effects of the most recent occupation. In a study of over 5,613 persons aged fifteen to seventy-five in Sweden, Lundberg[154] found that the physical working conditions were the major source of SES differences in physical illness, although economic hardship during upbringing and health-related behaviors also played a role. Bad working conditions were defined as heavy work and daily contact with poisons, dust, smoke, acid, explosives, vibration, and the like.

Environmental Exposure

Concerns have also been raised about the extent to which low-SES persons in general and racial minorities in particular are disproportionately exposed to environmental risks in residential environments. One early study found that treatment, storage, and disposal of hazardous waste sites were disproportionately located in areas where the surrounding residential population was black, and a study by the United Church of Christ[155] found that race was the strongest predictor of the location of hazardous waste sites in the United States. However, a recent industry-funded national study found that there is no significant relationship between the racial or ethnic composition of census tracts and the presence of commercial hazardous waste facilities.[156]

The Economy and Health

Brenner has recently reviewed the evidence linking changes in the economy to health status.[157] Rates of suicide and admissions to psychiatric hospitals increase during economic recessions. Cirrhosis mortality increases substantially one to two years after a national economic recession. Instructively, it is the consumption of distilled spirits, rather than wine or beer, that is a significant factor in the increase in cirrhosis mortality. Blacks are estimated to purchase half of all the rum sold in the United States, 41 percent of the gin, 50 percent of scotch whiskeys, and 77 percent of Canadian whiskeys.[158]

In Britain, higher mortality rates are also found for the unemployed compared to the employed.[157] The wives of unemployed men had higher mortality rates during the follow-up period in some studies. This literature also indicates that economic stress induces divorce and separation in families, and adversely affects friendship networks.

Personality

A number of personality variables have emerged as major risk factors for health status or as buffers or moderators of the impact of stressful experiences on health. These personality variables include self-esteem, perceptions of mastery or control, anger or hostility, feelings of helplessness and hopelessness, and repression or denial of emotions.[159] The distribution of at least some health-enhancing personality characteristics varies by SES,[5,144] and future research must seek to identify the ways in which individual dispositions are shaped by the larger social context. Research on John Henryism illustrates the interaction between personality characteristics and socioeconomic status.[160] The John Henryism scale measures an active predisposition to master stress. Research with this measure suggests that John Henryism acts to increase blood pressure among lower SES blacks while simultaneously decreasing it among their higher SES black counterparts. It is interesting that the limited evidence available indicates that John Henryism is unrelated to blood pressure in whites.

Early Life Conditions

Most studies of SES and racial differences in health focus on current socioeconomic status. However, an adult's health status is a function not only of current SES but of the SES conditions experienced over the life course.[5,12] Elo and Preston have provided a comprehensive review of the evidence suggesting that early life socioeconomic and health conditions have long-term consequences for an adult's health status.[161] Several mechanisms appear to be at work. It appears that some diseases acquired in childhood, such as tuberculosis and typhoid, can be harbored for decades and manifest themselves later in life. Infection with the hepatitis B virus can impair liver functioning and lead to cirrhosis of the liver and liver cancer. Living in a crowded household can increase one's risk of streptococcal infection and acute rheumatic fever, which in turn become major risk factors for rheumatic heart disease later in life. Infection plays a major role in growth retardation, and malnutrition as reflected in height may adversely affect the immune system. Diarrhea in childhood can also affect child growth.

In other instances a childhood disease may impair an individual's organ system, which can create a chronic debility that leads to worse health status and earlier mortality. Some childhood illnesses and conditions can lead to changes in adult health status. Nutritional intake in childhood and exposure to and host resistance to infections play a major role in determining adult height. Respiratory tract infections in childhood as well as height (a proxy for early environmental influences) are related to the development of chronic bronchitis, asthma, and emphysema in adulthood. Several studies have also noted an association between height and mortality. Shorter persons have higher mortality rates than do their taller counterparts. However, some of these connections between height and adult mortality can be linked indirectly through SES status achieved in adulthood. There is a positive relationship between height and SES.

There is growing evidence that conditions related to the intrauterine environment during the fetal period and/or patterns of behavior acquired in early childhood are major risk factors for cardiovascular disease in adulthood.[161] Several of these factors appear to have direct relevance for the health status of the African American population. For example, some studies have found that growth retardation during the fetal period or low birthweight is associated with high blood pressure in later life. Rates of low birthweight are twice as high for African Americans as for whites, and low birthweight is believed to be a crude indicator of growth retardation.

Using infant weight up to age one as a proxy for nutritional deprivation in early childhood, a study of over 5,000 British boys documented a strong association between nutritional deprivation in childhood and heart disease in adulthood.[162] Death rates for heart disease were 2.6 times higher for those in the lowest weight category at age one than for those in the highest category. Interestingly, breast-fed children were also at lower risk of heart disease. Breast-feeding is positively associated with SES, and blacks are less likely to breast-feed than whites; rates of breast-feeding also decline for Hispanic and Asian immigrants with assimilation.[163] Infant formula companies aggressively market their product to low-income and minority women, who may be less aware of the benefits of breast-feeding, and the WIC program (a federal program that provides nutritional support to poor women) accounts for 40 percent of the sale of infant formula in the United States.[163]

Power

The proliferation of studies of socioeconomic status and health needs to be placed in an appropriate framework to enhance our understanding of the underlying dynamics. Some studies tend to reify the categories of SES such as education or income by addressing what it is about these specific factors that is linked to health outcomes. Rather, SES measures are crude indicators of location in social structure. A return to the sociological construct of social class can serve to inform and structure our understanding of inequalities in health. Social classes are hierarchically arranged, socially meaningful groupings linked to the structure of society. Systematic inequality will flow from membership in one class rather than another. The Marxist view of class, in particular, emphasizes that antagonistic and contradictory relations will exist between classes as they mobilize and struggle over economic and political power. Class membership leads to differential political and economic power, and inequality in power is a neglected but important construct for enhancing our understanding of the consequences of class for health.[164]

Power is differentially distributed in society, and location in the social structure determines the degree of power and influence that social groups have with regard to the decisions that have a differential impact on all members of society. Good health status is one product of the power of the class to which one belongs. The power of social classes in a given community can be inferred from an analysis of which groups occupy important institutional positions, who takes part in important decisions made over private and public issues, and ultimately, who benefits or is harmed by these decisions and policies.[164] Packham illustrates this process in the case of the location of hazardous waste sites and hazardous production.[164] Similarly, Brenner argues that because of blue-collar workers' relative lack of power (knowledge of occupational health risks and political influence to change their work environments), they are less able to affect the development of occupational safety and health codes.[157] Also, Rice and Winn emphasize that those with the most power and influence have a greater impact on decision making and the allocation of benefits for themselves.[165] Groups with less influence are less competitive in policy and decision-making processes, and therefore they experience inequities in a broad range of societal outcomes linked to this deficit in power. Rice and Winn argue that governmental involvement and advocacy are necessary to reduce the natural tendency for the higher social classes to exert greater control and extract greater benefit from the allocation and distribution of valued benefits and services.

The concept of power along with the related concept of control can serve to integrate major findings in the literature on inequalities in health and can point to promising directions for future research. LaVeist found a strong inverse relationship between black political power and postneonatal mortality rates, and outlines some pathways through which political empowerment may enhance health.[166] Syme also indicates that control may be the key determinant of the SES gradient in health.[167] He argues that the effects of social support, Type A behavior, and stressful life events can all be interpreted to reflect the presence or absence of different aspects of control. Other evidence suggests that the ability to understand, predict, and control daily life experiences can determine both the level of stress to which persons are exposed and the impact of stress on them.[168] Control may facilitate the management of uncertainty, which can be a key determinant of the stressfulness of many social situations. Lack of control in occupational environments has also been shown to predict increased risks of disease.[169]

Differences in power may also undergird the greater awareness of health risks by higher SES persons and their greater responsiveness to health education campaigns. Coleman indicates that access to and control of valuable information in society is a key manifestation of power.[170] High-SES persons are among the first to be exposed to new information and have the necessary economic and other resources to capitalize on new information and to develop alternatives to behaviors that have been shown to be health damaging.

ARE INEQUALITIES IN HEALTH INEVITABLE?

International comparisons of inequality in health and trends in social inequalities over time provide compelling data to address the issue of reducing health inequalities. National mortality rates are not strongly related to a country's overall economic status but are closely linked to the level of inequality within each country.[171] Countries with the least inequality have the best health profiles.[172,173] Differences in income distribution alone account for two-thirds of the variation in national mortality rates for the twenty-three countries belonging to the Organization for Economic Cooperation and Development. Trends in income inequality are also related to SES variations in health over time within a given country. An analysis of SES differences in mortality in England and Wales between 1921 and 1981 revealed that they widened or narrowed to correspond with increases or decreases in relative poverty.[174]

A study of the relationship between education and mortality in nine industrialized countries also suggests that a country's level of egalitarian social and economic policy is linked to the nature of SES differentials in health within that country. Inequalities in mortality were twice as large in the United States, France, and Italy as in the Netherlands, Sweden, Denmark, and Norway.[30] Finland, England, and Wales occupied intermediate positions. Vagaro and Lundberg have shown that the lowest social classes in Sweden have lower mortality than the highest social classes in Great Britain.[175] Thus, the benefits of income redistribution within a society may affect the health status of the majority of the population.

A clear illustration of the link between economic inequality and health is found in the comparison of the trends in life expectancy and income for Japan and Great Britain over the past two decades.[173] In 1970, Japan and Great Britain were similar in average life expectancy and income distribution. During the last two decades SES differentials in Japan became the narrowest in the world, while the income distribution widened in Great Britain. During this same period Japan's life expectancy rapidly increased to become the highest in the world while Britain's relative international ranking in life expectancy has declined. Changes in Japanese nutrition, health services, or prevention policies do not account for these differences.[176]

Further evidence that the health status disadvantage of low-SES groups is not driven by an absolute standard of economic well-being comes from comparisons of the African American population in the United States with their counterparts in the Caribbean. Although the average annual income in Barbados is under US$3,000, life expectancy among black men in Barbados was seventy-one years in 1988, while it was sixty-five years for black men in the United States. Infant mortality in Barbados was similar to that of U.S. blacks—19 per 1,000 live births.[82]

The evidence is fairly clear that reductions in inequalities in health are closely linked to reductions in societal inequality. Factors such as medical care, even if equally provided to all, are unlikely to diminish SES differentials. Improved access to health-enhancing resources may improve health for both high and low social status groups without reducing the health disparity between them. Reducing the SES gradient in health will require more fundamental changes. Freeman suggests that Third World communities in the United States (geographically and culturally defined areas of extreme excess mortality) should be identified and designated as chronic disaster areas.[83] Special federal, state, and local resources should then be provided to such designated areas, as is done in the case of natural disasters. Conditions such as substandard housing, low education levels, poor social support, and unemployment, as well as insufficient access to preventive health services, should then be improved.

Income is probably the component of SES that is most amenable to change through redistributive policies such as tax credits or direct income supplementation. Two studies have documented that changes in household income can enhance health. In a study of expanded income support, Kehrer and Wolin[177] found that the birthweight of the infants of mothers in the experimental income group was higher than that for infants of mothers in the control group, although neither group experienced any experimental manipulation of health services. Improved nutrition, probably a result of the income manipulation, appeared to have been the key intervening factor. Similarly, Wilkinson found in an analysis of mortality over a ten-year period that changes in the proportion of workers with low earnings in specific occupational categories were significantly associated with changes in occupational mortality.[178]

CONCLUSION

One of sociology's most enduring contributions to the health field is the documentation that social class position is a key determinant of variations in the distribution of disease. Researchers in diverse disciplines recognize that SES is so strongly linked to health that they must statistically control for it in order to study their phenomena of interest. However, familiarity has bred complacency, and an opportunity exists for sociologists to provide leadership and direction to enhance understanding of the pathways by which social structure affects health.

The evidence reviewed indicates that large-scale societal factors are the primary determinants of health status. They determine not only the social categories to which people are assigned but their exposure to risk factors and resources. However, the ways in which location in social structure constrains and shapes daily life experiences in ways that adversely affect health is not well understood. Studies that seek to identify these pathogenic factors and mechanisms are urgently needed. Research on racism, acculturation, and power is a fruitful place to begin. However, research and policy aimed at understanding the determinants of and ensuring improvements in health must recognize that intervening mechanisms and risk factors can be understood and effectively modified only in the context of the larger social environment in which they occur.

For example, the high levels of low birthweight among African Americans are regarded as the prime risk factor for elevated rates of infant mortality. However, the mean birthweight for blacks in the United States is similar to mean birthweight in Japan—but Japan has the lowest rate of infant mortality in the world.[179] Not surprisingly, the available evidence indicates that interventions aimed at altering known risk factors without addressing fundamental social causes have had very limited success.[180] Thus, improvement in the health of vulnerable populations appears to be contingent on altering the fundamental macrosocial causes of inequalities in health.

Racial and socioeconomic inequality in health is arguably the single most important public health issue in the United States. The evidence reviewed indicates that SES inequalities in health are widening, and the health status of at least some racial groups has worsened over time. The ranking of the United States relative to other industrialized countries in terms of health has been declining over time, while America continues to spend more on medical care per capita than any other country in the world. The evidence reviewed suggests that a serious and sustained investment in reducing societal inequalities can enhance the quantity and quality of life of all Americans and create the necessary liberty for the pursuit of health and happiness.

Notes

1. Bunker, J. P., Gomby, D. S., & Kehrer, B. H. (Eds.). (1989). *Pathways to health: The role of social factors.* Menlo Park, CA: Kaiser Family Foundation.

2. Haan, M. N., & Kaplan, A. G. (1986). The contribution of socioeconomic position to minority health. In U.S. Department of Health and Human Services, *Report of the Secretary's Task Force on Black and Minority Health* (Vol. 2, pp. 69–103). Washington, DC: U.S. Government Printing Office.

3. Marmot, M. G., Kogevinas, M., & Elston, M. A. (1987). Social/economic status and disease. *Annu Rev Public Health, 8,* 111–135.

4. Wilkinson, R. G., (Ed.). (1986). *Class and health: Research and longitudinal data.* London: Tavistock.

5. Williams, D. R. (1990). Socioeconomic differentials in health: A review and redirection. *Soc Psychol Q, 53,* 81–99.

6. Adler, N. E., Boyce, T., Chesney, M. A., Folkman, S., & Syme, S. L. (1993). Socioeconomic inequalities in health: No easy solution. *JAMA, 269,* 3140–3145.

7. Adler, N. E., Boyce, T., Chesney, M. A., Folkman, S., et al. (1994). Socioeconomic status and health: The challenge of the gradient. *Am Psychol, 49,* 15–24.

8. Feinstein, J. S. (1993). The relationship between socioeconomic status and health. *Milbank Q, 71,* 279–322.

9. Krieger, N., & Fee, E. (1994). Social class: The missing link in U.S. health data. *J Health Serv, 24,* 25–44.

10. Krieger, N., Rowley, D. L., Herman, A. A., Avery, B., & Phillips, M. T. (1993). Racism, sexism, and social class: Implications for studies of health, disease, and well-being. *Am J Prev Med, 9*(Suppl.), 82–122.

11. Rogot, E. (1992). *A mortality study of 1.3 million persons by demographic, social and economic factors: 1979–1985 follow-up: U.S. National Longitudinal Mortality Study*. Bethesda, MD: National Institutes of Health, National Heart, Lung, and Blood Institute.

12. Mare, R. D. (1990). Socio-economic careers and differential mortality among older men in the United States. In J. Vallin, S. D'Souza, & A. Polloni (Eds.), *Measurement and analysis of mortality: New approaches* (pp. 362–387). Oxford, UK: Clarendon Press.

13. Feldman, J. J., Makuc, D. M., Kleinman, J. C., & Cornoni-Huntley, J. (1989). National trends in educational differentials in mortality. *Am J Epidemiol, 129*, 919–933.

14. Duleep, H. O. (1989). Measuring socioeconomic mortality differentials over time. *Demography, 26*, 345–351.

15. Pappas, G., Queen, S., Hadden, W., & Fisher, G. (1993). The increasing disparity in mortality between socioeconomic groups in the United States, 1960 and 1986. *N Engl J Med, 329*, 103–115.

16. Haan, M., Kaplan, G., & Camacho, T. (1987). Poverty and health: Prospective evidence from the Alameda County Study. *Am J Epidemiol, 15*, 989–998.

17. Dohrenwend, B. (1990). Socioeconomic status (SES) and psychiatric disorders. *Soc Psychiatry Psychiatr Epidemiol, 25*, 41–47.

18. Holzer, C., Shea, B., Swanson, J., Leaf, P., Myers, J., et al. (1986). The increased risk for specific psychiatric disorders among persons of low socioeconomic status. *Am J Soc Psychiatry, 6*, 259–271.

19. Robins, L. N., & Regier, D. A. (Eds.). (1991). *Psychiatric disorders in America: The epidemiologic catchment area study*. New York: Free Press.

20. Williams, D. R., Takeuchi, D., & Adair, R. (1992). Socioeconomic status and psychiatric disorder among blacks and whites. *Soc Forces, 71*, 179–194.

21. Power, C., Manor, O., Fox, A. J., & Fogelman, K. (1990). Health in childhood and social inequalities in health in young adults. *J Royal Statist Soc, 153*(Part I), 17–28.

22. Fox, A., Goldblatt, P. O., & Jones, D. R. (1985). Social class mortality differentials: Artefact, selection or life circumstances? *J Epidemiol Community Health, 39*, 1–8.

23. Kitagawa, E. M., & Hauser, P. M. (1973). *Differential mortality in the United States: A study in socioeconomic epidemiology*. Cambridge, MA: Harvard University Press.

24. Wagener, D. K., & Schatzkin, A. (1994). Temporal trends in the socioeconomic gradient for breast cancer mortality among U.S. women. *Am J Public Health, 84*, 1003–1006.

25. Mandinger, M. O. (1985). Health service funding cuts and the declining health of the poor. *N Engl J Med, 313,* 44–47.

26. Lurie, N., Ward, N. B., Shapiro, M. F., & Brook, R. H. (1984). Termination from Medi-Cal: Does it affect health? *N Engl J Medicine, 311,* 480–484.

27. Danziger, S., & Gottschalk, P. (Eds.). (1993). *Uneven tides: Rising inequality in America.* New York: Russell Sage Foundation.

28. Duncan, G. J., Smeeding, T., & Rodgers, W. (1993). W(h)ither the middle class? A dynamic view. In D. Papadimitriou & E. Wolff (Eds.), *Poverty and prosperity in the USA in the late twentieth century* (pp. 240–271). London: Macmillan.

29. Department of Health and Social Security. (1980). *Inequalities in health: Report of a research working group* (The Black Report). London: Author.

30. Kunst, A. E., & Mackenbach, J. P. (1994). The size of mortality differences associated with educational level in nine industrialized countries. *Am J Public Health, 84,* 932–937.

31. Mackenbach, J. P., Stronks, K., & Kunst, A. (1989). The contribution of medical care to inequalities in health: Differences between socio-economic groups in decline of mortality from conditions amenable to medical intervention. *Soc Sci Med, 29,* 369–376.

32. Marmot, M. G., Shipley, M. J., & Rose, G. (1984). Inequalities in death: Specific explanations of a general pattern? *Lancet, 1,* 1003–1006.

33. Marmot, M. G., Smith, G. D., Stansfeld, S., Patel, C., North, F., et al. (1991). Health inequalities among British civil servants: The Whitehall II Study. *Lancet, 337,* 1387–1393.

34. Goldblatt, P. (1990). *Longitudinal study: Mortality and social organisation.* London: Her Majesty's Stationery Office.

35. House, J. S., Kessler, R. C., Herzog, A. R., Mero, R. P., Kinney, A. M., & Breslow, M. J. (1990). Age, socioeconomic status, and health. *Milbank Q, 68,* 383–411.

36. McDonough, P., Duncan, G., Williams, D. R., & House, J. S. (1995). *Income dynamics and adult mortality in the U.S., 1972–1989.* Unpublished manuscript, Survey Research Center, Institute for Social Research, Ann Arbor, MI.

37. Liberatos, P., Link, B. G., & Kelsey, J. L. (1988). The measurement of social class in epidemiology. *Epidemiol Rev, 10,* 87–121.

38. Williams, D. R., Lavizzo-Mourey, R., & Warren, R. C. (1994). The concept of race and health status in America. *Pub Health Rep, 109,* 26–41.

39. Sheak, R. (1988). Poverty estimates: Political implications and other issues. *Sociol Spectrum, 8,* 277–294.

40. Ruggles, P. (1990). *Drawing the line: Alternative poverty measures and their implications for public policy.* Washington, DC: Urban Institute.

41. Duncan, G. (1988). The volatility of family income over the life course. In P. Bates, D. Featherman, & R. Lerner (Eds.), *Life span development and behavior* (Vol. 9, pp. 317–358). Hillsdale, NJ: Erlbaum.

42. Miller, J. E., & Korenman, S. (1994). Poverty and children's nutritional status in the United States. *Am J Epidemiol, 140*, 233–243.

43. Takeuchi, D. T., Williams, D. R., & Adair, R. K. (1991). Economic stress in the family and children's emotional and behavioral problems. *J Marriage Fam, 53*, 1031–1041.

44. Duncan, G. J., Brooks-Gunn, J., & Klebanov, P. K. (1994). Economic deprivation and early childhood development. *Child Dev, 65*, 296–318.

45. Hauser, R. M. (1993). Trends in college entry among blacks, Hispanics, and whites. In C. Clotfelter & M. Rothschild (Eds.), *Studies of supply and demand in higher education* (pp. 61–119). Chicago: University of Chicago Press.

46. Waitzman, N. J., & Smith, K. R. (1994). The effects of occupational class transitions on hypertension: Racial disparities among working class men. *Am J Public Health, 84*, 945–950.

47. Moore, D. E., & Hayward, M. D. (1990). Occupational careers and mortality of elderly men. *Demography, 27*, 31–53.

48. Krieger, N. (1991). Women and social class: A methodological study comparing individual, household, and census measures as predictors of black/white differences in reproductive history. *J Epidemiol Community Health, 45*, 35–42.

49. Townsend, P., Phillimore, P., & Beattie, A. (1988). *Health and deprivation: Inequality and the north.* London: Croom Helm.

50. Carstairs, V., & Morris, R. (1989). Deprivation and mortality: An alternative to social class? *Community Med, 11*, 210–219.

51. Baxter, J. (1994). Is husband's class enough? Class location and class identity. *Am Sociol Rev, 59*, 220–235.

52. Antonovsky, A. (1967). Social class, life expectancy and overall mortality. *Milbank Q, 45*, 31–73.

53. House, J. S., Lepkowski, J. M., Kinney, A. M., Mero, R. P., Kessler, R. C., & Herzog, A. R. (1994). The social stratification of aging and health. *J Health Soc Behav, 35*, 213–234.

54. Wu, C., & Ross, C. E. (1994). *Education, age, and health.* Paper presented at the annual meeting of the American Sociological Association, Los Angeles.

55. Arber, S. (1987). Social class, non-employment and chronic illness: Continuing the inequalities in health debate. *Br Med J, 294*, 1069–1073.

56. Arber, S. (1991). Class, paid employment and family roles: Making sense of structural disadvantage, gender and health status. *Soc Sci Med, 32*, 425–436.

57. Passannante, M. K., & Nathanson, C. (1985). Female labor force participation and female mortality in Wisconsin, 1974–78. *Soc Sci Med, 21*, 655–665.

58. Hibbard, J., & Pope, C. (1991). Effect of domestic and occupational roles on morbidity and mortality. *Soc Sci Med, 32*, 805–811.

59. Moen, P., Dempster-McClain, D., & Williams, R. (1989). Social integration and longevity: An event history analysis of women's roles and resilience. *Am Sociol Rev, 54*, 635–647.

60. Haug, M. (1977). Measurement on social stratification. *Annu Rev Sociol, 3,* 51–77.

61. Powers, M., & Holmberg, J. (1982). Occupational status scores: Changes introduced by the inclusion of women. In M. Powers (Ed.), *Measures of socioeconomic status: Current issues* (pp. 55–81). Boulder, CO: Westview Press.

62. Moser, K. A., Pugh, H., & Goldblatt, P. (1990). Mortality and the social classification of women. In P. Goldblatt (Ed.), *Longitudinal study: Mortality and social organization* (Ser. LS, No. 6, pp. 146–162). London: Her Majesty's Stationery Office.

63. Ellis, L. (Ed.). (1993). *Social stratification and socioeconomic inequality* (Vol. 1). Westport, CT: Praeger.

64. Rose, G. (1985). Sick individuals and sick populations. *Int J Epidemiol, 14,* 32–38.

65. Navarro, V. (1990). Race or class versus race and class: Mortality differentials in the United States. *Lancet, 336,* 1238–1240.

66. Braithwaite, R. L., & Taylor, S. E. (1992). *Health issues in the black community.* San Francisco: Jossey-Bass.

67. Furino, A. (Ed.). (1992). *Health policy and the Hispanic.* Boulder, CO: Westview Press.

68. Livingston, I. L. (1994). *Handbook of black American health: The mosaic of conditions, issues, policies, and prospects.* Westport, CT: Greenwood Press.

69. Zane, N.W.S., Takeuchi, D. T., & Young, K.N.S., (Eds.). (1994). *Confronting critical health issues of Asian and Pacific Islander Americans.* Thousand Oaks, CA: Sage.

70. National Center for Health Statistics. (1994). *Health, United States, 1993.* Hyattsville, MD: U.S. Department of Health and Human Services.

71. Sorlie, P. D., Backlund, E., Johnson, N. J., & Rogot, E. (1993). Mortality by Hispanic status in the United States. *JAMA, 270,* 2464–2468.

72. Vega, W. A., & Amaro, H. (1994). Latino outlook: Good health, uncertain prognosis. *Annu Rev Public Health, 15,* 39–67.

73. Fingerhut, L. A., & Makuc, D. M. (1992). Mortality among minority populations in the United States. *Am J Public Health, 82,* 1168–1170.

74. Lin-Fu, J. S. (1993). Asian and Pacific Islander Americans: An overview of demographic characteristics and health care issues. *Asian Am Pacific Islander J Health, 1,* 20–36.

75. Chen, M. S. (1993). A 1993 status report on the health status of Asian American and Pacific Islanders: Comparisons with *Healthy People 2000* objectives. *Asian Am Pacific Islander J Health, 1,* 37–55.

76. Crews, D. E. (1994). Obesity and diabetes. In N.W.S. Zane, D. T. Takeuchi, & K.N.J. Young (Eds.), *Confronting critical health issues of Asian and Pacific Islander Americans* (pp. 174–208). Thousand Oaks, CA: Sage.

77. Smith, E. M. (1993). Race or racism? Addiction in the United States. *Ann Epidemiol, 3,* 165–170.

78. Smith, J. P., & Welch, F. R. (1989). Black economic progress after Myrdal. *J Econ Lit, 27,* 519–564.

79. Hernandez, D. J. (1993). *America's children: Resources from family, government and the economy.* New York: Russell Sage Foundation.

80. National Center for Health Statistics. (1994). *Excess deaths and other mortality measures for the black population: 1979–81 and 1991.* Hyattsville, MD: U.S. Public Health Service.

81. Kochanek, K. D., Maurer, J. D., & Rosenberg, H. M. (1994). Why did black life expectancy decline from 1984 through 1989 in the United States? *Am J Public Health, 84,* 938–944.

82. Cooper, R. S. (1993). Health and the social status of blacks in the United States. *Ann Epidemiol, 3,* 137–144.

83. Freeman, H. P. (1993). Poverty, race, racism, and survival. *Ann Epidemiol, 3,* 145–149.

84. Rowley, D. L., Hogue, C.J.R., Blackmore, A. C., Ferre, C. D., Hatfield-Timajchy, K., et al. (1993). Preterm delivery among African-American women: A research strategy. *Am J Prev Med, 9*(Suppl.), 1–6.

85. Castro, K. G. (1993). Distribution of acquired immunodeficiency syndrome and other sexually transmitted diseases in racial and ethnic populations, United States: Influences of life-style and socioeconomic status. *Ann Epidemiol, 3,* 181–184.

86. Mullings, L. (1989). Inequality and African-American health status: Policies and prospects. In W. A. VanHome & T. V. Tonnesen (Eds.), *Twentieth century dilemmas—Twenty-first century prognoses* (pp. 154–182). Madison: University of Wisconsin, Institute on Race and Ethnicity.

87. Cooper, R. S., Steinhauer, M., Schatzkin, A., & Miller, W. (1981). Improved mortality among U.S. blacks, 1968–78: The role of antiracist struggle. *Int J Health Serv, 11,* 511–522.

88. Jackson, J. S., Brown, T. N., Williams, D. R., Torres, M., Sellers, S. L., & Brown, K. (1995). Perceptions and experiences of racism and the physical and mental health status of African Americans: A thirteen year national panel study. *Ethn Dis, 5*(1).

89. Williams, D. R. (1995). Poverty, racism and migration: The health of the African American population. In S. Pedraza & R. G. Rumbaut (Eds.), *Immigration, race, and ethnicity in America: Historical and contemporary perspectives.* Belmont, CA: Wadsworth.

90. Wilson, W. J. (1987). *The truly disadvantaged.* Chicago: University of Chicago Press.

91. Harburg, E., Erfurt, J., Chape, C., Havenstein, L., Scholl, W., & Schork, M. A. (1973). Sociological stressor areas and black-white blood pressure: Detroit. *J Chronic Dis, 26,* 595–611.

92. McCord, C., & Freeman, H. P. (1990). Excess mortality in Harlem. *N Engl J Med, 322,* 173–177.

93. Massey, D. S., & Gross, A. B. (1993). *Black migration, segregation, and the spatial concentration of poverty.* Irving B. Harris Graduate School of Public Policy Studies Working Paper, Ser. 93-3, University of Chicago.

94. Gabarino, J., Dubrow, N., Kostelney, K., & Pardo, C. (1992). *Children in danger: Coping with the consequences of community violence.* San Francisco: Jossey-Bass.

95. Williams, D. R. (1991). Social structure and the health behavior of blacks. In K. W. Schaie, J. S. House, & D. Blazer (Eds.), *Aging, health behaviors and health outcomes* (pp. 59–64). Hillsdale, NJ: Erlbaum.

96. Herd, D. (1985). Migration, cultural transformation and the rise of black liver cirrhosis mortality. *Br J Addict, 80,* 397–410.

97. Davis, R. M. (1987). Current trends in cigarette advertising and marketing. *N Engl J Med, 316,* 725–732.

98. Singer, M. (1986). Toward a political economy of alcoholism. *Soc Sci Med, 23,* 113–130.

99. Levin, M. (1988). The tobacco industry's strange bedfellows. *Bus Soc Rev, 65,* 11–17.

100. Wilson, T. W., & Grim, C. E. (1991). Biohistory of slavery and blood pressure differences in blacks today. *Hypertension, 17*(Suppl. I), 122–128.

101. Jackson, F.L.C. (1991). An evolutionary perspective on salt, hypertension, and human genetic variability. *Hypertension, 17*(1, Suppl. 1), 129–132.

102. Curtin, P. D. (1992). The slavery hypothesis for hypertension among African Americans: The historical evidence. *Am J Public Health, 82,* 1681–1686.

103. Williams, D. R. (1992). Black-white differences in blood pressure: The role of social factors. *Ethn Dis, 2,* 126–141.

104. Baquet, C. R., Horm, J. W., Gibbs, T., & Greenwald, P. (1991). Socioeconomic factors and cancer incidence among blacks and whites. *J Natl Cancer Inst, 83,* 551–557.

105. Rogers, R. G. (1992). Living and dying in the U.S.A.: Sociodemographic determinants of death among blacks and whites. *Demography, 29,* 287–303.

106. Greenberg, M., & Schneider, D. (1994). Violence in American cities: Young black males is the answer, but what was the question? *Soc Sci Med, 39,* 179–187.

107. Lillie-Blanton, M., Anthony, J. C., & Schuster, C. R. (1993). Probing the meaning of racial or ethnic group comparisons in crack cocaine smoking. *JAMA, 269,* 993–997.

108. Otten, M. C., Teutsch, S. M., Williamson, D. F., & Marks, J. S. (1990). The effect of known risk factors on the excess mortality of black adults in the United States. *JAMA, 263,* 845–850.

109. Schoendorf, K. C., Hogue, C.J.R., Kleinman, J. C., & Rowley, D. (1992). Mortality among infants of black as compared with white college-educated parents. *N Engl J Med, 326,* 1522–1526.

110. Kessler, R. C., & Neighbors H. W. (1986). A new perspective on the relationships among race, social class, and psychological distress. *J Health Soc Behav, 27,* 107–115.

111. Eller, T. J. (1994). *Household wealth and asset ownership, 1991* (U.S. Bureau of the Census, Current Population Reports, P70–34). Washington, DC: U.S. Government Printing Office.

112. Hogue, C.J.R., Buehler, J. W., Strauss, L. T., & Smith, J. C. (1987). Overview of the National Infant Mortality Surveillance (NIMS) project: Design, methods, results. *Pub Health Rep, 102,* 126–138.

113. King, G., & Williams, D. R. (1995). Race and health: A multi-dimensional approach to African American health. In S. Levine, D. C. Walsh, B. C. Amick, & A. R. Tarlov (Eds.), *Society and health: Foundation for a nation.* New York: Oxford University Press.

114. Williams, D. R. (Ed.). (1995). Special issue on racism and health. *Ethn Dis, 5.*

115. Maxwell, N. L. (1994). The effect on black-white wage differences in the quantity and quality of education. *Indust Labor Relations Rev, 47,* 249–264.

116. U.S. Bureau of the Census. (1991). *Money income of households, families, and persons in the United States* (Current Population Reports, Ser. P-60, No. 174). Washington, DC: U.S. Government Printing Office.

117. Dressler, W. W. (1993). Health in the African American community: Accounting for health inequalities. *Med Anthropol Q, 7,* 325–345.

118. Collins, S. M. (1983). The making of the black middle class. *Soc Problems, 10,* 369–382.

119. Wilhelm, S. M. (1987). Economic demise of blacks in America: A prelude to genocide? *J Black Studies, 17,* 201–254.

120. Cooper, R. (1984). A note on the biological concept of race and its application in epidemiologic research. *Am Heart J, 108,* 715–723.

121. Robinson, J. (1984). Racial inequality and the probability of occupation-related injury or illness. *Milbank Q, 62,* 567–590.

122. Polednak, A. P. (1993). Poverty, residential segregation, and black/white mortality rates in urban areas. *J Health Care Poor Underserved, 4,* 363–373.

123. LaVeist, T. A. (1989). Linking residential segregation and infant mortality in U.S. cities. *Sociol Soc Res, 73,* 90–94.

124. Polednak, A. P. (1991). Black-white differences in infant mortality in 38 standard metropolitan statistical areas. *Am J Public Health, 81,* 1480–1482.

125. Council on Ethical and Judicial Affairs, American Medical Association. (1990). Black-white disparities in health care. *JAMA, 263,* 2344–2346.

126. Klag, M. H., Whelton, P. K., Coresh, J., Grim, C. E., & Kuller, L. H. (1991). The association of skin color with blood pressure in U.S. blacks with low socioeconomic status. *JAMA, 265,* 599–602.

127. Keith, V. M., & Herring, C. (1991). Skin tone and stratification in the black community. *Am J Sociol, 97,* 760–778.

128. Kumanyika, S. K. (1987). Obesity in black women. *Epidemiol Rev, 9*, 31–50.

129. Geronimus, A. T. (1992). The weathering hypothesis and the health of African-American women and infants: Evidence and speculations. *Ethn Dis, 2*, 207–221.

130. Sorel, J. E., Ragland, D. R., Syme, S. L., & Davis, W. B. (1992). Educational status and blood pressure: The second National Health and Nutrition Examination Survey, 1976–1980, and the Hispanic Health and Nutrition Examination Survey, 1982–1984. *Am J Epidemiol, 135*, 1339–1348.

131. Collins, J. W., Jr., & Shay, D. K. (1994). Prevalence of low birthweight among Hispanic infants with United States–born and foreign-born mothers: The effect of urban poverty. *Am J Epidemiol, 139*, 184–192.

132. Jenkins, C.N.H., & Kagawa-Singer, M. (1994). Cancer. In N.W.S. Zane, D. T. Takeuchi, & K.N.J. Young (Eds.), *Confronting critical health issues of Asian and Pacific Islander Americans* (pp. 105–147). Thousand Oaks, CA: Sage.

133. James, S. A. (1993). Racial and ethnic differences in infant mortality and low birth weight. *Ann Epidemiol, 3*, 130–136.

134. Marmot, M. G., & Syme, S. L. (1976). Acculturation and coronary heart disease in Japanese-Americans. *Am J Epidemiol, 104*, 225–247.

135. Rogler, L. H., Cortes, D. E., & Malgady, R. G. (1991). Acculturation and mental health status among Hispanics. *Am Psychol, 46*, 585–597.

136. Jones, C. P., LaVeist, T. A., & Lillie-Blanton, M. (1991). Race in the epidemiologic literature: An examination of the *American Journal of Epidemiology,* 1921–1990. *Am J Epidemiol, 134*, 1079–1084.

137. Williams, D. R. (1994). The concept of race in *Health Services Research,* 1966–1990. *Health Serv Res, 29*, 261–274.

138. Hahn, R. A. (1992). The state of federal health statistics on racial and ethnic groups. *JAMA, 267*, 255–258.

139. Johnson, C. E. (1974). *Consistency of reporting ethnic origin in the current population survey* (U.S. Department of Commerce Technical Paper No. 31). Washington, DC: U.S. Bureau of the Census.

140. Massey, J. T. (1980). *A comparison of interviewer observed race and respondent reported race in the National Health Interview Survey.* Paper presented at the annual meeting of the American Statistical Association, Houston.

141. Census undercount and the quality of health data for racial and ethnic populations (Notes & Comments). (1994). *Ethn Dis, 4*, 98–100.

142. Morton, N. E., Chung, C. S., & Mi, M.-P. (1967). *Genetics of interracial crosses in Hawaii.* Basel, Switzerland: S. Karger.

143. Collins, J. W., Jr., & David, R. J. (1993). Race and birthweight in biracial infants. *Am J Public Health, 83*, 1125–1129.

144. Mirowsky, J., & Ross, C. E. (1989). *Social causes of distress.* New York: Aldine de Gruyter.

145. Kessler, R. C. (1979). Stress, social status, and psychological distress. *J Health Soc Behav, 20*, 259–272.

146. Blendon, R., Aiken, L., Freeman, H., & Corey, C. (1989). Access to medical care for black and white Americans. *JAMA, 261,* 278–281.

147. Woolhandler, S., Himmelstein, D. U., Silber, R., Bader, M., Harnly, M., & Jones, A. A. (1985). Medical care and mortality: Racial differences in preventable deaths. *Int J Health Serv, 15,* 1–11.

148. Schwartz, E., Kofie, V. Y., Rivo, M., & Tuckson, R. V. (1990). Black/white comparisons of deaths preventable by medical intervention: United States and the District of Columbia, 1980–1986. *Int J Epidemiol, 19,* 591–598.

149. U.S. Department of Health, Education, and Welfare. (1979). *Healthy people: The Surgeon General's report on health promotion and disease prevention.* Washington, DC: U.S. Government Printing Office.

150. U.S. Department of Health and Human Services. (1985). *Report of the Secretary's Task Force on Black and Minority Health.* Washington, DC: U.S. Government Printing Office.

151. Chen, V. W. (1993). Smoking and the health gap of minorities. *Ann Epidemiol, 3,* 159–164.

152. Sterling, T. D., & Weinkam, J. J. (1989). Comparison of smoking-related risk factors among black and white males. *Am J Industr Med, 15,* 319–333.

153. Engels, F. (1984). *The condition of the working class in England.* Chicago: Academy Chicago. (Original work published 1844.)

154. Lundberg, O. (1991). Causal explanations for class inequality in health: An empirical analysis. *Soc Sci Med, 32,* 385–393.

155. Commission for Racial Justice. (1987). *Toxic wastes and race in the United States: A national report on the racial and socioeconomic characteristics of communities with hazardous waste sites.* New York: United Church of Christ.

156. Anderton, D. L., Anderson, A. B., Oakes, J. M., & Fraser, M. R. (1994). Environmental equity: The demographics of dumping. *Demography, 31,* 229–248.

157. Brenner, M. H. (1995). Economy, society, and health: Theoretical links and empirical relations. In S. Levine, D. C. Walsh, B. C. Amick, & A. R. Tarlov (Eds.), *Society and health: Foundation for a nation.* New York: Oxford University Press.

158. Djata. (1987). The marketing of vices to black consumers. *Bus Soc Rev, 62,* 47–49.

159. Kessler, R. C., House, J. S., Anspach, R., & Williams, D. R. (1995). Social psychology and health. In K. Cook, G. Fine, & J. S. House (Eds.), *Sociological perspectives on social psychology* (pp. 548–570). Boston: Allyn & Bacon.

160. James, S. A. (1994). John Henryism and the health of African-Americans. *Cult Med Psychiatry, 18,* 163–182.

161. Elo, I. T., & Preston, S. H. (1992). Effects of early-life conditions on adult mortality: A review. *Popul Index, 58,* 186–212.

162. Barker, D.J.P., Osmond, C., Winter, P. D., Margetts, B., & Simmonds, S. J. (1989). Weight in infancy and death from ischaemic heart disease. *Lancet, 9,* 578–580.

163. Jeffrey, C. (1993). Formula for failure. *Chicago Reporter, 22,* 1, 6–11.

164. Packham, J. (1991). *Power as a neglected variable in the assessment of the class/health relation.* Paper presented at the annual meeting of the American Sociological Association.

165. Rice, M. F., & Winn, M. (1990). Black health care in America: A political perspective. *J Natl Med Assoc, 82,* 429–437.

166. LaVeist, T. A. (1992). The political empowerment and health status of African-Americans: Mapping a new territory. *Am J Sociol, 97,* 1080–1095.

167. Syme, S. L. (1991). Control and health: A personal perspective. *Advances, 7,* 16–27.

168. Sutton, R., & Kahn, R. L. (1987). Prediction, understanding and control as antidotes to organizational stress. In J. W. Lorsch (Ed.), *Handbook of organizational behavior* (pp. 272–285). Englewood Cliffs, NJ: Prentice Hall.

169. Karasek, R. A., & Theorell, T. (1990). *Healthy work.* New York: Basic Books.

170. Coleman, J. S. (1974). *Power and the structure of society.* New York: Norton.

171. Wilkinson, R. G. (1992). National mortality rates: The impact of inequality? *Am J Public Health, 82,* 1082–1084.

172. Smith, D. G., Bartley, M., & Blane, D. (1990). The Black Report on socioeconomic inequalities in health 10 years on. *Br Med J, 301,* 373–377.

173. Wilkinson, R. G. (1992). Income distribution and life expectancy. *Br Med J, 304,* 165–168.

174. Wilkinson, R. G. (1989). Class mortality differentials, income distribution and trends in poverty, 1921–81. *J Soc Policy, 18,* 307–335.

175. Vagaro, D., & Lundberg, O. (1989). Health inequalities in Britain and Sweden. *Lancet, II*(8653), 35–36.

176. Marmot, M. G., & Smith D. G. (1989). Why are the Japanese living longer? *Br Med J,* pp. 1547–1551.

177. Kehrer, B. H., & Wolin, C. M. (1979). Impact of income maintenance on low birth weight: Evidence from the Gary experiment. *J Hum Resour, 14,* 434–462.

178. Wilkinson, R. G. (1990). Income distribution and mortality: A "natural" experiment. *Soc Health Illness, 12,* 391–412.

179. Wise, P. H., & Pursley, D. M. (1992). Infant mortality as a social mirror. *N Engl J Med, 326,* 1558–1560.

180. Syme, S. L. (1994). The social environment and health. *Daedalus, 123,* 79–86.

CHAPTER TWENTY-THREE

The Relationship of Neighborhood Socioeconomic Characteristics to Birthweight Among Five Ethnic Groups in California

Michelle Pearl
Paula Braveman
Barbara Abrams

The association between lower socioeconomic status (SES) and poor birth outcomes has been well documented in the United States.[1-5] In recent years, several studies, after accounting for the personal socioeconomic characteristics of mothers, have reported an association between measures of neighborhood socioeconomic deprivation and poor birth outcomes.[6-12] These studies support a growing literature demonstrating increased risks of adult mortality,[8,13-16] long-term illness,[17] lower ratings for self-rated health,[18] cardiovascular disease,[19] and smoking[20] associated with poorer socioeconomic conditions of neighborhoods. Such studies highlight the importance of the social environment, in addition to individual socioeconomic standing, in shaping individual behaviors and health outcomes.[21-23]

Although some studies have shown that neighborhood effects on adult health vary by the individual's age, sex, and ethnicity,[22,23] ethnicity-specific findings

Michelle Pearl conceptualized and conducted the analysis and wrote the chapter. Paula Braveman designed and directed the maternity care survey and contributed to the writing of the paper. Barbara Abrams contributed to the analytical plan and interpretation of results. This work was supported in part by the Maternal and Child Health Bureau (Grant MCJ-067951). We wish to thank Steve Selvin and John Neuhaus for statistical guidance and Jeff Gould for analytical suggestions in preliminary analyses. We also wish to acknowledge Kristen Marchi and Susan Egerter, who played major roles in designing, conducting, and analyzing the maternity care survey. Approvals for these analyses were obtained from institutional review boards of the University of California, San Francisco and Berkeley, and the California Department of Health Services.

with respect to birth outcomes have been reported in only one study. That study found that the risk of low birthweight was lower among children born to white women and U.S.-born black women living in middle- or high-income census tracts in New York City relative to those living in low-income tracts, although the trend was reversed among foreign-born blacks.[11] The only study of birthweight that included ethnic groups other than whites and blacks did not present ethnicity-specific results.[6] Among U.S.-born, but not foreign-born, Mexican American mothers, those living in poor census tracts in Chicago had an increased risk of delivering low-birthweight infants compared with those living in less poor tracts; however, that study did not adjust for the mothers' socioeconomic characteristics.[24] No study adjusted for the mothers' personal or family income, leaving open the possibility that unmeasured socioeconomic characteristics of mothers might account for the observed associations.

In this study, we explored the relationship between selected neighborhood socioeconomic factors and birthweight among women delivering in California. The sample included sufficient numbers of Asians and Latinas as well as blacks and whites for subgroup analyses. We hypothesized that the magnitude of association between neighborhood socioeconomic factors and birthweight would vary by ethnicity, as in studies of individual-level socioeconomic measures.[1,25] Information was available on Medi-Cal (California Medicaid) coverage and educational attainment; a large subsample also provided information on family income, which was adjusted for family size, and other risk factors.

METHODS

Data Sources

The subjects were women delivering live infants at eighteen public and private hospitals in California selected for a statewide representative postpartum survey on access to maternity care.[26,27] Eligible hospitals were randomly selected within strata defined by geographic region, proportion of deliveries to black women, and prevalence of private health insurance. An additional hospital that participated in the survey was excluded from this analysis, because birth certificates in that hospital's county were unavailable for geocoding.

We obtained birth certificate data for all deliveries occurring at the eighteen hospitals during the interview phase of the study (August 1994 to July 1995). Of these 23,922 birth certificates, 94.3 percent were geocoded and subsequently linked to information from the 1990 Census of Population and Housing corresponding to census tract and block group areas. Excluding women with multiple births (229) and those whose children's birth certificates had geocodes that lacked valid census data (18), the final overall sample (hereafter referred to as the "overall sample") for this analysis was 22,304 women.

Of this overall sample, a subset of 8,457 women had participated in the face-to-face survey in English or Spanish during their postpartum stays and had records that could be linked with census data (hereafter referred to as the "survey subsample"). Compared with the overall sample, the subsample under-represented mothers younger than eighteen years and foreign-born Asian mothers, consistent with age and language inclusion criteria.

Variable Definitions

The main outcome for this study was infant birthweight, as recorded on birth certificates. We studied birthweight as a continuous variable because maternal education has been associated with birthweight along the entire birthweight continuum.[3] Use of birthweight as a continuous outcome also improves statistical power.[28] We also dichotomized birthweight, with weights of less than 2,500 g representing low birthweight.

We used census data at the tract and block group levels to characterize neighborhood socioeconomic conditions. Block groups typically include 1,000 residents; tracts include 2,500 to 8,000 residents. Census variables included poverty (percentage of residents whose family income was below the federal poverty level); unemployment (percentage of males sixteen years old or older who were unemployed); and low education (percentage of adults twenty-five years old or older with less than a high school education). We present results for measures at the level of block groups (referred to as "neighbor-hoods"); tract-level results were very similar and are available on request.

Individual or family socioeconomic measures included the mother's educational attainment; Medi-Cal coverage during pregnancy; and family income, adjusted for family size. Information on years of education was obtained from birth certificates and modeled as a continuous variable. Self-reported information on family income as a percentage of poverty level was available for the survey subsample only and was treated as a continuous variable. We assessed family income during the twelve months before the interview by using income categories that were specific to family size. Each income category consisted of a range of incomes that represented 50 percent increments of the federal poverty level in 1994 (for example, 0 percent to 50 percent, 51 percent to 100 percent). Less than 5 percent of women in the survey subsample were missing income information. For the overall sample, Medi-Cal coverage during pregnancy, as reported on birth certificates, was used as a measure of income. With rare exceptions, women with Medi-Cal have incomes at or below 200 percent of the poverty level; however, one-third of women in the postpartum survey with family incomes at or below 200 percent of the poverty level were privately insured.[27] Birth certificate reporting of Medi-Cal coverage has been shown to be very reliable.[26]

The mother's self-identified ethnicity and birthplace were defined according to survey responses for the survey subsample and according to birth certificates for the overall sample; agreement between these two sources is excellent.[29] Latinas were further grouped by nativity as foreign-born or U.S.-born, because these two groups showed distinct relationships between socioeconomic measures and birthweight in preliminary analyses. We also studied foreign-born Asians separately. Subgroup numbers were insufficient, however, to stratify by nativity status among blacks and whites (in the overall sample, 78 percent of Latinas, 10 percent of whites, 7 percent of blacks, and 87 percent of Asians were foreign born).

Potential explanatory factors for associations between neighborhood-level socioeconomic conditions and birthweight include the mother's age, parity, and receipt of first-trimester prenatal care, which were described on birth certificates for all study subjects. In addition, survey participants reported self-perceived health status before the pregnancy. Among women born outside the United States, two measures of acculturation were used: the number of years respondents had lived in the United States and speaking a language other than English at home. Women in the survey subsample with family incomes less than 400 percent of the poverty level also reported whether they had smoked during pregnancy, felt their neighborhood was unsafe, or lacked a supportive person to turn to during pregnancy.

Statistical Analyses

To minimize the contribution of individual-level socioeconomic factors in estimates of neighborhood-level associations, we used linear regression models that adjusted for the mother's education and family income or Medi-Cal status to examine the impact of neighborhood factors within each ethnic group. Preliminary analyses suggested nonlinear relationships between income and birthweight among whites, Asians, and foreign-born Latinas; therefore, we included quadratic and cubic terms for income in the models for more complete adjustment of income-birthweight relationships. We also used quadratic and cubic terms to investigate nonlinear relationships between neighborhood characteristics and birthweight. We use tables to present linear coefficients for neighborhood characteristics; we use figures to represent nonlinear models.

We used linear and logistic regression that incorporated generalized estimating equations to account for within-hospital correlation. Although correlation among study subjects may result from inclusion of neighborhood-level variables in regression models,[30] the majority of block groups we analyzed contained only one study participant, and there was no evidence that the independence assumption of ordinary least squares regression was violated by inclusion of block group–level variables.

RESULTS

Table 23.1 presents maternal, infant, and neighborhood characteristics for the overall sample and additional factors for the surveyed subsample, stratified by maternal ethnicity. White women lived in neighborhoods with less poverty, lower concentrations of residents with low education, and lower male unemployment rates than did blacks and Latinas. Foreign-born Latinas lived in neighborhoods with the highest concentration of residents with low education, but similarly high concentrations of poverty and unemployment were observed among neighborhoods of black women. The correlation coefficients for neighborhood-level factors ranged from 0.5 for education and unemployment to 0.7 for education and poverty. The individual- and neighborhood-level characteristics of the survey subsample were generally similar to those of the overall sample, except for expected differences deriving from the survey's exclusion of very young teens. There were fewer mothers with less than a high school education and fewer primiparous women in the survey subsample than in the overall sample.

Coefficients for neighborhood-level factors in Table 23.2 represent the average change in birthweight (in grams) associated with 10 percent increments of neighborhood-level variables, after adjustment for Medi-Cal and mother's education. These results for neighborhood and individual-level measures differed little from unadjusted results. Overall, increasing neighborhood poverty and unemployment were associated with decreasing birthweight. When stratified by ethnicity and birthplace, neighborhood socioeconomic characteristics were related to decreasing birthweight among blacks and Asians only (Figure 23.1). For example, among black women, living in block groups where 20 percent of males were unemployed was associated with smaller birthweight—on the order of 62 g—compared with living in block groups with 10 percent male unemployment. When the analysis was limited to foreign-born Asians, the negative associations between birthweight and neighborhood unemployment and education were similar in magnitude to those among Asians overall and remained statistically significant after all adjustments.

The linear estimates for foreign-born Latinas presented in Table 23.2 mask nonlinear associations between neighborhood-level measures and birthweight among foreign-born Latinas (Figure 23.2). Block group poverty and unemployment were unrelated to birthweight at low concentrations (<25 percent of

Table 23.1. Characteristics of Overall Sample and Surveyed Subsample of Women Delivering at 18 Hospitals, by Ethnicity: California, 1994–1995

	All Women, % (N = 22,304)	White, % (n = 5,666)	Black, % (n = 2,390)	Foreign-Born Latinas, % (n = 9,097)	U.S.-Born Latinas, % (n = 2,592)	Asians, % (n = 2,226)
Individual-level characteristics of overall sample						
Age, years						
<18	6	3	9	5	14	2
18–19	8	5	12	8	15	3
20–34	75	76	68	79	64	75
≥35	12	16	10	9	7	20
Mother's education						
<High school	39	10	19	70	36	13
High school completed	30	36	44	20	39	28
>High school	31	54	38	10	25	59
Medi-Cal coverage	47	18	42	71	45	27
Parity						
1	40	43	43	34	47	46
2–4	55	54	51	59	48	50
≥4	6	3	6	7	5	4
Received 1st trimester prenatal care	77	86	80	70	75	83
Infant birthweight, g (mean)	3,380	3,498	3,184	3,395	3,369	3,239
Low birthweight (<2500 g)	6	4	11	4	6	7

(Continued)

Table 23.1. Characteristics of Overall Sample and Surveyed Subsample of Women Delivering at 18 Hospitals, by Ethnicity: California, 1994–1995 (Continued)

	All Women, % (N = 22,304)	White, % (n = 5,666)	Black, % (n = 2,390)	Foreign-Born Latinas, % (n = 9,097)	U.S.-Born Latinas, % (n = 2,592)	Asians, % (n = 2,226)
Neighborhood* characteristics of overall sample						
>25% of residents were poor	21	4	33	32	21	10
>8% of adult men were unemployed	29	11	40	39	32	15
>40% of adults had less than high school education	37	5	34	62	40	14
Survey subsample characteristics		(n = 2,005)	(n = 907)	(n = 3,832)	(n = 950)	(n = 653)
Family income, % of poverty level						
≤100		19	54	71	50	18
101–200		18	17	21	22	18
201–400		37	21	7	21	35
>400		26	7	1	6	29
Self-rated prepregnancy health was fair or poor		6	13	18	18	9
Felt neighborhood was unsafe†		11	14	11	12	9
Had no supportive person†		3	4	5	3	4
Smoked during pregnancy†		23	17	4	10	6

Note: Characteristics are expressed as percentages, except for mean birthweight. Data are from birth records with linked census data of 22,304 women who delivered in 18 California hospitals chosen for a statewide postpartum survey between August 1994 and July 1995. Subsample data are from interview data from a subsample of 8,457 women whose records were linked with birth records and census data; differences between overall sample and survey subsample are noted in text.

*Census block group.

†Variable available for women in survey subsample with household income ≤ 400% poverty level.

Table 23.2. Change in Birthweight Associated with Mother's Individual and Neighborhood Socioeconomic Characteristics, by Ethnicity, Among 22,304 Women Delivering at 18 Hospitals: California, 1994-1995

	Overall (N = 22,304)	White (n = 5,666)	Black (n = 2,388)	Foreign-Born Latina (n = 9,097)	U.S.-Born Latina (n = 2,592)	Asian (n = 2,226)
	Coef. (SE)	Coef. (SE)	Coef. (SE)	Coef. (SE)	Coef. (SE)	Coef. (SE)
Model 1						
Neighborhood poverty	−12** (4)	−5 (13)	−24 (13)	5† (3)	2 (13)	−18 (16)
Mother's education	−5 (3)	14** (4)	34** (6)	−2 (1)	7 (7)	0 (4)
Medi-Cal coverage	−45* (19)	−50 (36)	−31 (18)	−20 (22)	−63 (37)	−64** (20)
Model 2						
Neighborhood unemployment	−23* (11)	20 (18)	−62* (31)	24*† (11)	−33 (33)	−82 (45)
Mother's education	−5 (3)	15** (4)	34** (6)	−2 (1)	5 (7)	0 (4)
Medi-Cal coverage	−47* (19)	−53 (36)	−43** (13)	−21 (22)	−59 (36)	−60** (20)
Model 3						
Low neighborhood education	−3 (3)	4 (8)	−24** (8)	0 (4)	−6 (6)	−19** (7)
Mother's education	−5* (2)	15** (4)	33** (7)	−2 (1)	5 (7)	−2 (4)
Medi-Cal coverage	−47* (19)	−53 (36)	−20 (21)	−20 (22)	−58 (37)	−60** (20)

Note: Coefficient (coef.) represents average increase or decrease in birthweight (g) associated with a 10 percentage point increase in the specified neighborhood (census block group) characteristic (for example, from 10% to 20% of neighborhood residents with income below poverty level). Coefficients and standard errors are from separate linear regression models of birthweight that used generalized estimating equations to account for hospital clustering. All models include mother's education and Medi-Cal coverage.

†Nonlinear relationships with birthweight were found for these neighborhood variables; see Figure 23.2.

*p < .05; **p < .01.

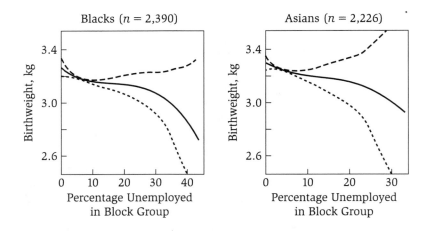

Figure 23.1 Relationship of Birthweight to Neighborhood Unemployment Among Blacks and Asians in the Overall Sample, After Adjustment for Medi-Cal and Mother's Education.

Note: Neighborhood unemployment modeled with quadratic and cubic terms. Data are from birth records with linked census data of women who delivered in 18 California hospitals chosen for a statewide postpartum survey between August 1994 and July 1995. Dotted lines represent 95% confidence bounds, including indicator variables for hospitals to reflect hospital sampling.

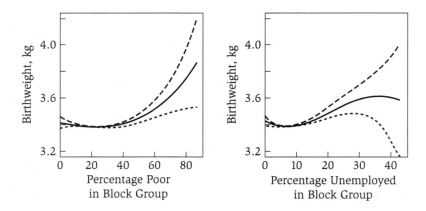

Figure 23.2 Relationship of Birthweight to Neighborhood Poverty and Unemployment Among Foreign-Born Latinas in Overall Sample, After Adjustment for Medi-Cal and Mother's Education.

Note: Neighborhood poverty and unemployment modeled with quadratic and cubic terms. Data are from birth records with linked census data of 9,097 Latinas born outside the United States who delivered in 18 California hospitals chosen for a statewide postpartum survey between August 1994 and July 1995. Dotted lines represent 95% confidence bounds, including indicator variables for hospitals to reflect hospital sampling.

persons with household incomes below the poverty level or <8 percent unemployment). At levels of neighborhood poverty above 25 percent and unemployment above 8 percent, however, birthweight unexpectedly increased linearly with increasing poverty ($\beta = 40$, SE $= 11$, $p < .01$) and unemployment ($\beta = 87$, SE $= 19$, $p < .01$), after adjustment for education and Medi-Cal.

Similar results for the survey subsample, adjusted for individual-level income, are presented in Table 23.3. Among blacks and Asians, lower birthweights were associated with increasing unemployment but not with other neighborhood measures. As observed in the overall sample, birthweights were unexpectedly higher among foreign-born Latinas living in neighborhoods with high concentrations of poverty or unemployment. Foreign-born Latinas in the subsample with higher education levels and those with family income less than 200 percent of the poverty level also delivered babies with lower birthweights.

Further adjustments for mother's age, parity, and timing of prenatal care initiation had little effect on the results presented in Tables 23.2 and 23.3. Among black women in the subsample with a full range of interview data, adjustment for income, education, age, timely prenatal care, fair or poor prepregnancy health, having a supportive person, living in a perceived unsafe neighborhood, parity, and smoking did not diminish the negative association between unemployment level and birthweight ($\beta = -88$, SE $= 38$, $p < .05$ versus $\beta = -86$ in the income- and education-adjusted model for the same subset). For foreign-born Latinas, adjustment for acculturation in addition to the foregoing factors did not appreciably affect the positive linear association between birthweight and increasing poverty or unemployment at higher concentrations of these neighborhood factors. The association between increasing neighborhood unemployment and lower mean birthweight among foreign-born Asians remained after adjustment for acculturation and the foregoing factors ($\beta = -131$, SE $= 63$, $p < .05$).

Results of logistic models predicting low birthweight mirror those for continuous birthweight. After adjustment for all factors among Asians in the overall sample, the odds ratio (OR) for low birthweight associated with a 10 percent increment in neighborhood unemployment was 1.8 (95% confidence interval [CI] $= 1.0, 2.8$; $p < .05$). The risk of low birthweight increased for blacks living in neighborhoods with higher unemployment, but the odds ratio was statistically significant only among the survey subsample (OR $= 1.8$, 95% CI $= 1.3$, 2.4; $p < .05$ for subsample; OR $= 1.3$, 95% CI $= 0.9, 1.7$; $p = .13$ overall). For foreign-born Latinas, the risk of low birthweight decreased at high levels of neighborhood unemployment. The positive association between increasing neighborhood unemployment and risk of low birthweight remained strong among blacks and Asians in the survey subsample after adjustment for potential explanatory factors.

Table 23.3. Change in Birthweight Associated with Mother's Individual and Neighborhood Socioeconomic Characteristics, by Ethnicity, Among the Survey Subsample of 8,457 Women Delivering at 18 Hospitals: California, 1994–1995

	White (n = 2005) Coef. (SE)	Black (n = 907) Coef. (SE)	Foreign-Born Latina (n = 3832) Coef. (SE)	U.S.-Born Latina (n = 950) Coef. (SE)	Asian (n = 653) Coef. (SE)
Model 1					
Neighborhood poverty	−1 (16)	−28 (20)	17** (7)	1 (15)	−56 (38)
Mother's education	11 (7)	−7 (14)	−11** (3)	8 (13)	−12 (12)
Household income†	↑ up to 400% poverty level	↑ up to 200% poverty level	↑ up to 200% poverty level**	Slight ↑ up to 200% poverty level	↑ up to 300% poverty level, then ↓**
Model 2					
Neighborhood unemployment	72 (38)	−104** (41)	32 (22)	−2 (45)	−163* (83)
Mother's education	12 (7)	−8 (14)	−11** (2)	8 (14)	−13 (12)
Household income†	↑ up to 400% poverty level	↑ up to 200% poverty level*	↑ up to 200% poverty level**	Slight ↑ up to 200% poverty level	↑ up to 300% poverty level, then ↓**
Model 3					
Low neighborhood education	7 (10)	−24 (12)	0 (4)	8 (8)	−25 (16)
Mother's education	12 (7)	−7 (15)	−12** (3)	8 (14)	−13 (13)
Household income†	↑ up to 400% poverty level	↑ up to 200% poverty level	↑ up to 200% poverty level**	Slight ↑ up to 200% poverty level	↑ up to 350% poverty level, then ↓**

Note: Coefficient (coef.) represents average increase or decrease in birthweight (g) associated with a 10 percentage point increase in the specified neighborhood (census block group) characteristic (for example, from 10 percent to 20 percent of neighborhood residents with income below poverty level). Coefficients and standard errors are from separate linear regression models of birthweight that used generalized estimating equations to account for hospital clustering. All models include mother's education and family income.

†Nonlinear relationships between family income as percentage of poverty and birthweight were modeled with quadratic and cubic terms. The ↑ and ↓ symbols describe direction of birthweight curve as income increases, after adjustment for mother's education and neighborhood characteristics (for example, ↑ indicates that birthweight increases with increasing income).

*$p < .05$; **$p < .01$.

DISCUSSION

This study indicates that the nature of the relationship between neighborhood socioeconomic characteristics and birthweights of infants born to California residents varies greatly, depending on the ethnicity of the mother and the area-level characteristic considered. Among white women and U.S.-born Latinas, the neighborhood socioeconomic characteristics we examined generally were unrelated to birthweight; among Asians and blacks, birthweight declined in a linear fashion with lower neighborhood SES, as measured by higher unemployment levels. Paradoxically, among foreign-born Latinas, living in the neighborhoods with the highest rates of poverty and unemployment was associated with higher mean birthweights and lower risk of low birthweight. Adjustment for family income and other individual-level factors available for the surveyed subsample did not account for the observed associations of neighborhood SES with mean birthweight or risk of low birthweight.

Previous studies have observed lower birthweights with greater neighborhood socioeconomic disadvantage, as well as with lower personal SES[6–8,11]; only one study reported findings by ethnicity, however.[11] Unlike that study, ours did not find a neighborhood association with birthweight among whites. This study is the first to report specifically on the nature of the relationship between socioeconomic characteristics measured at individual and neighborhood levels and birthweight among Asians and Latinas, among whom nativity status appears to play an important role.

Neighborhood-level characteristics measure a dimension of socioeconomic conditions that may not be captured by individual-level measures such as income or education. Among all ethnic groups, neighborhood-level results were largely unaffected by inclusion of individual-level socioeconomic measures and vice versa. Thus, it is likely that both community and individual pathways link socioeconomic conditions to birth outcomes. To some degree, these census-derived variables serve as surrogate measures for aspects of the social, service, and physical environments on which we might intervene,[31] with community support for health-promoting behaviors, for example, or access to health care or nutritious foods. Community joblessness itself may be a strong indicator of neighborhood deterioration as well as a key contributor to problems of social organization and isolation that can shape individual habits and behaviors.[32]

These findings also suggest that the meaning of aggregate measures may vary with ethnicity and nativity. Wilson has observed that blacks living in poor, inner-city neighborhoods are more likely to suffer discrimination and are more sensitive to exploitation than Mexican American immigrants who have come from areas of intense poverty. In addition, poor neighborhoods dominated by Mexican Americans tend to have more businesses and services.[32] Kinship ties within the community are an important support for Mexican Americans,[33] and these local kin networks may be stronger in poorer communities. Studies that seek to adjust for socioeconomic influences by using neighborhood measures should consider ethnic groups separately.

Neighborhood-level associations observed after adjustment for measured individual socioeconomic factors may reflect unmeasured socioeconomic influences at the individual level.[22,23] Recent family income, along with education and Medi-Cal coverage, may not adequately represent accumulated economic assets and socioeconomic conditions experienced early in life, which could have important health effects. To the extent that personal income and education result from socioeconomic conditions of neighborhoods, however,[34] adjustment for individual-level socioeconomic factors may remove part of the neighborhood effect. Therefore, the estimate of neighborhood-level effects may be conservative.

Low rates of low birthweight among Latina mothers in the United States in spite of low education levels and underutilization of prenatal care have been described as an epidemiologic paradox.[35] Foreign-born Mexican Americans have lower rates of low birthweight than U.S.-born Mexican Americans.[24,36,37] In addition, having a U.S. cultural orientation (defined by language preference, ethnic identification, and birthplace) has been associated with an increased risk of low birthweight relative to having a Mexican cultural orientation,[38] although speaking only Spanish as opposed to English has been associated with increased risk for preterm birth among Mexico-born women in California.[39] In the present sample of foreign-born Latinas, language spoken at home was not associated with birthweight; although time lived in the United States was associated with increasing birthweight in unadjusted analyses, this relationship was explained entirely by family income and parity. Acculturation did not appear to explain neighborhood-level findings among foreign-born Latinas.

Dietary factors were not measured in this study, but they provide another potential explanation for the paradoxical findings among foreign-born Latinas. The diets of Latinas born in Mexico are higher in calcium, folate, protein, vitamin A, and ascorbic acid than those of U.S.-born Latinas.[40] Among Mexican Americans, diets characterized as nutrient rich and protein dense are related to increased birthweight, whereas diets that are high in fat, sugars, and cereals are associated with lower birthweight.[41] To the extent that Latinas living in the poorest neighborhoods adhere to traditional diets, poor neighborhoods may be associated with higher birthweight.

The consistency of neighborhood-level socioeconomic differences in birth outcomes suggests a small but real effect among certain ethnic groups that is not explained by several known risk factors. Our findings suggest that regardless of individual financial resources, living in a community with high levels of poverty or unemployment can result in lower birthweight infants for black and Asian women. For these groups, neighborhood influences may compound individual socioeconomic disadvantages. In contrast, foreign-born Latinas appear to have more favorable birthweights in the most socioeconomically deprived neighborhoods. Searching for protective factors among those communities may strengthen our understanding of the factors that determine birthweight and aid in the development of policies and interventions to improve birthweight and birth outcomes generally.

Notes

1. Parker, J. D., Schoendorf, K. C., & Kiely, J. L. (1944). Associations between measures of socioeconomic status and low birthweight, small for gestational age, and premature delivery in the United States. *Ann Epidemiol, 4,* 271–278.

2. Wise, P. H., Kotelchuck, M., Wilson, M. L., & Mills, M. (1985). Racial and socioeconomic disparities in childhood mortality in Boston. *N Engl J Med, 313,* 360–366.

3. Cogswell, M. E., & Yip, R. (1995). The influence of fetal and maternal factors on the distribution of birthweight. *Semin Perinatol, 19,* 222–240.

4. Gould, J. B., & LeRoy, S. (1988). Socioeconomic status and low birthweight: A racial comparison. *Pediatrics, 82,* 896–904.

5. Gould, J. B., Davey, B., & LeRoy, S. (1989). Socioeconomic differentials and neonatal mortality: Racial comparison of California singletons. *Pediatrics, 83,* 181–186.

6. Roberts, E. M. (1997). Neighborhood social environments and the distribution of low birthweight in Chicago. *Am J Public Health, 87,* 597–603.

7. O'Campo, P., Xue, X., Wang M. C., & Caughty, M. (1997). Neighborhood risk factors for low birthweight in Baltimore: A multilevel analysis. *Am J Public Health, 87,* 1113–1118.

8. Sloggett, A., & Joshi, H. (1998). Deprivation indicators as predictors of life events 1981–1992, based on the UK ONS Longitudinal Study. *J Epidemiol Community Health, 52,* 228–233.

9. Morgan, M., & Chinn, S. (1983). ACORN group, social class, and child health. *J Epidemiol Community Health, 37,* 196–203.

10. Jarvelin, M. R., Elliott, P., Kleinschmidt, I., et al. (1997). Ecological and individual predictors of birthweight in a northern Finland birth cohort, 1986. *Paediatr Perinat Epidemiol, 11,* 298–312.

11. Fang, J., Madhavan, S., & Alderman, M. H. (1999). Low birthweight: Race and maternal nativity—impact of community income. *Pediatrics, 103,* E5.

12. Wasserman, C. R., Shaw, G. M., Selvin, S., Gould, J. B., & Syme, S. L. (1998). Socioeconomic status, neighborhood social conditions, and neural tube defects. *Am J Public Health, 88,* 1674–1680.

13. Waitzman, N., & Smith, K. (1998). Phantom of the area: Poverty-area residence and mortality in the United States. *Am J Public Health, 88,* 973–976.

14. Haan, M., Kaplan, G. A., & Camacho, T. (1987). Poverty and health: Prospective evidence from the Alameda County Study. *Am J Epidemiol, 125,* 989–998.

15. Kaplan, G. (1996). People and places: Contrasting perspectives on the association between social class and health. *Int J Health Serv, 26,* 507–519.

16. Anderson, R., Sorlie, P., Backlund, E., Johnson, N., & Kaplan, G. (1997). Mortality effects of community economic status. *Epidemiology, 8,* 42–47.

17. Shouls, S., Congdon, P., & Curtis, S. (1996). Modelling inequality in reported long term illness in the UK: Combining individual and area characteristics. *J Epidemiol Community Health, 50,* 366–376.

18. Humphreys, K., & Carr-Hill, R. (1991). Area variations in health outcomes: Artefact or ecology. *Int J Epidemiol, 20,* 251–258.

19. Diez-Roux, A. V., Nieto, F. J., & Muntaner, C., et al. (1997). Neighborhood environments and coronary heart disease: A multilevel analysis. *Am J Epidemiol, 146,* 48–63.

20. Duncan, C., Jones, K., & Moon, G. (1996). Health-related behaviour in context: A multilevel modelling approach. *Soc Sci Med, 42,* 817–830.

21. Diez-Roux, A. V. (1998). Bringing context back into epidemiology: Variables and fallacies in multilevel analysis. *Am J Public Health, 88,* 216–222.

22. Pickett, K., & Pearl, M. (2001). Multilevel analyses of neighbourhood socioeconomic context and health outcomes: A critical review. *J Epidemiol Community Health, 55,* 111–122.

23. Robert, S. A. (1999). Socioeconomic position and health: The independent contribution of community socioeconomic context. *Annu Rev Sociol, 25,* 489–516.

24. Collins, J. W., Jr., & Shay, D. K. (1994). Prevalence of low birthweight among Hispanic infants with United States–born and foreign-born mothers: The effect of urban poverty [see comments]. *Am J Epidemiol, 139,* 184–192.

25. Starfield, B., Shapiro, S., Weiss, J., et al. (1991). Race, family income, and low birthweight. *Am J Epidemiol, 134,* 1167–1174.

26. Braveman, P., Pearl, M., Egerter, S., Marchi, K., & Williams, R. (1998). Validity of insurance information on California birth certificates. *Am J Public Health, 88,* 813–816.

27. Braveman, P., Egerter, S., & Marchi, K. (1999). The prevalence of low income among childbearing women in California: Implications for the private and public sectors. *Am J Public Health, 89,* 868–874.

28. Selvin, S., & Abrams, B. (1996). Analysing the relationship between maternal weight gain and birthweight: Exploration of four statistical issues. *Paediatr Perinat Epidemiol, 10,* 220–234.

29. Baumeister, L., Marchi, K., Pearl, M., Williams, R., & Braveman, P. (2000). Validation of racial/ethnic information in California birth certificates. *Health Serv Res, 35,* 869–883.

30. Duncan, C., Jones, K., & Moon, G. (1998). Context, composition and heterogeneity: Using multilevel models in health research. *Soc Sci Med, 46,* 97–117.

31. Macintyre, S., Maciver, S., & Sooman, A. (1993). Area, class and health: Should we be focusing on places or people? *J Soc Policy, 22,* 213–233.

32. Wilson, W. J. (1996). *When work disappears: The world of the new urban poor.* New York: Knopf.

33. Keefe, S., Padilla, A., & Carlos, M. (1979). The Mexican-American extended family as an emotional support system. *Hum Organ, 38,* 144–152.

34. Garner, C.R.S. (1991). Neighborhood effects on educational attainment: A multi-level analysis. *Soc Educ, 64,* 251–262.

35. Markides, K. S., & Coreil, J. (1986). The health of Hispanics in the Southwestern United States: An epidemiologic paradox. *Public Health Rep, 101,* 253–265.

36. Singh, G. K., & Yu, S. M. (1996). Adverse pregnancy outcomes: Differences between U.S.- and foreign-born women in major U.S. racial and ethnic groups. *Am J Public Health, 86,* 837–843.

37. Balcazar, H., Cole, G., & Hartner, J. (1992). Mexican-Americans' use of prenatal care and its relationship to maternal risk factors and pregnancy outcome. *Am J Prev Med, 8,* 1–7.

38. Scribner, R., & Dwyer, J. H. (1989). Acculturation and low birthweight among Latinos in the Hispanic HANES. *Am J Public Health, 79,* 1263–1267.

39. English, P. B., Kharrazi, M., & Guendelman, S. (1997). Pregnancy outcomes and risk factors in Mexican Americans: The effect of language use and mother's birthplace. *Ethn Dis, 7,* 229–240.

40. Guendelman, S., & Abrams, B. (1995). Dietary intake among Mexican-American women: Generational differences and a comparison with white non-Hispanic women. *Am J Public Health, 85,* 20–25.

41. Wolff, C. B., & Wolff, H. K. (1995). Maternal eating patterns and birth weight of Mexican American infants. *Nutr Health, 10,* 121–134.

CHAPTER TWENTY-FOUR

Neighborhood Characteristics Associated with the Location of Food Stores and Food Service Places

Kimberly Morland
Steve Wing
Ana Diez Roux
Charles Poole

A growing number of articles in the medical literature indicate that individuals' health and behaviors are affected by their social and physical surroundings.[1-6] More than a decade ago, medical geographers found that physical proximity to a doctor or medical facility affected utilization of health care resources.[7] More recently, investigators in Canada found that in areas in which the number of places selling wine had increased, wine consumption by residents had also increased.[8]

The role that diet plays in the causation and prevention of heart disease has been studied for several decades. The relationship among serum cholesterol, high- and low-density lipoproteins, and heart disease has led researchers to suggest that the amount and type of fat consumed may influence risk for cardiovascular disease.[9] Although the mechanisms by which foods and nutrients interact to affect cardiovascular disease risk are not well understood, recommendations for the prevention of cardiovascular disease include diets low in fat and sodium, as well as diets high in fiber, fruits, and vegetables.[10,11]

This study was funded by the University of North Carolina School of Medicine, Women's Health Research Grant (KM); National Institute of Environmental Health Sciences, Grant No. 2 R25 ES08206-05 under the Environmental Justice: Partnerships for Communication program (SW); and National Heart, Lung and Blood Institute Grant No. R29 HL59386 (ADR). We are also grateful to Drs. Gerardo Heiss, Nancy Milio, Lori Carter-Edwards, Hermann A. Tyroler, and Paul Sorlie for their useful comments.

People's ability to meet these recommendations for a healthy diet has been a concern of public health researchers and practitioners for many years. Many intervention studies that focused on individuals' behavior did not result in long-term dietary changes that would affect risk for cardiovascular disease.[12-14] Dietary choices may be influenced by a variety of factors, such as taste, nutrition, weight control, convenience, and cost.[15]

Some studies show that cost is the most significant predictor of dietary choices, making healthy eating habits difficult to achieve for the poor.[16-18] Research indicates that low-income people generally cannot afford healthier foods.[19] Other research suggests that food costs more for people of low socio-economic status because purchases are made in smaller quantities and there is more reliance on processed food. It has been shown that urban dwellers pay 3 percent to 37 percent more for groceries in their local community compared to suburban residents who buy the same goods at large supermarkets.[20] Such findings led researchers to speculate that the migration of supermarkets to suburbs and the lack of transportation available to low-income communities are contributing to malnutrition among the poor.[21,22] Other studies concur with these findings, reporting that because of the sharp decline of supermarkets in low-income areas, residents are forced to depend on small stores with limited selections of foods at substantially higher prices.[23]

Although the cost of food is an important barrier, fewer studies have attempted to address locality as a factor that may hinder people's ability to achieve a healthy diet. A study that compared supermarkets, neighborhood groceries, convenience stores (such as 7-Elevens), and health food stores in San Diego, California, found that supermarkets had twice the average number of "heart-healthy" foods as neighborhood grocery stores had and four times the average number of such foods as convenience stores had.[24] Another study, conducted in Australia, found that an equal proportion of all income groups shopped at large supermarkets exclusively. However, the lowest socioeconomic group studied was least likely to have private vehicles to use for food shopping, making the location of food stores more critical for the poor.[25]

The impact that the location of food stores and food service has on individuals' diets remains unclear. The few studies that have addressed locality have not investigated the similarity of the numbers and types of food stores and food service places in American neighborhoods. Therefore, this study describes the prevalence of places where people can obtain food in their neighborhoods. In addition, we test the hypothesis that fewer supermarkets and more corner markets are located in low-wealth neighborhoods than in higher-wealth neighborhoods.

In addition to neighborhood wealth, residential racial and ethnic segregation are structural features of U.S. society.[26] Black Americans face barriers that prevent residential mobility at all income levels, resulting in racially distinct neighborhoods. For this reason, we also investigated whether the prevalence of food stores and food service places is associated with the proportion of black residents. We tested the hypothesis that fewer supermarkets and more corner markets are located in predominantly black neighborhoods than in racially mixed or predominantly white neighborhoods.

METHODS

Because U.S. census data for 2000 had not yet been released, 221 census tracts defined in the 1990 Census were used as proxies for neighborhoods in the following areas: Jackson City, Mississippi; Forsyth County, North Carolina; Washington County, Maryland; and selected suburbs of Minneapolis, Minnesota (Brooklyn Center, Brooklyn Park, Crystal, Golden Valley, New Hope, Plymouth, and Robbinsdale). This research is ancillary to the Atherosclerosis Risk in Communities (ARIC) study, an ongoing study of atherosclerosis based on sample populations from these areas.[27] Census tracts with ten or fewer housing units were excluded. Of the remaining 216 tracts, 56 were located in Mississippi, 78 in North Carolina, 28 in Maryland, and 54 in Minnesota.

Housing, transportation, and demographic characteristics of census tracts were obtained from the 1990 Census of Population and Housing Summary Tape Files 3A.[28] Block group data were summed for each census tract within places.

Measurement of the Local Food Environment

Business addresses of places where people can buy food were collected from the local departments of environmental health and state departments of agriculture. Of the 3,987 business addresses obtained, 99.5 percent (3,969) were geocoded to census tracts. Eighty businesses were excluded because the census tract for each of these businesses did not fall within the geographic boundaries of the study areas or the census tract had been excluded. Finally, 548 duplicate records were deleted, resulting in 3,341 businesses where people can obtain food in the four study areas (Mississippi, 871; North Carolina, 1,492; Maryland, 417; and Minnesota, 561).

Defining Types of Food Stores and Food Service Places

The 1997 North American Industry Classification System (NAICS) codes and definitions were modified to describe the types of food stores and food service places located in each census tract (Table 24.1).[29] For instance, in the "food and beverage stores" subsector, supermarkets are not distinguished from other grocery stores. Since supermarkets have been found to have the most healthy food items[24] at lower prices,[23] it is important to distinguish supermarkets from smaller food stores. Therefore, supermarkets were defined as large, corporate-owned "chain" stores (for example, Food Lion, Albertson's, Harris Teeter,

Table 24.1. North American Industry Classification System (NAICS) Codes and Examples of Food Stores and Food Service Places

Industry Group	1997 NAICS Definitions	NAICS Index	Examples
Supermarkets	445110 Supermarkets and other grocery (except convenience) stores	445110 Supermarkets	Food Lion, Albertson's, Kroger, Piggly Wiggly, Safeway
Grocery stores	445110 Supermarkets and other grocery (except convenience) stores	445110 Grocery stores 445110 Food stores	Beatty Street Grocery, Arkady's Market, West Side Market, Potomac Grocery, JC Morris Grocery, Ken's Grocery
Convenience stores	445120 Convenience stores	445120 Convenience stores	7-Eleven, 4 Brothers Convenience Store
Convenience stores with gas stations	447110 Gasoline stations with convenience stores	447110 Gasoline stations with convenience stores	Amoco, Chevron, Shell, Texaco, Sunoco, BP, Citgo, Mobile, Conoco, Exxon, Phillips 66
Specialty food stores	4452 Specialty food stores	445210 Meat markets 445220 Fish markets 445230 Fruit/vegetable markets 445291 Baked goods 445292 Confectionery/nut stores 445299 All other	Davis's Meat Market, Boonsboro Produce Market, Asia Market, 66 Produce, Holsinger's Meat Market, Baron's Gourmet, Valley Street Fish
Full-service restaurants	722110 Full-service restaurants	722110 Restaurants, full service 722110 Steak houses 722110 Pizzerias, full service 722110 Fine dining restaurants 722110 Family restaurants 722110 Diners, full service 722212 Cafeterias	Applebee's, Baker's Square, Benihana, Bennigan's, Bonsai Japanese Steakhouse, The Thai House, Ruby Tuesday, View Street Diner

(Continued)

Table 24.1. North American Industry Classification System (NAICS) Codes and Examples of Food Stores and Food Service Places (Continued)

Industry Group	1997 NAICS Definitions	NAICS Index	Examples
Fast-food restaurants	722211 Limited-service restaurants	722211 Fast-food restaurants 722211 Pizza parlor, limited service 722211 Pizza delivery shops	Arby's, Biscuitville, Bojangles, Burger King, Domino's, Blimpies, McDonald's, Wendy's, Krystal
Carryout eating places	722211 Limited-service restaurants	722211 Delicatessens 722211 Sandwich shops 722110 Bagel shops, full service	Carla's Deli, Harle's Subs, Silver Streak Sub & Deli, Bagel-Lisious, Mr. George's Sandwich World, Country Deli
Carryout specialty items	722213 Snack and nonalcoholic beverage bars	722213 Beverage (for example, coffee) bars (nonalcoholic) 722213 Doughnut shops 722213 Ice cream parlors 722213 Pretzel shops	Baskin Robbins, Colonial Bakery Store, Papa Vic's Gelato, Monroe's Donuts, Smoothie King, TCBY Yogurt, Dunkin Donuts, Starbucks Coffee, Gloria Jean's Coffee, Fanny Farmer's Candies
Bars and taverns	72241 Drinking places (alcoholic beverages)	722410 Alcoholic beverage drinking places	McBare's Public South End Tavern, Club City Lights, Eddie's Disco, Sportsmen's Den, Funktown Tavern

Kroger, and Piggly Wiggly), whereas grocery stores were defined as smaller, noncorporate-owned food stores. In addition, because convenience stores attached to gas stations contribute to the local food environment, we added this category to the food and beverage stores subsector. All specialty food stores (for example, meat markets and fruit and vegetable markets) were grouped together. In addition, within the NAICS subsector of "food service and drinking places," cafeterias were grouped with full-service restaurants. Franchised fast-food restaurants were not distinguished from other limited-service restaurants; however, because these fast-food establishments may offer foods different from those available at other limited-service restaurants, this food service category was added. Carryout eating places (for example, delicatessens, and bagel or sandwich shops) sell fast food but are not franchised fast-food places. Specialty carryout eating places (for example, smoothie shops and espresso bars) specialize in only one type of food. Each business was assigned to only one industry group.

Sixty-one percent (2,058) of the businesses were assigned an industry code based on name recognition. An additional 970 (29 percent) industry codes were assigned according to the category assigned to the business in the *Yellow Pages*.[30] Ten percent of the businesses had undefined industry codes and were excluded from the analysis.

We were interested in the availability of food stores and food service places through local, routine sources. Therefore, churches, community groups, hospitals, schools, and nursing homes (395) were excluded. Department stores (85) and places that exist primarily for entertainment (56), such as bowling alleys, may offer food that resembles carryout food. However, these places were also excluded because it was assumed that few people rely on these places for a significant portion of their diet. Catering businesses (41) were also excluded since they are not places where people regularly obtain food. Finally, liquor stores (14) were excluded because data collection was incomplete. Based on these criteria, an additional 591 businesses were excluded from the analysis.

Our analysis was based on 2,437 food stores and food service places in the 216 census tracts. Of these, 609 were located in Mississippi, 1192 in North Carolina, 315 in Maryland, and 321 in Minnesota.

Neighborhood Wealth and Racial Segregation

The median value for homes in each census tract was used as a measure of neighborhood wealth. We expected the wealth of the environment to be associated with the location of food stores and restaurants; therefore, we used home values to measure neighborhood wealth, instead of income, which is a measurement of individual wealth. The mean and range of home values varied by ARIC location, with Minnesota having the highest home values and Mississippi having the lowest (data not shown). Therefore, site-specific quintiles of wealth were averaged to create a measure of relative wealth. For instance, the lowest wealth category contains forty-four census tracts (twelve in Mississippi, fifteen in North Carolina, six in Maryland, and eleven in Minnesota), representing the lowest home values for each of those areas.

The proportion of black residents also varies by ARIC location. The analysis of neighborhood racial segregation was limited to North Carolina and Mississippi because <5 percent of residents in Maryland or Minnesota were black. The proportion of black residents within each census tract was used to define categories of segregation. Census tracts that had >80 percent black residents were defined as predominantly black (35 tracts). Census tracts that had <20 percent black residents were defined as predominantly white (69 tracts), and census tracts that had 20 percent to 80 percent black residents (30 tracts) were defined as racially mixed. Few people of racial groups other than black and white live in these locations (data not shown).

Statistical Analysis

Because the dependent variable is expressed as count data, Poisson regressions were used to evaluate the relationship between the number of stores (dependent variable) and neighborhood wealth and racial composition (independent variables).[31] The Poisson models were not overdispersed. Because the number of stores tended to be higher in more densely populated areas, a linear term for population density (persons/km^2) was included in separate models that focus on the effects of neighborhood wealth and racial segregation, which were represented as indicator variables corresponding to the categories described above. Indicator variables for each ARIC location were used to adjust for geographic difference. Prevalence of food stores (number of food stores/number of census tracts), adjusted prevalence ratios, and 95 percent confidence intervals (CIs) were calculated from regression coefficients using the lowest level of each dependent variable as the referent. All statistics were calculated using SAS GENMOD procedure.[32]

RESULTS

The means and standard deviations of census tract characteristics by neighborhood wealth are shown in Table 24.2. On average, the lower wealth groups contain the fewest people, and the areas of these tracts are the smallest. Nevertheless, the population density of the lowest wealth group is the highest. There are fewer housing units in low-wealth areas, and residents of the low-wealth neighborhoods are twice as likely as wealthy neighborhood residents to be renters. As the wealth of the neighborhoods decreases, the proportion of black residents increases, with over eight times as many black Americans living in the lowest wealth neighborhoods compared to the highest wealth areas. Furthermore, the proportion of households without a car or truck available is also higher among black Americans, regardless of wealth.

The number of food stores or food service places, prevalence of food stores or food service places, and population density– and site adjusted–prevalence

Table 24.2. Housing and Demographic Characteristics of Census Tracts by Neighborhood Wealth Category

	Neighborhood Wealth				
	Low (n = 44)	Low-Medium (n = 43)	Medium (n = 42)	High-Medium (n = 43)	High (n = 44)
Characteristics	**Mean (SD)**	**Mean (SD)**	**Mean (SD)**	**Mean (SD)**	**Mean (SD)**
Population	2,772 (1147)	3,745 (1448)	4,280 (1609)	3,868 (1762)	4,224 (1613)
Area (sq km)	8 (22)	7 (12)	19 (33)	15 (21)	20 (31)
Population density (persons/sq km)	1,456 (1012)	1,335 (1044)	895 (703)	588 (458)	619 (479)
Number of single family homes	1,169 (467)	1,578 (630)	1,716 (576)	1,642 (800)	1,687 (618)
Percentage of residents who are renters	0.46 (0.20)	0.41 (0.20)	0.29 (0.14)	0.30 (0.20)	0.22 (0.15)
Percentage of residents who are black Americans	0.53 (0.42)	0.36 (0.38)	0.18 (0.29)	0.13 (0.21)	0.06 (0.14)
Percentage of households without a vehicle					
White	0.19 (0.24)	0.17 (0.22)	0.06 (0.05)	0.05 (0.06)	0.03 (0.04)
Black	0.32 (0.26)	0.20 (0.17)	0.11 (0.19)	0.10 (0.13)	0.06 (0.11)

ratios by neighborhood wealth category are presented in Table 24.3. The types of food stores and food service places that exist in poor and wealthy neighborhoods are different. For instance, there are over three times as many supermarkets in the wealthier neighborhoods as there are in the lowest wealth areas. Convenience stores with gas stations are also more commonly found in wealthier areas, with the medium-wealth neighborhoods having the highest prevalence of these establishments. In contrast, the wealthier neighborhoods contain fewer small grocery stores, convenience stores (without gas stations), and specialty food stores than the lowest wealth neighborhoods do.

The most prevalent type of food service place is the full-service restaurant; on average three to four full-service restaurants are located in each neighborhood. Fast-food restaurants are more prevalent in the low-medium and medium-wealth neighborhoods and become less prevalent in the highest wealth neighborhoods. Carryout specialty eating places are 50 percent to 80 percent more prevalent in wealthier neighborhoods. As wealth increases, the number of bars and taverns declines.

Regarding neighborhood racial segregation, supermarkets and specialty food stores are more common in racially mixed and predominantly white neighborhoods (Table 24.4). The greatest difference is in the prevalence of supermarkets, which are four times more common in predominantly white neighborhoods than in predominantly black neighborhoods. Smaller grocery stores, convenience stores, and convenience stores attached to gas stations are less common in predominantly white neighborhoods. Mixed and predominantly white neighborhoods are similar in the prevalence of food store types compared to predominantly black neighborhoods. The only exception is convenience stores with gas stations, which are more prevalent in mixed neighborhoods than in predominantly white or black neighborhoods.

Compared to predominantly black neighborhoods, all food service places are more prevalent in racially mixed and predominantly white neighborhoods, except bars and taverns, which are less common in white neighborhoods. Full-service restaurants are two times more prevalent in white neighborhoods and three times more prevalent in racially mixed neighborhoods. Fast-food restaurants and carryout eating places are twice as common in white and racially mixed neighborhoods. Carryout eating places serving specialty items are nine to eleven times more prevalent in racially mixed and predominantly white areas.

DISCUSSION

This study shows that the locations of food stores and food service places are associated with the wealth and racial makeup of neighborhoods, and in the case of supermarkets and small corner grocery stores, this association is in

Table 24.3. Population Density– and Site Adjusted-Prevalence Ratios of Food Stores and Food Service Places by Neighborhood Wealth Category

	Neighborhood Wealth																			
	Low (n = 44)			Low-Medium (n = 44)				Medium (n = 41)				High-Medium (n = 43)				High (n = 44)			
Industry Group	n	P	PR	n	P	PR	95% CI	n	P	PR	95% CI	n	P	PR	95% CI	n	P	PR	95% CI
Food stores																			
Supermarkets	7	0.16	1.0	22	0.50	2.8	1.2, 6.7	20	0.49	2.6	1.1, 6.4	30	0.70	3.6	1.5, 8.7	27	0.61	3.3	1.4, 7.9
Grocery stores	45	1.02	1.0	38	0.86	0.9	0.6, 1.3	24	0.59	0.6	0.3, 0.9	25	0.58	0.6	0.3, 0.9	26	0.59	0.6	0.3, 0.9
Convenience stores	25	0.57	1.0	27	0.61	1.1	0.7, 1.9	35	0.85	1.4	0.9, 2.4	27	0.63	1.0	0.6, 1.7	29	0.66	1.0	0.6, 1.8
Convenience stores with gas stations	26	0.59	1.0	39	0.89	1.5	0.9, 2.5	53	1.29	2.0	1.2, 3.2	45	1.05	1.5	0.9, 2.5	37	0.84	1.2	0.7, 2.0
Specialty food stores	11	0.25	1.0	10	0.23	0.9	0.4, 2.1	10	0.24	0.9	0.4, 2.1	6	0.14	0.5	0.2, 1.3	10	0.23	0.8	0.3, 1.9
Food service																			
Full-service restaurants	149	3.39	1.0	197	4.48	1.2	1.0, 1.5	151	3.68	1.0	0.8, 1.2	194	4.51	1.2	0.9, 1.5	162	3.68	1.0	0.8, 1.2
Fast-food restaurants	63	1.43	1.0	97	2.20	1.4	1.0, 1.9	91	2.22	1.3	0.9, 1.8	87	2.02	1.1	0.8, 1.5	70	1.59	0.9	0.6, 1.3
Carryout eating places	26	0.59	1.0	44	1.00	1.7	1.0, 2.7	24	0.59	1.0	0.6, 1.8	41	0.95	1.6	0.9, 2.7	24	0.55	0.9	0.5, 1.7
Carryout specialty items	17	0.39	1.0	29	0.66	1.6	0.9, 3.0	26	0.63	1.5	0.8, 2.7	36	0.84	1.8	1.0, 3.2	33	0.75	1.6	0.9, 3.0
Bars/taverns	35	0.80	1.0	21	0.48	0.6	0.4, 1.0	22	0.54	0.7	0.4, 1.1	13	0.30	0.4	0.2, 0.7	11	0.25	0.3	0.1, 0.6

Note: CI = confidence interval; n = number of food stores or food service places; P = prevalence of food stores or food service places; PR = prevalence ratio.

Table 24.4. Population Density– and Site Adjusted-Prevalence Ratios of Food Stores and Food Service Places by Neighborhood Racial Segregation Category

					Neighborhood Racial Segregation						
	Predominantly Black (n = 35)			Racially Mixed (n = 30)				Predominantly White (n = 69)			
Industry Group	n	P	PR	n	P	PR	95% CI	n	P	PR	95% CI
Food stores											
Supermarkets	5	0.14	1.0	19	0.63	2.9	1.0, 8.6	68	0.99	4.3	1.5, 12.5
Grocery stores	44	1.26	1.0	27	0.90	0.8	0.4, 1.3	34	0.49	0.4	0.3, 0.7
Convenience stores	38	1.09	1.0	15	0.50	0.6	0.3, 1.1	21	0.30	0.4	0.2, 0.7
Convenience stores with gas stations	32	0.91	1.0	46	1.53	1.6	1.0, 2.6	69	1.00	1.0	0.6, 1.7
Specialty food stores	6	0.17	1.0	8	0.27	1.5	0.4, 5.2	13	0.19	1.1	0.3, 3.7
Food service											
Full-service restaurants	64	1.83	1.0	221	7.37	3.4	2.5, 4.7	374	5.42	2.4	1.8, 3.4
Fast-food restaurants	43	1.23	1.0	106	3.53	2.3	1.5, 3.4	163	2.36	1.5	1.0, 2.2
Carryout eating places	14	0.40	1.0	43	1.43	2.7	1.4, 5.4	76	1.10	2.0	1.0, 4.0
Carryout specialty items	4	0.11	1.0	23	0.77	8.9	2.8, 29.0	62	0.90	11.0	3.4, 39.2
Bars/taverns	17	0.49	1.0	23	0.77	1.7	0.8, 3.5	24	0.35	0.8	0.4, 1.7

Note: CI = confidence interval; n = number of food stores or food service places; P = prevalence of food stores or food service places; PR = prevalence ratio.

the expected direction. Diez Roux et al.[33] found variation in the dietary intake of neighborhood residents living in the same geographic locations. Therefore, results of this study support previous research that suggests people's dietary choices may be influenced by the availability of food stores and food service places.

Our analysis did not take into account the similarity of characteristics shared by neighboring census tracts, sometimes referred to as spatial autocorrelation. The clustering of census tracts along lines of race, ethnicity, and wealth means that the local food environment can be characterized at larger spatial scales. Information on membership of census tracts in larger neighborhood aggregations similar to the aggregation of census block groups into tracts was not available for this analysis. However, to the extent that census tracts with and without supermarkets are located in clusters of tracts with similar food environments, the impact of the presence or absence of supermarkets on residents was underestimated in our analysis because residents of tracts without supermarkets have access to few supermarkets in adjoining tracts, while residents of tracts with supermarkets have access to additional supermarkets in neighboring tracts.

Racial and wealth segregation remain prominent characteristics of U.S. neighborhoods even though the Fair Housing Act of 1968 prohibits racial discrimination in housing.[34] The Fair Housing Act does not govern the placement of food stores or restaurants by private industry. These environmental factors have not been traditionally considered as explanations for individuals' dietary choices. Our findings suggest that some people may be disadvantaged in terms of food availability within their local food environment. For example, five supermarkets are located in thirty-five predominantly black neighborhoods to provide service for nearly 118,000 people. In contrast, there are sixty-eight supermarkets to serve 259,500 residents of predominantly white neighborhoods. The ratio of supermarkets to residents for the predominantly white areas is 1:3,816, versus 1:23,582 for predominantly black neighborhoods. Our findings that supermarkets are more prevalent in predominantly white and wealthy neighborhoods, while small corner grocery stores are located in black and poor neighborhoods, support findings by previous researchers.[21–23]

In addition, our results show that fewer households in poor and black neighborhoods have access to private transportation, which support findings by Turrell[25] and suggest that residents of these neighborhoods have greater difficulty obtaining healthy food. The choices people make about what to eat are limited by the food available to them.[35] The lack of private transportation and of supermarkets in low-wealth and predominantly black neighborhoods suggests that residents of these neighborhoods may be at a disadvantage when attempting to achieve a healthy diet.

Our findings underscore the importance of including characteristics of individuals' local food environments in future studies to gain a better understanding of barriers to healthy eating. The retail sector has been affected by economic policies that support corporate retail chains, public and private sector loan policies that favor home ownership for whites, and land-use policies that facilitate development of predominantly wealthy and white suburban neighborhoods.[26] These economic trends, from which the race and class patterns of the local food environment observed in our study might be predicted, suggest that creation of more egalitarian local food environments will require fundamental changes in local, state, and national economic and land-use policies.

Notes

1. Yen, I. H., & Kaplan, G. A. (1999). Neighborhood social environment and risk of death: Multilevel evidence from the Alameda County Study. *Am J Epidemiol, 149,* 898–907.

2. Diez-Roux, A. V., Nieto, F. J., Muntaner, C., et al. (1997). Neighborhood environments and coronary heart disease: A multilevel analysis. *Am J Epidemiol, 146,* 48–63.

3. Stokols, D. (1992). Establishing and maintaining healthy environments: Towards a social ecology of health promotion. *Am Psychol, 47,* 6–22.

4. Sooman, A., & Macintyre, S. (1995). Health and perceptions of the local environment in socially contrasting neighborhoods in Glasgow. *Health & Place, 1,* 15–26.

5. Ellaway, A., & Macintyre, S. (1996). Does where you live predict health related behaviors? A case study in Glasgow. *Health Bull, 54,* 443–446.

6. O'Campo, P., Xue, X., Wang, M. C., & Caughy, M. (1997). Neighborhood risk factors for low birth weight in Baltimore City: A multilevel analysis. *Am J Public Health, 87,* 1113–1118.

7. Meade, M. S., & Earickson, R. J. (2000). *Medical geography* (2nd ed.). New York: Guilford Press.

8. Adrian, M., Ferguson, B. S., & Her, M. (1996). Does allowing the sale of wine in Quebec grocery stores increase consumption? *J Studies Alcohol, 57,* 434–448.

9. Gaziano, J. M., & Manson, J. E. (1996). Diet and heart disease: The role of fat, alcohol and antioxidants. *Cardiol Clin, 14,* 69–83.

10. Krichevsky, D. (1999). Diet and atherosclerosis. *Am Heart J, 138,* S426–S430.

11. American Heart Association. (2000). *An eating plan for healthy Americans: The new 2000 food guidelines.* Dallas, TX: American Heart Association.

12. Carleton, R. A., Lasater, T. M., Assaf, A. R., Feldman, H. A., & McKinlay, S. (1995). The Pawtucket Heart Health Program: Community changes in cardiovascular risk factors and projected disease risk. *Am J Public Health, 85,* 777–785.

13. Farquhar, J. W., Fortmann, S. P., Flora, J. A., et al. (1990). Effects of community-wide education on cardiovascular disease risk factors: The Stanford five-city project. *JAMA, 264,* 359–365.

14. Luepker, R. V., Rastam L., Hannan P. J., et al. (1996). Community education for cardiovascular disease prevention: Morbidity and mortality results from the Minnesota Heart Health Program. *Am J Epidemiol, 144,* 351–362.

15. Glanz, K., Basil, M., Maibach, E., Goldberg, J., & Snyder, D. (1998). Why Americans eat what they do: Taste, nutrition, cost, convenience, and weight control concerns as influences on food consumption. *J Am Diet Assoc, 98,* 1118–1126.

16. Sooman, A., Macintyre, S., & Anderson, A. (1993). Scotland's health: A more difficult challenge for some? The price and availability of healthy foods in socially contrasting localities in the West of Scotland. *Health Bull, 51,* 276–284.

17. Foley, R. M., & Pollard, C. M. (1998). Food cent$: Implementing and evaluating a nutrition education project focusing on value for money. *Aust N Z J Public Health, 22,* 494–501.

18. Mackerras, D. (1997). Disadvantaged, and the cost of food. *Aust N Z J Public Health, 21,* 218.

19. Mooney, C. (1986). Cost and the availability of healthy food choices in a London health district. *J Hum Nutr Diet, 86,* 1684–1693.

20. House Select Committee on Hunger. (1990, October). *Food security in the United States: Committee report.* Washington, DC: U.S. Government Printing Office.

21. House Select Committee on Hunger. (1987, December). *Obtaining food: Shopping constraints of the poor: Committee report.* Washington, DC: U.S. Government Printing Office.

22. House Select Committee on Hunger. (1992, October). *Urban grocery gap: Committee report.* Washington, DC: U.S. Government Printing Office.

23. Curtis, K. A., & McClellan, S. (1995). Falling through the safety net: Poverty, food assistance and shopping constraints in an American city. *Urban Anthropol, 24,* 93–135.

24. Sallis, J. F., Nader, R., & Atkins, J. (1986). San Diego surveyed for heart healthy foods and exercise facilities. *Public Health Rep, 101,* 216–218.

25. Turrell, G. (1996). Structural, material and economic influences on the food purchasing choices of socioeconomic groups. *Aust N Z J Public Health, 20,* 11–17.

26. Massey, D. S., & Denton, N. A. (1993). *American apartheid, segregation and the making of the underclass.* Cambridge, MA: Harvard University Press.

27. Atherosclerosis Risk in Communities Investigators. (1989). The Atherosclerosis Risk in Communities (ARIC) study: Design and objectives. *Am J Epidemiol, 129,* 687–702.

28. U.S. Bureau of the Census. (1990). *Population and housing summary tape files 3A* (Summary tape file 3 on CD-ROM). Washington, DC: U.S. Department of Commerce.

29. Economic Classification Policy Committee, U.S. Bureau of the Census. (1998). *NAICS: New data for a new economy.* Washington, DC: U.S. Bureau of the Census.

30. Verizon New Media Services, Inc. (1999). *Yellow Pages.* Retrieved October 19, 1999, from www.superpages.com

31. Selvin, S. (1995). *Practical biostatistical methods* (2nd ed.). Belmont, CA: Duxbury Press.

32. SAS Institute. (1990). *SAS/STAT User's Guide.* Cary, NC: Author.

33. Diez Roux, A. V., Nieto, F. J., Caulfield, L., Tyroler, H. A., Watson, R. L., & Szklo, M. (1999). Neighbourhood differences in diet: The Atherosclerosis Risk in Communities (ARIC) study. *J Epidemiol Community Health, 53,* 55–63.

34. Dobofsky, J. E. (1969). Fair housing: A legislative history and a perspective. *Washburn Law J, 8,* 149–166.

35. Milio, N. (1989). *Promoting health through public policy.* Ottawa, Canada: Public Health Association.

CHAPTER TWENTY-FIVE

"We Don't Carry That"

Failure of Pharmacies in Predominantly Nonwhite Neighborhoods to Stock Opioid Analgesics

R. Sean Morrison
Sylvan Wallenstein
Dana K. Natale
Richard S. Senzel
Lo-Li Huang

Pain is one of the most common and widely feared symptoms of illness.[1] Studies of diverse populations of patients have found that unrelieved pain is highly prevalent,[2-17] especially among minority groups.[18-20] We have observed that many of our patients, particularly those who are black or Hispanic, have substantial difficulty obtaining commonly prescribed opioids from their neighborhood pharmacies. We conducted a study to determine the availability of commonly prescribed opioids in New York City pharmacies.

METHODS

We surveyed a random sample of 30 percent of pharmacies listed in the 1998 NYNEX Yellow Pages for the five boroughs of New York City[21-25] in order to obtain information about their opioid stock. Using the 1998 *Physicians' Desk Reference*,[26] the Agency for Health Care Policy and Research (AHCPR) guidelines for the treatment of pain from cancer,[27] and advice from a panel of experts in palliative care, we developed a list of commonly prescribed oral and topical opioid analgesic agents, including doses for the treatment of moderate-to-severe pain (Table 25.1). Opioids were divided into four categories on the basis of the

We are indebted to Dante Tipiani and Grace Chow for assisting with the interviews and to Konheim & Ketcham, of Brooklyn, New York, for providing the census data.

Table 25.1. Opioid Agents and Doses

Opioid Category	Dose
Long-acting opioids	
Fentanyl transdermal patch	25 μg, 50 μg, 75 μg, and 100 μg
Delayed release	
Morphine	15 mg, 30 mg, 60 mg, 100 mg, and 200 mg
Oxycodone	10 mg, 20 mg, 40 mg, and 80 mg
Short-acting opioids—tablet	
Morphine	15 mg and 30 mg
Hydromorphone	2 mg, 4 mg, and 8 mg
Oxycodone	5 mg
Short-acting opioids—liquid	
Morphine	20 mg/ml, 10 mg/5 ml, 20 mg/5 ml, 100 mg/5 ml, and 20 mg/10 ml
Hydromorphone	5 mg/5 ml
Oxycodone hydrochloride	20 mg/ml
Combination products	
Acetaminophen and codeine	325 mg of acetaminophen and 15 mg of codeine, 325 mg of acetaminophen and 30 mg of codeine, and 325 mg of acetaminophen and 60 mg of codeine
Acetaminophen and oxycodone	325 mg of acetaminophen and 5 mg of oxycodone
Aspirin, oxycodone, and oxycodone terephthalate	325 mg of aspirin, 4.5 mg of oxycodone, and 0.38 mg of oxycodone terephthalate

AHCPR guidelines: combination products for the treatment of moderate pain, short-acting opioid tablets for dose-finding in patients with severe pain and for the treatment of breakthrough pain, short-acting opioids in liquid form for the treatment of severe pain in patients with swallowing difficulties or in those in whom precise dose adjustments are required, and long-acting opioids for the extended treatment of severe pain.

Pharmacy stock was categorized as complete, nearly complete, incomplete, or absent. We considered supplies complete if the pharmacy had in stock an agent in each of the four medication categories; nearly complete if the pharmacy had in stock sufficient medication to treat a patient in moderate or severe pain—that is, a long-acting opioid, a short-acting opioid (tablet or liquid), and an opioid combination product; incomplete if the pharmacy lacked either a long-acting or a short-acting opioid preparation; and absent if the pharmacy did not carry any opioids but did stock other prescription medications.

Research assistants contacted the pharmacists by telephone. They were assured that the information they provided would be used for research purposes only, that no record would be kept of the pharmacy's name, and that responses would be kept completely confidential. Information about the study, printed on official stationery of the Mount Sinai School of Medicine, was faxed to the individual pharmacies. Pharmacists were given the option of responding over the telephone or faxing their responses to the research office. To ensure the reliability of the results, ten responding pharmacists from each borough of New York City were randomly selected, contacted by telephone again, and questioned about a random sample of ten opioid agents. A comparison of these responses with the original responses yielded complete agreement in all fifty cases.

Pharmacists provided oral informed consent when they were contacted by the research assistant. The study was approved by the institutional review board of the Mount Sinai School of Medicine.

Pharmacists representing pharmacies with inadequate supplies (incomplete or absent supplies) were asked open-ended questions about why they did not carry a full stock of opioid agents. Two of us independently reviewed and classified the reasons given for inadequate supplies. There was complete agreement between the two sets of classifications.

For each of the pharmacies surveyed, we used 1997 U.S. Census block group estimates and mapping software (MapInfo Professional, version 4.0, MapInfo Corporation) to determine the racial and ethnic composition of the neighborhood in which the pharmacy was located (defined as the area within a 0.4-km (0.25-mile) radius of the pharmacy), as well as the median household income, education level of neighborhood residents, and proportion of persons over the age of sixty-five years in the neighborhood. We included the variable for age because the prevalence of terminal illness and of chronic painful conditions is higher among the elderly than among younger persons, and therefore the demand for analgesic medications may be associated with the age of the residents in a neighborhood. We chose a 0.4-km radius as the definition of a neighborhood because it represented a reasonable walking distance from a pharmacy. Since one reason for not stocking opioids may be concern about theft or drug abuse,[28] we obtained 1997 data on robberies, burglaries, and arrests involving illicit drugs from the New York City Police Department for the precinct in which each of the pharmacies was located.

Because of the extreme skewedness of crime rates, the data were analyzed by subdividing the rates for robbery, burglary, and illicit drug related arrests into four groups, which were then analyzed as unordered categorical variables. For the proportion of white residents in a neighborhood, data were divided into four categories on the basis of logical breaks in the histogram and a desire to use round numbers. A neighborhood was categorized as predominantly nonwhite if less than 40 percent of the residents were white, as mixed if 40 to 69 percent were white, as primarily white if 70 to 79 percent were white, and as predominantly white if 80 to 100 percent were white. For black, Hispanic, and Asian residents, the corresponding percentages for the four categories were less than 10 percent, 10 to 19 percent, 20 to 39 percent, and 40 percent or more. Neighborhoods could be categorized for two or more racial or ethnic groups.

The adequacy of opioid supplies was analyzed according to the categories of racial and ethnic composition. The Cochran-Armitage test for trend was used to determine whether differences in racial composition corresponded to differences in the availability of opioids. A generalized linear model for correlated data (constructed with the Proc Genmod procedure of the SAS software package, version 6.12) was used to analyze the data on the basis of a logit-link function, with the assumption that all census blocks within a precinct were equally correlated with each other. The dependent variable was a binary measure of the adequacy of opioid stock, with adequate stock defined as complete or nearly complete supplies and inadequate stock as incomplete supplies or none. Confidence intervals were based on asymptotic theory.

RESULTS

We identified 503 pharmacies (160 in Manhattan, 130 in Brooklyn, 114 in Queens, 72 in the Bronx, and 27 on Staten Island) from the NYNEX *Yellow Pages*. Seventy-two of these pharmacies were no longer in business, were duplicate establishments, were located outside the New York City limits, or did not carry prescription medications. Of the pharmacists who represented the remaining 431 pharmacies, 84 refused to participate in the study, leaving a sample of 347 (an 81 percent response rate). Seventy-six percent of the pharmacies represented by respondents were independent, as were 76 percent of the pharmacies represented by nonrespondents. There were no significant differences in opioid supplies between chain and independent pharmacies, and the pharmacists representing chain pharmacies reported no specific corporate policies with regard to stocking opioids. The pharmacies represented by nonrespondents did not differ from those represented by respondents in terms of characteristics of the neighborhood (racial or ethnic composition, median household income, or education level of residents), characteristics of the pharmacy (independent or chain), or precinct crime rates.

Of the 347 pharmacies, 176 (51 percent) did not have opioid supplies that were sufficient to provide adequate treatment for a patient with severe pain. Thirty-five pharmacies (10 percent) had complete supplies, 136 (39 percent) had nearly complete supplies, 122 (35 percent) had incomplete supplies, and 54 (16 percent) had no opioids in stock. Although 116 of the 122 pharmacies with incomplete supplies (95 percent) had a combination product in stock that could be used for the treatment of moderate pain, only 55 (45 percent) carried a strong opioid preparation that could be used for the treatment of severe pain.

Table 25.2 shows the adequacy of opioid supplies according to the racial and ethnic composition of the neighborhoods in which the pharmacies were located. The tests for trend for all four categories of opioid supplies were significant ($p \leq .01$). Twenty-five percent of pharmacies in predominantly nonwhite neighborhoods (those in which less than 40 percent of residents were white) had adequate opioid supplies, as compared with 72 percent of pharmacies in predominantly white neighborhoods (those in which at least 80 percent of residents were white) (odds ratio for adequate supplies in predominantly nonwhite neighborhoods, 0.13; 95% confidence interval, 0.07, 0.26). Sixty-six percent of pharmacies that had no supplies of opioids were in predominantly nonwhite neighborhoods.

Table 25.2. Adequacy of Opioid Supplies at 347 Pharmacies, According to the Racial and Ethnic Composition of the Neighborhood

Racial and Ethnic Composition of Neighborhood	Total Pharmacies (no.)	Pharmacies with Adequate Opioids (%)	p Value for Trend
White			<0.001
0–39%	110	25	
40–69%	72	56	
70–79%	72	50	
≥80%	93	72	
Black			<0.001
<10%	173	61	
10–19%	53	45	
20–39%	57	42	
≥40%	64	30	
Hispanic			0.002
<10%	89	56	
10–19%	108	54	
20–39%	70	50	
≥40%	80	34	
Asian			0.01
<10%	241	54	
10–19%	74	42	
20–39%	16	44	
≥40%	16	25	

The results of a separate analysis of each ethnic and racial group were similar. The proportion of pharmacies with adequate opioid stocks was 30 percent in predominantly black neighborhoods (those in which 40 percent or more of the residents were black) as compared with 61 percent in predominantly nonblack neighborhoods (those in which less than 10 percent of the residents were black) (odds ratio, 0.28; 95% confidence interval, 0.14, 0.54), 34 percent in predominantly Hispanic neighborhoods as compared with 56 percent in predominantly non-Hispanic neighborhoods (odds ratio, 0.38; 95% confidence interval, 0.19, 0.74), and 25 percent in predominantly Asian neighborhoods as compared with 54 percent in predominantly non-Asian neighborhoods (odds ratio, 0.29; 95% confidence interval, 0.07, 0.99). After adjustment for rates of burglary, robbery, and illicit drug related arrests at the precinct level and for the percentage of residents over the age of sixty-five years at the census block level, pharmacies in predominantly nonwhite neighborhoods were also significantly less likely to have adequate opioid supplies than were pharmacies in predominantly white neighborhoods (odds ratio, 0.15; 95% confidence interval, 0.07, 0.31). In addition, pharmacies in neighborhoods in the highest quartile of burglary rates were less likely to have adequate opioid supplies than were pharmacies in neighborhoods in the lowest quartile of burglary rates (odds ratio, 0.29; 95% confidence interval, 0.12, 0.71).

The pharmacists representing the 176 pharmacies with inadequate opioid supplies were asked why they did not have adequate supplies. Ninety-five pharmacists (54 percent) reported that they had little demand for these medications, 78 (44 percent) cited concern about disposal, 35 (20 percent) cited fear of fraud and illicit drug use that might result in investigations by the Drug Enforcement Administration, 34 (19 percent) cited fear of robbery, and 13 (7 percent) cited other reasons (for example, problems with reimbursement by health plans and Medicaid).

DISCUSSION

We found that more than 50 percent of a random sample of New York City pharmacies did not have adequate medication in stock to treat a person in severe pain. An analysis adjusted for age and rates of burglary, robbery, and drug-related arrests showed that pharmacies in predominantly nonwhite neighborhoods were significantly less likely to stock opioids than were pharmacies in predominantly white neighborhoods. Two-thirds of the pharmacies that did not carry any opioids were in neighborhoods where the majority of the residents were nonwhites. This finding, together with reports[18-20] that nonwhite patients are significantly less likely than white patients to receive prescriptions for analgesic agents recommended by the AHCPR,[27] suggests that members of racial and ethnic minority groups are at substantial risk for the undertreatment of pain.

Pharmacists gave three chief reasons for having inadequate supplies of opioids: regulations with regard to disposal, illicit use, and fraud; low demand; and fear of theft. Open-ended interviews revealed that a major reason for not stocking an adequate supply of opioids, apart from low demand, was the additional paperwork required by state and federal dug enforcement agencies, the regulatory oversight and monitoring of these medications, and fear of penalties imposed by state and federal agencies. Although this study was conducted in New York, which requires triplicate prescription forms for most opioids, pharmacists did not report that this requirement was a reason for stocking inadequate supplies of opioids. Pharmacists who reported a low demand for opioids or expressed concern about their disposal were most likely to be in predominantly nonwhite neighborhoods.

There are several limitations to this study. First, it was impossible to determine conclusively whether there were differences in pharmacy supplies across neighborhoods of differing ethnic compositions when all other variables were held constant. To the extent that other variables were held constant by means of statistical adjustment, the results suggest that large and statistically significant differences remain in pharmacies' opioid holdings in different ethnic neighborhoods.

Second, this study was conducted in New York City and the results may not be generalizable to other areas.

Third, pharmacists in predominantly nonwhite neighborhoods may not have provided accurate reports of their opioid supplies over the telephone. Although we considered using "professional shoppers" to validate our results, we decided that this was an impractical strategy, given the number of pharmacies, the number of agents, and the state requirement of triplicate prescriptions. Nevertheless, we believe that our results are valid because nonrespondents did not differ from respondents with regard to neighborhood characteristics or type of pharmacy (chain or independent), and follow-up telephone calls to a random sample of the respondents showed no discrepancies between their responses during the call and their responses to the original survey.

Fourth, we did not ask about all opioids but instead concentrated on those that have been recommended as appropriate first-line medications. Thus, it is possible, albeit unlikely, that some pharmacies carried opioids that are useful for the treatment of severe pain (for example, levorphanol or methadone) but that we did not inquire about. Finally, most of the pharmacists we surveyed stated that they could order and obtain the requested medication for a patient within seventy-two hours. For patients in severe pain, seventy-two hours is an unacceptably long period of time.

Our data demonstrate that many New York City pharmacies do not stock sufficient medication to treat patients with severe pain. Furthermore, pharmacies in predominantly nonwhite neighborhoods are significantly less likely to stock adequate supplies of opioids than are pharmacies in predominantly white neighborhoods. These results suggest that nonwhite patients may be at even greater risk for the undertreatment of pain than previously reported. The problem of inadequate supplies of opioids calls for a program to educate pharmacists about the safe and appropriate use of opioid analgesics, as well as an evaluation of regulations that may act as disincentives for pharmacists to stock controlled substances.

Notes

1. Meier, D. E., Morrison, R. S., & Cassel, C. K. (1997). Improving palliative care. *Ann Intern Med, 127,* 225–230.

2. Kelsen, D. P., Portenoy, R. K., & Thaler, H. T., et al. (1995). Pain and depression in patients with newly diagnosed pancreas cancer. *J Clin Oncol, 13,* 748–755.

3. Larue, F., Colleau, S. M., Brasseur, L., & Cleeland, C. S. (1995). Multicentre study of cancer pain and its treatment in France. *Br Med J, 310,* 1034–1037.

4. Tay, W. K., Shaw, R. J., & Goh, C. R. (1994). A survey of symptoms in hospice patients in Singapore. *Ann Acad Med Singapore, 23,* 191–196.

5. Zenz, M., Zenz, T., Tryba, M., & Strumpf, M. (1995). Severe undertreatment of cancer pain: A 3-year survey of the German situation. *J Pain Symptom Manage, 10,* 187–191.

6. Von Roenn, J. H., Cleeland, C. S., Gonin, R., Hatfield, A. K., & Pandya, K. J. (1993). Physician attitudes and practice in cancer pain management: A survey from the Eastern Cooperative Oncology Group. *Ann Intern Med, 119,* 121–126.

7. Twycross, R. G., & Fairfield, S. (1982). Pain in far-advanced cancer. *Pain, 14,* 303–310.

8. Bernabei, R., Gambassi, G., Lapane, K., et al. (1998). Management of pain in elderly patients with cancer. *JAMA, 279,* 1877–1882. (Erratum: *JAMA* (1999), *281,* 136.)

9. Lynch, E. P., Lazor, M. A., Gellis, J. E., Orav, J., Goldman, L., & Marcantonio, E. R. (1997). Patient experience of pain after elective noncardiac surgery. *Anesth Analg, 85,* 117–123.

10. Oates, J. D., Snowdon, S. L., & Jayson, D. W. (1994). Failure of pain relief after surgery: Attitudes of ward staff and patients to postoperative analgesia. *Anaesthesia, 49,* 755–758.

11. Cohen, F. L. (1980). Postsurgical pain relief: Patients' status and nurses' medication choices. *Pain, 9,* 265–274.

12. Breibart, W., McDonald, M. V., Rosenfeld, B., et al. (1996). Pain in ambulatory AIDS patients: I. Pain characteristics and medical correlates. *Pain, 68,* 315–321.

13. The SUPPORT Principal Investigators. (1995). A controlled trial to improve care for seriously ill hospitalized patients: The Study to Understand Prognoses and Preferences for Outcomes and Risks of Treatments (SUPPORT). *JAMA, 274,* 1591–1598. (Erratum: *JAMA* (1996), *275,* 1232.)

14. Cleeland, C. S., Gonin, R., Hatfield, A. K., et al. (1994). Pain and its treatment in outpatients with metastatic cancer. *N Engl J Med, 33,* 592–596.

15. Faherty, B. S., & Grier, M. R. (1984). Analgesic medication for elderly people postsurgery. *Nurs Res, 33,* 369–372.

16. Closs, S. J. (1990). An exploratory analysis of nurses' provision of postoperative analgesic drugs. *J Adv Nurs, 15,* 42–49.

17. Morrison, R. S., & Siu, A. L. (2000). A comparison of pain and its treatment in advanced dementia and cognitively intact patients with hip fracture. *J Pain Symptom Manage, 19,* 240–248.

18. Cleeland, C. S., Gonin, R., Baez, L., Loehrer, P., & Pandya, K. J. (1997). Pain and treatment of pain in minority patients with cancer: The Eastern Cooperative Oncology Group Minority Outpatient Pain Study. *Ann Intern Med, 127,* 813–816.

19. Todd, K. H., Samaroo, N., & Hoffman, J. R. (1993). Ethnicity as a risk factor for inadequate emergency department analgesia. *JAMA, 269,* 1537–1539.

20. McDonald, D. D. (1994). Gender and ethnic stereotyping and narcotic analgesic administration. *Res Nurs Health, 17,* 45–49.

21. *NYNEX Yellow Pages: Manhattan.* (1998). New York: NYNEX Information Resources.

22. *NYNEX Yellow Pages: Brooklyn.* (1998). New York: NYNEX Information Resources.

23. *NYNEX Yellow Pages: Staten Island.* (1998). New York: NYNEX Information Resources.

24. *NYNEX Yellow Pages: Bronx.* (1998). New York: NYNEX Information Resources.

25. *NYNEX Yellow Pages: Queens.* (1998). New York: NYNEX Information Resources.

26. *Physicians' desk reference* (52nd ed.). (1998). Montvale, NJ: Medical Economics.

27. Jacox, A., Carr, D. B., Payne, R., et al. (1994). *Management of cancer pain: Clinical practice guideline no. 9* (AHCPR publication No. 94-0592). Rockville, MD: Agency for Health Care Policy and Research.

28. Kanner, R. M., & Portenoy, R. K. (1986). Unavailability of narcotic analgesics for ambulatory cancer patients in New York City. *J Pain Symptom Manage, 1,* 187–189.

CHAPTER TWENTY-SIX

Solid Waste Sites and the Black Houston Community

Robert D. Bullard

Much attention in recent years has been devoted to the problem of equality and urban public services. Institutional racism and discrimination have been shown to greatly influence the quality of life in America's urban centers.[1,2] Wellman asserts that "racism can be seen to systematically provide economic, political, psychological, and social advantages for whites at the expense of blacks and other people of color" (p. 37).[3] Studies that focus on urban service allocation and delivery are inquiries into discrimination and equality (p. 15).[4] Lineberry describes the problem of differential public services in urban areas:

> That municipal governments may disadvantage the underclass through differential provision of public services is the more common focus. The other face of services equality, however, may be more important. It arises from the semimonopolistic character of public service delivery systems. . . . Escaping a deteriorating public school system, or a high crime rate or unsightly neighborhoods involves either moving or securing comfort and convenience from the private sector. . . . The ease of exit is roughly proportional to affluence. When racial barriers also exist, minority groups suffer a sort of double jeopardy in attempting to exit an unresponsive monopoly [pp. 174–175].[4]

Originally presented at the annual meeting of the Southwestern Sociological Association, March 17–20, 1982, San Antonio, Texas.

The idea that the poor and minority groups suffer a differential effect of inadequate public services is a widely held view.[5] The principal factors that contributed to the urban disturbances of the 1960s included dissatisfaction with municipal services in the urban ghettos (for example, policing, educational institutions, parks and recreational facilities, garbage and refuse collection, and so forth). The National Advisory Commission on Civil Disorders found that "inadequate sanitation services are viewed by many ghetto residents not merely as instances of poor public services but as manifestations of racial discrimination" (p. 148).[6] Low-income and minority neighborhoods in many urban areas are often less well served by municipal governments than are their high-income counterparts. Many of the early federal poverty programs were designed to combat these service inequities.[7,8]

Urban neighborhoods within America's municipalities are not randomly scattered over the urban landscape. Minority and lower income neighborhoods often occupy the "wrong side of the tracks" and subsequently may receive inadequate public services. The sociospatial groupings that emerge in urban areas are a result of "the distribution of wealth, patterns of racial and economic discrimination, access to jobs, housing, real estate practices, and a host of other variables" (p. 11).[4] While neighborhoods are not randomly located in the metropolitan complex, neither are nonresidential activities randomly scattered. David M. Smith contends that

> the location of every new facility favors or disfavors those nearby, and thus redistributes well-being or ill-being. Any development of land has similar effects. How people in different areas establish differential claims on society's resources depends upon the spatial exercise of political power. . . . Ultimately, who gets what *where* and how must be viewed as a question of equity or fairness [p. 294].[9]

Zoning has been the major land use control of external diseconomics and disamenities imposed by nonresidential activities on nearby residents. Externalities such as "polluting discharges to air and water, noise, vibrations, traffic congestion and hazard, and aesthetic disamenities" are often segregated from residential areas because of "public goods, or more commonly public bads." These activities are "spatially located, that is, their adverse effects fall off with distance from the source" (pp. 521–522).[10]

A great deal of attention in recent years has been devoted to the issues of pollution, waste disposal, and the possible health problems that may result from mismanagement of waste. The more than 20,000 active hazardous waste sites scattered across the United States were not publicized until the Love Canal incident made the news. The Environmental Protection Agency estimates that 90 percent of these sites do not meet the federal standards. Waste disposal sites cover more than 100,000 acres of land in the United States; many of these sites are located on prime real estate. As America has developed into a "throw away society," waste collection and disposal is big business. American consumers spend over $4 billion each year to collect and dispose of waste; it will cost consumers over $6 billion a year to collect and dispose of waste by 1985.[11]

The siting of waste disposal facilities has become a controversial issue in the Houston area. As one of the largest American cities without zoning, Houston's land use pattern is somewhat erratic. A proliferation of waste disposal facilities dots the Houston landscape. A liberal annexation policy has allowed the city to expand from a mere 9 square miles in 1850 to over 550 square miles in 1982. The city's lax enforcement of deed restrictions in many inner-city and minority neighborhoods has contributed to uneven growth and has accelerated neighborhood decline.[12] Industrial encroachment into residential areas has become an ever increasing problem in a number of minority neighborhoods. Lower income and minority neighborhoods (for example, "poverty pockets") lie in the path of expanding industrial markets.

The decisions to locate municipal waste disposal facilities near residential areas were political decisions made by local city council members. Prior to 1970, no black or Hispanic person had ever held a city council seat in Houston. Thus, Houston's all-white and all-male city council, with assistance from the city's planning and solid waste departments, made key decisions on where to dispose of the city's waste. As landfills and waste disposal sites are considered to be disamenities to residential areas, it seems plausible that white council members would locate these facilities *away* from their neighborhoods (that is, white neighborhoods).

The development of residential areas in Houston continues along racial and ethnic lines. Specifically, blacks remain segregated from both whites and Hispanics.[13–18] Over three-fourths of the city's blacks live in neighborhoods that are more than 70 percent black.[19] Houston's black population has had a steady increase over the past thirty years, growing from 125,000 in 1950 to 440,257, or 27.6 percent of the city's population, in 1980.[20]

Thus, the purpose of this study was to test the proposition that waste disposal siting has followed the "path of least resistance" in the Houston area. The research attempts to answer the following three questions:

1. Is there a relationship between the location of waste disposal facilities and racial composition of neighborhoods?

2. Is there a significant difference between the waste disposal siting patterns of municipalities and those of private sector disposal companies?

3. Are black children more likely to attend schools near municipal landfills than are their nonblack counterparts (for example, whites and Hispanics)?

THE POLITICS OF WASTE DISPOSAL AND THE ENVIRONMENT

Prior to 1976, the term "solid waste" meant only one thing to most people: namely, municipal garbage. However, the passage of the Resource Conservation and Recovery Act (RCRA) in 1976 directed the nation's attention to hazardous waste, industrial waste, and to all waste, solid or liquid, that is disposed of in landfills. Jorling has asserted that "prior to the passage of RCRA the effect of our public policy was to subsidize dumping" (p. 3).[21] There were over 14,000 "dumps" in the United States in 1972 that posed a serious environmental and health problem (pp. 21–22),[22] (pp. 41–42).[23]

Finding suitable sites for sanitary landfills has become a critical problem nationwide mainly because people are reluctant to live near a facility where garbage is dumped. The standard public reaction has been "not in my neighborhood" (p. 1).[24] Solid waste management and land disposal siting have become volatile political issues throughout the nation. There is a general consensus that "everyone wants you to pick up their garbage, but no one wants you to put it down" (p. 24).[25] The "politics of garbage" has plunged elected officials deeper into the collection and disposal problems associated with municipal waste. Political "fall guys" are often created, at whom elected officials can point their fingers. When a landfill site is located near a residential area, public officials often place the blame away from their offices and onto the federal government, state or other governmental jurisdiction, or private disposal companies.[25]

Christopher Lindley, a city council member from Rochester, New York, adequately summed up the political nature of landfill siting as follows:

> The political problem is not only that people do not like landfills around them anymore, but also the problem of the interrelationship among the communities in a metropolitan area. Traditionally, the public's view of their relationship with the central city has always been "what's ours is ours and what's yours we share." . . . The central cities have become the dumping grounds frequently for metropolitan social costs across the board. But when we raise the question of a landfill outside our jurisdiction, all of a sudden it becomes intolerable [p. 25].[25]

The differential quality of affluent and poor neighborhoods has long been documented. The quality of life in many lower- and working-class neighborhoods is far worse than that in middle- and upper-class neighborhoods (p. 436).[26] The various forms of pollution take a heavy toll on inner-city neighborhoods because "the poor or near poor are the ones most vulnerable to the assaults of air and water pollution, the stress and tension of noise and squalor" (p. 26).[27] Air pollution in inner cities can be found at levels up to five times greater than those in suburban areas; middle- and upper-class households can often shut out the noise, fumes, and odors with their air conditioning, grind up their garbage, and keep out the rats (p. 27).[27]

While lower and working classes are subjected to a disproportionately larger amount of pollution within their workplace as well as neighborhoods, these groups have been only marginally involved in the nation's environmental movement.[10,26–32] The historical development of the environmental movement in America emerged with agendas that were primarily supported by middle- and upper-middle-class people; the poor and working-class people who often have less favorable environments desire a better physical environment but have less basis to expect a more favorable setting.[30] Many environmental battles were waged that seemed only to affect the elites and to injure the poor. The mobility of middle-class people makes them less vulnerable to environmental problems than the poor. People and businesses that can afford to flee to the suburbs do so while the poor and the less advantaged stay behind and suffer from poverty and pollution (p. 27).[27]

RESEARCH PROCEDURE

This case study of Houston's municipal solid waste disposal system was developed from in-depth interviews with personnel from Houston's Solid Waste Management Division and the Houston Air Quality Board. Initial contacts were made by telephone with both city departments, and personal interviews were undertaken with key administrative personnel.* During these interviews field notes were taken, and they form the basis for this report. On-site visits were made to the solid waste disposal facilities to verify the data obtained from the interviews.

Secondary data were also used as a source for this study. The major sources of secondary data were (1) the Texas Department of Health Solid Waste Active Permit Sites in Harris County as of August 30, 1979; (2) the U.S. Bureau of the Census tract and block statistics for the Houston–Harris County area; and (3) pupil enrollment data for the Houston area public schools.

HOUSTON-OWNED GARBAGE INCINERATORS

The City of Houston operated its own garbage disposal facilities up until the early 1970s. The historical disposal approaches that have been used by Houston include incineration and landfills. One of the oldest city-owned incinerators was located in Houston's Fourth Ward (see Table 26.1). This site dates back to the

---

*Personal interviews were conducted between November 13, 1981, and February 10, 1982. Key City of Houston staff persons interviewed were Ta-Bin Yim, director of planning, Solid Waste Management Division; Anthony Lamott, an administrator in the Houston Solid Waste Management Division and city employee since 1956; and Carl Seltzer and Virgil Lehmburg, both of the Houston Air Quality Control Division.

Table 26.1. City of Houston Garbage Incinerators

Site of Incinerator	Neighborhood	Ethnicity	Location
Fourth Ward (Gillette and Hobson)	Fourth Ward	Black	Southwest
Patterson Street (2500 Patterson and Katy Freeway)	West End/ Cottage Grove	Black	Northwest
Kelly Street (North Loop and Eastex Freeway)	Kashmere Gardens	Black	Northeast
Holmes Road (Bellfort and South Freeway)	Sunnyside	Black	Southeast
Velasco (Velasco and Navigation)	Second Ward	Hispanic	Southeast

Note: These Houston-owned garbage incinerators were in operation from the 1920s to 1975.

1920s. Other city-owned incinerators include the Patterson Street site, the Kelly Street site, the Holmes Road site (located on Bellfort), and the Velasco site. The data in Table 26.1 clearly illustrate that the City of Houston historically located its incinerators in nonwhite neighborhoods. Specifically, four of the five incinerator sites were located in predominantly black neighborhoods; the fifth site was located in a predominantly Hispanic neighborhood. The five neighborhoods where Houston incinerators were operated were (1) Fourth Ward, (2) West End/Cottage Grove, (3) Kashmere Gardens, (4) Sunnyside, and (5) Second Ward, or "Segundo Barrio." The cost of operating these incinerators and the problems of pollution generated by these systems were major factors in their closing.

HOUSTON MINI-INCINERATOR PROJECT

The City of Houston contracted with a private company to conduct a "pilot project" of mini-incinerators that were supposed to be more efficient (that is, cost less to operate and burn cleaner). The City of Houston invested $1.9 million in a contractual agreement with Houston Natural Gas Company in 1972 for these mini-incinerators that were thought to be "pollution free." Three sets of incinerators were installed in the city (see Table 26.2). One site was located on Westpark, another site was located on Kelly Street near the North Loop, and the third site was located on Sommermeyer in northwest Houston. The Northwest Service

Table 26.2. Mini-Incinerators Operated by the City of Houston

Site of Mini-Incinerator	Neighborhood	Ethnicity	Location
Westpark (5900 Westpark)	Larchmont	White	Southwest
Kelly Street (North Loop and East Freeway)	Kashmere Gardens	Black	Northeast
Northwest Service Center (14300 Sommermeyer)	Carverdale	Black	Northwest

Note: The City of Houston contracted with a private firm, Houston Gas Company, to operate a "pilot" mini-incinerator project in 1972.

Center Incinerator site is the current site of Houston's first garbage transfer station. The incinerator and the present garbage transfer station are located in the Carverdale neighborhood, a predominantly black neighborhood. In addition, the Kelly Street mini-incinerators are also located in a predominantly black neighborhood (Kashmere Gardens). The Westpark mini-incinerator site, which is located on Westpark near the Southwest Freeway, was adjacent to a predominantly white neighborhood (Larchmont). Pilot tests of the mini-incinerators found them not to be "pollution free" because they performed with mixed results. The mini-incinerators did not meet the pollution standards of the Houston Air Quality Control Board and were shut down after a short period of operation in the mid-1970s.

CITY OF HOUSTON LANDFILLS

The City of Houston was in the landfill business for over fifty years. At least one of Houston's garbage dumpsites dates back to the 1920s. Table 26.3 is a listing of Houston landfill sites. The Fourth Ward dump was located on the site of present Jefferson Davis Hospital. That is, Jefferson Davis Hospital sits on top of Houston's Fourth Ward dump. The hospital was constructed in 1937 and 1938; the dumpsite was cleared and filled in for the building of the hospital. The Fourth Ward dumpsite extended from Taft Street on the west all the way to Lamb Street on the east. The Fourth Ward Incinerator on Gillette and Hobson was near the center of the dump.

Another Houston landfill that is over thirty years old is the Sunnyside site on Bellfort and Woodard, the Sunnyside Dump. Adjacent to the Sunnyside site on Bellfort is the Reed Road landfill. These two landfill sites are located just east of the Holmes Road Incinerator on Bellfort in southeast Houston. The landfill site on Bellfort and Woodard, the site on Reed Road, and the Holmes Road Incinerator—Houston's largest incinerator—are located in the heart of the predominantly black Sunnyside neighborhood. This area has a long and rich

Table 26.3. City of Houston Municipal Landfill Sites

Landfill Site	Neighborhood	Ethnicity	Location
Fourth Ward (Gillette and Allen Parkway)	Fourth Ward	Black	Southwest
Sunnyside (3500 Bellfort)	Sunnyside	Black	Southeast
Reed Road (2300 Reed Road and Kish)	Sunnyside	Black	Southeast
Kirkpatrick (Kirkpatrick and HB & T Railroad)	Trinity Gardens	Black	Northeast
West Donnovan (West Donnovan and Ella Boulevard)	Acres Homes	Black	Northwest

Note: These landfill sites were not permitted by the Texas Department of Health. The period of operation of the sites was from the 1920s to the early 1970s.

history as a semirural black community. The major business corridor in the Sunnyside neighborhood lies along Reed Road. Historically, Reed Road is to Sunnyside what Lyons Avenue is to Fifth Ward, Dowling Street is to Third Ward, and West Dallas is to Fourth Ward. The Sunnyside area developed as a "self-contained" segregated community in the 1940s. Much of the development of the neighborhood took place along Holmes Road. The placing of these waste disposal facilities along the major streets in this area is equivalent to such facilities being placed along Bellaire Boulevard in the City of Bellaire or along University Boulevard in the City of West University Place or along Main Street in the City of Houston.

The Kirkpatrick landfill in Trinity Gardens operated during 1970 and 1971. This landfill is also located in a predominantly black neighborhood. Residents in the neighborhood strongly protested the siting of the landfill in their neighborhood. However, the site was opened and operated for a short period of time.

The West Donnovan site off Ella Boulevard, or the Acres Homes Dump, has been an issue in this predominantly black neighborhood in northwest Houston. This northwest Houston neighborhood has four solid waste sites that were permitted by the Texas Department of Health from 1970 to 1975.

In tracing the historical development of Houston's waste disposal systems, the data revealed that Houston has operated incinerators and landfills, the earliest of which date back to the 1920s. Houston initiated a "pilot project" of mini-incinerators in the early 1970s that was not successful. Houston incinerators and landfills were more likely to be located in black Houston neighborhoods than nonblack Houston neighborhoods (see Table 26.4). Specifically, four (80 percent) of the five Houston-owned incinerators were located in black neighborhoods,

Table 26.4. Summary of City of Houston Solid Waste Disposal Sites

Waste Disposal Sites	Ethnicity		Total
	Black	Nonblack	
Incinerators	4	1	5
	(80.0%)	(20.0%)	(100.0%)
Mini-incinerators	2	1	3
	(66.7%)	(33.3%)	(100.0%)
Landfills	5	—	5
	(100.0%)	—	(100.0%)

while one incinerator (20 percent) was located in a nonblack neighborhood (that is, it was located in a Hispanic neighborhood); two (66.7 percent) of the three mini-incinerators Houston operated under its pilot program were located in black neighborhoods, while the third site was near a nonblack neighborhood. The data for Houston's landfill sites revealed that all five sites (100 percent) were operated in predominantly black neighborhoods.

TEXAS DEPARTMENT OF HEALTH PERMITTED HOUSTON LANDFILLS

Between 1970 and 1978, the Texas Department of Health permitted a total of twenty-one solid waste sites in the Houston area. Of the twenty-one solid waste sites permitted by the state, eleven (or 54.2 percent) were located in predominantly black neighborhoods (blacks constituted 26 percent of the Houston population in 1970 and 27.6 percent in 1980). The Texas Department of Health permitted a total of six landfill sites to receive municipal garbage from 1970 to 1978 in the Houston area; five of the six Houston landfills (83.3 percent) were located in predominantly black neighborhoods and the sixth landfill site was located near a predominantly white neighborhood undergoing racial transition (see Table 26.5).

The City of Houston was not alone in its siting of municipal landfills in predominantly black neighborhoods. The data in Table 26.5 indicate that the City of West University Place and the City of Bellaire both located their landfills during the mid-1950s in a predominantly black neighborhood in southwest Houston, namely, Riceville. The Riceville neighborhood dates back to the 1850s. The area was developed as a rural community surrounded by rice fields. The City of Houston annexed the Riceville community in 1965. However, the area is still without many neighborhood amenities such as paved streets, regular garbage pickup, running water, and sewer and gas hookups. It seems somewhat

Table 26.5. Texas Department of Health Permitted Municipal Landfill Sites, Houston, Texas, 1953–1978

Landfill Site	Year Permitted/ Opened	Neighborhood	Ethnicity
City of Bellaire (9792 Ruffino)	1953*	Riceville	Black
West University Place (9610 Ruffino)	1956†	Riceville	Black
American Refuse Systems (1140 Holmes Road)	1970	Almeda Plaza	Black
Browning-Ferris Industries (11013 Beaumont Highway)	1971	Chatwood	Nonblack‡
Browning-Ferris Industries (1140 Holmes Road)	1978	Almeda Plaza	Black
Southwestern Waste Management (11800 E. Houston Dyersdale Road)	1978	Northwood Manor	Black

*This date represents the year in which the City of Bellaire site opened; the site was later permitted in 1970.

†This date represents the year in which the West University Place site opened; the site was later granted a permit in 1970.

‡The Chatwood subdivision is a predominantly white area that lies within Houston's Community Development Program Settegast Target Area. The Settegast Target Area is a racial transitional area because its racial composition has increased from 40 percent black in 1970 to over 70 percent black in 1980.

ironic that two virtually all-white cities (Bellaire and West University) would select the nearby all-black Riceville neighborhood as the site to dispose of their garbage. On the other hand, the Riceville community, after nearly seventeen years since annexation, has yet to receive regular garbage pickup services on all of its streets.

When the City of Houston prepared to discontinue its own waste disposal facilities, private waste disposal companies were used to fill the void. The City of Houston contracted with a private waste disposal company (American Refuse Systems, Inc.) in 1968 to dispose of city waste by landfill. The city contract with American Refuse Systems was extended in 1971. From 1969 to 1972, American Refuse Systems operated five landfill sites: (1) Ella site, (2) Kirkpatrick site, (3) Almeda site, (4) Holmes Road site, and (5) Beaumont Highway site. American Refuse Systems was subsequently bought out by the Houston-based Browning-Ferris Industries (BFI), the "General Motors" of the garbage disposal business. Browning-Ferris Industries or its subsidiaries operated six state-permitted sites from 1970 to 1978. Five (83.3 percent) of the six landfill sites were located in predominantly black Houston neighborhoods; the sixth site was located in a nonblack transitional neighborhood, the Chatwood subdivision (see Table 26.6).

SOLID WASTE SITES AND NEIGHBORHOOD SCHOOLS

A great deal of public opposition to landfills has occurred in Houston neighborhoods. A central theme of this opposition seems to center on the location of landfill sites near neighborhood schools. The lack of city ordinances or restrictions on locating landfills has contributed to the siting concerns of residents of affected areas. Landfills located near schools can present special problems: (1) schools may not have air conditioning; (2) the neighborhood may not have sidewalks and the students may have to walk along the streets in going to and from school; and (3) increased truck traffic may present a special safety problem for elementary school age children.

The data in Table 26.7 reveal that solid waste sites are located near a significantly large number of Houston area schools. A disproportionately large number of predominantly black schools, compared to their nonblack counterparts, were found near solid waste sites. This was true for city-owned landfills as well as privately owned landfills. Specifically, the landfill sites that were operated by

Table 26.6. Browning-Ferris Industries Landfill Sites, Houston, Texas, 1970–1978

Site	Year of Permit	Neighborhood	Ethnicity	Location
American Refuse (1140 Holmes Road)	1970	Almeda Plaza	Black	Southeast
International Disposal (2100 Nieman Lane)	1970	Acres Homes	Black	Northwest
Browning-Ferris Industries (11013 Beaumont Highway)	1971	Chatwood	Nonblack	Northeast
Tex-Haul, Inc. (7200 Tidwell)	1972	Settegast	Black	Northeast
Browning-Ferris Industries (1140 Holmes Road)	1978	Almeda Plaza	Black	Southeast
Southwestern Waste Management (Whispering Pines) (11800 E. Houston Dyersdale Road)	1978	Northwood Manor	Black	Northeast

Note: These landfill sites are owned by Browning-Ferris Industries or its subsidiaries.

Table 26.7. Racial Composition of Area Schools Near Solid Waste Sites

| Solid Waste Sites | Ethnicity of Schools | | Total |
	Black	Nonblack	
City of Houston landfills	10	—	10
(1920–1976)	(100.0%)	—	(100.0%)
Texas Department of Health	31	16	47
permitted solid waste sites	(66.0%)	(34.0%)	(100.0%)
(1953–1978)			
Texas Department of Health	13	3	16
permitted municipal landfills	(77.0%)	(23.0%)	(100.0%)
(1953–1978)			
Browning-Ferris Industries	18	3	21
landfills in Houston	(85.7%)	(14.3%)	(100.0%)
(1970–1978)			

Note: These schools are located in the neighborhoods and census tracts where the solid waste sites were located.

the City of Houston were located near ten public schools; all ten schools were predominantly black schools. The twenty-one solid waste sites that were permitted by the Texas Department of Health between 1970 and 1978 were located near forty-seven schools of which thirty-one (66 percent) were predominantly black. The six Texas Department of Health municipal sites (licensed to receive municipal garbage) permitted in Houston were located near sixteen schools, over three-fourths (77 percent) of which were mostly black schools. And the six Browning-Ferris Industries landfill sites were located near twenty-one schools, 85.7 percent of which have a majority of black pupils. These data lend support to the notion that Houston's black schoolchildren are more likely to attend schools near landfills than are their nonblack counterparts.

CONCLUSION

The conclusion that can be drawn in this chapter reveals that the City of Houston located and operated solid waste disposal sites (incinerators and landfills) primarily in black neighborhoods. Thus, black Houston residents are more likely to live near Houston waste disposal sites than nonblacks are. This historical pattern of municipal waste disposal siting occurred over a fifty-year span.

The private waste disposal industry in Houston has followed the lead of local municipalities (the cities of Houston, Bellaire, and West University Place) in locating solid waste sites; that is, Houston solid waste disposal sites are more likely to be located in predominantly black neighborhoods than in nonblack neighborhoods. A disproportionately large percentage of waste disposal sites is located near predominantly black schools. Thus, the data indicate that black children are more likely to attend schools that are near solid waste sites than are their nonblack Houston counterparts.

The Texas Department of Health, a state permitting agency, has not deviated significantly from the long-established pattern of siting Houston municipal landfills in black neighborhoods. The state's record on Houston landfill permits clearly demonstrates that a significantly large percentage of such facilities are permitted in predominantly black neighborhoods.

Citizen opposition and environmental concerns over waste disposal are likely to increase and intensify in the future. Public opposition along with a shrinking pool of "cheap" land will force the adoption of alternative methods of waste disposal (for example, resource recovery). However, landfills are likely to be with us for some time as the chief method of waste disposal.

Finally, the jury is still out on the possible health hazards of municipal waste disposal sites on humans. That is, the long-term effects of municipal waste disposed of in landfills are not known. However, landfill sites are spatially localized; adverse effects decrease with distance from the landfill sites. Those neighborhoods and schools that are nearest to the waste disposal sites are likely to pay a significantly higher health price (that is, shorter lives, illnesses, and traffic hazards for children). It appears that institutionalized discrimination through the siting of waste disposal facilities has systematically provided social and economic advantages for whites at the expense of blacks, because whites do not live around waste disposal sites or send their children to schools near landfills.

Notes

1. Feagin, J. (1978). *Discrimination American style.* Englewood Cliffs, NJ: Prentice Hall.

2. Knowles, L., & Prewitt, K. (1970). *Institutional racism in America.* Englewood Cliffs, NJ: Prentice Hall.

3. Wellman, W. T. (1977). *Portraits of white racism.* Cambridge, UK: Cambridge University Press.

4. Lineberry, R. L. (1977). *Equality and urban policy: The distribution of municipal public services.* Beverly Hills, CA: Sage.

5. Fowler, F. J., Jr. (1974). *Citizen attitudes toward local government services and taxes.* Cambridge, MA: Ballinger.

6. National Advisory Commission on Civil Disorders. (1967). *Report of the National Advisory Commission on Civil Disorders.* Washington, DC: U.S. Government Printing Office.

7. Hallman, H. W. (1968). The community action program. In W. Bloomberg & H. Schmandt (Eds.), *Power, poverty and urban policy.* Beverly Hills, CA: Sage.

8. Lowry, I. S. (1968). Housing. In A. H. Pascal (Ed.), *Cities in trouble: An agenda for urban research*. Santa Monica, CA: Rand Corporation.

9. Smith, D. M. (1974, November). Who gets what where and how: A welfare focus for human geography. *Geography, 59,* 289–297.

10. Smith, J. N. (1974). *Environmental quality and social justice in urban America*. Washington, DC: The Conservation Foundation.

11. Purcell, A. H. (1980). *The wastewatchers: A citizen's handbook for conserving energy and resources*. New York: Anchor Books.

12. Bullard, R. D., & Tryman, D. L. (1981). *Strategies in neighborhood redevelopment: A case study of Houston's Fifth Ward*. Paper presented at the annual meeting of the Southwestern Sociological Association, Dallas.

13. Phillips, B. P. (1971). *Housing the poor: Dynamic factors*. Houston, TX: Southwest Center for Urban Research.

14. Davidson, C. (1972). *Biracial politics: Conflict and coalition in the metropolitan South*. Baton Rouge: Louisiana State University Press.

15. Bullard, R. D. (1978, July). Does Section 8 promote an ethnic and economic mix? *J Housing, 35,* 364–365.

16. Bullard, R. D., & Pierce, O. L. (1979, November–December). Black housing in a southern metropolis: Competition for housing in a shrinking market. *The Black Scholar, 11,* 60–67.

17. Bullard, R. D., & Tryman, D. L. (1980, Winter). Competition for decent housing: A focus on housing discrimination complaints in a sunbelt city. *J Ethn Studies, 7,* 51–63.

18. Bullard, R. D., & Tryman, D. L. (1980). *Housing mobility in the Houston metropolitan area: A survey of HUD assisted family developments* (Report prepared for the U.S. Department of Housing and Urban Development). Houston, TX: Demographic Environs Research, Inc.

19. Farrell, W. C., Johnson, J. H., & Johnson, P. A. (1978, March 4). The quality of Afro-American life in Houston, Texas: A geographic perspective. In J. Pilzer, W. Pindhur, & R. Proctor (Eds.), *Perspectives on the urban South: Selected papers from the Fourth Annual Urban South Conference* (pp. 207–221). Norfolk, VA: Norfolk State College and Old Dominion University.

20. U.S. Bureau of the Census. (1980). *Population and ethnicity 1980: Harris County Census Tracts* (1980 Census Data from PL 94-171 Tape). Houston, TX: Houston City Planning Department.

21. Jorling, T. C. (1977). *Balancing environment, economic, and resource conservation issues in the implementation of RCRA*. Paper presented at the meeting of the Sixth National Congress of Waste Management Technology and Resource and Energy Recovery of the National Solid Waste Management Association, Washington, DC.

22. Weddle, B. R., & Garland, G. A. (1974, October). Dumps: A potential threat to our ground water supplies. *Nation's Cities, 12,* 21–42.

23. Cimino, J. A. (1975, January). Health and safety in the solid waste industry. *Am J Public Health, 65,* 38–46.

24. Dunne, N. E. (1977). *Successful sanitary landfill siting: County of San Bernardino, California.* Washington, DC: U.S. Environmental Protection Agency.

25. Wahl, D., & Bancroft, R. L. (1975, August). Solid waste management today: Bringing about municipal change. *Nation's Cities, 13,* 18–32.

26. Buttel, F. H., & Flinn, W. L. (1978, September). Social class and mass environmental beliefs: A reconsideration. *Environ Behav, 10,* 433–450.

27. Zwerdling, D. (1973, January). Poverty and pollution. *The Perspective, 37,* 25–29.

28. Burch, W. R. (1971). *The peregrine falcon and the urban poor: Some ecological interrelations.* Paper presented at the annual meeting of the American Sociological Association, Denver.

29. Deutsch, S., & Van Houten, D. (1974, Fall–Winter). Environmental sociology and the American working class. *Humbolt J Soc Relations, 2,* 22–26.

30. Morrison, D. E. (1973, Spring). The environmental movement: Conflict dynamics. *J Voluntary Action Res, 2,* 78–85.

31. Tucker, L. (1978, September). The environmentally concerned citizen: Some correlates. *Environ Behav, 10,* 389–418.

32. Schnaiberg, A. (1980). *The environment: From surplus to scarcity.* New York: Oxford University Press.

CHAPTER TWENTY-SEVEN

Health Risk and Inequitable Distribution of Liquor Stores in African American Neighborhoods

Thomas A. LaVeist
John M. Wallace Jr.

It has been abundantly demonstrated that racial residential segregation is an enduring aspect of the urban landscape of the United States.[1,2] Some theorists have begun to link racial segregation to racial disparities to health status.[3-5] However, the pathways connecting racial segregation to health disparities remain largely untested empirically. In this analysis we examine the relationship between level of racial segregation within an urban area and the location of off-premises, packaged goods liquor stores. Such stores have been shown to be an important component of the "social infrastructure" that destabilizes communities.[6-10]

BACKGROUND

Alcohol use and alcohol-related problems have been found to be particularly high among African American men, the poor, and residents of large, highly segregated cities.[11-15] Alcohol sales, consumption, and various alcohol-related problems have all been found to relate to the physical availability of alcohol, where physical availability refers to "the location, number and density of retail outlets that sell alcoholic beverages," and "whether beverages are sold for off-premises use only, or for on-premises consumption."[16] Problems associated with the physical availability of alcohol include assaultive violence,[6] motor vehicle accidents,[7] a higher mortality rate from liver cirrhosis,[8] and alcoholism.[9,10]

It has been suggested that the relatively high number of alcohol-related problems that African Americans experience is due, at least in part, to the high level of alcohol availability in low-income urban African American communities.[17] Dawkins noted that "an often discussed but under analyzed phenomenon in the urban setting in terms of its policy implications is the high visibility of liquor establishments in and near black residential neighborhoods" (p. 214).[18] Although the physical availability of alcohol has received some attention in the popular press, our review of the scientific literature yielded only one study that empirically examined the physical availability of alcohol in African American communities.[19]

The disproportionate concentration of off-premise establishments such as package liquor stores is significant in that these outlets typically sell alcohol chilled, served in larger quantities than in taverns or restaurants (for example 40- and 64-ounce bottles), and ready for immediate consumption—on the street corner, in a nearby park, or in a motor vehicle. This drinking pattern is more likely to result in excessive drinking, public drunkenness, automobile crashes, and physical altercations that result in injury or death. These are all alcohol-related problems that have a substantial impact upon African American communities.[12,15,20]

Several scientific studies have examined the location, number, and density of alcohol outlets, whether their products are sold for on- or off-premises consumption, and the relationship of these characteristics to alcohol consumption and alcohol-related problems.[16,18,21–24] However, these issues, as they pertain to African American communities, have been largely ignored. In light of the relationship between the physical availability of alcohol outlets and negative social and physical health outcomes, the disproportionate share of alcohol-related problems experienced by African Americans, and the paucity of research on the availability of alcohol in African American communities, the purpose of the present research is threefold: (1) to examine empirically whether the physical availability of alcohol, through off-premises liquor stores is greater in predominantly black communities relative to predominantly white and racially integrated communities; (2) to investigate the extent to which the income status of the community residents mediates the relationship between community racial composition and alcohol availability; and (3) to explore whether the intersection of race and income status places low-income African American communities at greater risk for alcohol availability through off-premises package stores.

METHODS

We use census tract data from the city of Baltimore, Maryland, to examine the racial and socioeconomic status patterns in the physical availability of alcohol. Baltimore's population of 736,014 residents is distributed among 203 census tracts. Census tracts are geographic areas designated by the U.S. Census Bureau.

They range in population from about 1,200 to about 3,500 persons. Nine census tracts were primarily nonresidential areas (that is, the downtown business district, areas devoted to tourism, and industrial areas). Because these nine census tracts have an inordinately high number of liquor licenses and a relatively low number of residents, they have an excessively high per capita number of liquor licenses. In order to prevent the findings from being unduly biased by these nine tracts, they were eliminated from the analyses. Thus, the final sample consists of the 194 census tracts that are predominantly residential areas.

Data were abstracted from various official sources to produce the analytic database. Census tract data were based on 1990 U.S. Census designations. Data on liquor licenses were obtained from the Board of Liquor License Commissioners for Baltimore City (BLLCBC).

The other variables used in this analysis include census tract racial composition and median income. The racial composition of the census tract is specified as the percentage of black residents ("% black") in the census tract. As the racial composition of the entire city is 59.2 percent African American and 39.1 percent white, other racial and ethnic groups comprise less than 2 percent of the city's population. Thus, it can be stated that a lower percentage of blacks in a census tract indicates a higher percentage of whites. Median annual income is the aggregate median annual income of the residents of the census tract. It is specified as a continuous variable that ranges from $2,660 to $64,976.

RESULTS

Baltimore, like many of the nation's large cities, is highly segregated by race. Specifically, less than one-quarter (22 percent) of Baltimore's population lives in integrated (between 25 and 74 percent black) census tracts. In fact more than 45 percent of the population lives in predominantly (75 percent or more) black census tracts and nearly one-third (32 percent) lives in predominantly white census tracts.

In Table 27.1 we present results from regression analysis in which per capita off-premises liquor licenses was regressed on percentage black. The analysis is presented as Model 1 of Table 27.1. The model indicates a significant positive relationship. Thus, census tracts with higher percentages of black residents have significantly more liquor stores per capita than do census tracts with a lower percentage of black residents.

In Model 2 we test the hypothesis that controlling for the median income level of the residents of the census tract will eliminate the relationship between census tract racial composition and the per capita number of liquor stores. The model indicates that controlling for median income reduces the strength of the relationship between census tract racial composition and per capita number

Table 27.1. Linear Regression Model of Per Capita Liquor Stores Regressed on Percentage of African Americans Living in Tract and Median Income of Census Tract

Variable	Model 1	Model 2	Model 3
% black	0.267 $(p = 0.0002)$	0.176 $(p = 0.02)$	0.110 $(p = 0.1)$
Median income		-0.214 $(p = 0.005)$	-0.139 $(p = 0.08)$
Interaction			0.202 $(p = 0.01)$
Model statistics	R^2 (Adj) = 0.07	R^2 (Adj) = 0.10	R^2 (Adj) = 0.12
	$F = 14.80*$	$F = 11.68*$	$F = 9.95*$

$*p < .05.$

of liquor store licenses; however, it does not eliminate the relationship. Racial composition and income status of a census tract are both independent predictors of per capita number of liquor stores.

Finally, in Model 3 we test the hypothesis that it is neither race nor income status alone but rather their combination that is important as an explanation for the relatively higher concentration of liquor stores within a given area. The analyses designed to test this hypothesis are presented as Model 3. The model presents a regression analysis specifying a multiplicative interaction term between % black in the census tract and census tract median income. The significant effect of the interaction indicates that the effect of % black on per capita number of liquor stores differs by level of median income of the census tract.

To determine the nature of the income-race interaction, we present two models in Table 27.2. In Model 4, an interaction between a binary version of income status is multiplied by % black. To produce the binary variable the continuous version of census tract median income was divided at the 50th percentile into lower and higher income. The low-income binary variable is coded 1 for census tracts with median incomes below the 50th percentile and 0 for census tracts above. By multiplying the binary variable by % black, all higher income tracts are scored zero for the interaction; thus the interaction term in Model 4 produces a slope for the relationship between % black and per capita number of liquor stores among low-income census tracts. In Model 5 the binary variable is reversed (0 = below the 50th percentile; 1 = above) to produce a slope for the effect of % black among higher income tracts.

In Model 4 we find a significant direct effect indicating that among census tracts with a median income level below the 50th percentile for the city, a higher percentage of black residents is associated with a greater per capita number of liquor stores. In contrast, Model 5 finds a nonsignificant effect of the interaction, whereby a higher percentage of black residents is not associated with a higher per capita number of liquor stores.

Table 27.2. Linear Regression Model of Per Capita Liquor Stores Regressed
on Interaction Between Percentage of African Americans Living in Tract
and Median Income of Census Tract (Continuous Variable)

Variable	Model 4	Model 5
% black	0.123 ($p = 0.02$)	0.183 ($p = 0.03$)
Median income	-0.066 ($p = 0.2$)	-0.174 ($p = 0.05$)
Low income × % black	0.237 ($p = 0.01$)	
High income × % black		-0.058 ($p = 0.42$)
Model statistics	R^2 (Adj) = 0.12	R^2 (Adj) = 0.11
	$F = 9.1^*$	$F = 11.68$

$^*p < .05.$

SUMMARY AND CONCLUSIONS

In this study, we examined the extent to which liquor stores are more likely to be located in predominantly black census tracts. Our findings indicate that liquor stores are more likely to be located in predominantly African American communities. On the other hand, other research found that the more socially desirable establishments that sell alcohol (for example, restaurants) were more likely to be located in predominantly white communities.[18]

Given that African Americans in Baltimore are disproportionately poor and that liquor stores have been found to be concentrated in poor areas, analyses were performed to determine if community economic status, as well as racial composition, is an important predictor of the number of liquor stores. To test this hypothesis we examined the relationship between census tract racial composition and per capita number of liquor store licenses, adjusting for census tract aggregate median income status. Both income status and racial composition of the census tract are related, independently, to the number of liquor stores. Specifically, low-SES census tracts and predominantly black census tracts have significantly more liquor stores per capita than more affluent communities and predominantly white communities. Additionally, we hypothesized and confirmed that communities that are both low income and predominantly black have significantly more liquor stores compared to other communities.

Although it is beyond the scope of the present study, it should be noted that our data (not shown here) indicate significant associations between the per capita number of liquor store licenses in a census tract and other social problems, including assaults, rapes, and homicides. Clearly, it would be inappropriate to conclude on the basis of an ecological association that alcohol consumption is higher among African Americans in these communities. As we have demonstrated an association and not a cause-effect relationship, one may question the causal ordering of the relationships observed in our analysis. That is, could it be that demand for the products sold at these liquor stores is affecting supply, rather than supply inducing demand? Clearly, the answer to this question cannot be definitively determined without additional research. However, an example from research on crack cocaine use indicates that availability can increase use.[25,26] This seems a possible scenario in the case of alcohol as well.

There is also some speculation in the research literature that the relatively high availability of alcohol in low-income black communities may distort African American youths' perceptions surrounding appropriate levels of consumption of alcohol.[17] Future research on the impact of alcohol on the social, psychological, and physiological health of low-income urban African Americans should examine in greater detail the ecological conditions that expose them to significantly higher levels of alcohol availability compared to whites.

Although the data analyzed in this study are from a single city and although no direct causal conclusions can be made, these findings suggest that the relatively higher number of liquor stores in low-income African American communities may be tied to the disproportionate share of alcohol-related problems experienced by residents of these communities. Accordingly, the availability of alcohol in poor black communities is an issue that policymakers, health professionals, clergy, community activists, and other concerned citizens must address in their efforts to reduce alcohol abuse and its sequelae in African American communities.

Notes

1. Massey, D., & Denton, N. (1993). *American apartheid: Segregation and the making of the underclass.* Cambridge, MA: Harvard University Press.

2. White, M. J. (1983). The measurement of spatial segregation. *Am J Sociology, 88,* 1008–1018.

3. LaVeist, T. A. (1989). Linking residential segregation and the infant mortality race disparity. *Sociol Soc Res, 73,* 90–94.

4. LaVeist, T. A. (1992). The political empowerment and health status of African Americans: Mapping a new territory. *Am J Sociol, 97,* 1080–1095.

5. LaVeist, T. A. (1993). Separation, poverty and empowerment: Health consequences for African Americans. *Milbank Q, 73,* 41–64.

6. Scribner, R. A., MacKinnon, D. P., & Dwyer, J. H. (1995). The risk of assaultive violence and alcohol availability in Los Angeles County. *Am J Public Health, 85,* 335–340.

7. Scribner, R. A., MacKinnon, D. P., & Dwyer, D. H. (1994). Alcohol outlet density and motor vehicle crashes in Los Angeles County cities. *J Studies Alcohol, 55,* 447–453.

8. Colon, I. (1981). Alcohol availability and cirrhosis mortality rate by gender and race. *Am J Public Health, 71,* 1325–1328.

9. Harford, T. C., Parker, D., Paulter, C., & Wolz, M. (1979). Relationship between number of on-premise outlets and alcoholism. *J Studies Alcohol, 40,* 1053–1057.

10. Smart, R. G. (1977). The relationship of availability of alcohol beverages to per capita consumption and alcoholism rates. *J Studies Alcohol, 38,* 891–897.

11. Barr, K. E., Farrell, M. P., Barnes, G. M., & Welte, J. W. (1993). Race, class and gender differences in substance abuse: Evidence of middle class/underclass polarization among black males. *Soc Problems, 40,* 316–327.

12. Herd, D. (1989). The epidemiology of drinking patterns and alcohol-related problems among U.S. blacks. In D. L. Spielger, T. A. Tate, S. S. Aitken, & C. M. Christian (Eds.), *Alcohol use among U.S. ethnic minorities* (pp. 3–50). Washington, DC: National Institute on Alcohol Abuse and Alcoholism.

13. Lex, B. W. (1987). Review of alcohol problems in ethnic minority groups. *J Consult Clin Psychol, 55,* 293–300.

14. Moskowitz, J. M. (1989). The primary prevention of alcohol problems: A critical review of the research literature. *J Studies Alcohol, 50,* 54–88.

15. Herd, D. (1991). Drinking patterns in the black population. In E. B. Clark & M. E. Hilton (Eds.), *Alcohol in America: Drinking practices and problems* (pp. 308–328). New York: New York State University Press.

16. Wallace, J. M., & Brown, L. S. (1995). Alcohol abuse prevention in African American communities. In P. A. Lengton, *Alcohol prevention research in ethnic minority communities* (Office for Substance Abuse Prevention Cultural Competence Series Monograph). Rockville, MD: U.S. Department of Health and Human Services.

17. Harper, F. (1976). *Alcohol abuse and black America.* Alexandria, VA: Douglas.

18. Dawkins, M. P. (1983). Policy issues. In T. D. Watts & R. Wright (Eds.), *Black alcoholism: Toward a comprehensive understanding.* Springfield, IL: Thomas.

19. Dawkins, M., Farrell, W., & Johnson, J. (1979). Spatial patterns of alcohol outlets in the Washington, D.C., black community. *Proceedings of the Pennsylvania Academy of Science, 53,* 89–97.

20. Watts, T. D., & Wright, R. (Eds.). (1983). *Black alcoholism: Toward a comprehensive understanding.* Springfield, IL: Thomas.

21. Rabow, J., & Watts, R. K. (1982). Alcohol availability, alcoholic beverages sales and alcohol-related problems. *J Studies Alcohol, 43,* 767–801.

22. Macdonald, S., & Whitehead, P. C. (1983, Fall). Availability of outlets and consumption of alcoholic beverages. *J Drug Issues,* pp. 477–486.

23. Pfautz, H., & Hyde, R. (1960). The ecology of alcohol in the local community. *Q J Studies Alcohol, 21,* 447–456.

24. Gruenewald, P. J., Ponicki, W. R., & Holder, H. D. (1993, February). The relationship of outlet densities to alcohol consumption: A time series cross-sectional analysis. *Alcohol Clin Exp Res, 17*(1), 38–47.

25. Lillie-Blanton, M., Anthony, J. C., & Schuster, C. R. (1993). Probing the meaning of racial/ethnic group comparisons in crack cocaine smoking. *JAMA, 269*(8), 993–997.

26. Crum, R. M., Lillie-Blanton, M., & Anthony, J. C. (1996). Neighborhood environment and opportunity to use cocaine and other drugs in late childhood and early adolescence. *Drug Alcohol Depend, 43*(3), 155–161.

CHAPTER TWENTY-EIGHT

Probing the Meaning of Racial/Ethnic Group Comparisons in Crack Cocaine Smoking

Marsha Lillie-Blanton
James C. Anthony
Charles R. Schuster

Racial and ethnic group comparisons retain a central place in summaries of national data on the prevalence of illicit drug use. In some cases, these comparisons provide useful descriptive information on patterns of drug use specific to a racial/ethnic population group. In other cases, these basic comparisons by race/ethnicity can be misleading because they do not account for differences in the social environments experienced by community residents or for other determinants of illicit drug use. As a result, these basic comparisons sometimes reinforce racial prejudices and draw public attention away from community characteristics or other factors that may serve better to explain patterns of drug use.

In this study, we probe the meaning of a previous analysis of the 1988 National Household Survey on Drug Abuse (NHSDA) that reported that crack cocaine smoking is more common among African Americans and Hispanic Americans than among white Americans.[1] As shown in Figure 28.1, summary prevalence rates for lifetime (ever) use of crack cocaine were twice as high for African Americans and Hispanic Americans as for white Americans. This finding has been disseminated through a variety of reports, such as *Health Status of Minorities and Low-Income Groups* (3rd ed.),[2] and is becoming widely accepted as an accurate reflection of patterns of drug use in the household

---

This study was supported in part by Grant DA04392 from the National Institute on Drug Abuse.

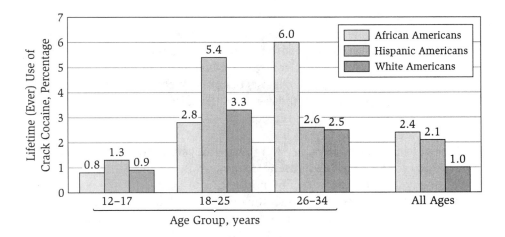

Figure 28.1 Summary Prevalence Rates for Lifetime (Ever) Use of Crack Cocaine by Age Group and Race/Ethnicity in 1988.

Source: Data drawn from National Institute on Drug Abuse. (1990). *National Household Survey on Drug Abuse: Main findings, 1988* (U.S. Dept of Health and Human Services Publication ADM 90-1692). Washington, DC: Author.

population. The survey findings deserve closer scrutiny because the analysis did not attempt to account for underlying community-level or macrosocial differences across racial/ethnic population groups. As a result, the previous analysis left ambiguous whether observed racial/ethnic differences in crack cocaine smoking should be understood in relation to individual personal or behavioral characteristics or in relation to characteristics that might be shared by residents of a community, no matter what the individual-level characteristics might be.

To examine this issue, we undertook a reanalysis of the original data from the 1988 NHSDA to assess whether crack cocaine smoking is associated with factors specific to race/ethnicity. We hypothesized that reported racial/ethnic group differences might be an artifact of macrosocial environmental risk factors or determinants of prevalence. Macrosocial factors, as defined by Henderson,[3] are social forces that "operate at a societal rather than an individual level . . . and have their origin in constructs such as what is valued by people as important, the strength of beliefs, and the extent to which individuals experience themselves as part of a larger social organism." Lesse[4] stresses the importance of understanding the interrelationships of macrosocial and microsocial forces in shaping intrapersonal development.

We compare racial/ethnic group differences in crack cocaine smoking using an epidemiologic strategy that holds constant macrosocial factors that might confound the analysis if left uncontrolled. The intent of the study is to clarify the magnitude of race-specific differences once these community-level and macrosocial factors are held constant. For example, differences in the availability of crack cocaine from neighborhood to neighborhood constitute one such community-level variable. Another array of theoretically important macrosocial factors associated with drug use consists of employment rates, premature death rates, community contact with the criminal justice system, socially acceptable mechanisms for coping with life stressors, the distribution of wealth, and access to social resources.

The epidemiologic strategy used in this investigation involves poststratification.[5] That is, after the 1988 household survey was completed, we grouped all of the survey respondents into more homogeneous strata, defined according to the local area segments from which they were sampled (that is, aggregates of city blocks or, in rural areas, census enumeration districts) and also according to age. As described elsewhere,[6] this procedure permits a sharpened focus on personal and behavioral risk factors while holding constant social and environmental risk factors that might vary from neighborhood to neighborhood. This strategy has been used in a number of studies to test hypotheses about risk factors for mental disorders[7,8] as well as other health problems.[9] Similar to neighborhood matching in epidemiologic case-control studies,[10] poststratification offers a way to control for factors such as the availability of crack cocaine within geographic areas and the influence of macrosocial factors on behavior.

MATERIALS AND METHODS

The 1988 NHSDA involved interviews with a total of 8,814 individuals residing in households in the coterminous United States. The subjects were selected using a multistage area probability sampling of all residents aged twelve years and older. After random selection of 100 primary sampling units, the survey team drew a sample of about 1,600 area segments within the sample primary sampling units. The area segments consisted of at least forty housing units, aggregated by grouping together adjacent city blocks or census enumeration districts. Across the area segments, approximately 40,000 households were listed, sampled, and classified as to their race/ethnicity and age composition; individuals within participating households were sampled to be interviewed. The 1988 NHSDA oversampled African Americans and Hispanic Americans to increase the reliability of estimates for these population groups. Response rates for the three racial/ethnic groups were 73 percent for white Americans, 75 percent for African Americans, and 78 percent for Hispanic Americans.

After the sampling, a trained interviewer conducted a structured interview using a questionnaire that included items on licit and illicit drug use. These interviews were conducted in each respondent's home. For sensitive questions, such as those concerning use of illicit drugs, respondents used a confidential (self-administered) answer sheet. Details of the survey design and data collection procedures are described elsewhere.[1]

In the original NHSDA reports and in this reanalysis of NHSDA data, crack cocaine use was operationally defined as self-reported use of cocaine in rock or chunk form one or more times ever in an individual's lifetime. This measure, referred to as the "lifetime" measure of use, includes individuals who reported current or past use of crack cocaine. To assess crack cocaine use, the NHSDA questionnaire first asked about use of cocaine in any form, such as powder, crack, freebase, and coca paste. A later question asked about the route of administration of cocaine as either "smoking or freebasing." Another series of questions asked specifically about crack, defined as cocaine in rock or chunk form. Race/ethnicity was defined using the four mutually exclusive categories reported in the original prevalence comparison analysis:[1] black non-Hispanic, white non-Hispanic, Hispanic, and other. The "other" category included Native Americans, Pacific Islanders, and Asians.

In the poststratification step of this reanalysis, respondents were grouped into strata, or risk sets, defined by the area segment, henceforth referred to as "neighborhoods," where they were living when sampled. This strategy deals with possible confounding that involves race/ethnicity and demographic variables such as income and education to the extent that neighbors are similar in their education and income levels. Within the neighborhood, respondents were further stratified by age (twelve through fourteen, fifteen through nineteen, twenty through twenty-four years, and so forth) to allow for the possibility that crack cocaine smoking varies across age strata.

After preparatory analyses, we used the conditional bivariate form of logistic regression and multiple logistic regression models to assess racial/ethnic variation in crack cocaine smoking. The conditional model took into account the poststratification of respondents into risk sets, while providing a statistical control for any residual confounding effects of age and gender.

In an analysis of this type, the maximum likelihood estimate for the degree of association depends only on sampled neighborhoods in which there is at least one crack cocaine smoker and at least one person who has not smoked crack cocaine. Neighborhoods where there is no crack cocaine smoking are not informative; since these neighborhoods show no variation in crack cocaine smoking, they do not permit a comparison of the odds of crack cocaine smoking while holding constant macrosocial characteristics of the community. Of the 1,532 neighborhoods, 128 had at least one crack cocaine smoker and at least one nonsmoker; in several neighborhoods there was more than one crack cocaine smoker. For this reason, the informative segment of the poststratified sample consisted of 128 risk sets, including a total of 939 respondents, 183 cases who had smoked crack cocaine and 801 nonsmokers (at least one case of crack cocaine smoking and up to fifteen noncases). In the sampled neighborhoods, only one sampled segment (that is, risk set) contained a crack cocaine smoker but no corresponding nonsmoker. Two-thirds of the 939 respondents resided in racially and ethnically heterogeneous neighborhoods with African Americans and either white or Hispanic Americans.

RESULTS

Table 28.1 compares the 138 crack cocaine smokers and 801 nonsmokers in the 128 informative neighborhoods, showing that crack cocaine smokers were more often men (58 percent) than women (42 percent). Also, crack cocaine smokers (mean age = 24 years) were on average younger than nonsmokers (mean age = 28 years). About 28 percent ($n = 39$) of the smokers of crack cocaine were

Table 28.1. Major Characteristics of Cases and Noncases in 128 Matched Sets Drawn from the 1988 National Household Survey on Drug Abuse, with Relative Odds Estimates Based on Bivariate Conditional Logistic Regression Analyses

Suspected Determinant	Cases ($n = 138$), No. (%)	Noncases ($n = 801$), No. (%)	Relative Odds (95% Confidence Interval)	p
Gender				
M	80 (58.0)	349 (43.6)	1.82 (1.24–2.65)	.002
F*	58 (42.0)	452 (56.4)	1.00	—
Age, years				
15–19	42 (30.4)	212 (26.5)	5.92 (2.25–15.54)	<.001
20–24	22 (15.9)	69 (8.6)	10.85 (3.80–30.94)	<.001
25–29	40 (29.0)	111 (13.9)	11.59 (4.25–31.62)	<.001
30–34	23 (16.7)	103 (12.9)	6.07 (2.15–17.14)	<.001
≥35	6 (4.4)	165 (20.6)	1.05 (0.31–3.56)	.93
12–14*	5 (3.6)	141 (17.6)	1.00	—
Race				
African American	39 (28.3)	227 (28.3)	0.99 (0.49–1.98)	.97
Hispanic American	40 (29.0)	271 (33.8)	0.96 (0.55–1.69)	.90
Other*†	0 (0.0)	25 (3.1)	—	—
White American	59 (42.8)	278 (34.7)	1.39 (0.80–2.43)	.25

*Reference category.

†There was no convergence because there were no crack smokers in this category.

Source: Data drawn from National Institute on Drug Abuse. (1990). National Household Survey on Drug Abuse: Main findings, 1988 (U.S. Dept of Health and Human Services Publication ADM 90-1692). Washington, DC: Author.

African Americans and 29 percent ($n = 40$) were Hispanic Americans, proportions about equal to their distribution in the analytic sample.

Under the conditional bivariate model, the relative odds (RO) of crack use did not differ significantly when African Americans were compared with all others (RO = 0.99; 95% confidence interval [CI], 0.49, 1.98) or when the Hispanic population groups were contrasted with all others (RO = 0.96; 95% CI = 0.55, 1.69) (Table 28.1). Comparable RO estimates were obtained when the model was changed to provide a more direct contrast of African Americans and Hispanic Americans with white Americans. Table 28.2 shows that the addition of age and gender to this model produced no more than a modest change in the estimate for the RO of crack cocaine use for African Americans (RO = 0.85; 95% CI = 0.37, 1.93) or for Hispanic Americans (RO = 0.88; 95% CI = 0.47, 1.67) compared with white Americans. However, terms for gender and age improved the fit of the regression model. Males were an estimated 1.8 times more likely to have been crack cocaine smokers than females (95% CI = 1.23, 2.72). The odds of crack cocaine smoking were greatest among persons aged twenty through twenty-four and twenty-five through twenty-nine years (Table 28.2), and there was considerable age-related variation in occurrence of crack cocaine smoking, as reflected in the different RO estimates for the five-year age groups.

The age-specific prevalence values shown in Figure 28.1 raised the possibility that crack cocaine smoking might have occurred with excess frequency

Table 28.2. Relative Odds of Crack Smoking Among 128 Risk Sets Based on Conditional Multiple Logistic Regression Analyses

Characteristic	Relative Odds (95% Confidence Interval)	p
Gender		
M	1.83 (1.23–2.72)	.003
F*	1.00	—
Age, years		
15–19	5.95 (2.26–15.63)	<.001
20–24	11.65 (4.05–33.60)	<.001
25–29	12.28 (4.48–33.70)	<.001
30–34	6.49 (2.29–18.37)	<.001
≥35	1.14 (0.34–3.88)	.83
12–14*	1.00	—
Race/ethnicity		
African American	0.85 (0.37–1.93)	.69
Hispanic American	0.88 (0.47–1.67)	.70
White American*	1.00	—

*Reference category.

among African Americans who were older (that is, twenty-six through thirty-four years) but not among younger African Americans. This possibility was tested in a supplementary analysis allowing for different associations within separate age strata. Consistent with the evidence shown in Tables 28.1 and 28.2, results from this supplementary analysis did not support the assertion that crack cocaine smoking occurred more frequently among African Americans. The only statistically significant association involved teens aged fifteen through nineteen years old; within this age group, African American youths were less likely to report crack cocaine smoking than were their white American counterparts (RO = 0.17; 95% CI = 0.04, 0.70). For twenty-five- to twenty-nine-year-olds, the estimated degree of association between crack cocaine smoking and being African American was close to the null value of 1.0 (RO = 0.97; 95% CI = 0.29, 3.20). For older adults, the point estimate for RO was greater than 1.0 but not reliably different from the null value, in that the 95 percent CI trapped the null value (data available on request from Marsha Lillie-Blanton).

In a supplementary analysis of the survey data on each neighborhood (Table 28.3), we explored the characteristics of neighborhoods with at least one crack cocaine smoker and found that, compared with neighborhoods that did not have any crack cocaine smokers, the population tended (1) to include a larger share of racial and ethnic minorities, (2) to have more young and middle-aged adults (ages twelve through thirty-nine years), and (3) to be more concentrated in large metropolitan areas and/or in the western parts of the United States. It is noteworthy that in aggregate, neighborhoods did not differ greatly in their distributions by education and income. This analysis, however, is only a beginning to this exploration. More detailed analyses would help to guide future investigations that seek to identify which characteristics of the social environment are important and potentially modifiable determinants of illicit drug use.

COMMENT

This reanalysis of national survey data raises questions about the meaning of a widely disseminated comparison of crack cocaine smoking by race/ethnicity. Once survey respondents were grouped into neighborhood clusters, in effect holding constant shared characteristics, such as drug availability and social conditions, the odds of crack cocaine use did not differ significantly by race/ethnicity. The analysis challenges us to think beyond race-specific personal factors (for example, biological factors) when we consider what might be determinants of crack cocaine use. It strengthens the evidence that given similar social conditions, crack cocaine smoking does not depend strongly on race per se as a personal characteristic of individuals. This finding, however, does not speak to the influence of social factors, such as racism, which may contribute to a

Table 28.3. Sociodemographic Characteristics of Respondents in Neighborhoods with at Least One Crack Cocaine Smoker and Neighborhoods with No Crack Cocaine Smokers (Unweighted Comparison)

Characteristic	Neighborhoods with at Least One Crack Cocaine User (128 Neighborhoods, 939 Residents)	Neighborhoods with No Crack Cocaine Users (1,404 Neighborhoods, 7,875 Residents)
All	100	100
Race/ethnicity		
White American	35.9	53.5
African American	28.3	20.6
Hispanic American	33.1	23.9
Other	2.7	2.0
Gender		
M	45.7	44.6
F	54.3	55.4
Education		
<High school	57.6	53.7
High school graduate	23.6	24.8
Some college	11.8	12.3
College graduate	7.0	9.2
Age, years		
12–14	15.6	16.4
15–19	27.1	23.3
20–24	9.7	9.9
25–29	16.1	12.1
30–34	13.4	12.2
35–39	4.3	4.8
≥40	14.0	21.3
Work status		
Full-time	45.9	49.1
Part-time	2.1	2.8
Nonwork income	8.8	7.5
Under age 18, not working	39.8	37.5
Population density		
Large metropolitan	62.3	46.9
Small metropolitan	23.6	30.1
Nonmetropolitan	14.1	23.0
Census region		
Northeast	16.7	19.4
North Central	12.8	20.9
South	39.9	37.9
West	30.6	21.8
Income (past annual), $		
No personal earnings	18.2	18.1
<5,000	16.8	16.6
5,000–8,999	9.5	10.2
9,000–19,999	20.8	17.0
20,000–29,999	8.6	8.9
≥30,000–40,000	7.0	7.9
Other*	18.7	21.3

Note: From the National Household Survey on Drug Abuse.

*Includes persons who refused to answer and those who provided unusable data.

disproportionate share of racial/ethnic minorities living in social environments where there is increased risk for crack cocaine use.

This study illustrates the need to give greater attention to the analysis and presentation of data by race/ethnicity. The findings do not refute the previous analysis but give evidence that unadjusted prevalence estimates may lead to misunderstanding about the role of race or ethnicity in the epidemiology of crack use. Shallow and possibly prejudiced misconceptions may be fostered by the presentation of basic racial/ethnic comparisons in prevalence of illicit drug use unless commentary about uncontrolled confounding is also presented. Also, reports generated from the NHSDA are a major source of information used for policy and planning purposes. Thus, reporting racial/ethnic differences in illicit drug use without commenting on factors that might account for the observed variations could lead to an erroneous assessment of causal factors and to ineffective preventive interventions.

It is important to note that this study is not without limitations. First, there are the obvious limitations of self-reported data. Second, individuals not residing in households are not represented in the data (for example, persons in prison or who are homeless). In addition, based on only 138 crack cocaine smokers, the study is but a first step in understanding the determinants of this important public health problem. Replication of this analysis with data from more recent surveys can help address this limitation. However, these limitations do not affect the present analysis any more than they affected the previous analysis.

Also, our poststratification strategy holds constant what neighbors have in common, including aspects of cultural life that are shared by persons residing within fairly homogeneous neighborhoods. In this respect, the reported lack of association does not provide evidence on all aspects of cultural life that can vary within or between racial/ethnic groups.

In relation to the generalizability of these findings, it is worth considering that the study's estimates depend on NHSDA respondents living in neighborhoods where at least one crack smoker was found and also on those living in racially mixed neighborhoods. It might be argued that individuals living in such neighborhoods differ from those living where there is total racial segregation. However, we are aware of no compelling evidence of intrinsic differences among African Americans or white Americans living under these varying circumstances. If such differences exist, they can become a focus of future research to determine whether they are important for the risk of crack cocaine smoking.

This study also raises new questions for investigation. Clustering the respondents provided a sharper focus on personal or behavioral characteristics; however, it also constrained the study's capacity to explore explicitly characteristics of the neighborhood that can be important in the epidemiology of crack cocaine smoking. Characteristics of the neighborhood environment that should be targeted in preventive interventions (for example, drug availability, shared hopes for the future) must be explored through primary research or experimental tests of interventions.

This analysis also has highlighted a need to make a more detailed study of age-related variation in occurrence of crack cocaine smoking across racial/ethnic subgroups. For example, we cannot say whether fifteen- through nineteen-year-old African Americans truly are at lower risk of smoking crack cocaine, as our analysis suggested, or whether this is an artifact created by some aspect of survey error (for example, error in sampling or measurement). In addition, the data indicate that African Americans aged thirty years or older might have had greater involvement in crack cocaine smoking than their nonblack age-mates in the population, although the observed differences did not achieve statistical significance. The appearance of this possible association involving race/ethnicity and age does not contradict our conclusion that race per se did not account for initially observed variation in prevalence, but it does raise issues about the epidemiology of crack cocaine smoking.

Given the sensitive nature of race/ethnicity in the United States, researchers have a responsibility to go beyond the reporting of racial/ethnic differences, particularly when population groups differ on attributes that can affect the comparison. The challenge to investigators is to make effective use of measures of race/ethnicity as fertile epidemiologic clues.[11] The findings of this study indicate that research on illicit drug use across racial/ethnic groups should include epidemiologic analyses with a renewed focus on neighborhood-level social conditions as a necessary complement to the search for individual-level explanations.

Notes

1. National Institute on Drug Abuse. (1990). *National Household Survey on Drug Abuse: Main findings, 1988* (U.S. Dept of Health and Human Services Publication ADM 90-1692). Washington, DC: Author.

2. U.S. Department of Health and Human Services. (1991). *Health status of minorities and low-income groups* (3rd ed.) (Publication HRS-P-DV-90-2). Washington, DC: Author.

3. Henderson, A. S. (1988). *An introduction to social psychiatry.* New York: Oxford University Press.

4. Lesse, S. (1987). Psychotherapy in a changing postindustrial society. *Am J Psychother, 41,* 336–348.

5. Schlesselman, J. J. (1982). *Case-control studies: Design, conduct, analysis.* New York: Oxford University Press.

6. Anthony, J. C., Tien, A. Y., & Petronis, K. R. (1990). Epidemiologic evidence on cocaine use and panic attacks. *Am J Epidemiol, 129,* 543–549.

7. Anthony, J. C., & Petronis, K. R. (1991). Epidemiologic evidence on suspected associations between cocaine use and psychiatric disturbances. In S. Schober &

C. Scoot (Eds.), *The epidemiology of cocaine use and abuse* (pp. 71–94) (U.S. Department of Health and Human Services Publication ADM 91-1787; National Institute on Drug Abuse research monograph 110). Washington, DC: National Institute on Drug Abuse.

8. Petronis, K. R., Samuels, J. F., Moscicki, E. K., & Anthony, J. C. (1990). An epidemiologic investigation of potential risk factors for suicide attempts. *Soc Psychiatry Psychiatr Epidemiol, 25,* 193–199.

9. Petronis, K. R., & Anthony, J. C. (1989). An epidemiologic investigation of marijuana- and cocaine-related palpitations. *Drug Alcohol Depend, 23,* 219–226.

10. Bassett, M. T., & Krieger, N. (1986). Social class and black-white differences in breast cancer survival. *Am J Public Health, 76,* 1400–1403.

11. Jones, C. P., LaVeist, T. A., & Lillie-Blanton, M. (1991). Race in the epidemiologic literature: An examination of the *American Journal of Epidemiology, 1921–1990. Am J Epidemiol, 134,* 1079–1084.

 PART FIVE

PROVIDER FACTORS

CHAPTER TWENTY-NINE

Ethnicity and Analgesic Practice

Knox H. Todd
Christi Deaton
Anne P. D'Adamo
Leon Goe

Oligoanalgesia, the inadequate prescribing of analgesics for patients in pain, is common among emergency department patients.[1-3] We previously reported that Hispanic patients with extremity fractures were less likely to receive analgesics than similar non-Hispanic white patients in the ED setting.[4] This disparity in analgesic practice could not be explained by patient characteristics (including gender, language, and insurance status), severity of injury, physician characteristics (including ethnicity, gender, or specialty), or a disparity in physicians' ability to assess pain in Hispanic as compared to non-Hispanic white patients.[5]

To determine whether our results are generalizable to different EDs and ethnic groups, we conducted a similar retrospective cohort study of analgesic practices comparing black and white ED patients with long-bone fractures.

MATERIALS AND METHODS

The study site was a community, university-affiliated ED serving urban Atlanta, Georgia. Board-certified emergency physicians staff the ED, although patients are at times seen primarily by their primary care physicians. The study protocol

Originally presented at the Society for Academic Emergency Medicine annual meeting, Washington, D.C., May 1997.

was approved by the Emory University School of Medicine Human Investigations Committee.

ED records were reviewed for a forty-month period (September 1, 1992, through December 31, 1995) to identify all black and white patients discharged from the ED with a diagnosis of isolated long-bone fracture. Patients with *International Classification of Diseases, Ninth Revision (ICD-9)* codes 812, 813, 821, and 823, comprising all humerus, radius, ulna, femoral shaft, tibia, and fibula fractures, were eligible for the study. Patients with fractures of the femoral neck (*ICD-9* code 820) were not included, nor were patients with additional discharge diagnoses. Patients were excluded if they presented for complications of previously treated fractures rather than for primary treatment.

We performed chart abstraction in a multistaged fashion. In the first stage, demographic information was obtained from the hospital's computerized database. This included patient age, gender, ethnicity, *ICD-9* code, and treating physician. Treating physicians were characterized by gender, ethnicity, and specialty.

Next, a trained research assistant reviewed the radiology report to confirm the presence of a fracture. Charts for which the radiology report did not confirm a fracture were excluded. The research assistant then reviewed the medical record, abstracting information on insurance, marital status, and employment status. At this point, all information indicating patient ethnicity was removed from the chart, blinding subsequent reviewers to patient ethnicity.

Next, an emergency physician reviewed the medical record, abstracting information on characteristics of the patient's presentation, including mode of arrival, mechanism of injury, time of presentation, time from initial injury, total time in the ED, and whether the presence of pain was explicitly recorded in nursing or physician notes.

Finally, a nurse reviewed the record, recording whether analgesics were administered in the ED, and if so, what type of analgesic was administered (for example, narcotic versus nonnarcotic) and what route was used (for example, parenteral versus oral). We did not abstract information regarding prescriptions for analgesics given at the time of ED discharge, as this information is not reliably recorded. A second reviewer confirmed all data abstracted from the medical record for each stage of the review process.

All data were entered onto a computerized spreadsheet and analyzed using Stata statistical software (*Stata Statistical Software: Release 5.0,* Stata Corp., College Station, TX). Baseline characteristics for black and white patients were compared using means, SDs, and proportions. The primary outcome measure for the study was the proportion of black patients versus white patients receiving ED analgesics. These proportions were compared using the χ^2 test, and we calculated black patients' relative risk (*RR*) of receiving no analgesic compared with white patients' risk. Multiple logistic regression was used to determine the effect of ethnicity on analgesic use while controlling for multiple potential confounders.

Using this model, we calculated odds ratios and estimated *RR*s with 95 percent confidence intervals (CIs).[6] The likelihood ratio test and the Hosmer-Lemeshow test were used to assess the strength of the model and goodness of fit.

RESULTS

During the forty-month study period, a total of 238 black and white patients were discharged from the ED with diagnoses limited to codes 812, 813, 821, or 823. Of these, fifteen cases were secondary presentations of previously treated fractures. In two cases, the fracture diagnosis was not confirmed by the radiology report, and in four cases, we could not locate the medical record. The remaining 217 patients were included in the study (Figure 29.1).

The 127 black patients and 90 white patients were managed by 37 different physicians. Baseline characteristics of the two patient groups are presented in Table 29.1. The groups were generally similar, although white patients were more likely to have private insurance. The presence of pain was explicitly noted in the medical record for similar proportions of black and white patients (54 percent versus 59 percent).

Fifty-seven percent of black patients with extremity fractures received analgesics compared with 74 percent of white patients ($p = .01$). The risk of

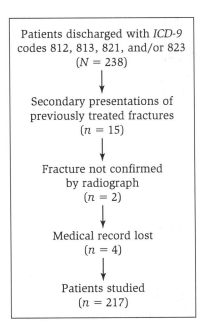

Figure 29.1 Study Exclusions.

Table 29.1. Baseline Characteristics

Characteristics	White Patients ($n = 90$)(%)	Black Patients ($n = 127$)(%)
Age, years (interquartile range)	35 (25–47)	33 (24–42)
Male	58	59
Married	36	32
Employed	77	67
Private insurance	88	74
Arrived by ambulance	12	14
Occupational injury	8	7
Mechanism of injury		
Fall	84	75
Assault	5	11
Motor vehicle crash	7	5
Other	5	10
Principal *ICD-9* code		
812 (humerus)	21	17
813 (radius/ulna)	70	69
821 (femoral shaft)	2	0
823 (tibia/fibula)	7	14
Time of presentation		
7 AM–3 PM	37	33
3 PM–11 PM	43	54
11 PM–7 AM	20	13
Time from fracture to presentation (hours)		
<3	61	51
3–6	8	8
6–12	11	5
12–24	9	15
>24	10	21
Total time in ED (hours) (SD)	3.6 (1.9)	3.6 (2.0)
Pain noted in medical record	59	54
Fracture reduction performed	9	10
White physician	83	89
Male physician	56	62
Emergency physician	95	90

receiving no analgesic was 66 percent greater for black patients than for white patients (crude *RR*, 1.66, 95% CI, 1.11–2.50; Table 29.2).

To control for potential confounders, multiple logistic regression analysis was performed. Analgesic administration was the dichotomous outcome variable, and patient ethnicity (black versus white race), time since injury (<3 hours

Table 29.2. Analgesic Use for White Versus Black Patients

	Ethnicity	
	White	Black
Variable	No. (%)	No. (%)
Analgesic given?		
Yes	67 (74)	73 (57)
No	23 (26)	54 (43)
Total	90	127

versus >3 hours), total time in the ED (in hours), shift of presentation (day versus night), need for fracture reduction (yes or no), and payer status (private insurance versus uninsured or public assistance) were included as potential predictor variables. Time since injury, total time in the ED, and need for fracture reduction were included in the model because they have been previously identified as predictors of analgesic use.[4] Payer status was included as a marker for socioeconomic status, a common confounder of ethnicity. Because analgesics are commonly dispensed to patients seen at times when pharmacies are closed, the shift of presentation was included as a potential confounder. After controlling for these covariates, black ethnicity remained predictive of no analgesic administration in the ED (estimated *RR*, 1.7; 95% CI, 1.1–2.3; likelihood ratio $\chi^2 = 5.99$; *df* = 1; *p* = .01). The Hosmer-Lemeshow goodness-of-fit test indicated that the logistic model suitably fit the data $\chi^2 = 5.15$, *p* = .74; Table 29.3).

Of the 140 patients receiving some form of analgesic, 114 (81 percent) received narcotics and 48 (34 percent) received some form of parenteral therapy. White and black patients received parenteral therapy in similar proportions. Black patients who were given analgesics were somewhat less likely to receive narcotics, although this difference was not statistically significant (87 percent versus 77 percent, *p* = .13; Table 29.4).

DISCUSSION

In this study, approximately two-thirds of our patients received analgesics in the ED. This proportion is similar to that found in our previous study, which reported ED analgesic administration to 68 percent of a group of Hispanic and white patients with extremity fractures. Our finding that black patients received analgesics less frequently than white patients is also similar to our previous finding that Hispanic patients received analgesics less often than white patients. Our findings are also consistent with those of two recent studies of cancer patients that found disparities in analgesic use between majority and minority

Table 29.3. Results of Multiple Logistic Regression Analysis

Independent Variables	Odds Ratio	Estimated RR	95% CI
Black race	2.1	1.7	1.1–2.3
Time since injury	2.4	1.8	1.2–2.4
Total time in ED	0.9	0.9	0.8–1.04
Time of presentation	0.7	0.8	0.5–1.2
Need for fracture reduction	0.4	0.5	0.1–1.2
Payer status	0.9	1.0	0.6–1.4

Note: In this model, a large odds or risk ratio denotes a lesser likelihood of analgesic administration. Likelihood ratio $\chi^2 = 25.1$; $df = 6$; $p = .0003$.

Table 29.4. Route and Class of Analgesic by Ethnicity for 140 Patients Receiving Analgesics

Variable	White Patients ($n = 67$) (%)	Black Patients ($n = 73$) (%)
Parenteral	23 (34)	25 (34)
Narcotic	58 (87)	56 (77)

ethnic groups.[7,8] The apparent disparity in analgesic administration to minority ethnic groups is of concern and requires further elucidation.

Our finding that time since injury predicted analgesic use was expected. The need for fracture reduction was associated with analgesic use; however, this association was not statistically significant, perhaps because of the small number of patients requiring reduction.

In interpreting our results, it is useful to consider the sequence of events that leads to treatment of pain and how each of these might be influenced by ethnicity (Figure 29.2). First, to ensure comparability of the source of each patients' pain experience, we included only subjects with specific, well-identified bone injuries. This increased the likelihood that our groups, on average, experienced similar trauma. Given similar injuries, there is no evidence from the literature that ethnicity differentially influences patients' experience of pain.[9,10]

Second, given a source of pain, the patient must express discomfort to gain the attention of health care workers. Ethnicity may indeed influence the patient's expression of pain.[11] We cannot be certain that some aspect of ethnicity, or an unmeasured confounder such as the presence of friends or family, might influence black patients' expression of pain to physicians and nurses. However, if present, this unmeasured confounder could only have biased the study against our findings, as explained in the following text.

Importantly, the medical records contained explicit notations of pain for nearly identical proportions of black and white patients. If some unmeasured confounder

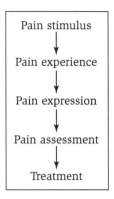

Figure 29.2 Steps Involved in the Patient-Physician Pain-Analgesic Process.

served to inhibit expressions of pain for black patients, it would follow that their pain experience could only have been more severe than that of white patients to result in this near identical assessment of pain by physicians and nurses.

We have previously examined health professionals' ability to assess pain in different ethnic groups, by testing physicians' skill in estimating pain severity among Hispanic and white patients with extremity trauma.[5] Although disparities between patient and physician pain scores were noted, they were identical for the two ethnic groups. This implies that any ethnic disparity in analgesic prescribing could not be attributed to differences in pain assessment.

We are left, then, with the final step, the physician's decision to administer analgesics. Our findings suggest that patient ethnicity affects decision making, independent of objective clinical criteria. Beyond this, we have no specific data to shed light on the reasons physicians order analgesics less frequently for minority patients than for white patients.

Our study is limited in several respects. Given its retrospective design, our study allows for potential misclassification of predictor or outcome variables, as well as potential confounders. Patient ethnicity was generally recorded by clerical personnel and is a potential source of error. It seems unlikely, however, that their perception of ethnicity differed from that of the physicians or nurses. Analgesic administration, particularly that of narcotics, tends to be well recorded in the medical record. However, it is possible that the administration of non-narcotic medications was recorded with less fidelity. If this did occur, we can see no reason that it should occur more commonly among black patients than white patients.

It is possible that our results are confounded by other factors, particularly alcohol or other drug use. Nursing staff often record information regarding mental status and intoxication on the medical record. In only two cases were patients noted to be less than "alert and oriented." In four additional cases, patients were judged "intoxicated." Of these six patients, two were white and four were black.

Although the infrequent notation of altered mental status and intoxication is somewhat reassuring, this information is inconsistently recorded by nursing personnel. However, time of day and occupational injury were two variables that were reliably recorded. These also correlate with alcohol and drug use, and may serve as partial proxies for intoxication. Black and white patients had similar proportions of occupational injuries, and their times of presentation, as well as the distribution of injury mechanisms, are similar; thus, we believe that unrecorded alcohol and drug use is unlikely to explain our findings.

Finally, although we found no association between physician ethnicity and analgesic prescribing patterns, the small numbers of minority physicians in this and our previous study preclude making definitive statements on this point. Future studies involving larger numbers of minority physicians will be required to assess the importance of physician-patient concordance in analgesic practice.

Oligoanalgesia is common in both outpatient and inpatient settings. Many authorities have implicated the lack of an adequate pain assessment as the primary barrier to the optimal treatment of pain. The primacy of pain assessment has been highlighted in a number of guides to improve analgesic practice, including the 1992 Agency for Health Care Policy and Research's *Clinical Practice Guideline: Acute Pain Management,* the 1994 Canadian Association of Emergency Physicians' consensus document *Emergency Pain Management,* and the American Pain Society's "Quality Improvement Guidelines for the Treatment of Acute Pain and Cancer Pain."[12-14]

A number of investigators have evaluated pain management interventions that include attempts to standardize pain assessment.[15-19] Unfortunately, none of these interventions have successfully altered physician practice or improved patients' pain experience.

Our findings suggest that it is not the failure of physicians to assess pain but the failure to administer analgesics that principally contributes to oligoanalgesia among Hispanic and black patients. Efforts to alter pain management practices may find better success with interventions targeting analgesic administration as well as standardized pain assessment, including clinical guidelines that couple pain ratings with specific recommendations for analgesic use.

Notes

1. Wilson, J., & Pendleton, J. (1989). Oligoanalgesia in the emergency department. *Am J Emerg Med, 7,* 620–623.

2. Selbst, S. M., & Clark, M. (1990). Analgesic use in the emergency department. *Ann Emerg Med, 19,* 1010–1013.

3. Ducharme, J., & Barber, C. (1995). A prospective blinded study on emergency pain assessment and therapy. *J Emerg Med, 13,* 571–575.

4. Todd, K. H., Samaroo, N., & Hoffman, J. R. (1993). Ethnicity as a risk factor for inadequate emergency department analgesia. *JAMA, 269,* 1537–1539.

5. Todd, K. H., Lee, T, & Hoffman, J. R. (1994). The effect of ethnicity on physician estimates of pain severity in patients with isolated extremity trauma. *JAMA, 271,* 925–928.

6. Zhang, J., & Yu, K. F. (1998). What's the relative risk? A method of correcting the odds ratio in cohort studies of common outcomes. *JAMA, 280,* 1690–1691.

7. Cleeland, C. S., Gonin, R., Baez, L., et al. (1997). Pain and treatment of pain in minority patients with cancer. *Ann Intern Med, 127,* 813–816.

8. Bernabei, R., Gambassi, G., Lapane, K., et al. (1998). Management of pain in elderly patients with cancer. *JAMA, 279,* 1877–1882.

9. Zatzick, D. F., & Dimsdale, J. E. (1990). Cultural variations in response to painful stimuli. *Psychosom Med, 52,* 544–557.

10. Pfefferbaum, B., Adams, J., & Aceves, J. (1990). The influence of culture on pain in Anglo and Hispanic children with cancer. *J Am Acad Child Adolesc Psychiatry, 29,* 642–647.

11. Greenwald, H. P. (1991). Interethnic differences in pain perception. *Pain, 44,* 157–163.

12. U.S. Department of Health and Human Services, Public Health Service, Agency for Health Care Policy and Research. (1992). *Clinical practice guideline: Acute pain management: Operative or medical procedures and trauma* (AHCPR Publication No. 92-0032). Silver Spring, MD: Center for Research Dissemination and Liaison, AHCPR Clearinghouse.

13. Ducharme, J. (1994). Emergency pain management: A Canadian Association of Emergency Physicians (CAEP) consensus document. *J Emerg Med, 12,* 855–866.

14. American Pain Society Quality of Care Committee. (1995). Quality improvement guidelines for the treatment of acute pain and cancer pain. *JAMA, 274,* 1874–1880.

15. Ward, S. E., & Gordon, D. B. (1996). Patient satisfaction and pain severity as outcomes in pain management: A longitudinal view of one setting's experience. *J Pain Symptom Manage, 11,* 242–251.

16. Bookbinder, M., Coyle, N., Kiss, M., et al. (1996). Implementing national standards for cancer pain management: Program model and evaluation. *J Pain Symptom Manage, 12,* 334–347.

17. Rhodes, D. J., Koshy, R. C., Waterfield, W., et al. (1997, November 12–15). *The feasibility and effectiveness of quantitative pain assessment in outpatient oncology practice* [Abstract]. Paper presented at the National Meeting of the Robert Wood Johnson Clinical Scholars Program, Fort Lauderdale, FL.

18. Kravitz, R. L., Delafield, J. P., Hays, R. D., et al. (1996). Bedside charting of pain levels in hospitalized patients with cancer: A randomized controlled trial. *J Pain Symptom Manage, 11,* 81–87.

19. Leapley, M., Watson, W. A., Todd, K. H., et al. (1996). Pain documentation and ED analgesic practice [Abstract]. *Acad Emerg Med, 3,* 475.

CHAPTER THIRTY

The Effect of Race and Sex on Physicians' Recommendations for Cardiac Catheterization

Kevin A. Schulman, Jesse A. Berlin, William Harless, Jon F. Kerner,
Shyrl Sistrunk, Bernard J. Gersh, Ross Dubé, Christopher K. Taleghani,
Jennifer E. Burke, Sankey Williams, John M. Eisenberg, and José J. Escarce

Epidemiologic studies have identified differences according to race and sex in the treatment of patients with cardiovascular disease in the United States.[1-18] Some studies have found that blacks and women are less likely than whites and men, respectively, to undergo cardiac catheterization or coronary artery bypass graft surgery when they are admitted to the hospital for treatment of chest pain or myocardial infarction.[1-5,7,8,10,11,13,14] In contrast, other studies were unable to confirm that invasive procedures are underused in women.[15,16]

Racial differences in the treatment of cardiovascular disease may be explained by financial and organizational barriers,[13] clinical differences among patients,[17] preferences of the patients,[7,8,10,12] and the amount of contact the patients have with the health care system or hospitals that offer invasive cardiovascular services.[18] Most studies that have controlled for the insurance status of patients[1,5,7,9-13] or have assessed patients already within the health care system[1-3,5,7-14] still found significant effects of race. However, one study has reported that there were no effects of race among patients with private insurance.[13]

William Ayers, M.D., Georgetown University Medical Center, Washington, D.C., was also an author. This study was supported by a grant (HS07315) from the Agency for Health Care Policy and Research. We are also indebted to Damon Seils for his assistance in the preparation of the manuscript and to Harry Glick for providing the risk profiles from the Framingham Study for use in this study.

Sex differences in the treatment of cardiovascular disease are less well established. Sex differences persist despite the poorer prognosis for women after myocardial infarction[19,20] and the higher likelihood that they will have had greater functional disability due to angina before myocardial infarction.[4] Differences in treatment may be related to a lack of research on cardiovascular disease in women,[21] differences in physicians' interpretations of women's and men's symptoms,[6] time of presentation for treatment with respect to the progression of disease,[22] or the recommendations of physicians.[23]

One question that has not been addressed directly by previous studies is the extent to which physicians are responsible for the differences in treatment recommendations with respect to race and sex. The goal of this study was to assess, in a controlled experiment, physicians' treatment recommendations for patients presenting with various types of chest pain. We hypothesized that the race and sex of the patients would influence the physicians' recommendations regarding cardiac catheterization.

METHODS

Survey Instrument

We developed a computerized survey instrument, incorporating video-recorded interviews and text, to present descriptions of patients with chest pain to clinicians and to assess clinicians' decisions about how to manage such symptoms. We constructed 144 descriptions using all possible combinations of six experimental factors: race (black or white), sex, age (fifty-five or seventy years), level of coronary risk (low or high), type of chest pain (definite angina, possible angina, or nonanginal pain), and the results of an exercise stress test with thallium (moderate inferolateral ischemia, moderate anterolateral ischemia, or multiple severe ischemic defects). In addition, each description included the same results of electrocardiography (nonspecific T wave changes).

The survey was administered by means of a multimedia computer program developed for this study. The instrument included a video-recorded interview of a patient with chest pain and was designed to assess the physicians' management recommendations and judgment of the characteristics of the patient, and to record the demographic characteristics of the physicians.

The recorded component consisted of a scripted interview with a patient. Three scripts were developed, one for each type of chest pain. Each script contained information on the presenting symptom, associated cardiac symptoms, relief of symptoms, and duration of symptoms. The scripts were reviewed by four cardiologists, who independently used established criteria to classify the features of the pain described in each interview as definite angina, possible angina, or nonanginal chest pain.[24] The rate of agreement among the classifications made by the cardiologists on the basis of the scripts was greater than 75 percent.

Eight actors, representing each of the possible combinations of race, sex, and age, were recruited to portray the patients in the interviews (Figure 30.1). Actors were used because they were considered better able than patients to express a consistent range of emotions and to read the scripts verbatim for recording. The interviews were recorded at a single studio, with the actors following a particular set of directions for each script. The hand motions used by the actors were identical for each script, the actors were dressed in identical gowns, and the camera position was the same for all interviews. The video recordings were produced by a company with experience in the production of educational medical video products (Interactive Drama, Bethesda, Maryland).

The video segment was introduced by a screen that listed the patient's type of insurance (Blue Cross–Blue Shield indemnity insurance for the fifty-five-year-old patients and Medicare and Blue Cross–Blue Shield supplemental insurance for the seventy-year-old patients) and occupation (assembly supervisor for the fifty-five-year-old patients, retired assembly supervisor for the seventy-year-old patients). The patients were considered to be at low risk or at high risk for coronary disease on the basis of blood pressure (low risk, 133/81 mmHg; high risk, 145/86 mmHg), blood cholesterol concentrations (low risk: low-density lipoprotein [LDL], 146 mg per deciliter [3.8 mmol per liter], and high-density lipoprotein [HDL], 59 mg per deciliter [1.5 mmol per liter]; high risk: LDL, 158 mg per deciliter [4.1 mmol per liter], and HDL, 46 mg per deciliter [1.2 mmol per liter]), and smoking history (low risk, no smoking; high risk, smoking one pack of cigarettes a day for thirty years). None of the patients had diabetes, and all had a father who had had a myocardial infarction at the age of seventy-five years. These characteristics were based on the characteristics of the subjects in the 20th to 30th percentiles for the risk of coronary artery disease (low risk) and the subjects in the 70th to 80th percentiles (high risk) in the Framingham Study.[25]

So that their decisions about management could be assessed, the physicians were asked to characterize the type of chest pain described by the patient and to estimate the probability that he or she had clinically significant coronary disease (defined as ≥70 percent narrowing of an epicardial coronary artery). The physicians were then asked if they wished to order further cardiac evaluations for the patient and were given four options: no stress test, regular stress test, stress test with thallium, and other types of functional cardiac assessment (for example, stress echocardiography). The physicians were then shown the results of one of three stress tests with thallium, asked to estimate the probability of coronary disease on the basis of the results of the stress test, and asked whether they wished to refer the patient for cardiac catheterization.

The section on patient assessment included a two-part survey to be completed by the physician, modified from the instrument developed by M. van Ryn

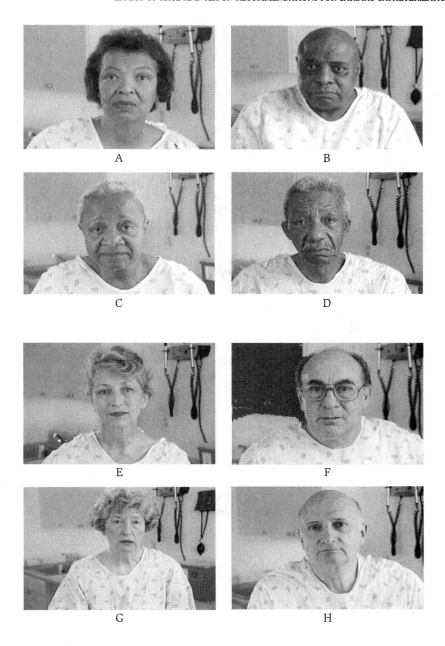

Figure 30.1 Patients as Portrayed by Actors in the Video Component of the Survey.

Panel A shows a fifty-five-year-old black woman, Panel B a fifty-five-year-old black man, Panel C a seventy-year-old black woman, Panel D a seventy-year-old black man, Panel E a fifty-five-year-old white woman, Panel F a fifty-five-year-old white man, Panel G a seventy-year-old white woman, and Panel H a seventy-year-old white man.

(personal communication). The first component of the survey was a ten-item scale, which included assessment items for the physicians' judgments of the emotional, intellectual, and communication characteristics of the patients; these factors are believed to be predictive of patient compliance and treatment outcomes. The personal characteristics of the patients were evaluated by the physicians on a 7-point Likert scale that rated the strength and direction of the attributes within the domain, with scores ranging from -3 (negative attributes) to 3 (positive attributes). The second component of the instrument included six individual assessment items evaluated on a 5-point Likert scale, with 1 representing "very unlikely" and 5 representing "very likely." The physicians were asked to predict the likelihood that the patient seen in the interview had overreported his or her symptoms, the likelihood that the patient would miss follow-up appointments, the likelihood that the patient would participate in treatment, the likelihood that the patient would sue for malpractice, the likelihood that the patient would comply with therapy, and the likelihood that the patient would benefit from a revascularization procedure (coronary angioplasty or coronary artery bypass surgery). Finally, the survey asked the physicians to report their age, race or ethnic group, sex, specialty and subspecialty, and year of graduation from medical school.

The software program required that all the components of the ten-minute survey instrument be presented to each physician and that the physician see the entire interview before answering questions. The interactive programs were developed with the use of Conversim, a proprietary software program designed by Interactive Drama for the creation of standardized multimedia patients on a personal computer for training purposes.

Study Subjects and Data Collection

Physicians who were in full-time clinical practice and who attended the 1997 annual meeting of the American College of Physicians (ACP) or the 1996 annual meeting of the American Academy of Family Practice (AAFP) were eligible to participate in the survey. Physicians who registered for these meetings in advance were mailed a postcard inviting them to participate in the survey, with the incentive of an offer of a food gift. The physicians were told they were participating in a study of clinical decision making but were not told that the primary purpose of the study was to assess the effects of patients' race and sex on decision making. The surveys were administered in a booth located in the main exhibit hall of each meeting with six individual computer stations. The computer stations were designed to offer privacy to the physicians and to prevent them from viewing other participants while they were completing the survey.

The physicians were randomly assigned to view 1 of 144 possible cases according to the full-factorial experimental design (that is, all the possible combinations of race, sex, age, risk level, type of chest pain, and stress test results). After each replication of the study design was completed, the randomized scheme began again for a new replicate of 144 cases. Sample size calculations required a minimum of two replicates (288 subjects) from each meeting for the study to achieve 80 percent power to detect a 15 percent difference in referral decisions at a level of significance of 0.05. We collected data for three replicates at the AAFP meeting (432 subjects) and for two replicates at the ACP meeting (288 subjects).

Statistical Analysis

We performed univariate analyses to assess differences in the physicians' responses when different values of the experimental factors were used to construct the case descriptions. Differences in the means of continuous variables were evaluated with t tests or analysis of variance, and differences in proportions were evaluated with chi-square tests.

In addition, we used multivariable logistic regression analyses to assess the effect of the race and sex of the patient on the decisions of physicians regarding referral for cardiac catheterization, with adjustment for the other experimental variables and additional potential confounding variables. We included the race and sex of the patient in the regression models, using two approaches: analyzing the main effects of race and sex only, and analyzing the main effects of race and sex plus a race–sex interaction. The second approach enabled us to assess treatment recommendations for four combinations of race and sex (white man, black man, white woman, and black woman).

In our main analyses, the covariates in the regression models were the age of the patient, the level of risk, the type of chest pain (as classified by the study cardiologists), the results of the exercise stress test with thallium, and the physician's estimate of the probability of coronary disease after the stress test. We also assessed whether the results remained robust after the following changes were made to the models: replacing the type of chest pain as classified by the study cardiologists with the type of chest pain as classified by the physicians; replacing the probability of disease after the results of the stress test were known with the probability before they were known; omitting estimates of the probability of disease altogether; adding the responses of the physicians regarding the personal characteristics of the patients to the covariates in the model; adding the physicians' responses regarding the individual assessment items to the covariates in the model; and adding the characteristics of the physicians, including race and sex, to the model.

Preliminary analyses showed no difference in survey responses between the physicians at the AAFP meeting and those at the ACP meeting and similar effects of the race and sex of the patient at the two meetings. Consequently, we pooled the data from both meetings in all subsequent analyses. We converted logistic regression coefficients to odds ratios and calculated 95 percent confidence intervals, using standard methods.

RESULTS

The only characteristic of the 720 physicians that differed with respect to the race and sex of the patient was the sex of the physician, with more female physicians assigned to black female patients ($p = .02$) (Table 30.1).

The physicians' estimates of the probability of coronary artery disease before the results of the stress test were known differed according to the sex, age, level of risk, and type of chest pain of the patient (Table 30.2). The patterns of the differences were consistent with the known prevalence of coronary disease in various groups of patients (for example, older patients have higher rates of coronary disease than younger patients). As expected, these estimates of probability did not differ according to the results of the stress test, which were unknown to the physicians at the time the assessments were made.

For all categories of all experimental factors, the probabilities of disease assigned after the results of the stress test were known were consistently greater than those assigned before the results were known (Table 30.2). This finding was expected, because all the patients had a positive stress test. The probabilities assigned after the results of the stress test were known differed according to age, the type of chest pain, and the results of the exercise stress test.

Table 30.1. Characteristics of the Physicians According to the Race and Sex of the Patient

Characteristic	White Male Patient	Black Male Patient	White Female Patient	Black Female Patient	p Value
No. of physicians	180	180	180	180	
Mean age, years	44.2	43.6	42.9	42.8	0.57
Sex, no. (%)					0.02
Male	130 (72.2)	131 (72.8)	126 (70.0)	107 (59.4)	
Female	50 (27.8)	49 (27.2)	54 (30.0)	73 (40.6)	
Race or ethnic group, no. (%)					0.41
White	148 (82.2)	136 (75.6)	139 (77.2)	137 (76.1)	
Black	7 (3.9)	8 (4.4)	7 (3.9)	11 (6.1)	
Hispanic	5 (2.8)	8 (4.4)	7 (3.9)	8 (4.4)	
Aleut	0	4 (2.2)	0	0	
Asian	16 (8.9)	13 (7.2)	20 (11.1)	17 (9.4)	
Don't know or no answer	4 (2.2)	11 (6.1)	7 (3.9)	7 (3.9)	
Specialty, no. (%)					0.97
Internal medicine	68 (37.8)	67 (37.2)	69 (38.3)	71 (39.4)	
Family medicine	104 (57.8)	106 (58.9)	101 (56.1)	103 (57.2)	
Other	8 (4.4)	7 (3.9)	10 (5.6)	6 (3.3)	
Board certified, no. (%)					0.63
Yes	164 (91.1)	166 (92.2)	159 (88.3)	162 (90.0)	
No	16 (8.9)	14 (7.8)	21 (11.7)	18 (10.0)	

Note: Because of rounding, percentages may not total 100.

Table 30.2. Physicians' Estimates of the Probability of Coronary Artery Disease According to Experimental Factors

Experimental Factor and Category	Estimate of Probability Before Stress Test %	p Value	Estimate of Probability After Stress Test %	p Value
Sex		<0.001		0.15
Male	69.2 ± 18.2		87.5 ± 13.7	
Female	64.1 ± 19.3		86.1 ± 13.3	
Race		0.120		0.26
White	65.5 ± 20.5		87.4 ± 13.7	
Black	67.7 ± 17.1		86.2 ± 13.3	
Age		<0.001		0.03
55 years	63.8 ± 19.5		85.7 ± 14.0	
70 years	69.5 ± 17.9		87.9 ± 12.9	
Risk level		<0.001		0.05
Low	63.5 ± 20.4		85.8 ± 14.0	
High	69.8 ± 16.8		87.8 ± 12.9	
Type of chest pain		<0.001		<0.001
Nonanginal pain	58.3 ± 19.0		84.5 ± 14.0	
Possible angina	64.4 ± 18.3		86.2 ± 13.7	
Definite angina	77.1 ± 14.0		89.7 ± 12.3	
Stress test result		0.77		<0.001
Inferolateral ischemia	67.3 ± 19.3		87.5 ± 15.9	
Anterolateral ischemia	66.1 ± 18.8		84.1 ± 11.7	
Multiple ischemic defects	66.5 ± 18.7		88.8 ± 12.1	

Note: The results of stress tests were not presented to the physicians for the initial assessment of the probability of disease but were presented for the final assessment. Plus–minus values are means ±SD.

Overall, the physicians classified 30.6 percent of the patients as having definite angina, 65.0 percent as having possible angina, and 4.4 percent as having nonanginal chest pain. There were no differences in the assessments of chest pain according to the combined race and sex of the patient ($p = .20$). The overall rate of agreement with the expert classification was 51 percent and varied from 48 percent to 55 percent for the various combinations of race and sex. Stress tests were recommended for 93.3 percent of white men and white women and for 97.8 percent of black men and black women ($p = .04$).

The physicians' perceptions of the personal characteristics of the patients differed significantly in seven of the categories measured on the ten-item scale according to the combined race and sex of the patient ($p < .05$). However, in no category was the difference greater than 0.87 point on the 7-point Likert scale (Table 30.3). In addition, the responses to the individual assessment of the predicted behavior of the patients differed significantly for three of the six categories according to the combined race and sex of the patient ($p < .02$); in no category was the difference greater than 0.27 point on a 5-point Likert scale (Table 30.3).

Table 30.3. Physicians' Assessments of the Characteristics of the Patients According to Category of Race and Sex

Characteristic	White Male Patient	Black Male Patient	White Female Patient	Black Female Patient	p Value
Personal characteristics*					
Hostile–friendly	1.81 ± 1.06	1.99 ± 1.06	1.66 ± 1.09	2.23 ± 0.90	0.001
Unintelligent–intelligent	1.91 ± 0.90	1.89 ± 0.97	2.05 ± 0.83	2.00 ± 0.84	0.29
Lacking self-control–self-controlled	2.17 ± 0.98	2.25 ± 0.95	2.28 ± 0.89	2.35 ± 0.79	0.31
Ignorant–knowledgeable	1.31 ± 1.13	1.56 ± 0.93	1.58 ± 1.08	1.51 ± 1.08	0.06
Poor communicator–good communicator	1.61 ± 1.40	1.94 ± 1.21	1.93 ± 1.20	1.94 ± 1.21	0.03
Dependent–independent	1.52 ± 1.20	1.91 ± 1.11	1.45 ± 1.35	1.83 ± 1.10	0.001
Sad–happy	0.24 ± 1.38	0.44 ± 1.50	−0.20 ± 1.45	0.67 ± 1.33	0.001
Negative affect–positive affect	0.14 ± 1.37	0.51 ± 1.44	−0.14 ± 1.54	0.51 ± 1.44	0.001
Worried–indifferent	−0.76 ± 1.65	−1.18 ± 1.58	−1.29 ± 1.42	−0.97 ± 1.49	0.005
Low socioeconomic status–high socioeconomic status	0.69 ± 1.06	−0.09 ± 1.03	0.76 ± 1.01	0.14 ± 1.04	0.001
Individual assessment of predicted behavior					
Likely to overreport symptoms[†]	2.04 ± 0.79	1.79 ± 0.60	2.05 ± 0.65	1.84 ± 0.51	0.001
Likely to miss appointments[†]	2.04 ± 0.79	2.21 ± 0.83	2.04 ± 0.84	2.04 ± 0.79	0.12
Likely to participate[†]	3.88 ± 0.98	3.78 ± 0.88	4.00 ± 0.90	3.81 ± 1.00	0.12
Likely to sue[†]	2.54 ± 0.85	2.27 ± 0.84	2.46 ± 0.81	2.32 ± 0.83	0.01
Likely to comply with treatment[†]	4.04 ± 0.80	3.97 ± 0.70	4.20 ± 0.63	4.06 ± 0.77	0.02
Likely to benefit from invasive procedure[‡]	3.47 ± 0.72	3.38 ± 0.65	3.44 ± 0.76	3.30 ± 0.75	0.12

Note: Plus–minus values are means ±SD.

*Patients' personal characteristics were rated on a 7-point Likert scale, with scores ranging from −3 to 3. A higher score indicates a stronger relation with the positive (second listed) characteristic.

†Physicians were asked to rate patients on a 5-point Likert scale, with 1 representing "very unlikely" and 5 representing "very likely."

‡Physicians were asked to rate patients on a 5-point Likert scale, with 1 representing "much less than average" and 5 representing "much greater than average."

In univariate analyses, the race and sex of the patient were significantly associated with the physicians' decisions about whether to make referrals for cardiac catheterization, with men and whites more likely to be referred than women and blacks, respectively (Table 30.4). For the other experimental factors, only the type of chest pain was a significant predictor of whether the patient would be referred for cardiac catheterization.

Table 30.5 shows the results of the multivariate logistic regression analyses. In the model that included only the main effects of race and sex, we found that both variables were significant predictors of rates of referral for cardiac catheterization. Men and whites were significantly more likely to be referred than women and blacks. These results indicate that the differences with respect to

Table 30.4. Referral for Cardiac Catheterization According to Experimental Factors

Experimental Factor and Category	Mean Referral Rate (%)	Odds Ratio (95% CI)*	p Value
Sex			
Male	90.6	1.0	
Female	84.7	0.6 (0.4–0.9)	0.02
Race			
White	90.6	1.0	
Black	84.7	0.6 (0.4–0.9)	0.02
Age			
55 years	89.7	1.0	
70 years	85.6	0.7 (0.4–1.1)	0.09
Risk level			
Low	88.9	1.0	
High	86.4	0.8 (0.5–1.2)	0.31
Type of chest pain			
Nonanginal pain	83.8	1.0	
Possible angina	90.0	1.7 (1.0–3.0)	0.04
Definite angina	89.2	1.6 (0.9–2.7)	0.08
Stress test result			
Inferolateral ischemia	86.3	1.0	
Anterolateral ischemia	86.7	1.0 (0.6–1.6)	0.89
Multiple ischemic defects	90.0	1.4 (0.8–2.5)	0.20

*CI = confidence interval.

race and sex were not due simply to the differences in the probabilities of disease assigned by the physicians. We then examined the interaction of race and sex in terms of referral for cardiac catheterization ($p = .06$ for the interaction). Black women were the only patients who were significantly less likely to be referred for cardiac catheterization than white men, who served as the reference category. In addition, age and the type of chest pain were significant predictors of referral for cardiac catheterization, with the odds ratios for all factors similar to those in the univariate results. Sensitivity analyses (alternative model specifications) did not change the results of the main analyses.

DISCUSSION

We found that the race and sex of the patient affected the physicians' decisions about whether to refer patients with chest pain for cardiac catheterization, even after we adjusted for symptoms, the physicians' estimates of the probability of

Table 30.5. Predictors of Referral for Cardiac Catheterization

Model and Variable	Odds Ratio (95% CI)*	p Value
Race and sex as separate factors		
Sex		
Male	1.0	
Female	0.6 (0.4–0.9)	0.02
Race		
White	1.0	
Black	0.6 (0.4–0.9)	0.02
Interaction of race and sex		
White male	1.0	
Black male	1.0 (0.5–2.1)	0.99
White female	1.0 (0.5–2.1)	>0.99
Black female	0.4 (0.2–0.7)	0.004

Note: Both models included all experimental factors as covariates, as well as the probability of coronary artery disease as estimated after the results of the stress tests were known. The first analysis included only the main effects. The second analysis explored a race-sex interaction.

*CI = confidence interval.

coronary disease, and clinical characteristics. Our findings are most striking for black women. Epidemiologic studies have reported differences in treatment according to race and sex,[1-18] but they could not assess whether these differences were due to differences in the clinical presentation of the patients. This study directly addressed this issue by using actors to represent patients with identical histories and controlling for characteristics reflective of their personalities. Our findings are consistent with the results of epidemiologic studies in which the lowest rates of cardiovascular procedures were among nonwhite women.[5,9]

The physicians' recommendations for cardiac catheterization could have reflected their perceptions of the personalities rather than the race or sex of the patients. To assess this possibility, we collected detailed information on the physicians' perceptions of the patients' personalities and other attributes with the use of a ten-item scale and six individual assessment questions. Incorporating this information into the analysis did not change the main results. Also, because we used a balanced, randomized design, the statistical tests of the experimental factors, including the race and sex of the patient, remain valid even if the patients' personality traits and attributes were imperfectly captured by our methods.[26]

Our findings suggest that a patient's race and sex may influence a physician's recommendation with respect to cardiac catheterization regardless of the patient's clinical characteristics. Alternatively, these findings may be the result of other factors not included in the information we presented to the physicians. For example, data on bypass surgery and angioplasty suggest that women may have worse outcomes than men,[27-30] although these effects may be due to differences in other confounding variables rather than to the sex of the patient.[28,30] Why these clinical effects would influence recommendations for black women and not white women is unclear. We did not find lower rates of referrals for stress tests among women or blacks.

Our study design has several strengths. By having actors pose as patients, clothed in an identical manner and having identical insurance and occupations, we removed the effects of differing socioeconomic status and insurance from our experiment. By providing the actors with identical scripts, by having them present in hospital gowns under identical direction, and by creating the program in a fixed format, we removed the effects of differences in the presentation of clinical symptoms by patients from our assessment. Finally, by asking the physicians for their estimates of the probability of coronary artery disease, we were able to control for differences in their perceptions of the prevalence of disease according to the race and sex of the patients. Although the physicians' estimates of the probability of disease before the results of the stress test were known were higher than the values for nonanginal pain reported in the literature,[31,32] these estimates are most relevant in the analysis of the treatment recommendations. Physicians' tendency to overestimate the probability of coronary artery disease in patients from groups with a low prevalence of disease has been documented previously.[33]

Our finding that the race and sex of the patient influence the recommendations of physicians independently of other factors may suggest bias on the part of the physicians. However, our study could not assess the form of bias. Bias may represent overt prejudice on the part of physicians or, more likely, could be the result of subconscious perceptions rather than deliberate actions or thoughts.[34,35] Subconscious bias occurs when a patient's membership in a target group automatically activates a cultural stereotype in the physician's memory regardless of the level of prejudice the physician has.[35]

Our study has two main limitations. First, we assessed the management decisions of physicians using video recordings of actors portraying patients and a computerized survey instrument. Several reports support the use of case vignettes to assess clinical decision making by physicians.[36-40] In two studies of the external validity of case vignettes, assessments made on the basis of written case descriptions correlated highly with those made on the basis of examinations of patients with equivalent symptoms seen in person.[37,38] Using video recordings rather than written case presentations may increase the accuracy of the probability estimates made by physicians.[40]

Second, the recruitment of physicians at national meetings of major professional organizations may have resulted in nonrepresentative samples. Physicians who attend professional meetings may be better informed than those who do not attend. Also, the physicians who volunteered for this project may have had a greater interest than others in coronary heart disease.

Our findings indicate that the race and sex of patients independently influence physicians' recommendations for the management of chest pain. They suggest that decision making by physicians may be an important factor in explaining differences in the treatment of cardiovascular disease with respect to race and sex.

Notes

1. Wenneker, M. B., & Epstein, A. M. (1989). Racial inequalities in the use of procedures for patients with ischemic heart disease in Massachusetts. *JAMA, 261,* 253–257.

2. Maynard, C., Litwin, P. E., Martin, J. S., et al. (1991). Characteristics of black patients admitted to coronary care units in metropolitan Seattle: Results from the Myocardial Infarction Triage and Intervention Registry (MITI). *Am J Cardiol, 67,* 18–23.

3. Johnson, P. A., Lee, T. H., Cook, E. F., Rouan, G. W., & Goldman, L. (1993). Effect of race on the presentation and management of patients with acute chest pain. *Ann Intern Med, 118,* 593–601.

4. Steingart, R. M., Packer, M., Hamm P., et al. (1991). Sex differences in the management of coronary artery disease. *N Engl J Med, 325,* 226–230.

5. Ayanian, J. Z., & Epstein, A. M. (1991). Differences in the use of procedures between women and men hospitalized for coronary heart disease. *N Engl J Med, 325,* 221–225.

6. Tobin, J. N., Wassertheil-Smoller, S., Wexler, J. P., et al. (1987). Sex bias in considering coronary bypass surgery. *Ann Intern Med, 107,* 19–25.

7. Peterson, E. D., Wright, S. M., Daley, J., & Thibault, G. E. (1994). Racial variation in cardiac procedure use and survival following acute myocardial infarction in the Department of Veterans Affairs. *JAMA, 271,* 1175–1180.

8. Peterson, E. D., Shaw, L. K., DeLong, E. R., Pryor, D. B., Califf, R. M., & Mark, D. B. (1997). Racial variation in the use of coronary-revascularization procedures: Are the differences real? Do they matter? *N Engl J Med, 336,* 480–486.

9. Giles, W. H., Anda, R. F., Casper, M. L., Escobedo, L. G., & Taylor, H. A. (1995). Race and sex differences in rates of invasive cardiac procedures in U.S. hospitals: Data from the National Hospital Discharge Survey. *Arch Intern Med, 155,* 318–324.

10. Whittle, J., Conigliaro, J., Good, C. B., & Lofgren, R. P. (1993). Racial differences in the use of invasive cardiovascular procedures in the Department of Veterans Affairs medical system. *N Engl J Med, 329,* 621–627.

11. Udvarhelyi, I. S., Gatsonis, C., Epstein, A. M., Pashos, C. L., Newhouse, J. P., & McNeil, B. J. (1992). Acute myocardial infarction in the Medicare population: Process of care and clinical outcomes. *JAMA, 268,* 2530–2536.

12. Gornick, M. E., Eggers, P. W., Reilly, T. W., et al. (1996). Effects of race and income on mortality and use of services among Medicare beneficiaries. *N Engl J Med, 335*, 791–799.

13. Carlisle, D. M., Leake, B. D., & Shapiro, M. F. (1997). Racial and ethnic disparities in the use of cardiovascular procedures: Associations with type of health insurance. *Am J Public Health, 87*, 263–267.

14. Laouri, M., Kravitz, R. L., French, W. J., et al. (1997). Underuse of coronary revascularization procedures: Application of a clinical method. *J Am Coll Cardiol, 29*, 891–897.

15. Bickell, N. A., Pieper, K. S., Lee, K. L., et al. (1992). Referral patterns for coronary artery disease treatment: Gender bias or good clinical judgment? *Ann Intern Med, 116*, 791–797.

16. Mark, D. B., Shaw, L. K., DeLong, E. R., Califf, R. M., & Pryor, D. B. (1994). Absence of sex bias in the referral of patients for cardiac catheterization. *N Engl J Med, 330*, 1101–1106.

17. Ferguson, J. A., Tierney, W. M., Westmoreland, G. R., et al. (1997). Examination of racial differences in management of cardiovascular disease. *J Am Coll Cardiol, 30*, 1707–1713.

18. Blustein, J., & Weitzman, B. C. (1995). Access to hospitals with high-technology cardiac services: How is race important? *Am J Public Health, 85*, 345–351.

19. Tofler, G. H., Stone, P. H., Muller, J. E., et al. (1987). Effects of gender and race on prognosis after myocardial infarction: Adverse prognosis for women, particularly black women. *J Am Coll Cardiol, 9*, 473–482.

20. Wenger, N. K., Speroff, L., & Packard, B. (1993). Cardiovascular health and disease in women. *N Engl J Med, 329*, 247–256.

21. Beery, T. A. (1995). Gender bias in the diagnosis and treatment of coronary artery disease. *Heart Lung, 24*, 427–435.

22. Newby, L. K., Rutsch, W. R., Califf, R. M., et al. (1996). Time from symptom onset to treatment and outcomes after thrombolytic therapy. *J Am Coll Cardiol, 27*, 1646–1655.

23. Ades, P. A., Waldmann, M. L., Polk, D. M., & Coflesky, J. T. (1992). Referral patterns and exercise response in the rehabilitation of female coronary patients aged greater than or equal to 62 years. *Am J Cardiol, 69*, 1422–1425.

24. Diamond, G. A. (1983). A clinically relevant classification of chest discomfort. *J Am Coll Cardiol, 1*, 574–575.

25. Abbott, R. D., & McGee, D. (1987). *The Framingham Study: An epidemiological investigation of cardiovascular disease: Section 37. The problem of developing certain cardiovascular diseases in 8 years at specific values of some characteristics* (NIH Publication No. 87-2284). Bethesda, MD: National Heart, Lung, and Blood Institute.

26. Begg, M. D., & Lagakos, S. (1993). Loss in efficiency caused by omitting covariates and misspecifying exposure in logistic regression models. *J Am Stat Assoc, 88*, 166–170.

27. Loop, F. D., Golding, L. R., MacMillan, J. P., Cosgrove, D. M., Lytle, B. W., & Sheldon, W. C. (1983). Coronary artery surgery in women compared with men: Analyses of risks and long-term results. *J Am Coll Cardiol, 1,* 383–390.

28. Kimmel, S. E., Berlin, J. A., Storm, B. L., & Laskey, W. K. (1995). Development and validation of a simplified predictive index for major complications in contemporary percutaneous transluminal coronary angioplasty practice. *J Am Coll Cardiol, 26,* 931–938.

29. O'Connor, G. T., Plume, S. K., Olmstead, E. M., et al. (1991). A regional prospective study of in-hospital mortality associated with coronary artery bypass grafting. *JAMA, 266,* 803–809.

30. Bell, M. R., Holmes, D. R., Jr., Berger, P. B., Garratt, K. N., Bailey, K. R., & Gersh, B. J. (1993). The changing in-hospital mortality of women undergoing percutaneous transluminal coronary angioplasty. *JAMA, 269,* 2091–2095.

31. Diamond, G. A., & Forrester, J. S. (1979). Analysis of probability as an aid in the clinical diagnosis of coronary-artery disease. *N Engl J Med, 300,* 1350–1358.

32. Pryor, D. B., Harrell, F. E., Jr., Lee, K. L., Califf, R. M., & Rosati, R. A. (1983). Estimating the likelihood of significant coronary artery disease. *Am J Med, 75,* 771–780.

33. Schulman, K. A., Escarce, J. J., Eisenberg, J. M., et al. (1992). Assessing physicians' estimates of the probability of coronary artery disease: The influence of patient characteristics. *Med Decis Making, 12,* 109–114.

34. Escarce, J. J., Epstein, K. R., Colby, D. C., & Schwartz, J. S. (1993). Racial differences in the elderly's use of medical procedures and diagnostic tests. *Am J Public Health, 83,* 948–954.

35. Devine, P. G. (1989). Stereotypes and prejudice: Their automatic and controlled components. *J Pers Soc Psychol, 56,* 5–18.

36. Wigton, R. J., Poses, R. M., Collins, M., & Cebul, R. D. (1990). Teaching old dogs new tricks: Using cognitive feedback to improve physicians' diagnostic judgments on simulated cases. *Acad Med, 65*(Suppl.), S5–S6.

37. Kirwan, J. R., Chaput de Saintonge, D. M., Joyce, C.R.B., & Currey, H.L.F. (1983). Clinical judgment in rheumatoid arthritis: I. Rheumatologists' opinion and the development of "paper patients." *Ann Rheum Dis, 42,* 644–647.

38. Kirwan, J. R., Bellamy, N., Condon, H., Buchanan, W. W., & Barnes, C. G. (1983). Judging "current disease activity" in rheumatoid arthritis: An international comparison. *J Rheumatol, 10,* 901–905.

39. Jones, T. V., Gerrity, M. S., & Earp, J. A. (1990). Written case simulations: Do they predict physicians' behavior? *J Clin Epidemiol, 43,* 805–815.

40. McNutt, R. A., O'Meara, J. J., de Bliek, R., et al. (1992). The effect of visual information and order of patient presentation on the accuracy of physicians' estimates of acute ischemic heart disease: A pilot study [Abstract]. *Med Decis Making, 12,* 342.

CHAPTER THIRTY-ONE

Patient Race and Psychotropic Prescribing During Medical Encounters

Betsy Sleath
Bonnie Svarstad
Debra Roter

There is a need to better understand what factors influence physician prescribing of psychotropic medications to patients with chronic illness during primary care medical visits. Researchers have suggested that the following four factors influence physician decision making: physicians, patients, the physician-patient encounter, and the political, economic, and cultural context in which health care is provided.[1,2] Gabe has argued that these same four variables are important influences on the prescribing of psychotropic medications and that more research especially needs to be conducted in the area of psychotropic prescribing during physician-patient encounters.[3] Perhaps better understanding the process of psychotropic prescribing during physician-patient encounters will help us better understand why nonwhites have consistently been found to have a lower rate of psychotropic drug use than whites.[4–8]

Most studies of psychotropic prescribing have examined the relationship between patient ratings of their physical and mental health status and psychotropic prescribing.[5,9–13] Both patient self-report of poor physical and mental

This research was supported by Agency for Health Care Policy and Research Grant No. R03 HS0749901. The authors would like to thank the members of the Collaborative Study Group of the Task Force on Doctor and Patient of the Society for General Internal Medicine for the use of the audiotapes. The authors would also like to thank Matthew Englerth for his assistance, and Betty Chewning, John Delamater, Emily Kane, and Jeanine Mount for comments on an earlier manuscript.

health status have been found to increase the likelihood that a psychotropic medication is prescribed.[5,9,10] Despite the fact that patients may rate their physical health, emotional health, and social problems poorly, they may not express all of their symptoms to their physicians during their medical visits. Patients may feel discouraged from talking about emotional or social problems because the problems may not seem appropriate or important enough to discuss during the medical visit.[14] Patient race or ethnicity may also influence whether individuals discuss emotional or social problems with their physicians.[15] Patients from certain ethnic groups may view mental health problems as a sign of weakness and therefore not discuss them with their physicians.[16,17]

Additionally, physicians may not be adequately trained on how to discuss emotional and social problems with patients. Family practice physicians cited inadequate education in treating emotional and psychiatric disorders as a major obstacle that prevents them from adequately treating patients' emotional and social problems.[18] Patient ethnicity may also influence how physicians interpret physical, emotional, or social problem symptoms expressed by patients from diverse cultural backgrounds.[19,20] There have not been many studies conducted that examine how patient ethnicity and symptom expression during physician-patient encounters influence psychotropic prescribing.[21]

Raynes did examine how patient symptom expression influenced physician prescribing of psychotropic medications during physician-patient encounters. She found that the major factors contributing to psychotropic prescribing were patient expression of psychological and social problems in addition to physical symptoms. She did not examine how physical, psychological, and social problems each respectively influenced psychotropic prescribing. Raynes found that treatment with psychotropic medications was more symptomatically than diagnostically based. During 59.5 percent of the encounters where a psychotropic medication was prescribed the patient expressed a psychosocial complaint, whereas in only 28.1 percent of the encounters where a psychotropic medication was prescribed the physician diagnosed the patient with a psychiatric condition. Raynes did not use multivariate analysis techniques in her research so future work could examine the relative impact of patient expression of symptoms and physician diagnoses of patients on psychotropic prescribing.[21]

There also have not been many studies conducted that examine how physician perceptions of patients' physical health, emotional health, and social problems influence psychotropic prescribing. Most studies of psychotropic prescribing relate only physician diagnoses and not physician perceptions of patients to psychotropic prescribing.[22,23] However, recognition of signs and symptoms of anxiety and/or depression may be sufficient justification for a prescription. For example, Wells, Goldberg, Brook, and Leake found that more than one-half of the patients who were prescribed minor tranquilizers had a diagnosis of anxiety disorder or signs and symptoms of anxiety written in their chart and more than

90 percent of patients on antidepressants had a diagnosis of depression or signs and symptoms of depression written in their chart.[4]

We conducted a content analysis of audiotapes of 508 primary care physician–chronic disease patient interactions to examine how patient ratings of their physical and emotional health; patient physical, emotional, and social problem symptom expression; and physician perceptions of patients' physical health, emotional health, and social problems influenced psychotropic prescribing to white and nonwhite patients. We conducted separate analyses for white and nonwhite patients because whites have consistently been found to use psychotropic medications more than nonwhites and we wanted to examine whether different factors influenced psychotropic prescribing to white and nonwhite patients. The following research questions were examined for both white and nonwhite patients: (1) Are patients who rate their physical and emotional health poorly more likely to receive a prescription for a psychotropic medication? (2) Are patients who express more physical, emotional, and social problem symptoms more likely to receive a prescription for a psychotropic medication? (3) Are patients who are perceived by their physicians as having more physical, emotional, and social problems more likely to receive a prescription for a psychotropic medication?

METHODS

Procedures

Data were collected as part of a larger study of 550 doctor-patient encounters in eleven U.S. and Canadian communities. The original data set, including audiotapes of physician-patient interactions and self-administered questionnaires from each participating physician and patient, has been described elsewhere.[24] The audiotapes of physician-patient interaction were obtained during regularly scheduled outpatient visits in academic and Veterans Administration centers, community hospitals, and private practices. Responsibility for data collection at each site was assumed by a local member of the Collaborative Study Group of the Task Force on Doctor and Patient of the Society for General Internal Medicine.

Research assistants at each site invited patients to participate in the study, obtained necessary consents, and made arrangements to audiotape one physician-patient encounter for each patient. They also administered a questionnaire to each patient immediately following the physician-patient encounter.

Study physicians were asked to complete a self-administered questionnaire for each enrolled patient immediately after the taped visit. The questionnaire, which was attached to the patient's chart, included a number of questions about the patient and the physician-patient visit. Researchers later obtained physician demographic information through a mailed questionnaire sent to study physicians.

Patients had to meet four criteria to be included in the study: (1) be eighteen years of age or older and give full consent; (2) have two or more previous visits with the study physician; (3) have one or more chronic medical conditions; and (4) have no language or communication difficulties that could interfere with physician-patient communication.

Audiotapes of adequate quality for transcription were obtained for 513 out of a sample of 550 physician-patient encounters. Twenty-four tapes were missing or damaged when the tapes were copied to be used in this analysis and thirteen tapes were inaudible. Physician or patient questionnaire data were missing for five encounters, yielding a final sample of 508 patients who were treated by 118 physicians. The unit of analysis used in this study is the doctor-patient encounter ($n = 508$).

Tapes were randomly assigned to trained transcriptionists who were blinded to the study hypotheses. They transcribed the tapes using rules adapted from other studies of physician-patient communication.[25,26] Trained coders then content analyzed and coded the transcriptions using the Patient Symptom Expression (PSE) coding tool (described below).

Coders recorded the name and/or type of each psychotropic medication mentioned during the physician-patient encounter, including psychotropic medications identified in general or lay terms (for example, "nerve pills," "tranquilizers," "pills for my depression"). Coders also recorded whether the medications were new or refill prescriptions.

Coders were blinded to patient race when coding the transcripts. A group of twenty-five randomly selected transcripts were double-coded to assess intercoder reliability. A kappa value was calculated to determine the level of agreement among the observers.[27,28] The kappa value for the observations recorded by the observers was 0.71.

Measurement

Patient questionnaire data were used to measure patient gender (female = 0, male = 1), race (0 = nonwhite, 1 = white), and family income per year (0 = less than $10,000, 1 = $10,000 to $19,999, 2 = $20,000 or more). Patient age was measured in years. The patient's perceived physical health and emotional health were obtained immediately after the physician-patient interaction. Both the patient's perceived physical health and the patient's perceived emotional health were measured using four response categories: poor, fair, good, and excellent. Number of previous visits to the physician was measured using four response categories: 1–3, 4–7, 7–10, and greater than 10. The physician's questionnaire provided information on physician gender, race, and physician age (years). However, only two patients in the sample saw African American physicians, so physician race was not used in any of the analyses.

The Patient Symptom Expression (PSE) coding tool measured the extent to which patients actually expressed various physical, emotional, and social problems during the taped encounter. The first section examined patient expression of *physical symptoms* and was adapted from the National Ambulatory Medical Care Survey (NAMCS) Reason for Visit Classification.[29] Physical symptoms were grouped into twelve categories: (1) general; (2) nervous system; (3) skin, hair, and nails; (4) circulatory; (5) respiratory; (6) musculoskeletal; (7) digestive system; (8) urinary tract; (9) reproductive; (10) eyes; (11) ears; and (12) endocrine. Definitions were obtained from the NAMCS Reason for Visit Classification and NAMCS Symptom Classification.[29,30] If the symptom category was uncertain, the symptom was placed in the "general" category.

For each category, the coder assessed whether there was no problem (0), a minor problem (1), or a major problem (2). A symptom was coded as being a major problem if the patient's statements indicated that it was bothering him or her a lot and a minor problem if it was bothering him or her somewhat. Because the physical categories were broad, we included space for coding up to two different problems for each category. A patient's total score on the physical symptom expression scale could range from 0 to 48. The second section of the PSE coding tool measured patient expression of *emotional symptoms* and also was adapted from the NAMCS Reason for Visit Classification.[29] Six categories were considered: (1) anxious/nervous, (2) worry/concern, (3) irritation/anger, (4) depression/sadness, (5) sleep disturbance, and (6) other (for example, antisocial behavior). Similar definitions were used for coding no problem, a minor problem, or a major problem. The total score on the emotional complaint expression scale could range from 0 to 12.

The third section contained eleven categories for coding patient expression of *social problems.* They were (1) financial difficulties, (2) marital/relationship difficulties, (3) difficulties with children, (4) difficulties with other relatives, (5) difficulties with friends, (6) difficulties in having sexual relations with others, (7) alcohol/drug abuse, (8) difficulties in finding or keeping housing, (9) problems at work, (10) difficulties in social life associated with aging, and (11) other (being under pressure, loneliness, and difficulties with activities of daily living). Coders again assessed whether there was no problem, a minor problem, or a major problem. Therefore, a patient's score on the social problem expression scale could range from 0 to 22.

We measured physician perception of patient emotional health using five items from the physician's questionnaire. The items asked the physician to rate the patient's level of anxiety, worry, irritation, depression, and sleep disturbance. The four response categories ranged from patient showing no signs (1) to patient showing many signs (4). Individual items were summed to obtain a summary score that could range from 4 to 20.

Physician perception of the patient's physical health was assessed by a single item that asked the physician to compare the patient's physical health to that of other patients of a similar age (less severe, the same, and more severe). Physician perception of the patient's social problems was assessed using a similarly worded item pertaining to the patient's social problems. Three response categories were again provided: less severe, the same, and more severe.

Prescribing of psychotropic medication was measured as a dichotomous variable. If the patient received a prescription for one or more psychotropic medications it was coded 1, and if the patient received no prescription for a psychotropic medication it was coded 0.

Data Analysis

First, descriptive statistics for all variables used in the analysis were calculated. Next, we compared the characteristics of our patient sample with patient characteristics of the 1990 National Ambulatory Medical Care Survey Sample.[31] Next, bivariate analyses between patient race and the other variables used in the analysis were conducted. Chi-square statistics for dichotomous variables and one-tail t tests for continuous variables were calculated for patient race and the other variables used in the analysis.

Finally, logistic regression techniques were used to predict psychotropic prescribing.[32,33] Physician prescribing of psychotropic medications to white and nonwhite patients were separately regressed on (1) demographic variables (patient gender, patient age, patient income, patient rating of own physical and emotional health, number of previous visits to the physician, physician age, and physician gender), (2) patient expression variables (patient physical, emotional, and social problem symptom expression), and (3) physician perception variables (physician perception of patient physical health, emotional health, and social problems). Ninety-five percent confidence intervals for the odds ratios were calculated using the exact method.[34]

RESULTS

Thirty-six percent of the eleven ambulatory care sites were private or small-group practice sites, whereas the other 64 percent of the sites were hospital-based clinics. All of the private or small-group practices were in suburban or urban areas, whereas all of the hospital-based clinics were in urban areas. The majority of the 118 physicians (79 percent) in the sample were male. The mean age of physicians was thirty-six years (range twenty-five to sixty-four).

The patient sample was 45 percent nonwhite. The nonwhite category contained primarily blacks (96 percent). A majority of patients were female (58 percent) and had a family income of less than $10,000 a year (68 percent). The mean age of patients was sixty-one years (range twenty to ninety-five). Forty-seven percent of the patients rated their physical health as fair or poor, and 32 percent rated their emotional health as fair or poor. The percentage of females in our sample was similar to the 61 percent figure in the 1990 NAMCS patient sample. Our sample had many more nonwhite patients than the 1990 NAMCS data set (45 percent as compared to 12 percent), possibly due to the location of our data collection sites in urban areas. Since the original study focused on patients with chronic conditions, it also yielded an older sample than the NAMCS sample. Only 18 percent of our patient sample was under forty-four years, whereas 57 percent of the NAMCS sample was under forty-four years. Our sample had roughly the same percentage of symptom visits and diagnostic, treatment, or test results visits as the NAMCS sample.[31]

Table 31.1 presents the cross-tabulation of patient race and patient and physician demographic variables. Nonwhite patients were significantly more likely to be female ($p < .01$) and poor ($p < .001$) than white patients. Nonwhite patients were also significantly more likely to see younger physicians ($p < .05$) than white patients. White and nonwhite patients were of similar ages, saw physicians of similar gender, had the same number of previous visits to their physicians, and rated their physical and emotional health similarly.

Table 31.2 presents the cross-tabulation of patient race and the patient expression, physician perception, and psychotropic prescription variables. White and nonwhite patients expressed similar levels of physical, emotional, and social problem symptoms. Also, physicians rated white and nonwhite patients' physical health, emotional health, and social problems similarly. However, white patients were almost twice as likely as nonwhite patients to receive a psychotropic prescription.

Twenty percent of white and 13.5 percent of nonwhite patients received one or more prescriptions for psychotropic medications. Seven percent of nonwhite and 10 percent of white patients received antidepressant medications whereas 11 percent of white and only 7 percent of nonwhite patients received anxiolytic, sedative, or hypnotic medications. The majority of patients who were prescribed psychotropic medications had already been on them. Of the eighty-eight patients who were prescribed psychotropic medications, only seventeen patients (six nonwhite and eleven white) were prescribed new psychotropic medications.

Table 31.3 contains the adjusted odds ratios and confidence intervals for the logistic regression equation predicting psychotropic prescribing to white patients. Both patient expression of emotional symptoms ($p < .01$) and the physician's rating of the patient's emotional health ($p < .01$) were significant predictors of psychotropic prescribing. Patient gender did not significantly influence psychotropic prescribing to white patients. Patient ratings of their physical and emotional health did not significantly influence psychotropic prescribing in the multivariate analysis. Patient expression of physical and social problem

Table 31.1. Patient and Physician Characteristics Among White and Nonwhite Patients

Variable	White ($n = 279$) Percentage (n)	Nonwhite ($n = 229$) Percentage (n)
Patient gender		
Female	52.0 (145)	65.0 (149)
Male	48.0 (134)	35.0 (80)**
Patient income		
$10,000 or less	56.3 (157)	82.5 (189)
$10,001–$20,000	18.3 (51)	9.2 (21)
More than $20,000	25.4 (71)	8.3 (19)***
Patient age		
20–39	12.5 (35)	14.0 (32)
40–59	24.0 (67)	31.0 (71)
60–69	25.8 (72)	27.5 (63)
70–79	26.9 (75)	21.0 (48)
80–95	10.8 (30)	6.6 (15)
Patient's rating of physical health		
Excellent	13.3 (37)	16.6 (38)
Good	38.7 (108)	38.0 (87)
Fair	31.9 (89)	33.6 (77)
Poor	16.1 (45)	11.8 (27)
Patient's rating of emotional health		
Excellent	20.8 (58)	20.5 (47)
Good	45.9 (128)	48.9 (112)
Fair	25.1 (70)	23.6 (54)
Poor	8.2 (23)	7.0 (16)
Physician gender		
Female	19.0 (53)	20.5 (47)
Male	81.0 (226)	79.5 (182)
Physician age		
25–30	19.0 (53)	20.5 (47)
31–35	33.7 (94)	28.4 (65)
36–40	29.4 (82)	24.9 (57)
41–64	17.9 (50)	16.2 (37)*
Number of previous visits		
1–3	12.9 (36)	23.1 (53)
4–6	28.3 (79)	34.1 (78)
7–10	19.7 (55)	22.7 (52)

Note: Significance level of the chi-square statistic for dichotomous variables and one-tail t test for continuous variables: *$p < .05$; **$p < .01$; ***$p < .001$.

Table 31.2. Patient Expression, Physician Perception, and Psychotropic Prescribing Among White and Nonwhite Patients

Variable	Whites ($n = 279$) Percentage (n)	Nonwhites ($n = 229$) Percentage (n)
Patient expresses physical symptom(s)		
0	4.3 (12)	7.0 (16)
1	12.2 (34)	11.4 (26)
2–3	39.1 (109)	41.4 (95)
4–5	26.9 (75)	25.8 (59)
6–13	17.6 (49)	14.4 (33)
Patient expresses emotional symptom(s)		
0	63.8 (178)	69.0 (158)
1	17.2 (48)	12.1 (28)
2	13.3 (37)	14.0 (32)
3–6	5.7 (16)	4.8 (11)
Patient expresses social problem(s)		
0	63.8 (178)	73.4 (168)
1	16.8 (470)	11.4 (26)
2	11.8 (33)	7.0 (16)
3–8	7.5 (21)	8.3 (19)
Physician's perception of patient's physical health		
Less severe	28.7 (80)	34.5 (79)
Same	40.1 (112)	42.0 (96)
More severe	31.2 (87)	23.6 (54)
Physician's perception of patient's emotional health		
4–8	27.2 (76)	33.6 (77)
9–11	38.4 (107)	32.3 (74)
12–13	20.0 (56)	18.3 (42)
14–19	14.3 (40)	15.7 (36)
Physician's perception of patient's social problems		
Less severe	36.9 (103)	35.8 (82)
Same	42.3 (118)	48.9 (112)
More severe	20.8 (58)	15.3 (35)
Psychotropic prescription		
Yes	20.4 (57)	13.5 (31)
No	79.6 (222)	86.5 (198)*

Note: Significance level of the chi-square statistic for dichotomous variables and one tail t test for continuous variables: *$p < .05$; **$p < .01$; ***$p < .001$.

Table 31.3. Logistic Regression Equation Results for Predicting Psychotropic
Drug Prescription for White Patients (n = 279)

Independent Variables	B (SE)	Odds Ratio	95% Confidence Interval
Patient gender male	0.40 (0.35)	1.49	(0.75, 2.97)
Patient age	0.16 (0.17)	1.17	(0.84, 1.63)
Patient income	0.33 (0.24)	1.39	(0.87, 2.23)
Patient rate physical health	−0.06 (0.24)	0.94	(0.59, 1.51)
Patient rate emotional health	0.15 (0.25)	1.16	(0.71, 1.90)
Physician gender male	0.32 (0.46)	1.37	(0.56, 3.39)
Physician age	−0.22 (0.20)	0.81	(0.54, 1.19)
No. previous visits	−0.08 (0.17)	0.92	(0.66, 1.28)
Patient expresses physical symptoms	−0.15 (0.17)	0.86	(0.62, 1.17)
Patient expresses emotional symptoms	0.91 (0.19)	2.48**	(1.72, 3.60)
Patient expresses social symptoms	−0.33 (0.20)	0.72	(0.49, 1.06)
Physician perception of physical health	0.03 (0.25)	1.03	(0.63, 1.68)
Physician perception of emotional health	0.59 (0.20)	1.81**	(1.22, 2.66)
Physician perception of social problems	0.08 (0.28)	1.08	(0.63, 1.88)
Constant	−4.08 (1.44)		
−2LL[†]	229.31***		
df	264		
Improvement of FIT	53.21/14*df****		

[†]−2LL = −2 log likelihood −2LL for intercept only 282.52.

*p < .05; **p < .01; ***p < .001.

symptoms and the physician's rating of the patient's physical health and social problems did not significantly influence psychotropic prescribing.

Table 31.4 contains the adjusted odds ratios and confidence intervals for the logistic regression equation predicting psychotropic prescribing to nonwhite patients. The only independent variable that significantly influenced physician psychotropic prescribing to nonwhite patients was patient expression of emotional symptoms (p < .001). The physician's rating of the patient's emotional

Table 31.4. Logistic Regression Equation Results for Predicting Psychotropic
Drug Prescription for Nonwhite Patients (n = 229)

Independent Variables	B (SE)	Odds Ratio	95% Confidence Interval
Patient gender male	1.02 (0.55)	2.79	(0.92, 8.33)
Patient age	−0.24 (0.24)	0.78	(0.49, 1.26)
Patient income	−0.56 (0.55)	0.57	(0.19, 1.72)
Patient rate physical health	0.64 (0.35)	1.89	(0.63, 5.70)
Patient rate emotional health	0.09 (0.33)	1.10	(0.57, 2.10)
Physician gender male	0.80 (0.73)	2.22	(0.53, 9.30)
Physician age	−0.04 (0.25)	0.96	(0.59, 1.57)
No. previous visits	0.37 (0.27)	1.45	(0.85, 2.46)
Patient expresses physical symptoms	0.31 (0.26)	1.36	(0.82, 2.27)
Patient expresses emotional symptoms	0.99 (0.27)	2.70***	(1.58, 4.57)
Patient expresses social symptoms	0.03 (0.24)	1.03	(0.64, 1.65)
Physician perception of physical health	0.15 (0.34)	1.16	(0.59, 2.27)
Physician perception of emotional health	0.40 (0.28)	1.50	(0.86, 2.59)
Physician perception of social problems	0.35 (0.41)	1.42	(0.64, 3.16)
Constant	−8.16 (2.0)		
−2LL†	112.13***		
df	214		
Improvement of FIT	69.45/14 df***		

†−2LL = −2 log likelihood −2LL for intercept only 181.58.

*p < .05; **p < .01; ***p < .001.

health did not significantly influence psychotropic prescribing as it did for white patients. Patient gender, patient ratings of their physical and emotional health, patient expression of physical and social problem symptoms, and the physician's rating of the patient's physical health and social problems did not significantly influence psychotropic prescribing.

The investigators also put interaction terms of (1) patient expression of emotional complaints and social problems, (2) patient expression of emotional complaints and physician rating of patient emotional health, (3) patient expression of social problems and physician rating of patient social problems, and (4) physician rating of patient emotional health and social problems into separate logistic regression equations for white and nonwhite patients. None of the interaction terms were significant or improved the overall fit of the models (results not shown).

DISCUSSION

A high percentage of our patient sample (17 percent) received one or more prescriptions for psychotropic medications. This finding could be due to the fact that all of the patients in our sample had chronic diseases. Previous research has shown that patients with chronic diseases are more likely to be on psychotropic medications.[9,10,35,36] Our finding that white patients were almost twice as likely as nonwhite patients to be prescribed one or more psychotropic medications is similar to the findings of other investigators.[4–7]

We found great similarities between white and nonwhite patients. White and nonwhite patients rated their physical and emotional health similarly. White and nonwhite patients also expressed similar levels of physical, emotional, and social problem symptoms. Additionally, physicians rated white and nonwhite patients' physical health, emotional health, and social problems similarly.

An interesting finding of our study is that patient expression of emotional symptoms influenced psychotropic prescribing to both white and nonwhite patients, but physician perceptions of patients' emotional health significantly influenced psychotropic prescribing only to white patients. Physician perceptions of nonwhite patients' emotional health did not significantly influence the prescribing of psychotropic medications to them. This finding suggests that physicians may not be perceiving and treating the mental health of nonwhite and white patients in a similar fashion, which might help explain why nonwhites have been found to have a lower rate of psychotropic drug use than whites. Future research needs to further explore how physician perceptions of the emotional health of patients from different cultures influences whether they prescribe psychotropic medications to these patients.

Another important finding of this study was that patients' emotional symptom expression was a significant predictor of psychotropic prescribing to both white and nonwhite patients whereas patient ratings of their emotional health were not. This suggests that physicians need to facilitate patient expression of emotional symptoms as much as possible so that patients' emotional problems (for example, depression, anxiety) can be diagnosed and treated. Another significant finding of the study was that patient expression of emotional symptoms was a significant predictor of psychotropic prescribing whereas patient expression of social problems was not. Although we examined psychotropic prescribing rather than psychotherapeutic drug use, this finding is similar to the results of Mellinger and associates who found that patient ratings of their emotional or psychic distress (for example, feel nervous, feel depressed) had a greater impact on psychotherapeutic drug use than patient ratings of their life or situational stress (for example, laid off, unable to pay bills, going through divorce, drug or alcohol abuse).[13] Our findings suggest that physicians do not prescribe psychotropic medications in an indiscriminate manner and rely heavily on patient symptoms (and explanations). Patients who complain about sleeplessness, anxiety, and other forms of distress and elaborate on the situational causes for their depression or anxiety may cause physicians to attribute the problem to environmental or social causes rather than biological processes, thereby decreasing reliance on medication.

These findings illustrate how critical it is for primary care physicians to probe and to provide patients with an opportunity to discuss their emotional symptoms and social problems. Physicians who do not adequately probe and discuss emotional symptoms may underprescribe medications to patients who are reluctant to express their anxiety or depression. In other cases, they may overprescribe psychotropic medications to patients who do not elaborate or articulate the alternative explanations or attributions for their emotional symptoms.

Communication skills are important not only in prescribing and diagnostic decisions but in the therapeutic value they provide to patients. Ormel and associates concluded that good patient outcomes cannot be wholly attributed to specific mental health treatments such as drugs.[37] Rather other effects of the recognition and treatment process, such as acknowledgment, reinterpretation of signs and symptoms, and social support also contribute to the "active element" of the recovery process. The mechanism by which even limited attention to psychosocial problems may alleviate distress is also proposed by Stoeckle and others.[38] The authors suggest that "active listening" can assist a patient in more appropriate attribution of distress, alleviate feelings associated with helplessness and isolation, and create a sense of support and partnership.

These types of communication skills can be taught. Roter et al. developed and evaluated a continuing medical education program for community-based, primary care physicians with the hope of improving their recognition and address of patients' psychosocial problems.[39] Physicians, in small groups in two four-hour sessions, were trained in interviewing skills that emphasized handling emotions or problem solving. Trained physicians were better than control physicians at recognizing which of their patients were emotionally distressed. Also, patients of trained physicians showed significantly greater improvement in their mental health than the control group patients for up to six months following the medical visit. Programs like the one developed by Roter and associates could be used to train already practicing physicians on how to better discuss patient emotional concerns.[39]

There are limitations to this study. First, the patient sample was low income and had a large proportion of nonwhite and elderly patients. Nevertheless, Roter et al.,[24] using this same data set, found that the average length of physician-patient interactions was very similar to the length of physician-patient interactions found by researchers using the NAMCS data set. Second, we did not have access to other potentially useful demographic information (for example, education level, marital status, medical diagnoses, employment status, psychiatric diagnoses), which could help us to understand the complex set of factors that can influence patient expression of somatic, emotional, and social problems.[24] Third, we could have missed cases where physicians and patients discussed medications in general terms without mentioning specific psychotropic medications, but our method of measuring psychotropic prescribing may be more sensitive than existing methods that rely on physician or patient report.

Finally, our results need to be interpreted with care, because the majority of psychotropic medications prescribed to our patient sample were repeat prescriptions. Only seventeen of the eighty-eight patients (six nonwhite and eleven white) who were prescribed psychotropics were prescribed new medications. We really may have found that overt expression of emotional symptoms by the patient is more likely to result in the physician continuing psychotropic medications rather than in the physician prescribing psychotropic medications to patients who have not used them previously. Future research could use a sample of patients receiving only new psychotropic prescriptions to examine whether our results would hold true when the majority of patients are receiving new rather than repeat prescriptions for psychotropic medications.

Notes

1. Eisenberg, J. M. (1979). Sociological influences on decision-making by clinicians. *Ann Int Med, 90*(6), 957.

2. Clark, J. A., Potter, D. A., & McKinlay, J. B. (1991). Bringing social structure back into clinical decision making. *Soc Sci Med, 32*(8), 853–866.

3. Gabe, J. (1990). Towards a sociology of tranquillizer prescribing. *Br J Addict, 85,* 41–48.

4. Wells, K. B., Goldberg, G., Brook, R., & Leake, B. (1988). Management of patients on psychotropic drugs in primary care clinics. *Med Care, 26*(7), 645–656.

5. Wells, K. B., Kamberg, C., Brook, R., Camp, P., & Rogers, W. (1985). Health status, sociodemographic factors, and the use of prescribed psychotropic drugs. *Med Care, 23*(11), 1295–1306.

6. Benson, P. R. (1983). Factors associated with antipsychotic drug prescribing by Southern psychiatrists. *Med Care, 21*(6), 639–654.

7. Seltzer, C., Friedman, G. D., & Siegelaub, A. B. (1974). Smoking and drug consumption in white, black, and Oriental men and women. *Am J Public Health, 64*(5), 466–473.

8. Cafferata, G. L., Kasper, J., & Bernstein, A. (1983). Family roles, structure, and stressors in relation to sex differences in obtaining psychotropic drugs. *J Health Soc Behav, 24,* 132.

9. Riska, E., & Klaukka, T. (1984). Use of psychotropic drugs in Finland. *Soc Sci Med, 19*(9), 983.

10. Ried, L. D., Christensen, D. B., & Stergachis, A. (1990). Medical and psychosocial factors predictive of psychotropic drug use in elderly patients. *Am J Public Health, 80*(11), 1349–1353.

11. Olfson, M., & Pincus, H. A. (1994). Use of benzodiazepines in the community. *Arch Int Med, 154,* 1235–1240.

12. Kessler, L. G., Amick, B. C., III, & Thompson, J. (1985). Factors influencing the diagnosis of mental disorder among primary care patients. *Med Care, 23*(1), 50–62.

13. Mellinger, G. D., Balter, M. B., Manheimer, D. I., Cisin, I. H., & Parry, H. J. (1978). Psychic distress, life crisis, and use of psychotherapeutic medications. *Arch Gen Psychiatry, 35,* 1045–1052.

14. Roter, D. L., & Hall, J. A. (1992). *Doctors talking with patients, patients talking with doctors: Improving communication in medical visits.* Westport, CT: Auburn House.

15. Angel, R., & Thoits, P. (1987). The impact of culture on the cognitive structure of illness. *Cult Med Psychiatry, 11,* 465–494.

16. Broadhead, W. E. (1944). Presentation of psychiatric symptomatology in primary care. In J. Miranda, A. A. Hohmann, C. C. Attkisson, & D. B. Larson (Eds.), *Mental disorders in primary care* (pp. 139–162). San Francisco: Jossey-Bass.

17. Katon, W., Kleinman, A., & Rosen, G. (1982). Depression and somatization: A review. *Am J Med, 72,* 127–135.

18. Orleans, C. T., George, L. K., Houpt, J. L., & Brodie, H. K. (1985). How primary care physicians treat psychiatric disorders: A national survey of family practitioners. *Am J Psychol, 142,* 52–57.

19. Ford, D. E. (1994). Recognition and underrecognition of mental disorders in adult primary care. In J. Miranda, A. A. Hohmann, C. C. Attkisson, & D. B. Larson (Eds.), *Mental disorders in primary care* (pp. 186–205). San Francisco: Jossey-Bass.

20. Jones, L. R., Mabe, P.A., & Riley, W. T. (1989). Physician interpretation of illness behavior. *Int J Psychiatry Med, 19*(3), 237–248.

21. Raynes, N. (1979). Factors affecting the prescribing of psychotropic drugs in general practice consultation. *Psychol Med, 9,* 671–679.

22. Hohmann, A. A. (1989). Gender bias in psychotropic drug prescribing in primary care. *Med Care, 27*(5), 478–490.

23. Hasday, J. D., & Karch, F. E. (1981). Benzodiazepine prescribing in a family medicine center. *JAMA, 246*(12), 1321.

24. Roter, D., Lipkin, M., & Korsgaard, A. (1991). Sex differences in patients' and physicians' communication during primary care medical visits. *Med Care, 29*(11), 1083–1093.

25. Waitkzin, H. (1991). *The politics of medical encounters: How patients and doctors deal with social problems.* New Haven, CT: Yale University Press.

26. Mishler, E. G. (1984). *The discourse of medicine: Dialectics of medical interviews.* Norwood, NJ: Ablex.

27. Fleiss, J. L. (1971). Measuring nominal scale agreement among many raters. *Psychol Bull, 6,* 378–381.

28. Altman, D. G. (1991). *Practical statistics for medical research.* New York: Chapman and Hall.

29. Schneider, D., Appleton, R., & McLemore, T. (1979). A reason for visit classification for ambulatory care. *Vital Health Stat, 10*(176).

30. Meads, S., & McLemore, T. (1974). The national ambulatory medical care survey: Symptom classification. *Vital Health Stat, 2*(63).

31. Schappert, S. M. (1992). *National ambulatory medical care survey: 1990 summary. Advance data from Vital and Health Statistics, No. 213* (U.S. Department of Health and Human Services Publication No. [PHS]92-1250). Hyattsville, MD: U.S. Public Health Service.

32. Cleary, P. D., & Angel, R. (1984). The analysis of relationships involving dichotomous dependent variables. *J Health Soc Behav, 25,* 334–348.

33. Agresti, A. (1990). *Categorical data analysis.* New York: Wiley.

34. Dawson-Saunders, B., & Trapp, R. (1990). *Basic and clinical biostatistics.* Norwalk, CT: Appleton and Lange.

35. Greenblatt, D. J., Shader, R. I., & Koch-Weser, J. (1975). Psychotropic drug use in the Boston area. *Arch Gen Psychiatry, 32,* 518–521.

36. Hemminki, E. (1974). Diseases leading to psychotropic drug therapy. *Scan J Soc Med, 2,* 129.

37. Ormel, J., VanDen Brink, W., Koeter, M.W.J., et al. (1990). Recognition, management and outcome of psychological disorders in primary care: A naturalistic follow-up study. *Psychol Med, 20,* 909–923.

38. Stoeckle, J., & Barsky, A. (1980). Attributions: Uses of social science knowledge in the doctoring of primary care. In Eisenberg & Kleinman (Eds.), *The relevance of social science for medicine* (pp. 223–240). New York: Reidel.

39. Roter, D. H., Hall, J. A., Kern, D. E., Barker, L. R., Cole, K. A., & Roca, R. P. (1995). Improving physicians' interviewing skills and reducing patients' emotional distress: A randomized clinical trial. *Arch Int Med, 155,* 1877–1884.

CHAPTER THIRTY-TWO

The Effect of Patient Race and Socioeconomic Status on Physicians' Perceptions of Patients

Michelle van Ryn
Jane Burke

There is considerable evidence that patient sociodemographic characteristics have an impact both on physician behavior during medical encounters[1-4] and on the diagnoses and treatments patients receive.[5-15] Furthermore, these differences persist even when patient income, insurance coverage (payer), and disease severity are controlled.[7,8,14,16-18] These studies suggest that the relationship between patient sociodemographic characteristics and physician behavior is at least partially mediated by differences in physicians' perceptions of and beliefs about patients. Physicians' perceptions of patients may systematically vary by patient race, socioeconomic status, or other demographic characteristics. In turn, these differences in perceptions may explain some of the variance in physician behavior toward and treatment of patients. Despite their potential influence on quality of care, there has been little research on the way physicians' perceptions of and beliefs about patients vary with patient race or socioeconomic status. The lack of research in this area creates a critical gap in our understanding of the mediating factors in the relationships between patient sociodemographic characteristics and encounter characteristics, diagnoses, treatment recommendations, and outcomes.

Physicians are generally expected and expect themselves to be unaffected by patients' social or demographic characteristics in forming judgments of patients.[19,20] Since perceptions of and beliefs about patients can have a significant impact on encounter characteristics and treatment recommendations, physicians are generally expected to view each patient objectively and impartially, using biomedical information obtained from physical examination and diagnostic test results to develop a diagnosis and effective treatment plan.[21] Unfortunately, the research on social categorization and stereotyping suggests that these expectations are unrealistic.

All humans share the generally adaptive strategy of making the world more manageable by using categorizing and generalizing techniques to simplify the massive amounts of complex information and stimuli to which they are exposed.[22-23] In order to make the social world more manageable, people often make judgments about categories or groups of people and generalize these judgments to all the individuals mentally assigned to that category or group.[22,24,25] This categorization strategy can lead to stereotype usage:[26] the generation of a widely held image of a group of people through which specific individuals are perceived, or the application of an attitude set based on the group or class to which the person belongs.[23,27,28] When individuals are mentally assigned to a particular class or group, the characteristics assigned to that group are unconsciously and automatically applied to the individual. Given that this type of strategy is common to all humans and cultures,[23] the expectation that physicians be immune is unrealistic. In addition, the very nature and context of physicians' work may enhance the likelihood of stereotype usage. There is evidence that time pressure, the need to make quick judgments, cognitive load, task complexity, and busyness increase the likelihood of stereotype usage.[29-34] Physicians may be especially vulnerable to the use of stereotypes in forming impressions of patients since time pressure, brief encounters, and the need to manage very complex cognitive tasks are common characteristics of their work.

This paper utilizes survey data provided by physicians on 618 postangiogram* physician-patient encounters to examine the way physician beliefs about patient personal and psychosocial characteristics, behavior, and likely role demands are affected by patient race and socioeconomic status.

METHODS

Sample

Physician survey data on patients and doctor-patient encounters were collected using a four-stage sampling plan.† In the first stage, ten New York State hospitals that perform angiograms were selected by a weighted random sample in which

---

*An invasive diagnostic test for coronary artery disease (CAD).

†This sampling scheme was developed for a larger ongoing research project examining the factors associated with race and sex differences in treatments.[14] Urban patients and CAD patients who are appropriate for aggressive treatment are overrepresented in the sample.

weights were assigned based on the number of minorities who received an angiogram at the facility in 1991. Eight of the ten hospitals agreed to participate in the study. In the second stage, a stratified random sample involving 16 percent of white men, 33 percent of white women, and all African Americans undergoing angiograms at the sampled hospitals was selected for clinical data abstraction. In the third stage, a stratified random sample of stage two patients was recruited into the survey portion of the study. These patients were asked to complete the survey questionnaire within two weeks of their postangiogram encounter. Strata were again based on the race and sex of patients as well as patients' appropriateness for aggressive cardiac treatments and the actual treatment they were to receive.[‡] Aggressive treatment is defined here as either of the revascularization procedures percutaneous transluminal coronary angioplasty (PTCA) or coronary artery bypass graft surgery (CABG). Patients recruited into the study included all African American patients who were appropriate for aggressive treatment; all white males and white females who were appropriate for aggressive treatment but did not receive it; 43 percent of white males and 51 percent of white females who were appropriate for aggressive treatment and did receive it, and 5 percent of all race-sex groups who were inappropriate for aggressive treatment. Patients with extensive cognitive disability, patients who did not speak English or Spanish, or, for the present study, who were not self-identified as either white or African American, were removed from the sample. Seventy-five percent of the patients surveyed (706) completed the questionnaire. In the fourth stage, physicians involved in postangiogram treatment determination encounters with patients sampled in stage three were also recruited into the survey portion of the study. Like their patient counterparts, they were asked to complete a questionnaire within two weeks of the sampled encounter. A total of 842 patient encounters were sampled, out of which 193 physicians provided data on 618 encounters, yielding data on 73 percent of the encounters sampled.

Clinical/Medical Record Data Collection Procedures

The site abstractor (either a research nurse, cardiology fellow, medical student, or physician's assistant) used medical records and angiography reports to enter data into a software program (adapted by study staff from software supplied by the Health Care Financing Administration (HCFA) for use in their Cooperative Cardiovascular Project (CCP), Edward Ellerbeck, M.D., personal communication). Data coding was based on criteria developed by the RAND Corporation.[35,36] The RAND methodology consists of first classifying patients into approximately 1,000 different categories, or "indications," consisting of

---

[‡]The RAND Corporation's criteria for determining a case as appropriate for CABG or PTCA were used.[35-38]

intersections of important clinical determinants of the need for aggressive intervention (for example, number of coronary arteries with stenosis greater than 70 percent, level of angina, recent myocardial infarction, ejection fraction, presence of left main disease, the extent of existing comorbidities). Each of the indications was rated either as appropriate, uncertain, or inappropriate for each of three interventions (CABG surgery, PTCA, and medical therapy), and then appropriate indications were rated either as necessary or as appropriate but not necessary for each intervention.

Sample Characteristics

Of the 618 encounters, 53 percent (328) were with male and 47 percent (290) with female patients, while 57 percent (353) were with white and 43 percent (265) with African American patients, yielding roughly similar cell sizes for the four race and sex combined categories. The mean patient age was sixty-five (SD = 11.33) with a range of twenty-eight to ninety-two years. The mean education level was twelve years of schooling (SD = 2.47) with a range of eight to seventeen-plus years of school completed. On average, patients reported an annual household income of US$27,363 (SD = US$21,852). The majority (84 percent, $n = 521$) of the encounters were with white physicians, with 11 percent (67) involving Asian physicians, 1 percent (9) involving African American physicians, 3 percent (17) Hispanic physicians, and 1 percent (4) physicians of other races/ethnicities. Of the Asian physicians, 60 percent described themselves as being from the Indian subcontinent (India, Pakistan or Burma), 15 percent were born in Malaysia, and the remainder had other origins, including Thailand, Japan, Korea, and the Philippines. Ninety-three percent (572) of the encounters involved male physicians. The mean physician age was forty-five (SD = 8.45), with a range of twenty-nine to seventy-nine years. The physicians were predominantly cardiologists ($n = 542$, 88 percent), with 21 (3 percent) being cardiac surgeons and 55 (9 percent) specializing in internal medicine, family practice, or another specialty.

MEASURES

Independent Variables

Patient Socioeconomic Status (SES). A three-category measure of SES was developed, with categories corresponding to three equal portions of a SES index distribution. The SES index was created by standardizing patient income and education and averaging the two together. Unfortunately, there were 153 cases in which medical record and physician encounter data were available, but the patient did not return the survey that provided education and income data, and so SES scores were missing. Thus, we performed two sets of analyses using two measures of SES. In the first measure, when data on education and/or income were missing, SES was coded as missing data, and as a result those cases were dropped from the analyses. In the second measure, missing data were replaced with imputed scores. The imputed score was the predicted SES score based on the predictors patient race, sex, age, and insurance (all obtainable from the medical record). This imputed score is essentially the mean SES score for each intersection of the four patient predictor variables (race, sex, payer, and age). Analyses were performed both with and without imputed cases. Since a large proportion of study participants were retired or working part-time jobs outside their main careers, occupational status was not included in this composite measure. The categorical SES measure was developed by splitting the SES index into three equal groups. Thus 33.3 percent of respondents were in the lowest SES group, 33.3 percent in middle SES group, and 33.3 percent in the highest third. The mean education level for the lowest SES group was 9.4 years of education (SD = 1.45), the middle SES group averaged 11.4 years of education (SD = 1.07), and the highest SES group had an average of 14.4 years of education (SD = 2.07). The mean income level for the lowest SES group was US$9,331 (SD = US$7,178), the mean income for the middle SES group was US$17,439 (SD = US$10,007), and the mean income for the highest SES group was US$41,886 (SD = US$25,753).

Patient Race. Patient race was identified as either "white" or "black" through the race recorded on the patient's medical record. Since it is the effect of physicians' perception of race that is of interest here, the patients' race as seen by the medical care organization is the most appropriate variable.[39]

Dependent Variables

The physician questionnaire contained twenty-four questions, developed for the present study, that were intended to assess physician perception of and attitudes toward patients. These measures were selected as a result of conversations with physicians during study development and a reading of the research literature on physician perceptions of patient characteristics. Due to both the lack of validated multi-item measures and the need to keep the questionnaire brief, these questions were single-item measures.

Physicians' perceptions of patients' abilities and personality characteristics were assessed through physician ratings on a series of bipolar measures including "intelligent–unintelligent," "self-controlled–lacking self-control," "pleasant–unpleasant," "educated–uneducated," "rational–irrational," "independent–dependent," and "responsible–irresponsible." For each item, the value 1 anchored one end of the scale (for example, "intelligent") and the value 7 anchored the opposite end of the scale (for example, "unintelligent").

Physicians' feeling of affiliation toward the patient was assessed with a single item: "This patient is the kind of person I could see myself being friends with," with five response options ranging from "strongly agree," to "strongly disagree."

Perceived behavioral likelihoods and role demands were assessed by asking physicians their opinion on how likely the patient was to behave in certain ways or to have certain role demands. Items were originally chosen based on their potential relevance for referral to aggressive treatments for coronary artery disease (CAD). Physicians rated patients on how likely they were to "lack social support," "overreport (exaggerate) discomfort," "fail to comply with medical advice," "abuse drugs, including alcohol," "strongly desire a very physically active lifestyle," "participate in cardiac rehabilitation (if it were prescribed)," "try to manipulate . . . physicians," "initiate malpractice litigation," "have a major responsibility for the care of a family member(s)," and "have significant and important career demands/responsibilities." Response options ranged from "not at all likely" to "extremely likely" on a 5-point scale.

Due to heavily skewed response distributions for most of the single-item ordinal measures, each was transformed into a dichotomous variable. Development of dichotomous dependent variables provided the opportunity for the use of logistic regression, a powerful multivariate technique without the violation of assumptions inherent in using other parametric techniques on ordinal or skewed dependent variables. The ordinal variables were split so that the 33 percent of the distribution (or as close to it as allowed by the distribution of responses) that was rated most positively on each characteristic was coded 1, and the 67 percent who were rated more negatively on the given characteristic, or less likely to have a desirable characteristic, were assigned a core of 0. Thus, the dependent variables allowed for comparison between patients who were perceived most positively by physicians and those perceived less positively on each measure. This choice of cut-points was based on the possibility that these positive characteristics increase the likelihood of being referred to cardiac treatments. Since the choice of cut-points is always somewhat arbitrary, analyses were repeated comparing the bottom, or least positively perceived, 33 percent with the most positive 67 percent with no change in pattern of findings. Table 32.1 presents the original response distribution of each item, as well as the distribution of the two-category measure used in the analyses presented. The items are presented as they appeared in the questionnaire.

Covariates

Standard Covariates. The purpose of the analyses was to identify the effect of patient sociodemographic characteristics on physicians' perceptions of patients. The analyses use physician self-reported data to understand differences in the way the race and SES of CAD patients in a postangiogram encounter are perceived by physicians. Thus, the unit of analysis is the postangiogram encounter with a patient. In order to control for the effect of physician characteristics, all

Table 32.1. Distribution of Ordinal Dependent Variables

In general, this patient is . . .	Very (1)	Somewhat (2)	A Little (3)	Neither/ Neutral (4)	A Little (5)	Somewhat (6)	Very (7)	
Intelligent	126 (21%)	239 (40%)	93 (16%)	84 (14%)	25 (4%)	14 (2%)	10 (2%)	Unintelligent
Dichotomous version for analysis	126 (21%)	465 (79%)						
Self-controlled	155 (26%)	241 (41%)	88 (15%)	79 (13%)	7 (1%)	17 (3%)	5 (1%)	Lacking self-control
Dichotomous version for analysis	155 (26%)	437 (74%)						
Unpleasant	3 (5%)	6 (1%)	6 (1%)	67 (11%)	53 (9%)	182 (31%)	272 (46%)	Pleasant
Dichotomous version for analysis	317 (54%)						272 (46%)	
Educated	53 (9%)	164 (28%)	87 (15%)	122 (21%)	61 (10%)	89 (15%)	16 (3%)	Uneducated
Dichotomous version for analysis	217 (37%)		375 (63%)					
Irrational	7 (1%)	14 (2%)	19 (3%)	74 (13%)	58 (10%)	189 (32%)	228 (39%)	Rational
Dichotomous version for analysis	361 (61%)						228 (39%)	
Controlling	32 (5%)	51 (9%)	55 (9%)	211 (36%)	33 (7%)	98 (17%)	110 (19%)	Not controlling
Dichotomous version for analysis	382 (65%)		208 (35%)					
Independent	99 (17%)	172 (29%)	71 (12%)	128 (22%)	51 (9%)	49 (8%)	21 (4%)	Dependent
Dichotomous version for analysis	271 (46%)	320 (54%)						
Responsible	169 (29%)	208 (35%)	75 (13%)	77 (13%)	20 (3%)	29 (5%)	13 (2%)	Irresponsible
Dichotomous version for analysis	169 (29%)	422 (71%)						

(Continued)

Table 32.1. Distribution of Ordinal Dependent Variables (Continued)

	Strongly Agree	Somewhat Agree	Uncertain	Somewhat Disagree	Strongly Disagree
This patient is the kind of person I could see myself being friends with	73 (12%)	121 (20%)	216 (36%)	102 (17%)	80 (14%)
Dichotomous version for analysis	194 (33%)		398 (67%)		

	Not at All Likely (1)	A Little Likely (2)	Somewhat Likely (3)	Very Likely (4)	Extremely Likely (5)
In your opinion, how likely is this patient to . . .					
. . . lack social support, that is someone to care for him or her?	343 (59%)	130 (23%)	69 (12%)	21 (4%)	13 (2%)
Dichotomous version for analysis	343 (59%)	233 (41%)			0.61
. . . overreport (exaggerate) discomfort?	322 (56%)	166 (29%)	66 (11%)	17 (3%)	
Dichotomous version for analysis	322 (56%)	255 (44%)			
. . . have a major responsibility for the care of a family member(s)?	179 (31%)	141 (25%)	136 (24%)	76 (13%)	36 (6%)
Dichotomous version for analysis	456 (80%)			112 (20%)	0.81
. . . fail to comply with medical advice?	311 (53%)	181 (31%)	60 (10%)	23 (4%)	

Dichotomous version for analysis	311 (53%)	272 (47%)			
. . have significant and important career demands/responsibilities?	261 (46%)	138 (24%)	96 (17%)	49 (8%)	30 (5%)
Dichotomous version for analysis	399 (70%)		175 (30%)		
. . . abuse drugs, including alcohol?	458 (79%)	81 (14%)	24 (4%)	8 (1%)	11 (2%)
Dichotomous version for analysis	458 (79%)	124 (21%)			
. . . initiate malpractice litigation?	381 (66%)	157 (27%)	32 (5%)	7 (1%)	2 (3%)
Dichotomous version for analysis	381 (66%)	189 (34.6%)			
. . . strongly desire a very physically active lifestyle?	159 (28%)	149 (26%)	141 (24%)	77 (13%)	53 (9%)
Dichotomous version for analysis	449 (78%)			130 (21%)	
. . participate in cardiac rehabilitation (if it were prescribed)?	55 (10%)	116 (20%)	150 (26%)	165 (28%)	92 (16%)
Dichotomous version for analysis	321 (56%)			257 (44%)	
. . . try to manipulate you or other physicians?	382 (66%)	128 (22%)	53 (9%)	14 (2%)	4 (7%)
Dichotomous version for analysis	382 (66%)	199 (34%)			

analyses assessing the effect of patient sociodemographic characteristics on physician perceptions and beliefs about patients were adjusted for characteristics that would be unique to individual physicians, including *physician age, sex, race,* and *specialty.* Patient age was identified from the medical record. Physician age was identified by asking each survey respondent his or her year of birth.

Physician race was identified by asking respondents what race they consider themselves, with the closed-ended choices being: "white (Caucasian)," "African American," "Hispanic," "Asian or Pacific Islander," or "other" (with the option to write in a response). For the analyses presented here, this covariate was reduced to a dichotomous variable (white or nonwhite), with 84 percent of physicians self-identifying as white.

Patient sex was identified from the medical record. Physician sex was assessed through a survey item in which respondents were asked to identify themselves as either male or female by checking the appropriate box. If physician sex was not available from the physician survey, data were obtained by contacting the respondent's office for information.

Physician specialty was measured by the item, "What is your medical specialty?" with response options "cardiology," "cardiac surgery," "general medicine," "family practice," and "other."

There is some evidence that physician positive affect toward patients is negatively associated with the degree of patient sickness.[40] Therefore, patients' risk status associated with cardiac procedures was used as the best available proxy control for patient *frailty* or *sickness.* This variable has three levels, comprising normal to low risk (healthiest), moderate risk (somewhat frail), and high risk (sickest). This variable was developed with an expert panel that identified intersections of patient characteristics that influence risk of surgery, including the presence and severity of comorbidities (for example, having had a prior stroke or related event, diabetes, chronic obstructive pulmonary disease, paraplegia or quadriplegia, aortic aneurysm, renal disease), whether previous surgery had occurred, and prior and evolving acute myocardial infarction.[35,36,41] In addition, the effect of each independent variable was adjusted for *patient age* and *sex* as well as the other independent variables.

Extended Set of Covariates. It is always possible that any observed associations between physician ratings of patients and patient race or socioeconomic status are due to patient characteristics correlated with race and SES. These characteristics may, in turn, influence patient behavior and thus physician perception of the patient. In order to provide the most conservative test of race and SES effects available with this data set, all analyses were repeated with patient self-reported depressive symptoms, mastery, and social assertiveness as additional controls. The test for effects while controlling for this extended set of covariates was conducted after testing for effects with the standard covariates, since analyses involving the extended covariates required that data from the patient survey, physician survey, and medical record be present. This dropped the number of cases to 465 for these analyses.

Depressive symptoms was assessed using a subscale based on the Hopkins Symptom Checklist.[42,43] The subscale was a six-item scale asking respondents to indicate how much (1 = "not at all," 5 = "extremely") they had been bothered in the last two weeks by things like "feeling blue," "feeling lonely," and "feeling no interest in things" (Cronbach's α = 0.84).

Social assertiveness was measured by a four-item index based on instruments by Galassi et al.[44] and Jones and Russell.[45] Respondents were asked to respond to the items: "I feel tense when I'm with people I don't know well," "I feel nervous when speaking to someone in authority," "It is difficult for me to continue a conversation with someone who disagrees with me," and, "When talking I worry about saying something dumb," by selecting from five response options ranging from "strongly agree" to "strongly disagree" (α = 0.79).

Generalized self-efficacy or mastery was assessed with a combination of seven items tapping both self-concept and feelings of control ("On the whole, I am satisfied with myself," "I wish I could have more respect for myself," "There is really no way I can solve some of the problems I have," "I can do just about anything I really set my mind to," "I often feel helpless in dealing with the problems of life," "What happens to me in the future mostly depends on me," and "There is little I can do to change many of the important things in my life"). Again, the response scale had five possible responses ranging from "strongly agree," to "strongly disagree." These items were combined because they are consistent with the concept of generalized "mastery" as discussed by Pearlin and Schooler[46] and because factor analyses revealed that they belong to a common underlying factor rather than separate self-esteem and locus of control factors (α = 0.74).

Additional patient covariates were applied to analyses when relevant. These included patient self-reported *perceived social support, education* (number of years in school), *occupational status* (defined as blue-collar, sales and service, or professional and managerial), *number of hours working per week,* and *number of people who rely on you to do things for them every day.* All of these items were identified through the patient survey. *Number of hours working* and *number of people relying* were both open, write-in responses, while years in school were identified by circling a choice, in annual increments, from "8 or less" to "17+." *Occupational status* was identified through three questions ("What is/was your occupation in your most recent job?" "What kind of work do/did you do in that occupation?" and, "What does the business or industry you were/are in make or do?"). These three items were coded into a ten-item occupation status variable which was then collapsed into the categories: blue-collar, sales and service, and professional and managerial.

Social support was assessed using the Medical Outcomes Study social support scale.[47] This is a twelve-item scale in which the respondent uses a 5-point response set ranging from "none of the time" to "all of the time" to indicate how often each of a variety of types of support is available to them if they need it. Representative items include "someone you can count on to listen to you when you need to talk," "someone to give you good advice about a crisis," "someone who shows you love and affection," and "someone to take you to the doctor."

Analytic Strategy. The bivariate relationships between patient race and socioeconomic status and each of the dependent variables were estimated using contingency tables and the chi-square test of association for categorical variables and Student's *t* test or ANOVA for interval level variables. Logistic regression was used to regress each of the dichotomous dependent variables on patient race and SES while controlling for the other as well as standard covariates including patient age, patient sex, patient sickness/frailty, physician age, physician sex, physician specialty, and physician race. Then the effect of the extended covariates, including patient self-reported depressive symptoms, mastery, and social assertiveness, on the main effects were examined. In addition, interaction effects between patient SES, race/ethnicity, and patient sex were tested.

Since the sample is the result of a disproportionate stratified sample intended to oversample blacks and those appropriate for revascularization, analyses were also performed with cases weighted back to their original proportion in the population sampled. The pattern of results remained the same with and without case weighting. Since the sampling scheme was designed to capture a representative sample within strata, the unweighted results are presented here for ease of interpretation.

RESULTS

The effects of patient race and socioeconomic status on physician perceptions of patients are presented in Tables 32.2 and 32.3, respectively. For each level of the independent variable, the bivariate response distribution and chi-square (χ^2) test of statistical significance is presented. The last column in all tables presents the odds ratio and statistical significance of each effect, controlling for the standard set of covariates (patient age, sex, race, SES, sickness/frailty, and overall health status, and physician age, sex, race/ethnicity, and specialty) and other relevant covariates (as indicated). All results remain the same when the extended set of covariates (depression, mastery, social assertiveness) are entered into the equation, unless otherwise noted. In addition, all results remained the same regardless of whether the SES variable in the analyses included cases with imputed means or whether cases missing SES scores were dropped from the analyses.

The results presented in Table 32.2 reveal that physicians are somewhat less likely to have positive perceptions of black than white patients on a number of dimensions. Only 67 percent of blacks versus 79 percent of whites are rated by physicians as having no risk for substance abuse. Only 42 percent of blacks versus 57 percent of whites are rated as having no risk for noncompliance with medical advice. As indicated by the odds ratios, even when controlling for the standard and the extended set of covariates, blacks are about half as likely (OR = 0.58) as whites to be rated as at no risk for substance abuse and only two-thirds as likely (OR = 0.62) as whites to be rated as at no risk for noncompliance. In addition, they are only half as likely (OR = 0.47) to be perceived by physicians as desiring an active lifestyle (26 percent of whites versus 14 percent of blacks) and being likely to participate in cardiac rehabilitation if it were prescribed (47 percent of whites versus 34 percent of blacks, OR = 0.66). In addition, they are about half as likely as whites (OR = 0.57) to be perceived as having no risk of low social support.

Black patients were somewhat less likely to get reports of physician feelings of affiliation with the patient. Physicians were less likely to agree that black patients, as compared with white patients, were the kind of person "I could see myself being friends with" (34 percent of white versus 27 percent of black patients). Controlling for the standard and extended sets of covariates, blacks were around two-thirds as likely as whites to be perceived as the kind of person the physician could see himself or herself being friends with.

Physicians rate blacks as less intelligent and educated than whites, even controlling for SES, other standard covariates, and an additional measure of patient self-reported years of education. Blacks are only half as likely as whites to be considered "very" intelligent and less than two-thirds as likely as whites to be considered "very" or "somewhat" educated.

Socioeconomic status moderates the relationship between patient race and physicians' rating of an interpersonal and personality characteristic. Among the patients in the lowest 33 percent of the SES distribution, physicians perceive blacks to be less pleasant and rational than whites. Blacks are only one-third as likely as whites to be rated "very" pleasant. As with all analyses discussed, this difference persists even when patient depressive symptoms, social assertiveness, and feelings of mastery are controlled for in addition to the standard covariates. In addition, low SES blacks are less than half as likely as their low SES white counterparts to be considered "very" rational by physicians. In this case, physicians' perceptions of patient rationality may be partially mediated through patient characteristics associated with race such as depression and levels of mastery. When these additional covariates were added, the odds ratio increased to 0.62 and was not statistically significant, although the lack of statistical significance may be more a result of the small n and large number of variables than an indication of a lack of relationship.

Table 32.2. The Effect of Patient Race/Ethnicity on Physicians' Ratings of Patients

Independent Variable	Race/Ethnicity	Bivariate Results		Multivariate Results (reference category; adjusted odds ratio, Significance)
		Percentage	χ^2, Significance	
Physician perception that patient is . . .				
"Not at all likely" to abuse alcohol or other drugs ($n = 582$)	White/Black	79/67	11.65, $p \leq 0.001$	58, $p \leq 0.02$
"Not at all likely" to fail to comply with medical advice ($n = 583$)	White/Black	57/42	13.02, $p \leq 0.001$	62, $p \leq 0.01$
"Very" to "extremely likely" to participate in cardiac rehabilitation ($n = 578$)	White/Black	47/34	11.09, $p \leq 0.001$	66, $p \leq 0.02$
"Very" to "extremely likely" to strongly desire a very physically active lifestyle ($n = 579$)	White/Black	26/14	13.97, $p \leq 0.001$	47, $p \leq 0.01$
"Not at all likely" to lack social support* ($n = 576$)	White/Black	63/45	19.61, $p \leq 0.001$	57*, $p \leq 0.01$
Physician feelings of affiliation with patient ("agree" with statement ["This patient is the kind of person I can see myself being friends with"]) ($n = 592$)	White/Black	34/27	3.56, $p \leq 0.06$	68, $p \leq 0.05$
"Very" intelligent (versus unintelligent)[†] ($n = 438$)	White/Black	26/13	16.32, $p \leq 0.0001$	51*, $p \leq 0.01$

"Very" to "somewhat" educated (versus uneducated)[†] ($n = 438$)	White/Black	41/31	8.61, $p \leq 0.02$	63[†], $p \leq 0.01$
"Very" pleasant. Significant interaction w/SES such that there are race differences at lowest level of SES only (no race effects at other levels) ($n = 113$)	Low SES White/ Low SES Black	53/27	8.26, $p \leq 0.01$	32, $p \leq 0.01$
"Very" rational. Significant interaction w/SES such that there are race differences at lowest level of SES only (no race effects at other levels)[‡] ($n = 113$)	Low SES White/ Low SES Black	37/20	3.76, $p \leq 0.05$	0.43, $p \leq 0.05$[†]

Note: Logistic regression results adjusted (controlled) for SES as well as for a set of standard covariates including patient age, sex, and health risk status, and physician age, race, sex, and specialty. Additional covariates indicated in the following notes. Pattern of results is identical when patient self-reported education, depressive symptoms, social assertiveness, and feelings of mastery are controlled for, unless otherwise noted.

*In addition to standard covariates, results controlled for patient self-reported availability of social support.

[†]In addition to standard covariates, results controlled for patient self-reported education level.

[‡]Multivariate results fail to reach significance when patient self-reported depressive symptoms and feelings of mastery are entered into the equation.

Table 32.3. The Relationship Between Patient Socioeconomic Status and Physicians' Perceptions of Patients

Independent Variable	Bivariate Results			Multivariate Results (adjusted odds ratio, statistical significance)
	SES Category	Percentage	χ^2, Significance	
Physician perception that patient is . . .				
"Somewhat–very" independent (versus dependent) ($n = 581$)	Lowest 33%	32	8.35	(Reference cat.)
	Middle 33%	45	$p \leq 0.02$	$1.76, p \leq 0.02$
	Highest 33%	48		$1.94, p \leq 0.01$
"Very" responsible (versus irresponsible)* ($n = 581$)	Lowest 33%	19	5.61	(Reference cat.)
	Middle 33%	28	$p \leq 0.06$	$1.73*, p \leq 0.05$
	Highest 33%	30		$1.73, p \leq 0.05$
"Very" rational (versus irrational) ($n = 582$)	Lowest 33%	27	6.43	(Reference cat.)
	Middle 33%	41	$p \leq 0.05$	$1.78, p \leq 0.02$
	Highest 33%	37		$1.48, p \leq 12$
"Very" intelligent (versus unintelligent) ($n = 609$)	Lowest 33%	10	15.92	(Reference cat.)
	Middle 33%	18	$p \leq 0.001$	$2.03, p \leq 0.05$[†]
	Highest 33%	27		$2.79, p \leq 0.01$
"Very" to "extremely likely" to participate in cardiac rehabilitation (if it were prescribed) ($n = 578$)	Lowest 33%	30	11.02	(Reference cat.)
	Middle 33%	40	$p \leq 0.01$	$1.49, p \leq 0.10$
	Highest 33%	48		$1.85, p \leq 0.02$

Note: Logistic regression results adjusted (controlled) for race as well as for a set of standard covariates including patient age, sex, and health risk status, and physician age, race, sex, and specialty. Additional covariates indicated in the following notes. Pattern of results is identical when patient self-reported education, depressive symptoms, social assertiveness, and feelings of mastery are controlled for, unless otherwise noted.

*Odds ratios drop to 1.58 and 1.52 when patient score on the mastery scale is controlled for.

[†]Odds ratio drops to 1.60 and fails to reach statistical significance for middle SES but is unchanged for highest SES patients when patient education, social assertiveness, and depression are additional covariates.

Table 32.3 presents the main effects of patient SES on physicians' perceptions of patients. The results presented in Table 32.3 suggest that patient SES had an impact on physician perceptions in a number of domains including personality, cognitive ability, behavioral tendencies, and role demands. Patients in the middle and high SES categories were more likely to be perceived as independent (OR = 1.76, 1.94), responsible (OR = 1.73, 1.73), and rational (OR = 1.78, 1.48) than are their lowest SES counterparts. For these personality ratings, only the lowest SES patients were at a disadvantage, with no clear distinction between the middle and highest SES groups. SES appears to have a fairly linear relationship with physician ratings of patient intelligence. Middle SES patients are two times as likely as the lowest SES patients to be rated "very" intelligent, while the highest SES patients were almost three times as likely as their lowest SES counterparts to be rated "very" intelligent.

Patient SES had an impact on physicians' perceptions of patient likelihood of participating in cardiac rehabilitation, if it were prescribed, with 30 percent of low SES, 40 percent of middle SES, and 48 percent of high SES patients being rated as likely to do so. The multivariate analyses indicate a clear highest-lowest SES difference (OR = 1.85, $p \le .02$) and a borderline middle-lowest SES relationship (OR = 1.49, $p \le .10$) when the standard and extended sets of covariates are controlled for. In addition, SES appears to have a relatively linear effect on physicians' rating of patients' likelihood of desiring a very physically active lifestyle, with 9 percent of the lowest SES patients, 17 percent of the middle SES patients, and 29 percent of the highest SES patients receiving this rating.

Patient SES also influences physicians' ratings of patients' likely role demands. Lower SES patients are seen as less likely to have responsibility for care of a family member (11 percent) than are their middle (17 percent) or highest (22 percent) SES counterparts. This relationship persisted even when the patients' self-report on the number of people who depend on them to do things for them every day is controlled for along with the standard and extended sets of covariates. In addition, higher and middle SES patients are perceived to be more likely to have significant career demands than their lower SES counterparts, even controlling for patients' report of the number of hours working per week. This relationship persists for both men and women, although women in the middle and highest SES groups are clearly rated as less likely to have significant career demands than their male counterparts, creating a significant interaction effect.

SUMMARY OF RESULTS

The results support the hypothesis that physicians' perceptions of patients are influenced by patients' race and socioeconomic status. Black CAD patients were more likely to be seen as at risk for noncompliance with cardiac rehabilitation, substance abuse, and having inadequate social support. In addition, physicians rated black patients as less intelligent than white patients, even when patient sex, age, income, and education were controlled. Physicians also report fewer affiliative feelings toward black patients.

In general, physicians gave lower SES patients more negative ratings on personality characteristics (lack of self-control, irrationality) and level of intelligence. In addition, lower SES patients were rated as less likely to be compliant with cardiac rehabilitation, less likely to desire a physically active lifestyle, less likely to have significant career demands, less likely to have responsibility for the care of a family member, and more likely to be judged to be at risk for inadequate social support. Again, the effect of patient SES on physician perception remained when patient age, sex, race, frailty/sickness, depression, mastery, and social assertiveness as well as physician characteristics were controlled.

DISCUSSION

The results support the hypothesis that physicians' perceptions of patients are influenced by patients' sociodemographic characteristics. Physicians tend to perceive African Americans and members of low-SES groups more negatively on a number of dimensions than they do whites and members of the middle and highest third in SES. Furthermore, although there is considerable shared variance, each characteristic is associated with a unique set of perceptions. Patient race is associated with physicians' assessment of patient intelligence, feelings of affiliation toward the patient, and beliefs about patient likelihood of high-risk behaviors (substance abuse) and noncompliance. Patient SES, on the other hand, seems to have the broadest effect on physician perceptions, indicating that SES is associated with generalized perceptions in a wider array of domains than race.

One possible explanation for these findings is that sociodemographic characteristics are associated with true differences on these dimensions and that physicians, rather than being prone to using stereotypes in forming impressions of patients, are accurate observers of individual patient differences. For example, physicians perceive lower SES patients as being less likely to desire a very physically active lifestyle. This perception is consistent with research indicating a direct relationship between SES and exercise behavior,[48-50] and thus may be an accurate reflection of true patient differences. Other observed differences however, are harder to accept as accurate. For example, black patients are rated as significantly less educated than white patients, even controlling for their actual level of education.

An alternate explanation is that epidemiologic evidence is incorporated into physicians' general belief systems in such a way that population-based likelihoods are applied to individuals even in the presence of disconfirming information. Physicians may fail to correctly incorporate individual diagnostic data, instead being swayed by their beliefs regarding the probabilities of individuals in a sociodemographic category having a given characteristic.[13] In this way, physicians' understanding of epidemiologic evidence regarding population-based likelihoods may function as a set of stereotypes and be applied to assessments and perceptions of individuals regardless of actual individual characteristics. It is possible that this is especially likely when population-based statistics are consistent with dominant biases. For example, physicians were more likely to rate whites than blacks as "somewhat" or "very" educated. In fact, black patients who report a lower average number of years of schooling (black number of years of education $\bar{x} = 11.4$, SD = 2.4 versus white $\bar{x} = 13.0$, SD = 2.9, $t = 6.20$, $p \leq .000$) than white patients. However, even when patients' actual education level was adjusted for, physicians were still statistically more likely to rate whites than blacks as educated. This suggests that physicians are applying general race differences to their impressions of individual patients and failing to incorporate disconfirming individual information. In considering the problem of group differences and stereotyping, it is important to distinguish between content accuracy (the accuracy of a generalized belief about a group of people) and application accuracy. This refers to the fact that the inappropriate use of stereotypic beliefs as a basis for responding to others, even if these beliefs are entirely accurate, is potentially damaging to the stereotyped individual.[51]

There is substantial evidence that people process disconfirming information in a variety of ways that leave their stereotypical beliefs untouched.[52–57] Stereotypic expectancies can bias the way information is interpreted, an effect that is magnified if the information is in any way ambiguous.[58–60] This may be more likely to occur in encounters with minority and lower SES patients, since communication barriers increase with physician-patient sociodemographic disparity due to differences in illness beliefs,[61–63] differences in general perceptions due to differences in social and cultural backgrounds,[64–66] and/or differences in styles and patterns of communication.[67,68]

Compounding these problems, physicians in this sample had less time to incorporate individuating information for their minority patients. Average postangiogram encounter length, as reported by physicians, was significantly shorter for black CAD patients than for white patients (number of minutes with black patients $\bar{x} = 12$, SD 6.6 versus white patients $\bar{x} = 14$, SD $= 7.3$, $t = 3.57$, $p \leq .000$).

The finding that physicians have lower feelings of affiliation toward black patients may be connected to their beliefs about the degree to which patients are rational or intelligent. This characteristic was found, in one sample of physicians, to be significantly associated with physicians' positive attitudes toward patients, along with perceptions of self-control.[69] This suggests that physicians in our sample may feel less liking for lower SES and black patients, who are less likely to be rated by these physicians as intelligent and rational.

There is substantial reason to be concerned about physicians' likelihood of perceiving African American and lower SES patients more negatively than white or upper SES patients. Differences in feelings of affiliation toward patients, perceptions of patient intelligence, and perceptions of patient characteristics may, in part, explain some of the treatment differences observed in other studies. Physician attitudes, perceptions, and beliefs about patients have been shown to influence physician behavior in medical care encounters[40,70-73] and treatment decisions.[74-78] Gerbert found that physicians varied treatment decisions based on their perceptions of the likability and competence of simulated patients.[76] Similarly, persons considered deviant[75] or less likable[74] have been found to receive less medical attention and follow-up care.

Even assuming that physicians' treatment decisions are unaffected by their perceptions of patients, physician attitudes toward patients are of concern because of their potential impact on patients' satisfaction and behavior. When patients perceive that physicians like them, care about them, and are interested in them as persons, they are likely to volunteer more information and be more active in the encounter, more satisfied, and more compliant with medical regimens.[40,79-84]

In addition, differences in perceptions of low-SES and minority patients on intelligence, education, and rationality may partially explain why physicians deliver less information to minorities and patients of lower economic class than they do to their white or higher SES counterparts.[20,71,85,86] In addition, they may be less likely to listen to or respect the contributions of patients who are perceived as less intelligent or rational.

There is evidence that working-class patients (corresponding to low-SES patients in this study) are more diffident in asking their physicians questions,[87-89] which may both result from and reinforce physician judgments regarding their intelligence and rationality; they may ask fewer questions because physician affect and behavior toward them is discouraging (perhaps unintentionally), and physicians may develop or reinforce beliefs about patients' cognitive ability or information needs based on their question-asking behavior. This dynamic is especially worrisome because information flow and physician affective and affiliative behavior has been found to influence patient satisfaction,[83,90-93] trust in physician competence,[94,95] and the level of stress or anxiety experienced during the encounter.[96,97] These factors, in combination with physician information and affect, are associated with patient adherence.[91,98,99]

Lastly, it is important to note that although race and SES each have independent and individual effects on physicians' perceptions, considering them separately may result in an underestimation of the effect of sociodemographic characteristics on physician perceptions and quality of care. Race is highly correlated with SES, with blacks having a lower average SES than whites (in this sample, black $\bar{x} = 7.0$ (1.4) versus white $\bar{x} = 8.2$ (2.0), $t = 8.78$, $p \leq .000$). Thus, physicians' negative attributions for blacks and those of lower SES may have a powerful cumulative effect in the clinical setting. For example, the results presented above suggest that lower SES African Americans consulting a cardiologist are more likely than affluent whites to be perceived as lacking intelligence, lacking self-control, irrational, unlikely to have significant career demands, at risk for inadequate social support, unlikely to desire a physically active lifestyle, at risk for substance abuse, and likely to be noncompliant with cardiac rehabilitation.

LIMITATIONS

There are a number of limitations that could suggest alternate interpretations of the findings presented. First, there is a possibility that social desirability effects biased physician ratings of patients. Physicians may have been mindful of the purpose of the research project, which was to identify factors associated with underuse of aggressive treatments for CAD among minorities and women. They received questionnaires on patients sporadically (as patients they treated were sampled) over a two-year period. If a social desirability bias was in effect, we would expect to see ratings of blacks that are more favorable than physicians actually believe them to be. If this is the case, the differences in perceptions reported here are underestimated.

Second, it is possible that race and SES differences in physician perceptions of patients are due to some other characteristic(s) associated both with race and/or SES and with physicians' perceptions. Although every possible effort was made to control for this possibility through adding covariates assessing patient sickness/frailty, mental health status through depression, and interpersonal behavior through social assertiveness and mastery, it is possible that some unmeasured factor is at play. In addition, the measure of patient sickness may be inadequate. As mentioned earlier, a few studies have found that sicker patients are liked less by physicians[40] and, in turn, are less satisfied with medical care.[100–102] Both Hall et al.[102] and Greenley et al.[100] theorize that physicians have more negative affect when dealing with sicker patients and that they unintentionally communicate this reaction to the patient, causing the patient to experience more dissatisfaction.[40] Alternately, sicker patients may be dissatisfied for other reasons, and their dissatisfaction may be conveyed to physicians, resulting in greater physician negative affect.

The findings here are limited to physicians in New York State treating a sample of postangiogram CAD patients and may not generalize to other types of physicians or encounters with other types of patients. Although other studies of this kind are scarce, the findings from this and another study of physician perceptions and affect are not entirely consistent. Hall et al. did not find patient SES to be associated with physicians' liking for patients,[40] while we found significant SES effects on physician ratings of patients. The discrepancy in findings could be due to different measures or different patient and physician populations.

We obtained data on 73 percent of the patient encounters sampled, which raises the possibility that physician perceptions of patients in the 27 percent of encounters for which data were missing differed systematically from the 73 percent of the encounters with available data. However, the results of a phone call follow-up to nonresponding physician offices suggest that nonresponse was unrelated to patient or physician sociodemographic characteristics, being instead a function of physician busyness and physician office mail processing procedures. It should be noted, however, that in 60 percent of the follow-up phone calls our data on causes of nonresponse are limited to office staff reports.

An additional limitation of the study is the potential for measurement error. The need to maximize physician response rate forced the use of single-item measures. It is important to note, however, that the measures used were identical across race, sex, and SES. Thus, the observed differences in physician perceptions of patients of differing sociodemographic characteristics are unlikely to be due to measurement error. The findings described here indicate that replication studies using multiple-item measures are warranted.

Lastly, this study does not provide direct evidence regarding quality of care, and it is unclear whether these differences in perceptions are associated with differences in care or outcome. Further research testing the degree to which physician perceptions are related to actual differences in care is needed.

CONCLUSION

In conclusion, the results of this study provide significant evidence for the effect of patient race and SES on physician perceptions of patients. These findings suggest that further exploration with multi-item measures and additional controls for physician perception accuracy is warranted. Most important, these results highlight the need for studies of variations in physician perceptions of patients in a wide variety of settings and with different physician and patient populations, as well as examination of the way physician perceptions affect the effectiveness of the helping relationship and resulting quality of care.

In addition, if perceptions of patients do affect quality of care as the existing literature suggests, these findings point to the need for interventions. The literature on stereotype usage suggests that it is unrealistic to expect physicians to be able to avoid using stereotypes at will. Rather, physicians need more supports in terms of training and structural factors for incorporating individuating patient information into their perceptions of patients. Possible interventions to be explored include consciousness-raising and training on the use and effect of stereotypes; training in eliciting, absorbing, and incorporating individual patient information in the therapeutic encounter; organizational interventions that allow for more time in encounters; and individual and organizational interventions aimed at decreasing physician stress and cognitive load.

Notes

1. Armitage, K., Schneidermann, L., & Bass, R. (1979). Response of physicians to medical complaints in men and women. *JAMA, 241*(20), 2186–2187.

2. Wallen, J., Waitzkin, H., & Stoecke, J. (1979). Physician stereotypes about female health and illness: A study of patient's sex and the informative process during medical interviews. *Women Health, 4*(2), 135–146.

3. Ventres, W., & Gordon, P. (1990). Communication strategies in caring for the underserved. *J Health Care Poor Underserved, 1*, 305–314.

4. Bertakis, K. D., Callahan, E. J., Helms, E. J., Azari, R., & Robbins, J. A. (1993). The effect of patient health status on physician practice style. *Fam Med, 25*(8), 530–535.

5. Perkoff, G. T., & Anderson, M. (1970). Relationship between demographic characteristics, patient's chief complaint and medical care destination in an emergency room. *Med Care, 8,* 309.

6. Tobin, J. N., Wasserheil-Smoller, S., Wexler, J. P., Steingart, R. M., Budner, N., Lense, L., & Wachspress, J. (1987). Sex bias in considering coronary bypass surgery. *Ann Intern Med, 107,* 19–25.

7. Ayanian, J., & Epstein, A. (1991). Differences in the use of procedures between women and men hospitalized for coronary artery disease. *N Engl J Med, 325*(4), 221–225.

8. Hannan, E., Kilburn, H., O'Donnell, J., Lukacik, G., & Shields, E. (1991). Interracial access to selected cardiac procedures for patients hospitalized with coronary artery disease in New York State. *Med Care, 29,* 430–441.

9. Redman, S., Webb, G. R., Hennrikus, D. J., Gordon, J. J., & Sanson-Fisher, R. W. (1991). The effects of gender on diagnosis of psychological disturbance. *J Behav Med, 14*(5), 527–540.

10. Steingart, R. (1991). Sex differences in management of coronary artery disease. *N Engl J Med, 325*(4), 221–225.

11. Majeroni, B. A., Karuza, J., Wade, C., McCreadie, M., & Calkins, E. (1993). Gender of physicians and patients and preventative care for community based older adults. *J Am Board Fam Pract, 6*(4), 359.

12. Todd, K. H., Samaroo, N., & Hoffman, J. R. (1993). Ethnicity as risk factor for inadequate emergency department analgesia. *JAMA, 269*(12), 1537–1539.

13. McKinlay, J. (1996). Some contributions from the social system to gender inequalities in heart disease. *J Health Soc Behav, 37*(1), 1–26.

14. Hannan, E., van Ryn, M., et al. (1998). Access to coronary artery bypass surgery by race/ethnicity and gender among patients who are appropriate for surgery. *Med Care, 37*(1), 68–77.

15. Martin, R., Gordon, E. E., & Lounsbury, P. (1998). Gender disparities in the attribution of cardiac-related symptoms: Contribution of common sense models of illness. *Health Psychol, 17*(4), 346–357.

16. Wenneker, M., & Epstein, A. (1989). Racial inequalities in the use of procedures for patients with ischemic heart disease in Massachusetts. *JAMA, 261*(2), 253–257.

17. Okelo, S., Mohan, G., Rosenthal, G., Lesnefsky, E., Wright, J., & Taylor, A. (1995). Racial variation in treatment recommendations for coronary artery disease in a VA population. *Circulation, 92*, 1–437.

18. Peterson, E., Shaw, L., DeLong, E., Pryor, D., Califf, R., & Mark, D. (1997). Racial variation in the use of cardiac revascularization procedures: Are the differences real? Do they matter? *N Engl J Med, 336*, 480–486.

19. Daniel, J. (1970). The poor: Aliens in an affluent society: Cross-cultural communication. In *Today's speech.*

20. Hooper, E. M., Comstock, L. M., Goodwin, J. M., & Goodwin, J. S. (1982). Patient characteristics that influence physician behavior. *Med Care, 20*, 630–638.

21. Eisenberg, J. M. (1979). Sociologic influences on decision making by clinicians. *Ann Intern Med, 90*, 957–964.

22. Hamilton, D. L. (Ed.). (1981). *Cognitive processes in stereotyping and intergroup behavior.* Hillsdale, NJ: Erlbaum.

23. Klopf, D. W. (1991). *Intercultural communication* (2nd ed.). Englewood, CO: Morton.

24. Hamilton, D. L., & Trolier, T. K. (1986). Stereotypes and stereotyping: An overview of the cognitive approach. In J. F. Dovidio & S. L. Gaetner (Eds.), *Prejudice, discrimination and racism* (pp. 127–163). San Diego, CA: Academic Press.

25. Andersen, S. M., Klatzky, R. L., & Murray, J. (1990). Traits and social stereotypes: Efficiency differences in the social information processing. *J Pers Soc Psychol, 59*, 192–201.

26. Lalonde, R. N., & Gardner, R. C. (1989). The intergroup perspective on stereotype organization and processing. *Br J Soc Psychol, 28*(4), 289–303.

27. Vassiliou, V., Trandis, H., Vassiliou, G., & McGuire, H. (1972). In H. Triandis (Ed.), *The analysis of subjective culture.* New York: Wiley.

28. Devito, J. A. (1982). *Communicology: An introduction to the study of communication* (2nd ed.). New York: Harper and Row.

29. Bodehausen, G. V., & Lichtenstein, M. (1987). Social stereotypes and information-processing strategies: The impact of task complexity. *J Pers Soc Psychol, 52*, 871–880.

30. Gilbert, D. T., & Hixon, J. G. (1991). The trouble of thinking: Activation and application of stereotypic beliefs. *J Pers Soc Psychol, 60*(4), 509–517.

31. Pratto, F., & Bargh, J. (1991). Stereotyping based on apparently individuating information: Trait and global components of sex stereotypes under attention overload. *J Exp Soc Psychol, 27*(1), 26–47.

32. Macrae, N. C., Hewstone, M., & Griffiths, R. J. (1993). Processing load and memory for stereotype based information. *European J Soc Psychol, 23*(1), 77–87.

33. Macrae, N. C., Milne, A. B., & Bodenhausen, G. V. (1994). Stereotypes as energy saving devices: A peek inside the cognitive toolbox. *J Pers Soc Psychol, 66*(1), 37–47.

34. Gordon, R. A., & Anderson, K. (1995). Perceptions of race stereotypic and race nonstereotypic crimes: The impact of response time instructions on attributions and judgements. *Basic Appl Soc Psychol, 16*(4), 455–470.

35. RAND Corporation. (1991a). *Coronary artery bypass graft surgery: A literature review and ratings of appropriateness and necessity.* Santa Monica: RAND.

36. RAND Corporation. (1991b). *Percutaneous transluminal coronary angioplasty: A literature review and ratings of appropriateness and necessity.* Santa Monica: RAND.

37. Winslow, C., Kosecoff, J., Chassin, M., et al. (1988). The appropriateness of performing coronary artery bypass surgery. *JAMA, 260,* 505–509.

38. Hilbome, L., Leape, L., Bernstein, S., Park, R., Fiske, M., Kamberg, C., Roth, C., & Brook, R. (1993). The appropriateness of use of percutaneous transluminal coronary angioplasty in New York State. *JAMA, 269*(6), 761–765.

39. LaVeist, T. A. (1994). Beyond dummy variables and sample selection: What health services researchers ought to know about race as a variable. *Health Ser Res, 29*(1), 1–16.

40. Hall, J. A., Epstein, A. M., DeCiantis, M. L., & McNeil, B. J. (1993). Physicians' liking for their patients: More evidence for the role of affect in medical care. *Health Psychol, 12*(2), 140–146.

41. Leape, L., Hilborne, L., Park, R., Bernstein, S., Kamberg, C., Sherwood, M., et al. (1993). The appropriateness of use of coronary artery bypass graft surgery in New York State. *JAMA, 269*(6), 753–760.

42. Derogatis, L. R., et al. (1974). The Hopkins Symptom Checklist (HSCL). In P. Pichot et al. (Eds.), *Modern problems in pharmacopsychiatry: Psychological measurements in psychopharmacology* (Vol. 7). New York: Karger.

43. Derogatis, L. R., & Melisaratos, N. (1983). The Brief Symptom Inventory: An introductory report. *Psychol Med, 13,* 595–605.

44. Galassi, J. P., Pelo, J. S., Galassi, M. D., & Bastien, S. (1977). The College Self-Expression Scale: A measure of assertiveness. *Behav Therapy, 5,* 165–171.

45. Jones, W. H., & Russell, D. (1982). The Social Reticence Scale: An objective instrument to measure shyness. *J Pers Assess, 46,* 629–631.

46. Pearlin, L., & Schooler, C. (1978). The structure of coping. *J Health Soc Behav, 19,* 2–21.

47. Sherbourne, C., & Stewart, A. (1991). The MOS social support survey. *Soc Sci Med, 32,* 705–714.

48. Matthews, K. A., Kelsey, S. F., Meilahn, E. N., Kuller, L. H., & Wing, R. R. (1989). Educational attainment and behavioral and biological risk factors for coronary heart disease in middle-aged women. *Am J Epidemiol, 129,* 1132–1144.

49. Ford, E. S., Merritt, R. K., & Heath, G. W. (1991). Physical activity behaviors in lower and higher socio-economic status populations. *Am J Epidemiol, 133,* 1246–1256.

50. Kaplan, G. A., Lazarus, N. B., Cohen, R. D., & Leu, D. J. (1991). Psychosocial factors in the natural history of physical activity. *Am J Prev Med, 7*(1), 12–17.

51. Stangor, C. (1996). Content and application inaccuracy in social stereotyping. In Y. Lee, L. J. Jussim, & C. R. McCauley (Eds.), *Stereotype accuracy: Toward appreciating group differences.* Washington, DC: American Psychological Association.

52. Macrae, N. C., & Shepherd, J. (1989). Stereotypes and social judgements. *Br J Soc Psychol, 28*(4), 319–325.

53. Jackson, L., Sullivan, L., & Hodge, C. (1993). Stereotype effects of attributions, predications, and evaluations: No two social judgements are quite alike. *J Pers Soc Psychol, 65.*

54. Seta & Seta, C. (1993). Among other mechanisms for maintaining stereotypes: Stereotypes and the generation of compensatory and noncompensatory expectancies of group members. *Pers Soc Psychol Bull, 19*(6), 722–731.

55. Ben-Ari, R., Schwarzwald, J., & Horiner-Levi, E. (1994). The effects of prevalent social stereotypes on intergroup attribution. *J Cross Cult Psychol, 25*(4), 489–500.

56. Krueger, J., Heckhausen, J., & Hundermark, J. (1995). Perceiving middle aged adults: Effects of stereotype-congruent and incongruent information. *J Gerontol, Series B, Psychological Sciences and Social Sciences, 50B*(2), 82–93.

57. Kunda, Z., & Oleson, K. C. (1995). Maintaining stereotypes in the face of disconfirmation: Constructing grounds for subtyping deviants. *J Pers Soc Psychol, 68*(4), 565–579.

58. Duncan, B. L. (1976). Differential social perception and attribution of intergroup violence: Testing the lower limits of stereotyping of blacks. *J Pers Soc Psychol, 34,* 590–598.

59. Sagar, H. A., & Schofield, J. W. (1980). Racial and behavioral cues in black and white children's perceptions of ambiguously aggressive acts. *J Pers Soc Psychol, 39,* 590–598.

60. Darley, J. M., & Gross, P. H. (1983). A hypothesis-confirming bias in labeling effects. *J Pers Soc Psychol, 44,* 20–33.

61. Kleinman, A., Eisenberg, L., & Good, B. (1978). Culture, illness and care: Clinical lessons from anthropologic and cross-cultural research. *Ann Med, 88,* 251–258.

62. Helman, C. G. (1990). *Culture, health and illness* (2nd ed.). London: Butterworth.

63. Allhouse, K. D. (1993). Treating patients as individuals. In M. Geirteis, S. Edgman-Levitan, J. Daley, & T. Delbanco (Eds.), *Through the patient's eyes: Understanding and promoting patient-centered care.* San Francisco: Jossey-Bass.

64. Huby, G., & Salkind, M. R. (1989). General medical practice in a multicultural and multiracial environment: Report from a multidisciplinary casework seminar. *Health Trends, 21,* 86–88.

65. Rothenburger, R. L. (1990). Transcultural nursing. *AORN J, 51,* 1349–1363.

66. Weddington, W. H., & Gabel, L. L. (1991). Racial differences in physicians and patients in relationship to quality of care. *JAMA, 83*, 569–572.

67. Fisher, S. (1988). *In the patient's best interest: Women and the politics of medical decisions*. New Brunswick, NJ: Rutgers University Press.

68. Muller, C. (1990). *Health care and gender*. New York: Russell Sage Foundation.

69. Briggs, G. W., & Replogle, W. H. (1991). Effect of communication skills training on residents' attitudes toward their patients. *Acad Med, 66*, 243.

70. Sheehan, T., et al. (1985). Structural equation models of moral reasoning and physician performance. *Eval Health Professions, 8*(4), 379.

71. Roter, D. L., Hall, J. A., & Katz, N. R. (1988). Doctor-patient communication: A descriptive summary of the literature. *Patient Educ Couns, 12*, 99–119.

72. Hall, J. A., Roter, D. L., & Katz, N. R. (1988). Meta-analysis of correlates of provider behavior in medical encounters. *Med Care, 26*(7), 657–675.

73. Kaplan, S., Gandek, B., Greenfield, S., Rodgers, W., & Ware, J. (1995). Patient and visit characteristics related to physicians' participatory decision making style. *Med Care, 33*, 1176.

74. Tishler, G. (1966). Decision making process in the emergency room. *Arch Gen Psychiatry, 14*, 69.

75. Sudnow, D. (1967). *Passing on*. Englewood Cliffs, NJ: Prentice Hall.

76. Gerbert, B. (1984). Perceived likability and competence of simulated patients: Influence on physicians' management plans. *Soc Sci Med, 18*, 1053–1059.

77. Stern, M., Ross, S., & Bielass, M. (1991). Medical students' perceptions of children: Modifying a childhood cancer stereotype. *J Pediatr Psychol, 6*(1), 27–38.

78. Schulman, K. A., Berlin, J. A., Harless, W., Kerner, J. F., Sistrunk, S., Gersh, B. J., Dubé, R., Taleghani, C. K., Burke, J. E., Wiliams, S., Eisenberg, J. M., & Escarce, J. J. (1999). The effect of race and sex on physicians' recommendations for cardiac catheterization. *N Engl J Med, 340*(8), 618–626.

79. Ben-Sira, Z. (1976). The function of the professional's affective behavior in client satisfaction: A revised approach to social interaction theory. *J Health Soc Behav, 17*, 3–11.

80. DiMatteo, M. R., & Friedman, H. S. (1980). *Social psychology and medicine*. Cambridge, MA: Oelgeschlager, Gunn and Ham.

81. Hall, J. A., & Dornan, M. C. (1988). Meta-analysis of satisfaction with medical care: Description of research domain and analysis of overall satisfaction levels. *Soc Sci Med, 27*(6), 637–644.

82. Ross, C. E., & Duff, R. S. (1982). Physician status characteristics and client satisfaction in two types of medical practices. *J Health Soc Behav, 23*, 317–329.

83. Buller, M. D., & Buller, D. B. (1987). Physicians' communication style and patient satisfaction. *J Health Soc Behav, 28*, 375–388.

84. Roter, D. L., Hall, J. A., & Katz, N. R. (1987). Relations of physicians' task and socio-emotional behaviors to analogue patients' satisfaction, recall and impressions. *Med Care, 25*, 437–451.

85. Epstein, A. M., Taylor, W. C., & Seage, G. R. (1985). Effects of patient's socio-economic status and physician's training and practice on doctor-patient communication. *Am J Med, 78,* 101–106.

86. Waitzkin, H. (1985). Information giving in medical care. *J Health Soc Behav, 26,* 81–101.

87. Cartwright, A. (1964). *Human relations and hospital care.* London: Routledge & Kegan Paul.

88. Boreham, P., & Gibson, D. (1978). The informative process in private medical consultations: A preliminary investigation. *Soc Sci Med, 12,* 409.

89. Matthews, J. (1983). The communication process in clinical settings. *Soc Sci Med, 17,* 1371.

90. Stewart, M. A. (1984). What is a successful doctor-patient interview? A study of interactions and outcomes. *Soc Sci Med, 19,* 167–175.

91. Roter, D. L. (1988). Reciprocity in the medical encounter. In D. S. Gochman (Ed.), *Health behavior: Emerging research perspectives.* New York: Plenum.

92. Bensing, J. (1991). Doctor-patient communication and the quality of care. *Soc Sci Med, 32,* 1301–1310.

93. Geirteis, M., Edgman-Levitan, S., Daley, J., & Delbanco, T. (1993). *Through the patient's eyes: Understanding and promoting patient-centered care.* San Francisco: Jossey-Bass.

94. Kasteler, J., Kane, R. L., Olsen, D. M., & Thetford, C. (1976). Issues underlying prevalence of "doctor shopping" behavior. *J Health Soc Behav, 17,* 328–339.

95. Ben-Sira, Z. (1982). Lay evaluation of medical treatment and competence: Development of model of the function of the physicians' affective behavior. *Soc Sci Med, 16,* 1013–1019.

96. Kosa, J., & Robertson, L. S. (1969). The social aspects of health and illness. In J. Kosa, A. Antonovsky, & L. K. Zola (Eds.), *Poverty and health: A sociological analysis* (pp. 35–68). Cambridge, MA: Harvard University Press.

97. Ben-Sira, Z. (1982b). Stress potential and esotericity of health problems: The significance of the physician's affective behavior. *Med Care, 20,* 414–424.

98. Hall, J. A., Roter, D. L., & Rand, C. S. (1981). Communication of affect between patient and physician. *J Health Soc Behav, 22,* 18–30.

99. Donovan, J. L., & Blake, D. R. (1992). Patient noncompliance: Deviance or reasoned decision making? *Soc Sci Med, 34*(5), 507–513.

100. Greenley, J. R., Young, T. B., & Schoenherr, R. A. (1982). Psychological distress and patient satisfaction. *Med Care, 20,* 373–385.

101. Pascoe, G. C. (1983). Patient satisfaction in primary health care: A literature review and analysis. *Eval Program Plan, 6,* 185–210.

102. Hall, J. A., Feldstein, M., Fretwell, M. D., Rowe, J. W., & Epstein, A. M. (1990). Older patients' health status and satisfaction with medical care in an HMO population. *Med Care, 28,* 261–270.

PART SIX

PATIENT FACTORS

CHAPTER THIRTY-THREE

Do Patient Preferences Contribute to Racial Differences in Cardiovascular Procedure Use?

Jeff Whittle
Joseph Conigliaro
C. B. Good
Monica Joswiak

Coronary artery disease (CAD) is the leading cause of death among blacks in this country.[1,2] The risk of death from CAD in blacks is similar to that in whites for all ages combined and exceeds that of whites between the ages of twenty-five and sixty-four.[2,3] Further, a recent widening of the difference in life expectancy between whites and blacks has been tied to an increasing difference between races in rates of death due to heart disease.[4] Despite this, numerous studies have shown that blacks are considerably less likely than whites to undergo invasive cardiovascular procedures, especially revascularization.[5–8] Whites are up to 50 percent more likely to undergo percutaneous transluminal coronary angioplasty (PTCA),[5] and three times as likely to undergo coronary artery bypass grafting (CABG).[8] These results are consistent in studies using administrative and clinical data,[9] in studies with prospective and retrospective data collection, and in studies of specialized populations such as that served by the Department of Veterans Affairs (VA) medical system. The differences are large, reproducible, and of unexplained origin.

Presented in part at the national meeting of the Society of General Internal Medicine, May 1995. Supported in part by the Department of Veterans Affairs HSR&D Investigator Initiated Research Award 93-107 (to Joseph Conigliaro), "Relationship of Race to Cardiovascular Procedure Use at VA Hospitals," and by a Department of Veterans Affairs Development Grant (92-006) (awarded to David S. Macpherson, M.D.). Barbara Hanusa helped us with the analysis of the data and performed the factor analyses.

As many revascularization procedures are elective, it is possible that a systematic racial difference in patient preferences for procedure use contributes to this difference. Data on the likelihood that a patient will accept a recommendation to undergo a revascularization procedure are scarce. In the Coronary Artery Surgery Study (CASS), physicians recommended CABG to 46.5 percent of blacks and 59.4 percent of whites. However, only 80.5 percent of blacks for whom CABG was recommended actually had the procedure as compared with 90.4 percent of whites. Moreover, of the 4,652 whites for whom medical management was recommended, 11.6 percent later underwent CABG, compared with only 1 percent of the 100 blacks.[10] Analysis of data from the weekly joint cardiology–cardiothoracic surgery conference of one VA referral center for CABG found that black patients were twice as likely as white patients to refuse a procedure when recommended (23 percent versus 10 percent) (S. Sedlis, personal communication).

Although limited, these data suggest that the racial differences in revascularization rates may, at least in part, reflect a tendency for blacks to decline these procedures or for whites to pursue them. The studies to date,[10] however, have compared patients who may have had dissimilar clinical situations when they accepted or declined procedures (S. Sedlis, unpublished results). We sought to compare the attitudes toward revascularization procedures among blacks and whites when presented with identical hypothetical clinical situations.

METHODS

Survey

A survey was developed that assessed attitudes toward procedure use as well as variables we believed would predict those attitudes. The survey, written in lay terms, was refined by pilot testing, first among black and white VA employees and then among black and white volunteer patients. Patients participating in pilot testing were not included in the final analysis. The survey included questions regarding participant age, race, education level, employment status, living arrangements, and health status, all of which may influence health behaviors. In addition, on the basis of the Health Belief Model for patient behavior and personal clinical experience,[11] we believed that patient familiarity with revascularization procedures should influence attitudes toward revascularization. Therefore, familiarity was measured by asking participants to report how many family members or friends had undergone CABG, participants' own estimate of operative mortality for CABG, and their self-reported familiarity with CABG, phrased two ways ("Are you familiar with bypass surgery?" and, "Do you have a good idea what happens to a person who has bypass surgery?"). Similar questions were asked about PTCA, except that an estimate of the risk of having complications requiring CABG was substituted for the estimate of operative mortality.

We believed that patients' decisions to undergo a cardiovascular procedure would involve both the patients' tendency to follow their doctors' recommendations and their attitudes toward the procedure. Therefore, attitudes toward procedure use were assessed using two approaches. First, a question concerning CABG was asked, as follows, "If your doctor recommended that you have bypass surgery to improve the blood flow to your heart, would you do so?" This was followed by a similar question about PTCA. Second, two scenarios were presented in which a man had suffered a myocardial infarction and was left with class II-III angina. In one, CABG was said to be likely to improve symptoms but not survival. In the second, CABG was said to be likely to improve both symptoms and survival. Both scenarios included an estimated operative mortality of 2.5 percent. The participant was then asked to comment regarding whether he would want bypass surgery if he were that person. The full scenarios, which were read aloud verbatim by a research assistant (RA), are shown in Table 33.1.

Table 33.1. Scenarios Used in the Survey

Scenario 1

Imagine a man who had a heart attack. After the heart attack, his chest pain prevents him from doing activities that he used to do. Walking up hills causes him shortness of breath, and he must often stop. He takes pills to help prevent the chest pain. His doctors do a catheterization and find that he has several blockages of the arteries to his heart. They tell him that if they do a bypass surgery that they are pretty sure that his pain will become less frequent, and that there is a pretty good chance it will go away completely. However, there is a one in forty chance he could die from the operation. Overall, the doctors think the chance of being alive in 5 years is the same whether or not he has surgery. In other words, the surgery will not make him live any longer but it will probably make him have less pain and need fewer medicines.

Scenario 2

Now imagine another man who had a heart attack. After the heart attack, his chest pain prevents him from doing activities that he used to do. Walking up hills causes him shortness of breath, and he must stop often. He takes pills to help prevent the chest pain. His doctors do a catheterization and find that he has several blockages of the arteries to his heart. They tell him that if he does not have surgery, he is very likely to die in the next year or two. They also say that if he has surgery, he is much less likely to die from heart disease, although he still could. The surgery is also likely to make his chest pain get better. In other words, he is more likely to live a long time, and have less chest pain, if he has the surgery, but there is a one in forty chance he could die from the operation.

Patients

The study population included three categories of male patients treated at the Pittsburgh VA Medical Center, a large, university-affiliated, acute care VA hospital: (1) ambulatory patients without a diagnosis of CAD ($n = 216$), (2) ambulatory patients who had previously undergone either PTCA or CABG ($n = 77$), and (3) hospitalized patients who were awaiting a scheduled cardiac catheterization (CATH) for known or suspected CAD ($n = 80$). Ambulatory patients were approached while they awaited appointments in the internal medicine clinic. Inpatients awaiting CATH were identified from the CATH schedule and approached in their rooms. All other inpatients awaiting CATH were asked to participate if they were not in an intensive care setting and not undergoing clinical care when approached by the RA. Trained RAs reviewed charts to identify eligible male veterans. Surveys were performed by three RAs, one black and two white. The RAs attempted to enroll all eligible blacks and as many whites as could be accommodated. Participants provided oral informed consent after being asked to participate in a survey to learn why some patients are more or less likely to agree to revascularization. As requested by the Pittsburgh VAMC's Subcommittee on Human Studies, which approved the study, patients did not provide their names or other unique identifiers when completing the survey.

Analysis

Simple descriptive statistics were used to describe the study population. The four dependent variables (willingness to undergo PTCA if recommended, willingness to undergo CABG if recommended, and two scenarios) were categorized into "yes" responses and "no/not sure" responses. Similar results were obtained when the not sure responses were excluded. Age was examined as a continuous and categorical variable in exploratory analyses, but was dichotomized at age sixty-five for the final analysis.

Because the responses to the questions measuring familiarity were highly correlated with one another, factor analysis was used to determine whether a summary variable would capture the meaning in these. However, no clear summary factor was found, so each question was treated as a separate measure. Similarly, although the measures of attitude toward revascularization were correlated, we elected to report separate analyses using each of these measures as the dependent variable.

Characteristics of the black and white populations were compared using χ^2 tests and Student's t tests, as appropriate. Then χ^2 tests were used to examine the association of each independent variable within the measures of attitude toward revascularization. Variables that approached ($p \leq .1$) significance in univariate analyses were entered into a logistic regression, using stepwise forward selection. This analysis was repeated with race forced into the model. It was also repeated with race, inpatient/outpatient status, and previous revascularization forced into the model. We also performed univariate and multivariable analyses of each of the independent and dependent variables stratified by category (inpatient, outpatient with CAD, and outpatient without CAD). We found that these analyses yielded no evidence of heterogeneity across categories, so only the analyses of all three categories combined are presented.

Because of concern that the race of the person administering the survey might affect patient responses, we compared attitudes toward revascularization among participants who were interviewed by black and white RAs, using χ^2 testing.

Survey data were entered into a computerized database, then verified after they had been converted into an SAS file. All statistical analyses were carried out using SAS statistical software in a Windows 3.11 environment (PC SAS for Windows 3.11, version 6.08).[12]

RESULTS

Overall, 373 patients were interviewed. Patients who could not be classified as either white or black were excluded, as were those whose interview was discontinued before at least one of the outcome variables had been answered, usually to avoid interfering with clinical care ($n = 21$). The characteristics of the remaining 352 patients are presented in Table 33.2. Blacks and whites were similar in age, working status, and education, but black patients reported worse health status, were more likely to live alone, and were less familiar with each of the revascularization procedures. Black patients were also less likely to have had a previous revascularization or to be awaiting CATH.

Overall, 65.7 percent of participants said they would choose CABG given the scenario in which it would improve symptoms but not survival, compared with 84.4 percent who would choose it if CABG improved both symptoms and survival. When asked whether they would undergo a PTCA if their doctor recommended it, 64.2 percent said yes. The comparable number for doctor-recommended CABG was 72.1 percent.

In univariate comparisons (Table 33.3), whites were generally more inclined to undergo procedures than blacks for each of the outcome variables. Each of the measures of increased patient familiarity with revascularization (self-report as "familiar" with the procedure, having a "good idea" what happens when one undergoes it, having a family member or friend who had a procedure, or having a realistic estimate of risk) was correlated with a more positive attitude toward revascularization, frequently to a significant degree (Table 33.3). However, none of the characteristics of age, education, employment, living situation, health status, history of previous revascularization, or being in the hospital awaiting CATH predicted responses favoring revascularization.

Table 33.2. Characteristics of the Study Population by Race

Patient Characteristic	n	Whites, n (%)	Blacks, n (%)
Number	352	234	118
Mean age, years	352	65.6	63.9
Inpatients awaiting CATH*	352	65 (28)	15 (13)
Inpatients with prior revascularization*	351	75 (32)	14 (12)
Working	352	48 (21)	25 (21)
Education	351		
High school graduate		78 (33)	31 (26)
At least some post–high school		76 (33)	41 (35)
Living alone*	351	62 (27)	44 (37)
Health status*	352		
Poor		33 (14)	18 (15)
Fair		86 (37)	58 (49)
Good		86 (37)	28 (24)
Very good/excellent		29 (12)	14 (12)
Familiarity with bypass surgery*			
States he is familiar with CABG	351	191 (82)	72 (62)
Has a good idea what happens	349	156 (68)	56 (47)
Knows someone who had CABG	351	149 (64)	53 (45)
Estimate of perioperative mortality	347		
0–10%		107 (47)	29 (25)
11% or more		78 (34)	46 (39)
Could not guess		45 (20)	42 (36)
Familiarity with PTCA*			
States he is familiar with PTCA	349	146 (63)	36 (31)
Has a good idea what happens	347	133 (57)	41 (36)
Knows someone who had PTCA	348	119 (52)	27 (23)
Estimate of need for urgent CABG	346		
0–10%		67 (29)	19 (16)
11% or more		76 (33)	34 (29)
Could not guess		87 (38)	63 (54)

Note: CATH = cardiac catheterization; CABG = coronary artery bypass grafting; PTCA = percutaneous transluminal coronary angioplasty.

*$p < .05$ for the difference between blacks and whites.

In the multivariate analysis (Table 33.4), measures of familiarity with the procedure were the most important predictors of attitude toward revascularization. For each of the dependent variables the pattern of predictors was slightly different, but one of the questions we have devised to measure familiarity was always the more powerful predictor. Race did enter the model predicting willingness to undergo PTCA if the patient's doctor so advised. When race was

Table 33.3. Patients with Various Characteristics Who Gave Positive Responses Regarding Procedure Use, Measured with Four Responses

Characteristic	PTCA If Recommended, n (%)	CABG If Recommended, n (%)	CABG for Pain, n (%)	CABG for Life, n (%)
Race				
Black	61 (52)	77 (65)	71 (61)	91 (78)
White	163 (70)	176 (76)	157 (68)	201 (87)
CAD				
Yes	98 (64)	117 (76)	100 (66)	132 (87)
No	125 (64)	135 (69)	127 (66)	158 (82)
Inpatient				
Yes	51 (64)	60 (75)	51 (65)	70 (89)
No	173 (64)	193 (71)	177 (66)	222 (83)
Prior procedure				
Yes	58 (66)	69 (78)	58 (66)	75 (85)
No	165 (64)	183 (70)	169 (66)	215 (84)
Working				
Yes	44 (60)	53 (73)	55 (75)	69 (95)
No	180 (65)	200 (72)	173 (63)	223 (82)
Living alone				
Yes	69 (65)	76 (72)	70 (67)	89 (85)
No	154 (64)	176 (72)	157 (65)	202 (84)
Education				
<High school grad.	76 (62)	91 (73)	71 (59)	95 (79)
High school grad.	67 (62)	75 (67)	72 (67)	96 (89)
>High school grad.	81 (69)	87 (74)	85 (73)	101 (87)
Health status				
Poor	26 (51)	33 (66)	30 (59)	37 (73)
Fair	91 (64)	102 (71)	94 (66)	118 (84)
Good	79 (70)	88 (77)	74 (67)	98 (88)
Very good+	28 (65)	30 (70)	30 (70)	39 (91)
Age group				
<65	91 (64)	100 (69)	99 (69)	130 (91)
65+	133 (65)	153 (74)	129 (63)	162 (80)
Familiar				
Yes	120 (66)	190 (73)	176 (68)	227 (88)
No	103 (62)	62 (70)	51 (58)	64 (73)
Has an idea				
Yes	126 (72)	164 (77)	153 (73)	191 (91)
No	96 (56)	87 (64)	73 (55)	100 (76)

(Continued)

Table 33.3. Patients with Various Characteristics Who Gave Positive Responses
Regarding Procedure Use, Measured with Four Responses (Continued)

Characteristic	PTCA If Recommended, n (%)	CABG If Recommended, n (%)	CABG for Pain, n (%)	CABG for Life, n (%)
Family/friend				
Yes	110 (76)	156 (77)	127 (64)	173 (87)
No	113 (56)	97 (66)	100 (68)	119 (82)
Risk estimate				
Realistic	71 (83)	111 (82)	100 (74)	124 (93)
High	68 (62)	96 (77)	79 (64)	107 (87)
None	84 (56)	43 (50)	46 (55)	58 (69)

Note: CABG = coronary artery bypass grafting; CAD = coronary artery disease; PTCA = percutaneous transluminal coronary angioplasty; $p < .05$, for the difference between the different groups in willingness to have procedures.

forced into the other models, it did not approach statistical significance, although in each case the responses of black participants tended to be less favorable toward procedure use. In addition, veterans less than sixty-five years of age were more likely to choose CABG given the scenario in which it improved both survival and symptoms, even after controlling for familiarity with the procedure. When these analyses were repeated with inpatient status and history of previous procedure use forced into the model, the results were unchanged.

In univariate analysis, race of the interviewer also appeared to have some influence on black participants' preferences for opting for revascularization procedures. For each dependent variable, black patients were more likely to state they would opt for a procedure when surveyed by a black RA rather than a white RA. These differences ranged from 20 percent for having a PTCA if the doctor recommended one to 12 percent for having a CABG when presented with a scenario in which it would improve survival as well as symptoms. These differences approached, but did not achieve, statistical significance. White participants had similar responses whether they were interviewed by a white or a black RA (data not shown).

DISCUSSION

In this survey of more than 350 black and white patients, we found that whites were more likely to say they would undergo revascularization if recommended by their physician and to say they would elect CABG if they were in a situation in which it would be likely to improve symptoms and long-term survival. This finding is consistent with previous work that has found that among patients offered CABG, blacks are less likely to actually undergo the procedure.[10] Unlike

Table 33.4. Multivariate Analyses of Factors Predicting Attitude Toward Revascularization, Measured by Four Outcome Variables

Outcome Variable	Multivariable Predictors of Attitude		Multivariate Odds Ratio (95%)
	Respondent Characteristic	Odds Ratio (95%)	Whites versus Blacks
Willing to have recommended CABG	Can estimate CABG risk	3.79 (2.25–6.30)	1.39 (0.84–2.35)
Willing to have recommended PTCA	Can estimate PTCA risk	2.52 (1.37–4.77)	1.69 (1.03–2.79)
	Knows someone post-PTCA	1.98 (1.18–3.35)	
	White race	1.69 (1.03–2.79)	
Desire for CABG for symptoms	Idea what CABG is	2.14 (1.35–3.39)	1.17 (0.72–1.89)
Desire for CABG for symptoms and improved survival	Can estimate CABG risk	3.13 (1.59–6.17)	1.59 (0.83–3.04)
	Idea what CABG is	2.10 (1.06–4.14)	
	Age less than 65	2.49 (1.22–5.09)	

Note: CABG = coronary artery bypass grafting; PTCA = percutaneous transluminal coronary angioplasty.

these previous findings, which may have reflected differences in clinical characteristics among blacks and whites offered CABG, our study design controls for different clinical scenarios by providing all patients with identical situations. In addition, we were able to show that much of the black-white difference in patient preferences seemed to be explained by questions that addressed familiarity with the procedures in different ways. When these questions are included in multivariate models, race is a significant predictor of only one of four measures of attitudes. Finally, although these findings are based on small numbers of patients, it is also interesting that these differences were smaller when the interviewer was also black.

We have been unable to identify analogous studies of patient preferences for procedure use in the literature. However, several studies have found that blacks are more likely to delay seeking care for chest pain than whites, although at least one study suggested this may reflect primarily socioeconomic differences.[13-15] Several authors have suggested that this may be because black patients are less familiar with the signs and symptoms of coronary heart disease.[16,17] Lack of knowledge concerning heart disease symptoms might lead to different responses to symptoms of chest pain, but it is not clear how this would result in different attitudes toward revascularization among black patients.[16,18] Another possibility is that blacks are more averse to using the medical system in general, perhaps reflecting previous negative experiences with it.[19,20] Our survey did not address this possibility.

Other factors that may be important for understanding racial differences in the decision to accept or elect revascularization procedures are identified in the Health Belief Model.[11] This model suggests that decision making is affected by a number of factors including beliefs about individual vulnerability to disease and the seriousness of disease and confidence in treatment efficacy, balanced against perceived barriers to care.[21] Our finding that familiarity with the procedure was associated with procedure use would seem consistent with this model.

We should note that the grouping of our questions measuring familiarity is based on our theoretical perception that these questions would all measure the same construct in different ways. Our inability to group them with factor analysis, despite their having significant collinearity, suggests that more than one construct is being measured by these questions. More detailed studies using larger numbers of patients and different formulations of these questions may clarify the constructs that are truly important to the decision-making process.

The consistent trend for black patients to be more likely to say they would choose revascularization when surveyed by a black RA as opposed to a white RA is also consistent with earlier reports. Brooks reported that 24 percent of black patients are dissatisfied with clinic visits, and attributed this to communication barriers, use of medical jargon, lack of warmth and friendliness in physicians, and perhaps a distrust of whites.[22] As blacks make up 12 percent of the U.S. population but only 3 percent of physicians,[23] and even fewer subspecialists, most black patients facing an invasive cardiac procedure will be counseled by a physician who is not black. Thus, it is plausible that racial incongruity between patient and physician may contribute to the lower revascularization rates among blacks. One should consider that this analysis was not a part of our original study design. It also should be noted that the RAs, who did not have medical training, simply posed the two questions and read the scenarios verbatim, as they appear in Table 33.1, a much different situation than that of a physician counseling a patient. Nonetheless, our results raise the possibility that increasing the number of minority physicians in the workforce, particularly in subspecialty positions, may decrease differences in procedure use between blacks and whites.

There are several limitations to this study. Most important, answers were purely hypothetical. Actual decision making, for example in the setting of an acute ischemic event, might be considerably different as this situation would presumably lead to marked changes in one's perceived susceptibility to disease, as well as disease seriousness. However, it is interesting that the 10 percent higher proportion of whites who said they would agree to CABG if their doctor recommended it is similar to the difference in acceptance rates of CABG among patients in the CASS registry.[10]

Second, although we asked participants to answer questions about a hypothetical situation, they may have considered their own condition in deciding whether or not to elect CABG in the scenarios presented. It is possible that the racial differences in responses that we found reflected differences in the participants' clinical situation, rather than differences in attitudes.

Third, because all participants were patients at the Pittsburgh VAMC, they may not be representative of blacks and whites across the country. For example, patients who use the VA medical system are more likely than other Americans to be male, poor, and have a lower level of education.[24] A population that included women, had higher incomes, or was more highly educated might have given different responses. On the other hand, by studying men who use the VA, we minimize the potential confounding of race by differences in income and education. Moreover, it is unlikely that the physicians caring for black and white participants in this study had made systematically different attempts at patient education, as the same internal medicine and cardiology faculty supervise or provide directly the primary and cardiac care for these patients.

In addition, the fact that we used a convenience sample, rather than a truly random sample, may have yielded an unrepresentative population. Patients who were available for an interview may be more or less willing to undergo procedures than the population in general. However, it is our impression that the vast majority of patients in this VA clinic arrive significantly in advance of their scheduled appointment, in time to be a candidate for the present study. Fewer than 5 percent of patients who were approached did not agree to be interviewed.

Finally, our study did not address whether increasing patient familiarity with the procedures would have led to changes in attitudes. Indeed, because our study relied on self-report, we cannot be sure whether we measured familiarity with a procedure or simply the desire to appear knowledgeable. Similarly, our study could not determine whether the lack of familiarity with procedures was secondary to other attitudes such as fear or distrust of invasive procedures or the medical system in general, which might have prevented gaining familiarity with CABG or PTCA.

We believe these results provide direction for researchers and clinicians concerned about patterns of use of revascularization procedures. First, the present results should be replicated in patients who are actually facing a decision whether or not to proceed to a revascularization procedure, as well as in a more scientifically selected sample of the general population. This is particularly important for patients for whom revascularization would be medically necessary—that is, for whom revascularization is clearly beneficial and better than any other alternative.

Second, clinicians should be careful to ensure that lower levels of familiarity with CABG and PTCA at baseline do not lead to uninformed decision making, regardless of patient race. Unfortunately, physicians may spend more time explaining risks and benefits of procedures to patients who are well educated and, paradoxically, give less information to those patients who are least familiar with proposed treatments.[22] Thus, clinicians should be careful to assess baseline levels of familiarity with procedures when discussing recommendations with patients. If unfamiliar with the procedure, patients could be exposed to tailored educational programs before being asked to make a decision. This might be especially important if the patients have not been exposed to such decision making, for example among friends and relatives, in the past.

Notes

1. Oberman, A., & Cutter, G. (1984). Issues in the natural history and treatment of coronary heart disease in black populations: Surgical treatment. *Am Heart J, 108,* 688–694.

2. Gillum, R. F. (1982). Coronary heart disease in black populations: 1. Mortality and morbidity. *Am Heart J, 104,* 839–851.

3. Watkins, L. O. (1984). Epidemiology of coronary heart disease in black populations: Methodological proposals. *Am Heart J, 108,* 635–640.

4. Kochanek, K. D., Maurer, J. D., & Rosenberg, H. M. (1994). Why did black life expectancy decline from 1984 through 1989 in the United States? *Am J Public Health, 84,* 938–944.

5. Whittle, J., Conigliaro, J., Good, C. B., & Lofgren, R. P. (1993). Racial differences in the use of invasive cardiovascular procedures in the Department of Veterans Affairs medical system. *N Engl J Med, 329,* 621–627.

6. Wenneker, M. B., & Epstein, A. M. (1989). Racial inequalities in the use of procedures for patients with ischemic heart disease in Massachusetts. *JAMA, 261,* 253–257.

7. Hannan, E. L., Kilburn, H., Jr., O'Donnell, J. F., Lukacik, G., & Shields, E. P. (1991). Interracial access to selected cardiac procedures for patients hospitalized with coronary artery disease in New York State. *Med Care, 29,* 430–441.

8. Goldberg, K. C., Hartz, A. J., Jacobsen, S. J., Krakauer, H., & Rimm, A. A. (1992). Racial and community factors influencing coronary artery bypass graft surgery rates for all 1986 Medicare patients. *JAMA, 267,* 1473–1477.

9. Johnson, P. A., Lee, T. H., Cook, E. F., Rouan, G. W., & Goldman, L. (1993). Effect of race on the presentation and management of patients with acute chest pain. *Ann Intern Med, 118,* 593–601.

10. Maynard, C., Fisher, L. D., Passamani, E. R., & Pullum, T. (1986). Blacks in the Coronary Artery Surgery Study (CASS): Race and clinical decision making. *Am J Public Health, 76,* 1446–1448.

11. Rosenstock, I. M. (1974). Historical origins of the Health Belief Model. *Health Educ Monographs, 2,* 328–335.

12. SAS Institute Inc. (1989). *SAS Language and Procedures: Usage, Version 6.* Cary, NC: Author.

13. Cooper, R. S., Simmons, B., Castaner, A., Prasad, R., Fanklin, C., & Ferlinz, J. (1986). Survival rates and prehospital delay during myocardial infarction among black persons. *Am J Cardiol, 57,* 208–211.

14. Ell, K., Haywood, L. J., Sobel, E., deGuzman, M., Blumfield, D., & Ning, J.-P. (1994). Acute chest pain in African Americans: Factors in the delay in seeking emergency care. *Am J Public Health, 84,* 965–970.

15. Strogatz, D. S. (1990). Use of medical care for chest pain: Differences between blacks and whites. *Am J Public Health, 80,* 290–294.

16. Raczynski, J. M., Taylor, H., Cutter, G., Hardin, M., Rappaport, N., & Oberman, A. (1994). Diagnoses, symptoms, and attribution of symptoms among black and white inpatients admitted for coronary heart disease. *Am J Public Health, 84,* 951–956.

17. Folsom, A. R., Sprafka, J. M., Luepker, R. V., & Jacobs, D. R., Jr. (1988). Beliefs among black and white adults about causes and prevention of cardiovascular disease: The Minnesota Heart Survey. *Am J Prev Med, 4,* 121–127.

18. Davis, I. J., Brown, C. P., Allen, F., Davis, T., & Waldron, D. (1995). African-American myths and health care: The sociocultural theory. *J Natl Med Assoc, 87,* 791–794.

19. Blendon, R. J., Aiken, L. H., Freeman, H. E., & Corey, C. R. (1989). Access to medical care for black and white Americans: A matter of continuing concern. *JAMA, 261,* 278–281.

20. Bailiey, E. J. (1987). Sociocultural factors and health care–seeking behavior among black Americans. *J Natl Med Assoc, 79,* 389–392.

21. Horner, R. D., Oddone, E. Z., & Matchar, D. B. (1995). Theories explaining racial differences in the utilization of diagnostic and therapeutic procedures for cerebro-vascular disease. *Milbank Q, 73,* 443–462.

22. Brooks, T. R. (1992). Pitfalls in communication with Hispanic and African-American patients: Do translators help or harm? *J Natl Med Assoc, 84,* 941–947.

23. King, G., & Bendel, R. (1994). A statistical model estimating the number of African-American physicians in the United States. *J Natl Med Assoc, 86,* 264–272.

24. Assistant Secretary for Finance and Planning, Office of Planning and Management Analysis, U.S. Department of Veterans Affairs. (1990). *Survey of medical system users.* Washington, DC: U.S. Department of Veterans Affairs.

CHAPTER THIRTY-FOUR

Racial Differences in Attitudes Toward Professional Mental Health Care and in the Use of Services

Chamberlain Diala
Carles Muntaner
Christine Walrath
Kim J. Nickerson
Thomas A. LaVeist
Philip J. Leaf

There is evidence that African Americans use fewer health services than do whites, and are less likely to use mental health services (MHS).[1-4] Some studies have examined racial variation in the use of services by focusing on regional populations,[5,6] while others have examined racial differences in utilization across a number of health services.[7] Demographic and economic factors are known to contribute in varying proportions to such differences; for example, African Americans with fewer resources and jobs lack the employment-based health insurance benefits that serve as the backbone of the health care system in the United States.[8] While poor families rely exclusively on public programs (Medicaid), families with higher incomes have private health insurance and can either co-pay or self-pay for services.[9,10] Inadequate resources create barriers to use of health services by poor families with limited health insurance benefits.[11]

Factors associated with racial differences in the use of MHS include wealth[12] and racial differentials in diagnosis.[13] In addition to economic barriers, social attitudes and perceptions effect the pursuit of mental health care and might be important in predicting use of mental health services. Among these attitudes and perceptions are cultural mistrust,[14] differences in attitudes and knowledge,[15] and differences in perspectives on seeking care.[4] Exploring racial differences in these perceptual and attitudinal considerations is the focus of the study reported here, which attempts to expand the scope of research on racial differences in attitudes toward seeking psychiatric care[16-18] in a nationally representative sample.

Research has consistently shown lower use of MHS by African Americans than by whites.[1,2] This may be because African Americans have different perceptions of psychiatric disorders or different attitudes toward seeking psychiatric care. As research on African American patterns of mental health service utilization evolves, however, conflicting results are emerging. For example, some studies have revealed practitioner bias against African Americans in diagnosis and treatment,[13,19,20] or differences between blacks and whites in treatment duration and utilization.[20] Others have found no racial differences in diagnoses or utilization of MHS.[16] Some of these inconsistencies may be explained by differences in methods of sampling study populations. They also suggest the necessity of examining issues unique to race by means of standardized methods of psychiatric assessment.

The present study sought to address this need by exploring racial differences in attitudes toward seeking professional care and their association with the use of MHS in a representative sample of the U.S. population. Based on previous findings, the following hypotheses were examined: (1) African Americans in general have less positive attitudes toward seeking professional mental health care than do whites; (2) African Americans with major depression (incidence is similar to that of whites) also have less positive attitudes toward seeking such care; and (3) as a result of their less positive attitudes, African Americans use fewer mental health services than do whites.

METHOD

Analysis was based on data from the National Comorbidity Survey (NCS). The NCS was designed to study the distribution, correlates, and consequences of psychiatric disorders in the United States,[1] and data were collected between 1990 and 1992 by the Institute for Social Research at the University of Michigan. As the first (and thus far only) national sample in which psychiatric disorders have been ascertained, the NCS data remain pertinent to present study purposes.

The diagnostic interview used by the NCS to generate *DSM-III-R* diagnoses[21] was a modified version of the Composite International Diagnostic Interview (CIDI),[22] which was designed for use by trained interviewers who are not clinicians.[23] Interviewers went through seven days of training specific to the use of CIDI and were closely monitored throughout the data collection period. The NCS did not attempt racial matching between interviewer and respondent. This is a limitation, since it could influence self-disclosure, particularly in light of the stigma associated with mental disorders.

The NCS interview was administered in two parts to respondents aged fifteen to fifty-four years, in the forty-eight contiguous states. Part I ($n = 8,098$) included the core diagnostic interview, a brief risk-factor battery of tests, and an inventory of sociodemographic information, and the response rate was 82.4 percent.[1] Part II ($n = 5,877$), which served as the basis for the present study, included a more detailed risk-factor test battery, plus secondary diagnoses. A nonresponse adjustment weight was constructed for the main survey data to compensate for systematic nonresponses. Households were selected at random. A second weight was constructed to adjust for probabilities of selection between and within households. The sample was then weighted (see Table 34.1) to approximate the U.S. population distribution for age, sex, race/ethnicity, and education, as defined by the 1989 National Health Interview Survey (NHIS).[1,24]

The dependent variable for the current study was use of MHS. For present study purposes, this was measured as any visits to a psychologist or psychiatrist (selected from other service providers as specifically and primarily trained in the treatment of mental and emotional disorders) during the twelve months prior to data collection.

Andersen's model of health services utilization guided selection of independent variables regarding familial and individual factors evaluated prior to care seeking.[25] The Andersen model considers the impact of three factors—predisposing, enabling, and need—on utilization of services. Data gathered via the NCS were not sufficient for the model's complete test, but along with predisposing (gender, age) and enabling (income, wealth, and health insurance) factors, respondents diagnosed with major depression could be stratified in the multivariate regressions to form the need component of the model.

Respondents' predispositions to seek care were measured in the NCS by responses to a question asking whether, if the respondents had a serious emotional problem, they would "definitely," "probably," "probably not," or "definitely not" go for help. Their attitudes toward seeking professional services were measured via responses to two questions: the first asked how comfortable they would feel talking about personal problems with a professional—"very," "somewhat," "not very," or "not at all" comfortable; the second asked how embarrassed they would be if their friends knew they were getting professional help for an emotional problem—"very," "somewhat," "not very," or "not at all" embarrassed.

Assessments of respondents' ability to seek care for mental and emotional disorders were not problem specific because identification of the origin (workplace, family) of the problems is difficult to obtain objectively from self-reports. However, while ethnic groups perceive and present problems differently, their ability to seek care is important, notwithstanding the origin of the problems.

The social stratification variables measured were race, gender, education, occupation, income, and wealth. Education, a common measure of social stratification,[26] represents knowledge that might have an influence on health-related behavior[27] and is stable and reliable over adult life.[28] In this study it was measured as years of formal education, using four categories (see Table 34.1).

Table 34.1. Characteristics of Non-MDE and MDE Respondents to the National Comorbidity Survey

	Non-MDE ($n = 5159$)		MDE ($n = 504$)	
	White ($n = 4479$)	Afr. Am. ($n = 680$)	White ($n = 441$)	Afr. Am. ($n = 63$)
Characteristic	%	%	%	%
Sex				
Males	48.2	40.2	31.6	23.1
Females	51.8	59.8	55.4	76.8
Age, years				
15–24	22.3	22.5	27.1	16.8
25–34	31.0	35.3	23.1	50.0
35–44	29.3	24.4	23.6	23.3
45–54	17.4	13.8	13.2	9.7
Education				
Less than high school	19.7	27.3	22.8	26.7
High-school graduate	37.8	37.6	31.7	37.6
Some college	21.4	24.4	20.2	29.4
College graduate+	21.1	10.5	12.5	6.1
Occupation				
Not in labor force	27.5	45.1	28.7	32.8
Professional	24.6	14.1	18.5	19.7
Sales	18.2	15.3	15.0	18.8
Services	9.6	4.3	5.1	8.2
Crafts	10.1	8.9	8.3	8.8
Laborer	10.0	12.4	11.4	11.4
Household Income				
$0–$12,499	10.2	28.7	10.3	39.9
$12,500–$24,999	18.5	15.3	20.0	10.3
$25,000–$34,999	16.3	12.9	11.6	23.2
$35,000–$49,999	21.0	12.2	16.5	18.1
$50,000+	33.7	17.6	22.6	6.6
Household Wealth				
$0–$9,999	35.6	56.5	40.4	68.7
$10,000–$19,999	9.2	10.5	6.4	6.0
$20,000–$49,999	12.6	8.1	8.4	3.5
$50,000–$99,999	12.4	11.2	9.5	12.2
$100,000+	27.6	11.9	18.0	8.4
Health Insurance				
None	12.2	15.3	13.7	17.5
Public	4.8	19.2	5.5	31.9
Private	81.8	64.6	67.5	50.4

Note: MDE = major depressive episode; weighted percentages.

Occupation in the NCS identified hierarchy, job autonomy, and technical aspects of work based on current employment status. Occupation is a major indicator of social classification, associated with skills, prestige, wealth, and working conditions.[29] Survey questions on occupation determined occupational or industry status, using categories similar to those of the Index of Industries and Occupations from the 1996 Bureau of the Census Occupation Code. Six categories (see Table 34.1) were analyzed in the present study.

Household income, which represents economic resources that enable health services utilization, was grouped in five annual levels (see Table 34.1). Household wealth is more unequally distributed than household income,[30,31] and factors like inheritance can mean that wealth does not show a strong positive correlation with income, education, or occupation. A single question in the survey asked respondents how much money they would realize if they (and their husband/wife/partner) cashed in all their checking and savings accounts, stocks and bonds, and real estate, and sold their home (after paying off the mortgage). They were asked to identify their level on a list of nine possible household wealth categories, which was then collapsed into five (see Table 34.1).

As can be seen in Table 34.1, health insurance, probably the most critical enabling factor for familial or individual MHS utilization, was represented in this study by three categories, while analysis also included four variables for age.

Statistical Analysis

Multiple logistic regression was conducted with the Statistical Analysis System (SAS). First, responses to various attitudes toward seeking professional care were assessed before and after respondents sought care. Attitude variables were grouped according to positive or negative response. Because African Americans were the reference category for the regression, a positive attitude for which the odds ratio (OR) was above 1 meant that African Americans had the more positive attitude to the specific variable, while a negative attitude with an OR above 1 meant that they had the more negative attitude. Use of mental health services by whites was then assessed, using African Americans as reference; here, ORs less than 1 meant that African Americans were using fewer services than their white counterparts. The entire SAS program model was then reanalyzed, using SUDAAN[32] to account for the complex sample design and weights employed in the NCS and to obtain more accurate standard estimates generalizable to the U.S. population. Marginally significant SAS results were not statistically significant when applied to SUDAAN and therefore are not reported in the final models presented here. SUDAAN adjustments thus meant that certain positive attitude variables prior to use of services were omitted in the after-services use section.

Data were stratified by means of an iterative procedure to approximate the national population distributions of cross-classifications of age, sex, race, ethnicity, education, household income and wealth, and health insurance status, as defined by the 1989 NHIS.[24] Multivariate results are presented in the form of prevalence and ORs, the latter obtained by exponentiating the regression coefficients from logistic models. Although household income and wealth were positively correlated, the rate (less than 0.5) was insignificant, making it unlikely to be problematic in the multivariate models.

Consistent with previous studies, such as Kohn and Schooler's study,[33] the three social class indicators measured in ordinal scales (education, income, and wealth) were not highly correlated. Other researchers have found that these indicators have unique effects on health outcomes. For example, Sorlie et al. reported that common social class indicators (education, income, and occupation) differentially predicted mortality in a probability sample of the U.S. population.[34]

RESULTS

Attitudes Toward MHS

General Population. The existence of an association between race and attitudes toward use of MHS was supported in the study findings, though not in the expected direction. African Americans, in fact, reported more positive attitudes toward use of MHS than did whites, a pattern holding true in both behavioral (predisposition to seek care) and emotional (level of comfort about seeking care) responses about use of MHS.

As can be seen in Table 34.2, prior to use of services, African Americans were more likely than whites in the general population to report positive attitudes toward seeking professional care. They were also more predisposed to seek care if they had serious emotional problems, to feel comfortable talking about personal problems with a professional, and to be less embarrassed about friends' knowing they were seeking professional help for emotional problems.

Attitudes among the general population after use of MHS are also shown in Table 34.2. Among users, African Americans were more likely than whites to report negative attitudes and less likely to return to MHS if their illness persisted. Furthermore, African Americans who had used MHS were less likely than whites to have positive attitudes toward their friends' knowing they had sought help. Finally, African Americans had significantly lower odds for using MHS than did Caucasians.

Population With Major Depressive Episodes. This analysis stratified respondents (African Americans and whites) by need, in this case, major depression. Attitudes of respondents with major depression were assessed regardless of services use status. African Americans with major depressive episodes (MDE) were more likely to report positive attitudes toward seeking care prior to use of services (see Table 34.3). Specifically, depressed African Americans were more likely than depressed whites to seek care and less likely to be embarrassed if

Table 34.2. Attitudes to Use of MHS by White (n = 4,479) and African American (n = 680) Respondents to the National Comorbidity Survey

Attitude	OR*	p	95% CI
Prior to MHS			
Positive attitude			
Definitely go	1.5	0.0001	1.3–1.8
Very comfortable	1.2	0.030	1.01–1.4
Somewhat comfortable	1.3	0.002	1.1–1.5
Not at all embarrassed	2.1	0.0001	1.7–2.4
Negative attitude			
Probably not go	0.5	0.001	0.3–0.6
Not very comfortable	0.4	0.001	0.3–0.5
Somewhat embarrassed	0.4	0.001	0.3–0.5
After MHSS†			
Positive attitude			
Probably go	0.3	0.005	0.1–0.7
Somewhat comfortable	0.2	0.001	0.1–0.6
Not very embarrassed	0.3	0.050	0.1–0.9
Not at all embarrassed	0.1	0.020	0.01–0.7
Use of MHSS	0.4	0.004	0.3–0.7

Note: OR = odds ratio; CI = confidence interval.

*Analyses regressed on African Americans.

†Within the 12 months preceding data collection.

their friends knew they had sought professional help for their emotional problems. No significant racial differences were evident in attitudes among those with MDE after they had used MHS. Finally, despite similar prevalence of MDE in both races (9.8 percent and 9.3 percent, respectively), African Americans in the NCS had significantly lower odds of using MHS than did whites.

Actual Use of MHS

General Population. In the final regression model (see Table 34.4), results confirmed that African Americans had lower odds of using MHS than did whites, and that respondents' attitudes had a significant impact on use of MHS (only significant SUDAAN variables were included in the analysis). Specifically, among respondents who had used MHS, those not comfortable about seeking care were five times less likely to use MHS than were those who were very comfortable about doing so. Similarly, those who would be very embarrassed if friends knew they had sought care were three times less likely to seek it than were those who would not be at all embarrassed. Females in the general population were more likely to use MHS than were males; high school graduates were less likely to use

Table 34.3. Use of MHS by Respondents to the National Comorbidity Survey with MDE

Attitude	OR*	p	95% CI
Prior to MHS			
Positive attitude			
Definitely go	1.8	0.020	1.08–3.1
Very comfortable	1.0	0.901	0.70–1.9
Somewhat comfortable	1.2	0.303	0.80–2.3
Not at all embarrassed	1.6	0.050	1.00–2.2
Negative attitude			
Probably not go	0.8	0.802	0.50–1.6
Not very comfortable	1.0	0.901	0.80–2.1
Somewhat embarrassed	0.4	0.020	0.20–0.9
After MHSS[†]			
Positive attitude			
Probably go	0.4	0.041	0.30–0.9
Somewhat comfortable	0.3	0.090	0.60–1.5
Negative attitude			
Not very comfortable	0.3	0.200	0.10–0.3
Not at all comfortable	2.1	0.026	1.40–3.2
Use of MHSS	0.4	0.040	0.20–0.9

Note: OR = odds ratio; CI = confidence interval; MDE = major depressive episodes; $n = 504$ (441 white, 63 African American).

*Analyses regressed on African Americans.

†Within the 12 months preceding data collection.

MHS than were those with college degrees or more education; respondents at the second lowest level of household income were less likely to use MHS than were those at the highest level; and those with no health insurance benefits or with public health insurance benefits were less likely to use MHS than were those with private health insurance coverage.

Respondents with MDE. In the NCS, education was a weaker predictor of major mental disorders than income or wealth,[1,35] while health insurance status (excluded in this final model) was not a predictor of either attitudes or use of services among those diagnosed with MDE. Preliminary findings of interaction of attitudes, race, and social class were not significant[36] and were not associated with use of MHS.

The regression models for the use of MHS among those diagnosed with MDE (see Table 34.5) confirmed that African Americans were only half as likely to use MHS as were whites. Respondents' attitudes had a significant impact on their use of MHS; specifically, those with MDE who were not very or not at all comfortable seeking professional help for their emotional problems were less likely to use

Table 34.4. Use of MHS by White (n = 4,479) and African American (n = 680) Respondents to the National Comorbidity Survey, Multiple Regression Model

Variable	β	SE	OR	p	95% CI
Race					
White	—	—	—	—	—
African Americans	−0.93	0.28	0.3	0.001	0.2–0.7
Comfortable seeking care					
Very	—	—	—	—	—
Somewhat	−0.52	0.17	0.6	0.002	0.4–0.8
Not very	−0.84	0.28	0.4	0.003	0.2–0.7
Not at all	−1.41	0.42	0.2	0.001	0.1–0.5
Embarrassed friends knew					
Very	−1.09	0.43	0.3	0.011	0.1–0.8
Somewhat	−0.77	0.28	0.4	0.005	0.2–0.8
Not very	−0.53	0.21	0.5	0.012	0.3–0.9
Not at all	—	—	—	—	—
Gender					
Males	—	—	—	—	—
Females	0.52	0.17	1.6	0.001	1.2–2.3
Education					
Less than high school	−0.34	0.29	0.7	0.243	0.3–1.2
High school graduate	−0.70	0.31	0.5	0.021	0.2–0.9
Some college	−0.54	0.28	0.5	0.052	0.3–1.0
College graduate +	—	—	—	—	—
Household income					
$0–$12,499	0.08	0.26	1.0	0.748	0.6–1.8
$12,500–$24,999	−0.72	0.22	0.4	0.001	0.3–0.7
$25,000–$34,999	−0.42	0.39	0.6	0.279	0.3–1.4
$35,000–$49,999	−0.15	0.25	0.8	0.567	0.5–1.4
$50,000 or more	—	—	—	—	—
Household wealth					
$0–$12,499	0.78	0.26	2.1	0.002	1.2–3.7
$12,500–$24,999	−0.04	0.33	0.9	0.896	0.5–1.8
$25,000–$34,999	−0.24	0.30	0.7	0.425	0.4–1.4
$35,000–$49,999	0.19	0.30	1.2	0.523	0.5–1.4
$50,000 or more	—	—	—	—	—
Health insurance					
None	−0.53	0.28	0.5	0.050	0.3–1.0
Public	−0.70	0.33	0.5	0.032	0.2–0.9
Private	—	—	—	—	—

Note: OR = odds ratio; CI = confidence interval.

Table 34.5. Use of MHS by White (n = 441) and African American (n = 63) Respondents to the National Comorbidity Survey with MDE, Multiple Regression Model

Variable	β	SE	OR	p	95% CI
Race					
White	—	—	—	—	—
African Americans	−0.68	0.36	0.4	0.048	(0.2–0.9)
Comfortable seeking care					
Very	—	—	—	—	—
Somewhat	0.66	0.31	0.5	0.033	(0.2–0.9)
Not very	−1.25	0.51	0.2	0.014	(0.1–0.8)
Not at all	−2.05	0.77	0.1	0.007	(0.03–0.6)
Embarrassed friends knew					
Very	−1.09	0.43	0.3	0.011	0.1–0.8
Somewhat	−0.77	0.28	0.4	0.005	0.2–0.8
Not very	−0.53	0.21	0.5	0.012	0.3–0.9
Not at all	—	—	—	—	—
Household income					
$0–$12,499	0.49	0.44	0.6	0.272	(0.2–1.5)
$12,500–$24,999	−1.05	0.51	0.3	0.039	(0.1–0.9)
$25,000–$34,999	−1.31	0.45	0.2	0.003	(0.1–0.6)
$35,000–$49,999	0.19	0.35	0.8	0.598	(0.4–1.6)
$50,000 or more	—	—	—	—	—
Household wealth					
$0–$12,499	0.03	0.46	0.9	0.956	(0.3–2.4)
$12,500–$24,999	−0.09	0.57	0.9	0.871	(0.2–0.8)
$25,000–$34,999	−0.04	0.58	0.9	0.939	(0.3–3.0)
$35,000–$49,999	1.16	0.51	3.1	0.023	(1.1–8.8)
$50,000 or more	—	—	—	—	—

Note: OR = odds ratio; CI = confidence interval; MDE = major depressive episodes.

MHS than were those who were very comfortable doing so. Respondents with MDE with household incomes at the second lowest level were less likely to use MHS than were those with incomes at the highest level. Thus, level of comfort, as well as household fiscal resources, played a significant role in the use of MHS among respondents with MDE.

DISCUSSION

Counter to the study hypotheses, African Americans, both those in the general population and those diagnosed with depression, displayed more positive attitudes than did whites toward seeking care, yet used fewer services. Although the negative attitudes reported among African Americans who had used MHS remain largely unexplained, the findings contribute to an understanding of attitudes and use of MHS among African Americans. They replicate other study findings of relative underuse of MHS by African Americans, both in the general population and among those identified as being in need of services.[3] The results also support earlier studies that relied on smaller, nonrepresentative samples of the U.S. population. For example, Hall and Tucker surveyed 513 black and white teachers in Alachua County, Florida, and found similarly positive attitudes toward seeking professional psychological help among African American teachers;[17] as did the present study, they also found that more of the white respondents than the black had actually been in therapy with a mental health professional.

The NCS made possible these inquiries into African Americans' attitudes toward seeking care and how these attitudes might affect use of MHS. The findings provide new insights on the evolution of attitudes and healthy behavior among African Americans using MHS. For example, it had been assumed that existing negative attitudes held by African Americans accounted for their lower use of MHS at times of need.[37] The present results, however, suggest alternative explanations. Prior to their actual use of services, African Americans' attitudes toward seeking MHS were comparable to, and in some instances more favorable than, those of whites. The study also found that African Americans who had demonstrated need for services and received them held more negative attitudes about MHS and were less likely to use them again than were whites with comparable needs and usage. This has implications not only for follow-up care among those with mental disorders but also for mental health outcomes. Thus, it is vital to probe more deeply into factors other than prior attitudes related to lower use of MHS among African Americans (for example, exposure to discrimination or judgmental attitudes on the part of providers).

Factors related to the current findings include how services are organized or structured (system-based factors), how they are delivered (provider-based factors), and individual orientations or dispositions (consumer-based factors). Among system-based factors is access to quality services located in the community. Difficulties in locating and traveling to quality MHS are barriers to access, as are burdens related to costs. Many ethnic minorities express a preference for receiving MHS from professionals of their own ethnic backgrounds,[14,38] and the lack of patient-provider matching is a limitation of the NCS. Given the low numbers of ethnic minorities trained to deliver medical services[39] many systems are unable to deliver racially matched services. However, interest has been increasing over the last few years in making mental health care more culturally appropriate and responsive.[6,40,41]

African Americans who rely on racially different providers may face underdeveloped interracial skills or discrimination, and this may negatively influence their attitudes toward MHS. Several studies have suggested the need to understand better how referrals are made, diagnoses rendered, and treatment delivered by providers.[13,19,20,42-44] This notion is supported by the present study findings, inasmuch as African Americans' attitudes toward MHS were more negative after they had experienced them.

It is also important to consider patient-based factors that contribute to disparities in attitudes and utilization of MHS. For example, race-specific beliefs[45] and knowledge[15] about mental illness might influence help-seeking behavior. How African Americans view mental health and how those views are associated with their help-seeking behavior and perceptions about treatment might be important determinants of differences in MHS utilization.[2] For example, Nickerson et al. found that African Americans who were more mistrustful of whites were less willing to seek mental health treatment from white therapists, and expected less satisfaction from such therapeutic encounters.[14] Mental illness and mental health treatment continue to be plagued by a stigma that inhibits help-seeking behavior. How labeling and stigma differentially affect racial groups needs to be better understood. Exploration of changes in patients' attitudes over time would help to determine the impact of attitudes on use of services, and vice versa.

System-, provider-, or consumer-based factors that affect attitudes about use of MHS should be considered in future research. Factors that change attitudes of African Americans toward seeking MHS from positive to negative can cause delay in seeking follow-up care, nonadherence to a medication regimen, or use of alternative nontraditional care, with unpredictable outcomes and accountability.[2]

The present study has certain limitations. Both the African Americans and the whites in the sample might be ethnically heterogeneous, and this might have influenced some of the study findings. There are also limitations associated with the social stratification variables and the exploration of their relationships with respondents' attitudes toward MHS. For instance, the size of households supported by income and wealth was not considered; yet this factor may widen the disparity between blacks and whites in use of MHS because, on average, African Americans tend to have larger households but fewer economic resources.[30,46,47] The NCS did not capture the extremes of the U.S. wealth spectrum, thereby diminishing the scope of wealth inequity and its association with study outcomes.[48] The cross-sectional nature of the NCS limited determination of changes in attitudes among respondents over time. Selective memory of significant life experiences may trigger the mentally ill to associate bad experiences with providers as justification of the chronicity of their mental disorder.[49] Finally, since the racial background of providers was not captured in the NCS, it was impossible to ascertain to what extent respondents' experiences were racially or ethnically based.

Its limitations notwithstanding, this study reveals the need for further investigation by researchers and policymakers into the help-seeking attitudes and behavior of African Americans in MHS utilization. Given the range of help-seeking patterns documented among African Americans,[2,50] and findings that suggest comparable[16] or overrepresentation of African Americans in some mental health care settings,[19,51] many unanswered questions remain. Future studies should follow African Americans over time to monitor their attitudes and changes in those attitudes with actual use of MHS. The results of this study suggest that underuse of MHS by African Americans is due not to intrinsic negative attitudes but to problems in the health services delivery systems that have a negative impact on those attitudes following the use of MHS. The fact that African Americans with experience of MHS utilization have more negative attitudes than do whites with such experience should be viewed as a critical problem, with public health consequences that require further investigation.

Notes

1. Kessler, R., McGonagle, K. A., Zhao, S., Nelson, C., Hughes, M., Eshleman, S., Wittchen, H. U., & Kendler, K. S. (1994). Lifetime and 12-month prevalence of *DSM-III-R* psychiatric disorders in the U.S.: Results from the National Comorbidity Survey. *Arch Gen Psychiatry, 51,* 8–19.

2. Neighbors, H. W. (1988). Help-seeking behavior of black Americans: A summary of findings from the National Survey of Black Americans. *J Natl Med Assoc, 80,* 1009–1012.

3. Regier, D. A., Narrow, W. E., Rae, D. S., Manderscheid, R. W., Locke, B. Z., & Goodwin, F. K. (1993). The de facto U.S. mental and addictive disorders service system: ECA prospective 1-year prevalence rates of disorders and services. *Arch Gen Psychiatry, 50,* 85–94.

4. Wallen, J. (1992). Providing culturally appropriate mental health services for minorities. *J Ment Health Admin, 19,* 288–293.

5. Bruce, M. L., Takeuchi, D. T., & Leaf, P. J. (1991). Poverty and psychiatric status: Longitudinal evidence from the New Haven epidemiologic catchment area study. *Arch Gen Psychiatry, 48,* 470–474.

6. Takeuchi, D. T., & Uehara, E. S. (1996). Ethnic minority mental health services: Current research and future conceptual directions. In B. L. Levin & J. Petrila (Eds.), *Mental health services: A public health perspective* (pp. 63–79). New York: Oxford University Press.

7. Eaton, W., Anthony, J., Gallo, J., Cai, G., Tien, A., Romanoski, A., & Lyketsos, C. (1997). The Baltimore ECA follow-up. *Arch Gen Psychiatry, 54,* 993–999.

8. Muntaner, C. (1999). Social mechanisms, race, and social epidemiology. *Am J Epidemiol, 150*(2), 121–126.

9. Holzer, C. E., Shea, B., Swanson, J. W., Leaf, P. J., Myers, J. K., George, L., Weissman, M. M., & Bednarski, P. (1986). The increased risk for psychiatric disorders among persons of low socio-economic status. *Am J Psychiatry, 6,* 259–271.

10. Muntaner, C., & Parsons, P. E. (1996). Income, stratification, class and health insurance. *Int J Health Serv, 26,* 655–671.

11. Carrasquillo, O., Himmelstein, D., Woolhandler, S., & Bor, D. (1999). Going bare: Trends in health insurance coverage, 1989 through 1996. *Am J Public Health, 89*(1), 36–42.

12. Mutchler, J. E., & Burr, J. A. (1991). Racial differences in health and health care services utilization in later life: The effect of socioeconomic status. *J Health Soc Behav, 32,* 342–356.

13. Flasker, J. H., & Li-Tze, H. (1992). Relationship of ethnicity to psychiatric diagnosis. *J Nerv Ment Dis, 180,* 296–303.

14. Nickerson, K. J., Helms, J. E., & Terrell, F. (1994). Cultural mistrust, opinions about mental illness, and black students' attitudes toward seeking psychological help from white counselors. *J Couns Psychol, 41,* 378–385.

15. Delphin, M. E., & Rollock, D. (1995). University alienation and African American ethnic identity as predictors of attitude about and likely use of psychological services. *J College Student Develop, 36,* 337–346.

16. Broman, C. L. (1987). Race differences in professional help-seeking. *Am J Community Psychol, 15,* 473–489.

17. Hall, L. E., & Tucker, C. M. (1985). Relationships between ethnicity, conceptions of mental illness, and attitudes associated with seeking psychological help. *Psychol Rep, 57,* 907–916.

18. Leaf, P., Bruce, M., Tischler, G., & Holzer, C. (1988). The relationship between demographic factors and attitudes towards mental health specialist services. *J Community Psychol, 15,* 275–284.

19. Adebimpe, V. R., & Cohen, E. (1989). Schizophrenia and affective disorder in black and white patients: A methodologic note. *J Natl Med Assoc, 81,* 761–765.

20. Scheffler, R. M., & Miller, A. B. (1991). Differences in mental health service utilization among ethnic sub-populations. *Int J Law Psychiatry, 14,* 363–376.

21. American Psychiatric Association. (1987). *Diagnostic and statistical manual of mental disorders* (3rd ed., rev.). Washington, DC: Author.

22. World Health Organization. (1990). *Composite International Diagnostic Interview (CIDI) (Version 1.0).* Geneva, Switzerland: Author.

23. Robins, L. N., Wing, J., Wittchen, H.-U., Helzer, J. E., Babor, T. F., Burke, J., Farmer, A., Jablenski, A., Pickens, R., Regier, D. A., Satorius, N., & Towle, L. H. (1988). The CIDI: An epidemiological instrument suitable for use in conjunction with different diagnostic systems and in different cultures. *Arch Gen Psychiatry, 45,* 1069–1077.

24. U.S. Department of Health and Human Services. (1992). *National Health Interview Survey.* Hyattsville, MD: National Center for Health Statistics.

25. Andersen, R. M. (1995). Revisiting the behavioral model and access to medical care: Does it matter? *J Health Soc Behav, 36,* 1–10.

26. Liberatos, P., Link, B. G., & Kelsey, J. L. (1988). The measurement of social class in epidemiology. *Epidemiol Rev, 10,* 87–121.

27. Blane, D. (1995). Social determinants of health: Socioeconomic status, social class and ethnicity [Editorial]. *Am J Public Health, 85,* 903–905.

28. Kaplan, G. A., & Keil, J. E. (1993). Socioeconomic factors and cardiovascular diseases: A review of the literature. *Circulation, 88,* 1973–1998.

29. Muntaner, C., Eaton, W. W., & Diala, C. (2000). Social inequities in mental health: A review of concept and underlying assumptions. *Health, 4*(1), 89–113.

30. Oliver, M. O., & Shapiro, T. M. (1995). *Black wealth/white wealth: A new perspective on racial inequality.* New York: Routledge.

31. Wolff, E. N. (1996). *Top heavy: A study of wealth inequity in America.* New York: Twentieth Century Fund.

32. Shah, B. V., Barnwell, B. G., & Bieler, G. S. (1996). *SUDAAN user's manual: Software for analysis of correlated data (Release 7.0).* Research Triangle Park, NC: Research Triangle Institute.

33. Kohn, M., & Schooler, C. (1983). *Work and personality. An inquiry into the impact of social stratification.* Norwood, NJ: Ablex.

34. Sorlie, P., Backlund, E., & Keller, J. (1995). U.S. mortality by economic, demographic and social characteristics: The National Longitudinal Mortality Study. *Am J Public Health, 85,* 949–956.

35. Muntaner, C., Eaton, W. W., Diala, C., Kessler, R. C., & Sorlie, P. (1998). Social class, assets, organizational control and the prevalence of common groups of psychiatric disorders. *Soc Sci Med, 47,* 243–253.

36. Diala, C. C. (1997). *Race differences in attitudes toward seeking professional care and use of health services.* Unpublished doctoral dissertation, School of Public Health, Johns Hopkins University, Baltimore.

37. Mouton, C. P., Harris, S., Rovi, S., Solorzano, P., & Johnson, M. S. (1997). Barriers to black women's participation in cancer clinical trials. *J Natl Med Assoc, 89,* 721–727.

38. Sue, S., Zane, N., & Young, K. (1993). Research on psychotherapy with culturally diverse populations. In A. Bergin & S. Garfield (Eds.), *Handbook on psychotherapy and behavior change* (4th ed., pp. 783–817). New York: Wiley.

39. Sue, S. (1988). Psychotherapeutic services for ethnic minorities: Two decades of research findings. *Am Psychol, 42,* 37–45.

40. Cross, T., Bazron, B., Dennis, K., & Isaacs, M. (1989). *Towards a culturally competent system of care* (Vol. 1). Washington, DC: Georgetown University Child Development Center.

41. Isaacs, M. R., & Benjamin, M. P. (1991). *Towards a culturally competent system of care* (Vol. 2). Washington, DC: Georgetown University Child Development Center.

42. Angell, M. (1997). The ethics of clinical research in the Third World. *N Engl J Med, 337,* 847–849.

43. Coleman, D., & Baker, F. M. (1994). Misdiagnosis of schizophrenia in older, black veterans. *J Nerv Ment Dis, 182,* 527–528.

44. Strakowski, S. M., Shelton, R. C., & Kolbrener, M. L. (1993). The effects of race and co-morbidity on clinical diagnosis in patients with psychosis. *J Clin Psychiatry, 54,* 96–102.

45. Silva-de-Crane, R., & Spielberger, C. D. (1981). Attitudes of Hispanic, black, and Caucasian university students toward mental illness. *Hispanic J Behav Sci, 3,* 241–255.

46. Conley, D. (1999). *Being black, living in the red: Race, wealth and social policy in America.* Berkeley: University of California Press.

47. Farley, R. (1997). Racial trends and differences in the U.S., 30 years after the civil rights decade. *Soc Sci Res, 26,* 235–262.

48. Wright, E. O. (1997). *Class counts.* New York: Cambridge University Press.

49. Niesbert, R., & Ross, R. (1980). *Human inference.* Englewood Cliffs, NJ: Prentice Hall.

50. Neighbors, H. W. (1985). Seeking professional help for personal problems: Black Americans' use of health and mental health services. *Community Ment Health J, 21,* 156–166.

51. Snowden, L., & Cheung, F. (1990). Use of inpatient mental health services by members of ethnic minority groups. *Am Psychol, 45,* 347–355.

PART SEVEN

PROVIDER-PATIENT INTERACTION FACTORS

CHAPTER THIRTY-FIVE

Race, Gender, and Partnership in the Patient-Physician Relationship

Lisa Cooper-Patrick
Joseph J. Gallo
Junius J. Gonzales
Hong Thi Vu
Neil R. Powe
Christine Nelson
Daniel E. Ford

Studies have shown that African Americans and other minority patients often receive differential and less optimal technical health care than white Americans.[1-16] It is uncertain how much of this racial difference in health care and outcomes can be explained by patient cultural factors, health care professional biases, or health care system biases. Differences in socioeconomic status and health insurance coverage between patients only partially explain the observed racial differences in health care.[7,17,18]

Race and ethnicity have been cited as important cultural barriers in patient-physician communication.[19-22] However, cross-cultural factors in patient-physician communication are largely unexplored. Problems in communication due to cultural differences between patients and physicians often contribute to a disparity in the understanding that patients and physicians have regarding the cause of disease and the effectiveness of available treatments.[23,24] One study showed some enhancement of communication when physicians and patients belonged to the same ethnic group; however, the match between the physician and patient with

Originally presented at the twenty-first annual meeting of the Society of General Internal Medicine, Chicago, April 24, 1998. The work was partially supported by research grants from the Bayer Institute for Health Care Communication (West Haven, Connecticut), the Robert Wood Johnson Foundation (Princeton, New Jersey) Minority Medical Faculty Development Program (Dr. Cooper-Patrick), and grant 5U01MH54443 from the National Institute of Medical Health (Bethesda, Maryland).

respect to the explanatory model of illness and expectations for the visit were equally important in determining outcome.[25]

Few studies have related differences in the quality of interpersonal health care to patients' and physicians' ethnicity or to ethnic concordance or discordance in the patient-physician relationship. These studies have found that racial and ethnic differences between physicians and patients do influence physicians' communication and decision making.[8,26-29] In the Medical Outcomes Study, minority patients rated their physicians' decision-making styles as less participatory than nonminority patients did.[30]

Studies investigating the influence of patient gender on communication in the medical visit show that female patients generally receive more information, ask more questions, and have more partnership building with physicians than male patients.[28,31-33] Less is known about the communication style of female physicians. A few recent studies have shown that female physicians exhibit more empathy and engage in more positive talk, partnership building, question asking, and information giving compared with their male counterparts.[30,34-36]

The quality of interpersonal care is important to patients. Studies have shown that increasing patient involvement in care via negotiation and consensus seeking improves patient satisfaction and outcomes.[37-39] Specifically, visits in which the physician uses a participatory decision making (PDM) style are associated with higher levels of patient satisfaction.[40] Recent studies of patient-physician communication in primary care show the highest levels of patient satisfaction and the lowest levels of malpractice claims with the psychosocial pattern, which is characterized by psychosocial exchange and an almost equal distribution of patient and physician talk.[41-43]

Our study questions were as follows: (1) Do minority patients rate their physicians' decision-making styles as less participatory than white patients do? (2) Do the patients of minority physicians rate their physicians' decision-making styles as less participatory than the patients of white physicians do? and (3) What is the association between race and gender concordance or discordance in the patient-physician relationship and PDM style?

METHODS

Study Design and Population

The data for this analysis were collected in the baseline survey for a randomized clinical trial evaluating an intervention to improve care of primary care patients with depression. We identified all primary care practices with more than 200 enrollees from a large mixed-model independent practice association and network-style managed care organization (NYLCare) with primary care captivation in the Washington, DC, metropolitan area for our sample target. Washington, DC, and its Maryland suburbs have a large percentage of minorities compared with the national average. Additionally, this managed care organization has historically served geographic areas that have high African American patient and physician populations. Two-thirds of the practices agreed to participate, and 85 percent of those actually provided data. Patients from a total of thirty-two practices, representing general internal medicine and family practice, were interviewed. Most practices had fewer than five physicians. For larger practices, a maximum of five physicians was included. The physician sample included sixty-four primary care physicians. There were thirty-six white physicians (56 percent), sixteen African American physicians (25 percent), ten Asian physicians (15 percent), and two Latino physicians (3 percent). The physician sample included forty men (63 percent) and twenty-four women (37 percent).

The original sampling procedure for patients was for the office receptionist to identify all consecutive NYLCare patients who came to see the physician on recruitment days. Race and other patient demographics were not included in the sampling scheme. The mean and median number of patients contributed per physician was twenty-eight.

The study procedures were reviewed and approved by the Johns Hopkins Medical Institutions Joint Committee on Clinical Investigation. After giving informed consent, 2,481 patients (87 percent of those eligible) who were insured by the managed care organization, aged eighteen years or older, and had visited their primary care physician within the preceding two weeks were interviewed on the telephone between November 1996 and June 1998. No Medicare or Medicaid patients were enrolled in this managed care organization at the time of this study. Patients had to respond to the question about self-defined race/ethnicity and all three questions regarding PDM style to be included in this analysis. Of the 2,481 patients, 665 patients did not answer all three of the questions regarding PDM style or did not self-identify into a racial group. Therefore, there were 1,816 patients in our main analyses. Individuals with incomplete responses were slightly younger than the study respondents, more educated, less likely to have known their physician for at least one year, and had higher self-rated overall health status. Additionally, incomplete response rates were lower for African Americans (21 percent) than for whites (26 percent) and other races (26 percent) (χ^2, $p < .01$). There were no gender differences between the study respondents and those responding to fewer than three questions. More than 4,300 of the incomplete responders answered "I don't know" or "I am not sure" to at least one of the three questions. None of the characteristics of incomplete responders suggests these individuals did not understand the questions. Since our incomplete responders were more healthy and less likely to have known their physician for at least one year, it is likely that these patients did not have enough experiences with medical decisions upon which to base an evaluation of their physicians' partnership style. Fewer than ten patients refused to answer all three questions.

Study Variables

Our main independent variables included patient race/ethnicity, physician race/ethnicity, physician gender, and race and gender concordance or discordance in the patient-physician relationship. Covariates for the analyses included factors related to race and to PDM style in previous studies. Patient factors included age, gender, education, marital status, self-rated perceived health (using a 5-point scale from "poor" to "excellent"), and length of the patient-physician relationship.

Because patient satisfaction and PDM style have been highly associated in previous studies, we wanted to see if the association would be similarly strong within each racial group. The measure of patient satisfaction included questions about the patients' level of satisfaction with the following: (1) overall health care; (2) their physician's technical skills, such as thoroughness, carefulness, and competence; (3) their physician's explanation of their problem and its treatment; and (4) their physician's personal manner, including such things as courtesy, respect, sensitivity, and friendliness. Each question was scored on a scale from 0 to 4, from "not at all satisfied" to "extremely satisfied." The scores were added together, divided by 16, and multiplied by 100 to arrive at the satisfaction score.

Our main dependent variable was PDM style, originally described in 1995 by Kaplan and colleagues.[30] The PDM style is defined as the propensity of physicians to involve patients in treatment decisions and is measured as the aggregate of three items, each rated on a 5-point scale from 0 ("never") to 4 ("very often"), as follows: (1) "If there were a choice between treatments, how often would this doctor ask you to help make the decision?" (2) "How often does this doctor give you some control over your treatment?" and (3) "How often does this doctor ask you to take some of the responsibility for your treatment?" The highest possible score is 12. By convention, the raw score is divided by 12 and multiplied by 100 to arrive at a 0- to 100-point scale. A higher score means the visit was more participatory.

Analyses

Generalized estimating equations (GEEs) were used to analyze the relationships among PDM style and patient race/ethnicity, physician race/ethnicity, race and gender concordance or discordance in the patient-physician relationship, and all other covariates. The GEE method was preferred over linear regression because of its ability to account for the clustering effects of any existing within-physician correlation and the different number of patients per physician while producing valid and robust results.[44,45] In the multivariate model, we adjusted for patient age, gender, education, marital status, health status, and length of the patient-physician relationship. In subsequent models, we also included physician gender and race.

We also used GEEs to study the relationship between patient satisfaction and PDM style for the overall sample and by patient race/ethnicity. We explored unadjusted and adjusted models.

RESULTS

Characteristics of Study Sample

Characteristics of the patient sample are shown in Table 35.1. About half the patients had been seeing their physician for more than three years. The mean overall health status was 77.2 on a 0- to 100-point scale, with approximately 60 percent reporting that they felt their health was very good or excellent. Approximately 60 percent of the patients were seeing a male physician and 40 percent were seeing a female physician. Almost half the patients were seeing white physicians, 27 percent were seeing African American physicians, and 26 percent were seeing physicians of other races. There were statistically significant differences among patient race/ethnic groups in several variables. Compared to white patients, African American patients were slightly older, more likely to be women, less likely to be married, less educated, had poorer perceived health, and were more likely to see African American physicians (Table 35.1).

Relationship of Patient Characteristics to PDM Style

Several patient factors were associated with PDM style in unadjusted analyses. Patients aged forty to sixty-five years rated their visits as more participatory than patients younger than thirty years did. Patients with a graduate school education had more participatory visits than those with a high school education or less. Patients with better ratings of their own health status had more participatory visits with physicians. Patients who knew their physician for three years or longer rated their visits as more participatory than patients who knew their physician for less than one year. In this sample, there were no differences in PDM style ratings by patient gender or marital status (Table 35.2).

Relationship of Patient Race to PDM Style

There were significant differences in PDM scores among patient racial groups in unadjusted analyses. African Americans and other minority patients rated their physicians as having lower PDM scores than did white patients. In models adjusting for patient age, gender, education, marital status, health status, and length of the patient-physician relationship, African Americans had significantly

Table 35.1. Characteristics of Patient Sample

	Total (N = 1816)	Race/Ethnic Group		
		White (n = 784)	African American (n = 814)	Other (n = 218)
Age, years				
18–29	15	19	12	16*
30–39	28	25	29	31
40–49	32	30	33	31
50–65	25	26	25	22
Gender				
Male	34	39	28	41†
Female	66	61	72	59
Education				
High school or less	36	27	45	35†
Some college	24	22	27	22
College graduate	21	26	15	26
Graduate school	19	25	13	17
Marital status				
Married	55	60	47	68†
Separated/divorced/ widowed	19	15	24	12
Never married	26	24	29	20
Self-rated health status				
Poor/fair	11	7	14	8†
Good	28	26	31	30
Very good	40	43	37	39
Excellent	21	24	18	23
Length of relationship with primary care physician, years				
<1	20	18	20	25†
1–3	28	26	28	37
>3	52	55	52	38
Race of physician seen				
White	47	67	30	39†
African American	27	13	43	16
Other	26	19	26	46
Gender of physician seen				
Male	61	66	56	61
Female	39	34	44	39

Note: All data are percentages.

*Differences among racial/ethnic groups, χ^2, $p \leq .01$.

†Differences among racial/ethnic groups, χ^2, $p \leq .001$.

Table 35.2. Relationship of Patient Characteristics to Participatory Decision-Making (PDM) Style

	No. of Patients	PDM Style Score, Mean (SE)	p
Age, years			
18–29	278	72.7 (1.3)	Reference
30–39	514	73.5 (1.6)	.61
40–49	577	76.8 (1.5)	.008
50–65	433	77.5 (1.6)	.003
Gender			
Male	626	75.2 (1.0)	Reference
Female	1,190	75.4 (1.0)	.84
Education			
High school or less	653	74.2 (1.0)	Reference
Some college	438	74.8 (1.3)	.63
College graduate	381	75.8 (1.4)	.25
Graduate school	338	77.9 (1.4)	.008
Marital status			
Married	1,003	75.6 (0.8)	Reference
Separated/divorced/ widowed	338	76.5 (1.2)	.51
Never married	469	73.8 (1.3)	.13
Self-rated health status			
Poor/fair	194	71.4 (1.6)	Reference
Good	517	73.8 (1.8)	.004
Very good	720	76.2 (1.7)	.001
Excellent	379	77.9 (1.9)	.001
Length of relationship with primary care physician, years			
<1	360	73.9 (1.2)	Reference
1–3	516	74.0 (1.5)	.95
>3	933	76.8 (1.4)	.04

Note: The PDM style score is based on 3 questions and ranked on a 0- to 100-point scale. Higher scores mean the physician is more participatory. *p* values are from generalized estimating equations.

less participatory visits than whites. Asian, Latino, and other minority patients also rated their physicians as less participatory, but the results did not achieve statistical significance. Adding physician gender and physician race to the model attenuated the relationship between PDM style and patient race; however, African American patients still rated their visits as less participatory than white patients did (Table 35.3).

Table 35.3. Relationship of Patient Race to Participatory Decision-Making (PDM) Style

Patient Race	No. of Patients	Model 1* Unadjusted Score, Mean (SE)	p	Model 2† Adjusted Score, Mean (SE)	p	Model 3‡ Adjusted Score, Mean (SE)	p	Model 4§ Adjusted Score, Mean (SE)	p
White	784	77.1 (0.9)	Reference	60.6 (3.3)	Reference	59.3 (3.3)	Reference	59.8 (3.4)	Reference
African American	814	73.9 (1.2)	.007	58.0 (1.2)	.03	56.6 (1.2)	.02	57.5 (1.2)	.07
Other minority	218	73.8 (1.7)	.05	58.3 (1.7)	.17	56.9 (1.7)	.17	57.9 (1.7)	.26

Note: The PDM style score is based on 3 questions and ranked on a 0- to 100-point scale. Higher scores mean the physician is more participatory. *p* values are from generalized estimating equations.

*PDM score by patient race (unadjusted).

†Adjusted for patients' age, gender, education, marital status, and length of the patient-physician relationship.

‡Adjusted for patients' age, gender, education, marital status, health status, length of the patient-physician relationship, and physician gender.

§Adjusted for patients' age, gender, education, marital status, health status, length of the patient-physician relationship, physician gender, and physician race.

Relationship of Physician Race and Gender to PDM Style

There were no significant differences between minority and white physicians with respect to patient ratings of PDM style in unadjusted analyses. Similarly, in analyses adjusting for patients' age, education, health status, and length of the patient-physician relationship, there were no significant differences between minority and white physicians with respect to PDM style. However, physician gender was related to PDM style. Female physicians had more participatory visits with their patients than male physicians in adjusted analyses (Table 35.4).

Relationship of Race and Gender Concordance or Discordance to PDM Style

To study the potential influence of race concordance or discordance between physicians and patients on PDM style, we stratified patients according to the race/ethnicity of their physicians and measured the relationship between PDM style and patient race within each physician race group, adjusting for patient age, gender, education, marital status, health status, and length of the relationship. African American patients had significantly less participatory visits with white physicians than white patients did ($\beta = -4.3$, SE $= 1.7$, $p < .02$, adjusted). Asian and Latino patients had less participatory visits with African American physicians than African American patients did; however, these results were based on very small sample sizes. There were no significant racial differences in PDM scores among patients seeing Asian or Latino physicians.

Table 35.4. Relationship of Physician Characteristics to Participatory Decision-Making (PDM) Style

Characteristic	No. of Patients	Model 1* Unadjusted Score, Mean (SE)	*p*	Model 2† Adjusted Score, Mean (SE)	*p*
Physician race					
White	860	76.3 (1.0)	Reference	61.7 (3.1)	Reference
African American	489	74.2 (1.7)	.23	59.2 (1.7)	.13
Other minority	467	74.3 (1.8)	.28	59.9 (1.7)	.30
Physician gender					
Female	707	76.9 (1.4)	.09	62.4 (1.3)	.03
Male	1,109	74.5 (0.8)	Reference	59.5 (3.1)	Reference

Note: The PDM style score is based on 3 questions and ranked on a 0- to 100-point scale. Higher scores mean the physician is more participatory. *p* values are from generalized estimating equations.

*PDM score by physician race or physician gender (unadjusted).

†Adjusted for patients' age, gender, education, marital status, health status, and length of the patient-physician relationship.

However, there were only two Latino physicians in the study sample; therefore, reliable conclusions regarding the PDM style of Latino physicians cannot be drawn (data not shown).

To explore the overall significance of racial and ethnic concordance in the patient-physician relationship, we conducted an analysis to assess the relationship between race/ethnic concordance between physicians and patients and PDM style. Because of previously described relationships between physician gender and PDM style, we looked at the effect of both race and gender concordance or discordance. Patients in race-concordant relationships with their physicians rated their physicians as significantly more participatory than patients in race-discordant relationships ($\beta = +2.6$, SE $= 1.1$, $p < .02$, adjusted). Gender concordance between physicians and patients was not significantly related to PDM style (Table 35.5). Participatory decision-making style was highest in relationships that were race and gender concordant ($\beta = +4.3$, SE $= 1.5$, $p < .01$, adjusted) compared with relationships that were race and gender discordant (data not shown).

Patient Satisfaction and PDM Style

Patient satisfaction with technical and interpersonal aspects of care was highly associated with PDM score ($\beta = +0.5$, SE $= 0.02$, $p < .001$, adjusted). The relationship between patient satisfaction ratings and PDM style was similar for all racial groups. Asian and Latino patients, but not African American patients, were significantly less satisfied than whites. Patient gender was not related to satisfaction. Both race concordance and gender concordance were significantly and positively associated with patient satisfaction.

COMMENT

In this study, African American patients had significantly less participatory visits with their physicians than white patients did. This finding persisted after adjusting for potential confounders in the relationship between patient race and physician decision-making style. There were no significant differences between minority and white physicians with respect to patient ratings of PDM style. Female physicians had more participatory visits with patients than male physicians. Patients in race-concordant relationships with their physicians rated their physicians as significantly more participatory than patients in race-discordant relationships. Gender concordance was not significantly related to PDM style. The data suggest that all patients prefer participatory visits, as patient satisfaction was highly associated with PDM score for patients in all ethnic groups.

This study adds to a growing body of research indicating that ethnic differences between physicians and patients are often barriers to partnership and

Table 35.5. Relationship of Race and Gender Concordance in the Patient-Physician Relationship to Participatory Decision-Making (PDM) Style

Concordant Status	No. of Patients	Model 1*		Model 2†		Model 3‡	
		Unadjusted Score, Mean (SE)	p	Adjusted Score, Mean (SE)	p	Adjusted Score, Mean (SE)	p
Race concordant	958	76.6 (1.1)	.02	62.6 (1.1)	.05	61.1 (1.1)	.02
Race discordant	858	74.0 (0.9)	Reference	60.4 (2.9)	Reference	58.5 (3.0)	Reference
Gender concordant	949	76.0 (1.0)	.12	62.2 (1.0)	.12	63.3 (1.0)	.11
Gender discordant	867	74.5 (0.9)	Reference	60.7 (3.2)	Reference	61.7 (3.0)	Reference

Note: The PDM style score is based on 3 questions and ranked on a 0- to 100-point scale. Higher scores mean the physician is more participatory. *p* values are from generalized estimating equations.

*Adjusted for patients' age, gender, education, marital status, health status, and length of the patient-physician relationship.

†Adjusted for patients' age, gender, education, marital status, health status, and length of the patient-physician relationship.

‡Adjusted for patients' age, gender, education, marital status, health status, length of the patient-physician relationship, and physician gender (race-concordant analysis) or physician race (gender-concordant analysis).

*PDM score by race- or gender-concordant status (unadjusted).

effective communication.[19–22,30] A number of physician factors may account for these problems. First, physicians may unintentionally incorporate racial biases, such as racial and ethnic stereotypes, into their interpretation of patients' symptoms, predictions of patients' behaviors, and medical decision making.[46] Second, physicians may lack understanding of patients' ethnic and cultural disease models or attributions of symptoms. A third possibility is that physicians are often not aware of or have expectations of the visit that differ from patients' expectations. There are also patient factors that might contribute to less participatory visits. Factors such as language barriers, low health literacy and educational status, and lack of self-efficacy regarding managing one's health may be more prevalent among ethnic minority patients.

Why do patients seeing physicians of the same ethnic background as themselves rate their physicians as more participatory? Physicians and patients belonging to the same race or ethnic group are more likely to share cultural beliefs, values, and experiences in the society, allowing them to communicate more effectively and to feel more comfortable with one another. Previous research has suggested that socioeconomic differences, rather than racial or ethnic differences, might serve as more important communication barriers between physicians and patients.[31,36] Our study does not support this finding, since African American and other minority patients had less participatory visits with white physicians, regardless of educational level. It is possible that shared cultural experiences and values between patients and physicians offset the effects of differences in socioeconomic status on communication. The physicians in race-concordant visits may have actually used more partnership-building communication in their encounters with patients, or the patients may have simply perceived the communication that way. Regardless of the objective findings, patient perceptions are still important and do influence patient behavior. Since communication is both verbal and nonverbal, analyzing audiotapes and videotapes of racially concordant and discordant visits might help to further clarify this issue.

In our study, patients of female physicians had more participatory visits than patients of male physicians; however, gender concordance between physicians and patients was not significantly related to PDM style. It is unclear whether these findings are the results of patient selection or socialization of women physicians. Previous work has shown that both physician and patient gender may be important determinants of PDM style, other aspects of interpersonal care, and medical decision making.[30–32,34,35,46–48]

Small numeric differences in adjusted style scores of the magnitude presented in this study are likely to be meaningful with respect to patient care. Previous studies have shown that small differences in patient ratings of care can have an important impact on patient behavior. In the Medical Outcomes Study, differences of 2 points in the PDM style score were related to a 10 percentage point difference in the likelihood that patients would leave a physician's practice in the next twelve months.[30] Our study showed differences in PDM scores between minority and white patients, patients of female and male physicians, and race-concordant and race-discordant relationships, of between 2 and 4 points. Based on results from previous studies, it is likely that these differences would be related to important differences in patient behavior.

This study has several strengths. First, the percentage of middle-class African American patients and physicians is larger than in previous studies. Second, all the study subjects had the same managed care insurance coverage, which minimizes the possibility of confounding due to racial and ethnic differences in socioeconomic status. Third, we had good measures of potential confounders between PDM style and patient race, such as patient age, gender, education, health status, and length of the patient-physician relationship.

There are also limitations. First, this was an observational study, and patients were not assigned to physicians in a randomized fashion. For example, patients who favor a more participatory decision-making style might be more likely to choose female physicians or physicians of their own ethnicity. Second, PDM style relies on patient self-report, and a high percentage of patients did not respond to all three questions. However, in a recent study, physician conversation styles measured by audiotape corresponded with patient measures of PDM style.[49] In separate analyses that included individuals who answered at least two questions (giving them a PDM score based on 8 points), our results were not changed. Third, it would have been useful to have other physician or practice measures known to affect physician communication, such as the practice volume. Unfortunately, this information was not available for most of the physicians in our sample.

What are the implications of this study for clinical practice, medical education, and health policy? One strategy to improve access to care for ethnic minority patients is to increase their participation in care. A multifaceted approach should include patient and physician interventions to improve cross-cultural communication in primary care settings. Interventions that empower ethnic minority patients to become more informed and active consumers of health care should be developed and evaluated. Additionally, since minority physicians are more likely to practice in areas with a high concentration of poor and minority patients, the study supports the argument for increasing the numbers of minority physicians in the workforce.[50-52] Furthermore, communication training programs for medical students, residents, practicing physicians, and health professionals of all ethnic backgrounds should include an emphasis on understanding and addressing the needs of a patient population that is becoming more culturally diverse. Cultural competence is described as the demonstrated awareness, inclusion, and integration of three population-specific issues in the delivery of health care: (1) health-related beliefs and cultural values, (2) disease incidence and prevalence, and (3) treatment efficacy.[53] Health care organizations interested in fostering cultural competence should incorporate evidence-based medicine as well as the viewpoints of ethnic minority patients, patients with low levels of education and literacy, patients with poor health status, and other vulnerable populations. Improving cross-cultural communication in health care settings may lead to more patient involvement in care, more adherence to recommended treatment, higher quality of care, and better health outcomes.

Notes

1. Wenneker, J. B., & Epstein, A. M. (1989). Racial inequalities in the use of procedures for patients with ischemic heart disease in Massachusetts. *JAMA, 261,* 253–257.

2. Carlisle, D. M., Leake, B. D., & Shapiro, M. F. (1995). Racial and ethnic differences in the use of invasive cardiac procedures among cardiac patients in Los Angeles County, 1986 through 1988. *Am J Public Health, 85,* 352–356.

3. Kjellstrand, C. M. (1988). Age, sex, and race inequality in renal transplantation. *Arch Intern Med, 148,* 1305–1309.

4. Yergan, J., Flood, A. B., LoGerfo, J. P., & Diehr, P. (1987). Relationship between patient race and intensity of hospital services. *Med Care, 25,* 592–603.

5. Blendon, R. J., Aiken, L. H., Freeman, H. E., & Corey, C. R. (1989). Access to medical care for black and white Americans: A matter of continuing concern. *JAMA, 261,* 278–281.

6. Schwartz, E., Kofie, V. Y., Rivo, M., & Tuckson, R. V. (1990). Black/white comparisons of deaths preventable by medical intervention: United States and the District of Columbia, 1980–1986. *Int J Epidemiol, 19,* 591–598.

7. Weissman, J. S., Stern, R., Fielding, S. L., & Epstein, A. M. (1991). Delayed access to health care: Risk factors, reasons, and consequences. *Ann Intern Med, 114,* 325–331.

8. Pappas, G., Queen, S., Hadden, W., & Fisher, G. (1993). The increasing disparity in mortality between socioeconomic groups in the United States, 1960 and 1986. *N Engl J Med, 329,* 103–109.

9. Scheffler, R. M., & Miller, A. B. (1989). Demand analysis of mental health service use among ethnic subpopulations. *Inquiry, 26,* 202–215.

10. Hu, T. W., Snowden, L. R., Jerrell, J. M., & Nguyen, T. D. (1991). Ethnic populations in public mental health: Services choice and level of use. *Am J Public Health, 81,* 1429–1434.

11. Williams, S. J., Diehr, P., & Ducker, W. L. (1979). Mental health services: Utilization by low-income enrollees in a prepaid group practice plan and in an independent practice plan. *Med Care, 17,* 139–151.

12. Sussman, L. K., Robins, L. N., & Earl, F. (1987). Treatment-seeking for depression by black and white Americans. *Soc Sci Med, 24,* 187–196.

13. Vernon, S. W., & Roberts, R. E. (1982). Prevalence of treated and untreated psychiatric disorders in three ethnic groups. *Soc Sci Med, 16,* 1575–1582.

14. Whittle, J., Conigliaro, J., Good, C. B., & Lofgren, R. P. (1993). Racial differences in the use of invasive cardiovascular procedures in the Department of Veterans Affairs Medical System. *N Engl J Med, 329,* 621–627.

15. Kahn, K. L., Pearson, M. L., Harrison, E. R., et al. (1994). Health care for black and poor hospitalized Medicare patients. *JAMA, 271,* 1169–1174.

16. Lee, J. A., Gehlbach, S., Hosmer, D., Reti, M., & Baker, C. S. (1997). Medicare treatment differences for blacks and whites. *Med Care, 35,* 1173–1189.

17. Rask, K. J., Williams, M. V., Parker, R. M., & McNagny, S. E. (1994). Obstacles predicting lack of a regular provider and delays in seeking care for patients at an urban public hospital. *JAMA, 271,* 1931–1933.

18. Hayward, R. A., Bernard, A. M., Freeman, H. E., & Corey, C. R. (1990). Regular source of ambulatory care and access to health services. *Am J Public Health, 81,* 434–438.

19. Kleinman, A., Eisenberg, L., & Good, B. (1978). Culture, illness, and care: Clinical lessons from anthropologic and cross-cultural research. *Ann Intern Med, 88,* 251–258.

20. Lurie, N., & Yergan, J. (1990). Teaching residents to care for vulnerable populations in the outpatient setting. *J Gen Intern Med, 5,* S27–S34.

21. Mull, J. D. (1993). Cross-cultural communication in the physician's office. *West J Med, 159,* 609–613.

22. Quill, T. E. (1989). Recognizing and adjusting to barriers in doctor-patient communication. *Ann Intern Med, 111,* 51–57.

23. Roter, D. L., & Hall, J. (1992). *Doctors talking with patients, patients talking with doctors: Improving communication in medical visits.* Westport, CT: Auburn House.

24. Mathews, J. J. (1983). The communication process in clinical settings. *Soc Sci Med, 17,* 1371–1378.

25. Lin, E. H. (1983). Intraethnic characteristics and the patient-physician interaction: "Cultural Blind Spot Syndrome." *J Fam Pract, 16,* 91–98.

26. Levy, D. R. (1985). White doctors and black patients: Influence of race on the doctor-patient relationship. *Pediatrics, 75,* 639–643.

27. Eisenberg, J. M. (1979). Sociologic influences on decision-making by clinicians. *Ann Intern Med, 90,* 957–964.

28. Hooper, E. M., Comstock, L. M., Goodwin, J. M., & Goodwin, J. S. (1982). Patient characteristics that influence physician behavior. *Med Care, 20,* 630–638.

29. McKinlay, J. B., Potter, D. A., & Feldman, H. A. (1996). Nonmedical influences on medical decision-making. *Soc Sci Med, 42,* 769–776.

30. Kaplan, S. H., Gandek, B., Greenfield, S., et al. (1995). Patient and visit characteristics related to physicians' participatory decision-making style: Results from the Medical Outcomes Study. *Med Care, 33,* 1176–1187.

31. Pendleton, D. A. (1980). The communication of medical information in general practice consultations as a function of patients' social class. *Soc Sci Med, 14A,* 669–673.

32. Hall, J. A., Roter, D. L., & Katz, N. R. (1988). Meta-analysis of correlates of provider behavior in medical encounters. *Med Care, 26,* 657–675.

33. Verbrugge, L. M., & Steiner, R. P. (1981). Physician treatment of men and women patients: Sex bias or appropriate care? *Med Care, 19,* 609–632.

34. Roter, D., Lipkin, M., & Korsgaardt, A. (1991). Sex differences in patients' and physicians' communication during primary care medical visits. *Med Care, 29,* 1083–1093.

35. van den Brink-Muinen, A., Bensing, J. M., & Kerssens, J. J. (1998). Gender and communication style in general practice: Differences between women's health care and regular health care. *Med Care, 36,* 100–106.

36. Wasserman, R. C., Inui, T. S., Barriatua, R. D., Carter, W. B., & Lippincott, P. (1984). Pediatric clinicians' support for parents makes a difference: An outcome-based analysis of clinician-parent interaction. *Pediatrics, 74,* 1047–1053.

37. Barsky, A. J., Kazis, L. E., Freiden, R. B., et al. (1980). Evaluating the interview in primary care medicine. *Soc Sci Med, 14A,* 653–658.

38. Greenfield, S., Kaplan, S., & Ware, J. E. (1985). Expanding patient involvement in care. *Ann Intern Med, 102,* 520–528.

39. Kaplan, S. H., Greenfield, S., & Ware, J. E. (1989). Assessing the effects of physician-patient interactions on the outcomes of chronic disease. *Med Care, 27,* S110–S127.

40. Kaplan, S. H., Greenfield, S., Gandek, B., et al. (1996). Characteristics of physicians with participatory decision-making styles. *Ann Intern Med, 124,* 497–504.

41. Bertakis, K. D., Roter, D., & Putnam, S. M. (1991). The relationship of physician medical interview style to patient satisfaction. *J Fam Pract, 32,* 175–181.

42. Roter, D. L., Stewart, M., Putnam, S. M., Lipkin, M., Stiles, W., & Inui, T. S. (1997). Communication patterns of primary care physicians. *JAMA, 277,* 350–356.

43. Levinson, W., Roter, D. L., Mullooly, J. P., Dull, V. T., & Frankel, R. M. (1997). Physician-patient communication: The relationship with malpractice claims among primary care physicians and surgeons. *JAMA, 277,* 553–559.

44. Zeger, S. L., & Liang, K. (1986). Longitudinal data analysis for discrete and continuous outcomes. *Biometrics, 42,* 121–130.

45. Liang, K., & Zeger, S. L. (1986). Longitudinal data analysis using generalized linear models. *Biometrika, 73,* 13–22.

46. Schulman, K. A., Berlin, J. A., Harless, W., et al. (1999). The effect of race and sex on physicians' recommendations for cardiac catheterization. *N Engl J Med, 340,* 618–626.

47. Roter, D. L., Hall, J. A., & Katz, N. R. (1988). Patient-physician communication: A descriptive summary of the literature. *Patient Educ Couns, 12,* 99–119.

48. Elderkin-Thompson, V., & Waitzkin, H. (1999). Differences in clinical communication by gender. *J Gen Intern Med, 14,* 112–121.

49. Kaplan, S. H., Greenfield, S., & Montminy, J. (1992). Training private practice physicians to negotiate treatment decisions: Results of a randomized controlled trial [Abstract]. *Clin Res, 40,* 614A.

50. Komaromy, M., Grumbach, K., Frake, M., et al. (1996). The role of black and Hispanic physicians in providing health care for underserved populations. *N Engl J Med, 334,* 1305–1310.

51. Moy, E., & Bartman, B. A. (1995). Physician race and care of minority and medically indigent patients. *JAMA, 273,* 1515–1520.

52. Carlisle, D. M., & Gardner, J. E. (1998). The entry of African-American students into U.S. medical schools: An evaluation of recent trends. *J Natl Med Assoc 90,* 466–473.

53. Lavizzo-Mourey, R., & Mackenzie, E. R. (1996). Cultural competence: Essential measurements of quality for managed care organizations. *Ann Intern Med, 124,* 919–921.

CHAPTER THIRTY-SIX

Patient-Physician Racial Concordance and the Perceived Quality and Use of Health Care

Somnath Saha
Miriam Komaromy
Thomas D. Koepsell
Andrew B. Bindman

Numerous studies have demonstrated racial inequalities in health care in the United States. Specifically, minority populations have less access to care,[1-6] use fewer health care resources,[6-8] and are less satisfied with the care they receive[3,5] than the majority white population. Differences in health insurance coverage do not fully explain these disparities.[1,4,8]

Racial inequalities in health care may be partly attributable to racial, cultural, and communication barriers between minority patients and white health care providers.[9-12] Such barriers might arise from cultural or linguistic incongruity between patient and physician, from lack of mutual trust, or from racial discrimination. If these barriers existed, one might expect patients and physicians of similar racial or ethnic background to have better communication and more salubrious relationships than those of dissimilar background. Better relations might in turn lead to greater patient satisfaction and more effective use of the health care system. While this reasoning seems plausible, little empirical evidence exists to support it. We therefore sought to determine the extent to which racial concordance between patient and physician affects patients' ratings and reported use of health care.

This work was supported by the Robert Wood Johnson Clinical Scholars Program and the Department of Veterans Affairs.

METHODS

Data Source

We analyzed data from the Commonwealth Fund's Minority Health Survey, a telephone survey of noninstitutionalized adults in the forty-eight contiguous United States. Interviews were conducted between May and July 1994 in six different languages, using an interviewer-administered, computer-assisted telephone interviewing system. Data from this survey contained information regarding individuals' health care access and utilization, regular physicians, health status, and demographics.

Sampling was designed to obtain approximately 1,000 white, 1,000 black, and 1,000 Hispanic subjects. Random digit dialing using a three-stage, stratified-sampling process was used to ensure proper representation of households in different regions of the country and in central-city, suburban, and rural areas. After achieving the desired number of white respondents in initial cross-sections, oversamples of black and Hispanic Americans were obtained by screening additional national cross-sections and interviewing only members of those minority groups, until the desired sample sizes had been achieved. Additionally, interviews were conducted with Chinese, Vietnamese, and Korean Americans drawn from list samples, based on surnames listed in telephone directories.[13]

Of 10,576 individuals contacted, 5,776 (55 percent) agreed to participate. The eligibility status and characteristics of nonparticipants were not known. Of those agreeing to participate, 1,684 (29 percent) were ineligible either because they were not among the targeted racial groups or because the quota for their racial groups had been filled. Of 4,092 respondents known to be eligible, 3,789 (93 percent) completed interviews.

The 626 Asian respondents consisted, by sampling design, almost exclusively of Chinese, Vietnamese, and Korean Americans, and were not representative of Asian Americans in general. They were therefore excluded from our analysis, as were the 19 American Indians and the 24 respondents who did not identify their race.

Predictor Variable

Racial Concordance. After classifying themselves as Hispanic or non-Hispanic, respondents were asked to indicate their race as well as their national origin. Respondents were also asked if they had a regular physician to whom they usually went when they needed health care. Those who responded affirmatively identified their physicians' race. Based on these responses, we categorized individuals and their physicians into the following groups: non-Hispanic white, non-Hispanic black, and Hispanic. We considered racial concordance to be present when respondent and physician were in the same group.

Response Variables. We examined the association of racial concordance with responses to questions in the following four categories: ratings of physician, satisfaction with health care, receipt of preventive care, and receipt of needed medical care (Table 36.1).

Covariates. We examined potential confounding variables in four domains: sociodemographic factors, access to care, sources of care, and health and well-being. Sociodemographic variables included age, sex, marital status, urbanicity, geographic region, education, employment status, household income, home ownership, receipt of public assistance, primary language (English versus other), birthplace (United States versus other), and number of years in the United States (for immigrants). Access variables included health insurance type, convenience of physician's office hours and location, and major barriers faced when seeking medical care: transportation, cost, waiting time, difficulty getting an appointment, and poor access to specialty care. Variables related to sources of care included usual care site, ability to choose one's care site, health maintenance

---

Table 36.1. Questions Assessing Patient Satisfaction and Use of Health Care

Ratings of Physician
    How would you rate your regular physician on the job he or she is doing in
        Providing you with good health care overall?*
        Treating you with dignity and respect?*
        Making sure you understand what you have been told about your medical
            problems or medication?*
        Listening to your health concerns and taking them seriously?*
        Being accessible either by telephone or in person?*
        Overall, how satisfied are you with your regular physician?[†]
        All things considered, would you recommend your physician to a friend?[‡]
Satisfaction with health care
    Overall, how satisfied are you with the quality of your health care services?[†]
Receipt of preventive care
    In the past 12 months have you received preventive care (such as blood
        pressure tests, Papanicolaou smears, or cholesterol level readings)?[§]
Receipt of needed medical care
    In the past 12 months
        Was there a time when you needed medical care but did not get it?[§]
        Have you ever put off or postponed seeking health care which you felt you
           needed?[§]

---

*"Excellent," "good," "fair," or "poor."

[†]"Very satisfied," "somewhat satisfied," "somewhat dissatisfied," or "very dissatisfied."

[‡]"Very strongly," "somewhat strongly," or "not at all."

[§]"Yes" or "no."

organization membership, number of physicians seen over the last year, physician specialty (generalist versus other), ability to choose one's regular physician, physician sex, and patient-physician sex concordance. Variables related to health and well-being included self-perceived health status, number of health care visits during the last year, hospitalization within the last year, and a psychological score derived from five questions measuring psychological distress and well-being.[14]

Data Analysis

For bivariate comparisons of respondents with racially concordant versus non-concordant physicians, we used t tests for continuous variables and the Pearson χ^2 test for binary and categorical variables. Ordered response variables were dichotomized between the highest rating and all other ratings (for example, excellent versus other).

To adjust for covariates we used logistic regression analysis. We selected a uniform set of covariates for all responses within a given category (for example, ratings of physician) through the following model-building strategy. We built regression models for the association between racial concordance and each response variable within each racial group. All models included age, sex, insurance type, primary care site, and self-perceived health status. Other covariates were included if their elimination from a model containing other variables in the same covariate domain (for example, sociodemographic factors) changed the odds ratio (OR) estimate for the association being examined by 10 percent or more. Covariates that changed the OR estimate for one response variable within a category were used in the final models for all response variables in that category, and covariates that changed the estimate for one racial group were used for all racial groups. Interactions of racial concordance with respondents' education, income, language, and nationality were examined. All analyses were stratified by respondents' race.

We also conducted further analyses to explore potential reasons for observed associations. We first repeated all our analyses while adjusting for respondents' reported experience of racial discrimination within and outside medical are settings. Next, we repeated our analyses after excluding those respondents who stated that their choice of regular physician was influenced by the physician's race or ethnicity. We conducted these analyses to determine whether respondents who were "race-conscious," and who therefore might be expected to have better relationships with physicians of their own race, accounted for observed associations between racial concordance and our response variables.

To address the possibility that any observed associations were confounded by differences in health plans or in physicians' office staffs, we repeated our analyses adjusting for respondents' satisfaction with their health plans and with the helpfulness of their physicians' office staff.

Finally, to address the concern that significant associations between racial concordance and our ordered response variables might be a result of our dichotomizations, we used linear regression analysis to test the relationship between racial concordance and our ordered measures modeled as continuous variables. (All data were analyzed using SPSS for Windows [Release 7.0; SPSS Inc., Chicago].)

RESULTS

Characteristics of Respondents

A total of 3,120 white, black, and Hispanic individuals completed the survey. Nine percent of black respondents were of Caribbean heritage. Hispanics were primarily of Mexican (53 percent) and Puerto Rican (16 percent) descent.

A total of 2,331 respondents (75 percent) had a regular physician. Whites were more likely than nonwhites to have a regular physician (82 percent versus 71 percent; $p < .001$). Among the 2,201 respondents who were able to identify their physician's race, whites were much more likely than nonwhites to have a racially concordant physician (88 percent versus 22 percent; $p < .001$) (Figure 36.1). Nonconcordant physicians for blacks and Hispanics were primarily white (82 percent) and Asian (14 percent).

Within each racial group, respondents with racially concordant and nonconcordant physicians were similar with regard to most of our covariates (Table 36.2). We used multivariate analysis to adjust for differences.

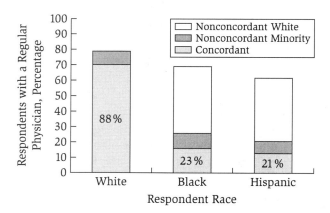

Figure 36.1 Racial Concordance Between Respondents and Their Regular Physicians.

Note: Percentages shown within bars indicate proportions of regular physicians who are racially concordant with respondents.

Table 36.2. Characteristics of Respondents by Racial Concordance with Physician

Characteristics	White		Black		Hispanic	
	Yes (n = 779)	No (n = 102)	Yes (n = 162)	No (n = 534)	Yes (n = 133)	No (n = 491)
Mean age, years	49.1	52.4	43.8	46.3	40.7	40.7
Male	50	46	45	46	38	47*
Married/live with partner	64	58	47	48	59	64
High school graduate	91	87	83	85	79	87*
Household income ≤$15,000	17	19	20	24	24	18
Homeowner	77	77	56	58	59	63
On public assistance	4	7	7	10	9	8
Unemployed	2	3	4	4	5	6
Region						
West	19	27	7	11	26	43*
Midwest	26	29	15	15	2	9
South	32	20	47	50	56	28
Northeast	23	25	31	23	17	20
Urbanicity						
Urban	30	23	64	48*	64	48*
Suburban	44	52	24	29	25	39
Rural	26	26	12	23	11	14
English as primary language	99	99	98	98	52	75*
Born in United States	97	95	93	93	57	70*
In United States <10 years	0	0	1	1	3	2

(Continued)

Table 36.2. Characteristics of Respondents by Racial Concordance with Physician (Continued)

Characteristics	White		Black		Hispanic	
	Yes (n = 779)	No (n = 102)	Yes (n = 162)	No (n = 534)	Yes (n = 133)	No (n = 491)
Insurance type						
Private	69	62	70	66	68	76
Medicare	25	30	20	22	9	9*
Medicaid	7	11	10	15	11	8
None	5	3	7	6	17	9
Physician's office hours/location very convenient	70	64	75	68	73	67
Major access barriers						
Transportation	3	5	3	5	5	6
Cost	21	19	19	27	33	28
Waiting time	13	13	17	17	24	20
Getting appointments	7	7	6	10	12	13
Poor access to specialists	6	9	9	9	13	14
Primary care site						
Physician's office or HMO	88	84	81	78	84	83
Hospital OPD or public clinic	9	8	11	13	13	13
Emergency department	4	8	8	9	4	4
Chose primary care site	88	88	82	77	78	83
HMO member	23	39*	39	29*	20	36*

	2.2	2.3	2.0	2.0	2.1	2.0
No. of physicians seen, last 12 months mean	2.2	2.3	2.0	2.0	2.1	2.0
Chose regular physician	94	90	92	88	93	88
Choice influenced by physician's race/ethnicity	3	5	25	10*	21	5*
Female physician	13	18	20	17	13	19
Patient-physician gender concordance	55	50	50	53	46	57*
Generalist physician[†]	82	86	83	83	77	81
Fair/poor health status	16	24*	18	24	25	19
Health care visits, last 12 months mean	5.5	5.8	4.8	6.0*	4.4	5.7
Hospitalized, last 12 months	16	16	11	15	12	11
Psychological distress[‡]						
Low	33	36	33	37	32	30
Medium	38	33	41	31	31	36
High	29	30	27	32	38	35

Note: Values are percentages, unless otherwise indicated; HMO = health maintenance organization; OPD = outpatient department.

*$p < .05$ for comparison between race-specific concordant and nonconcordant groups.

[†]Internal medicine, family practice, or obstetrics/gynecology.

[‡]Possible scores from responses to 5 items, ranging from 0 (low distress, high sense of well-being) to 25 (high distress, low sense of well-being). Cutoff points for low, medium, and high distress categories were determined by tertiles of score for the entire sample.

Satisfaction with Physicians and Health Care

In unadjusted comparisons, blacks with racially concordant as opposed to non-concordant physicians more often rated their physicians as excellent in providing health care, in treating them with respect, in explaining their medical problems, in listening to their concerns, and in being accessible (Table 36.3). Similar results were seen for other measures of satisfaction with physicians. White respondents gave higher ratings to white physicians than to nonwhite physicians on treating them with respect, explaining medical problems, and listening to their concerns. Hispanics with Hispanic physicians were found not to differ significantly from those with non-Hispanic physicians in rating their physicians, but were more likely to be very satisfied with their health care overall. Multivariate analyses revealed similar patterns, although after adjusting for confounders, racial concordance among whites was no longer significantly associated with excellent ratings of physicians in treating patients with respect or in explaining patients' medical problems (Table 36.4).

Reported Use of Health Care

In unadjusted analyses, blacks with racially concordant physicians were more likely than those with nonconcordant physicians to report receiving preventive care and always receiving needed medical care (Table 36.3). These findings persisted after adjusting for confounders (Table 36.4). Racial concordance was not significantly associated with differences in delaying care seeking for any of the racial groups.

Secondary Analyses

Restricting the sample to respondents who said that their choice of regular physician was not influenced by the physician's race or ethnicity altered our results in two ways. The effect of racial concordance among whites on rating physicians as excellent in listening to concerns was substantially reduced (OR, 1.34; 95% confidence interval [CI], 0.80–2.24), as was the effect among blacks on receiving preventive care (OR, 1.21; 95% CI, 0.65–2.25). Adjusting for respondents' reported experience of discrimination did not materially change our results.

Adjusting for respondents' satisfaction with their health plans also had little effect on our results. However, adjusting for satisfaction with the helpfulness of physicians' office staffs reduced the magnitude of the effect of racial concordance on satisfaction with health care among Hispanics (OR, 1.40; 95% CI, 0.78–2.51).

When we used linear regression to model our ordered response variables as continuous measures, the results of significance tests were generally similar to those obtained in our logistic regression analyses (data not shown). The only differences were that (1) among whites, the association between racial concordance

Table 36.3. Unadjusted Association of Patient-Physician Racial Concordance with Patient Satisfaction and Use of Health Care

	Concordance with Physician								
	White			Black			Hispanic		
Variable	Yes ($n = 779$)	No ($n = 102$)	p	Yes ($n = 162$)	No ($n = 534$)	p	Yes ($n = 133$)	No ($n = 491$)	p
Patient satisfaction									
Excellent rating of physician									
Overall	60	57	.59	67	51	<.001	58	54	.33
Treating with respect	73	63	.04	78	61	<.001	71	67	.41
Explaining problems	68	56	.02	70	61	.04	63	59	.44
Listening	64	51	.008	70	54	<.001	62	60	.65
Being accessible	53	47	.20	57	42	.001	52	45	.13
Very satisfied with physician	81	78	.53	87	76	.005	78	72	.17
Very strongly recommend physician	68	69	.80	81	71	.02	71	65	.17
Very satisfied with health care	69	64	.29	61	58	.48	66	55	.03
Use of health care									
Received preventive care	79	87	.09	87	80	.05	69	75	.19
Received all needed care	90	92	.56	95	90	.04	90	87	.43
Never delayed seeking care	72	73	.78	72	72	.96	71	70	.73

Note: Values are percentages.

Table 36.4. Multivariate Association of Patient-Physician Racial Concordance with Patient Satisfaction and Use of Health Care

	Odds Ratio (95% CI)*		
Variable	White	Black	Hispanic
Patient satisfaction			
Excellent rating of physician[†]			
Overall	1.11 (0.69–1.78)	2.40 (1.55–3.72)	0.91 (0.57–1.45)
Treating with respect	1.53 (0.93–2.52)	2.75 (1.70–4.46)	1.09 (0.65–1.83)
Explaining problems	1.47 (0.91–2.42)	1.62 (1.05–2.51)	1.08 (0.67–1.75)
Listening	1.63 (1.01–2.62)	1.95 (1.27–3.00)	0.91 (0.56–1.46)
Being accessible	1.28 (0.80–2.04)	1.66 (1.11–2.47)	1.21 (0.77–1.93)
Very satisfied with physician[†]	1.02 (0.56–1.86)	2.62 (1.44–4.76)	1.34 (0.76–2.37)
Very strongly recommend physician[†]	0.94 (0.56–1.56)	1.97 (1.19–3.28)	1.43 (0.85–2.40)
Very satisfied with health care[‡]	1.49 (0.89–2.51)	1.04 (0.67–1.62)	1.74 (1.01–2.99)
Use of health care			
Received preventive care[§]	0.76 (0.39–1.46)	1.74 (1.01–2.98)	0.90 (0.54–1.50)
Received all needed care**	0.62 (0.25–1.55)	2.94 (1.10–7.87)	1.11 (0.52–2.36)
Never delayed seeking care**	0.78 (0.45–1.34)	1.01 (0.64–1.61)	0.98 (0.59–1.61)

*Odds ratios represent odds of given response among respondents with racially concordant physicians versus respondents with racially nonconcordant physicians. CI = confidence interval.

[†]Odds ratios adjusted for age, sex, education level, insurance type, primary care site, health maintenance organization membership, ability to choose physician, number of physicians seen, health status, and psychological score.

[‡]Odds ratios adjusted for age, sex, language, insurance type, difficulty with access to specialty care, difficulty with waiting for medical care, satisfaction with physician's office hours/location, number of physicians seen, primary care site, health status, and psychological score.

[§]Odds ratios adjusted for age, sex, language, education level, household income, insurance type, primary care site, number of health care visits, number of physicians seen, physician gender, and health status.

**Odds ratios adjusted for age, sex, household income, region, insurance type, difficulty getting appointments, convenience of physician's office hours/location, primary care site, and health status.

and ratings of physicians on listening to concerns was not significant, and (2) among blacks, the associations between concordance and ratings of physicians on explaining problems and on listening to concerns were also no longer significant.

No significant interactions were found between racial concordance and education, income, language, or nationality.

COMMENT

Our findings indicate the importance of racial and cultural factors in the patient-physician relationship. They also suggest that the importance of these factors differs across racial groups. We found that blacks were more satisfied with the care they received from black as opposed to nonblack physicians. This finding was consistent across several measures of satisfaction. In addition, blacks with black physicians were more likely to report receiving preventive care and necessary medical care than were blacks with other-race physicians. Whites rated white physicians more often than nonwhite physicians as excellent in listening to patients' concerns but not in the overall provision of health care. Finally, Hispanic individuals with Hispanic as opposed to non-Hispanic physicians were more likely to be very satisfied with their health care overall but not with their physicians. All these findings persisted after controlling for sociodemographic characteristics and factors related to health care access, sources of care, and health status.

Prior studies[15-18] have demonstrated that minority populations receive a disproportionately large amount of their care from racially concordant physicians. Our data corroborate this finding. For instance, although black physicians account for less than 5 percent of the total U.S. physician workforce,[19] they served as regular health care providers for 23 percent of black individuals in our sample (Figure 36.1). While this observation may simply reflect the fact that many black individuals live in areas with high concentrations of black physicians,[17] our findings suggest that black patients prefer the care they receive from black physicians. Racial matching between minority patients and physicians may result, therefore, not only from the geographic distribution of minority physicians but also from the nature of the care they provide as well.

We believe that our findings reflect important differences in health care quality and access for individuals with racially concordant versus nonconcordant physicians. Patient satisfaction with interpersonal care as assessed in our study is an important aspect of health care quality that influences whether a patient continues to see a particular physician or remains enrolled in a health care plan.[20-22] Use of preventive services and the ability to obtain needed care are recognized indicators of access to health care.[23,24] While self-reported preventive care probably overestimates actual use,[25] unless the reports of respondents with racially concordant physicians were more or less accurate than those with nonconcordant physicians, our results are likely to represent conservative estimates of true differences in utilization.[26]

We dichotomized our satisfaction variables between the highest and all other ratings. This raises the concern that our findings may reflect differences of subtle, perhaps unimportant, degrees of patient satisfaction. However, we believe our dichotomizations were appropriate for several reasons. First, most survey respondents, including ours, express high levels of satisfaction with their health care, possibly because those who are not satisfied tend to shop around for different physicians or health plans until they are satisfied.[27] Most detectable differences in satisfaction, therefore, fall between the highest rating and all others. Second, differences between excellent and lower ratings of health care are associated with important patient behaviors, such as remaining with one's physician.[28] Finally, we repeated our analyses using linear regression to eliminate the effects of dichotomization, and the results were largely unchanged.

To add further perspective to our statistically significant results, we compared unadjusted estimates of the effect of racial concordance on some of our response variables to the effect of other predictors within our data set. Among blacks, the effect of racial concordance on ratings of physicians as excellent overall was similar to the effect of respondents' ability to choose their physician (absolute difference [AD], 16 percent versus 19 percent; OR, 1.94 versus 2.14), a factor associated with high levels of patient satisfaction.[29] The effect among blacks of racial concordance on receiving preventive care was similar to the effect of uninterrupted health insurance coverage during the previous two years (AD, 7 percent versus 6 percent; OR, 1.64 versus 1.75). The effect of racial concordance for blacks on receiving needed care was similar to the effect of having any health insurance at all (AD, 5 percent versus 6 percent; OR, 2.23 versus 2.56). Among Hispanics, the effect of racial concordance on overall satisfaction with health care was also similar to the effect of having any health insurance (AD, 10 percent versus 11 percent; OR, 1.56 versus 1.56).

Why might racial concordance between patients and physicians affect patients' assessments of their health care? Our analyses provide some insight. Among blacks, the strongest association between racial concordance and the several response variables measuring patient satisfaction was with respondents' ratings of their physicians in treating them with respect. This finding suggests that black physicians may have more harmonious interpersonal relationships with their black patients than do physicians of other races. Better relations may be a product of cultural and experiential similarities that promote mutual understanding and trust.[30] Alternatively, since many black physicians see large numbers of black patients, it is possible that better relationships are due to cultural competence acquired through practice rather than to factors more directly attributable to racial concordance.

The effect of black patient-physician racial concordance on reported use of preventive care diminished after the exclusion of respondents whose choice of physician was influenced by physician race. This suggests that for the majority of blacks, physician race did not appear to influence the likelihood of receiving preventive care. However, for a substantial minority of blacks, race was important, affecting not only their choice of physician but perhaps also their likelihood of using physician services.

Our findings among Hispanic respondents were more difficult to explain. It is puzzling that patient-physician racial concordance affected patients' satisfaction with health care without affecting their satisfaction with physicians. However, it is noteworthy that adjustment for satisfaction with the physicians' office staff significantly reduced this effect. It is possible that Hispanics are more satisfied with their health care when the office staff, including the physician, provide a more culturally and linguistically congruent setting. Future studies should address this possibility.

Our results should be viewed in light of several limitations. First, participation in the survey was incomplete, raising the concern of selection bias. However, for our results to be biased in this respect, the effects of self-selection would have had to be unevenly distributed between those with racially concordant and nonconcordant physicians.[31] Second, nonparticipation resulted in a sample of subjects with higher levels of education, income, and insurance coverage than the population from which the sample was drawn (Table 36.2).[32] Also, the Hispanic group had few recent immigrants, limiting the generalizability of our results. Third, we did not have detailed information on the ethnicity, or nationality, of physicians. We were therefore not able to test the effects of finer degrees of patient-physician ethnic concordance on our response variables. This may explain the paucity of observed associations among Hispanics, who were more ethnically diverse than the black respondents in our sample. It is possible, for instance, that Hispanic individuals of Puerto Rican heritage are more satisfied with physicians who are also Puerto Rican and not necessarily more satisfied with physicians who are Mexican American. We could not address this hypothesis with our data. Fourth, we relied on respondents' assessments of physician race, which may not always accurately reflect the physician's true race. However, it is likely that the mechanisms by which racial concordance affects patient satisfaction and use of health care depend more on patients' perceptions of the physician's race than on the physician's true race.

Finally, because of the observational nature of our study, the possibility exists that our findings do not reflect true associations but are the result of confounding. We adjusted for numerous variables associated with satisfaction and use of health care, including age, sex, education, income, insurance, language, primary care site, physician sex, access barriers, and psychological distress.[20,33-40] Furthermore, we attempted to adjust for illness severity through variables in our data set, including health status, number of health care visits, and hospitalization. It remains possible, however, that unmeasured differences across our comparison groups in illness severity or other factors may have partially accounted for our findings.

These limitations notwithstanding, we believe our results confirm the importance of racial and cultural factors in the patient-physician relationship. The finding that racial concordance affected patients' perceptions of their health care in measurable ways suggests that there is room for improvement in the relationships that physicians have with patients of nonconcordant backgrounds and supports efforts to increase cultural competence among physicians caring for diverse populations.

Our findings may also help predict the likely effects of policies influencing the recruitment of minorities into the U.S. physician workforce. In the wake of recent trends in policies regarding affirmative action and international medical graduates, a decline in the proportion of physicians from racial and ethnic minorities is expected.[41,42] Studies[15-18] showing that minority physicians provide care for a large proportion of the rapidly growing minority communities in the United States suggest that with fewer minority physicians, the physician supply for many already underserved communities may diminish even further. Selectively admitting medical students with an interest in primary care of underserved communities may mitigate this problem. However, in light of our finding that physician race may affect black and Hispanic patients' satisfaction with and use of health care, such admissions policies, without the specific aim of recruiting black and Hispanic students, would serve as only a partial solution.

Our findings point to unique benefits that black and Hispanic individuals may experience when receiving health care from black and Hispanic physicians. When considering policy changes likely to reduce the number of underrepresented minorities in the physician workforce, governments and educational institutions should be mindful of the detrimental impact that such changes may have on health care for minority populations.

Notes

1. Council on Ethical and Judicial Affairs, American Medical Association. (1990). Black-white disparities in health care. *JAMA, 263*, 2344–2346.

2. Ginzberg, E. (1991). Access to health care for Hispanics. *JAMA, 265*, 238–241.

3. Blendon, R. J., Aiken, L. H., Freeman, H. E., & Corey, C. R. (1989). Access to medical care for black and white Americans: A matter of continuing concern. *JAMA, 261*, 278–281.

4. Lieu, T. A., Newacheck, P. W., & McManus, M. A. (1993). Race, ethnicity, and access to ambulatory care among U.S. adolescents. *Am J Public Health, 83,* 960–965.

5. Andersen, R. M., Giachello, A. L., & Aday, L. A. (1986). Access of Hispanics to health care and cuts in services: A state-of-the-art overview. *Public Health Rep, 101,* 238–252.

6. Lillie-Blanton, M., & Alfaro-Correa, A. (1995). *In the nation's interest: Equity in access to health care.* Washington, DC: Joint Center for Political and Economic Studies.

7. Gornick, M. E., Eggers, P. W., Reilly, T. W., et al. (1996). Effects of race and income on mortality and use of services among Medicare beneficiaries. *N Engl J Med, 335,* 791–799.

8. Escarce, J. J., Epstein, K. R., Colby, D. C., & Schwartz, J. S. (1993). Racial differences in the elderly's use of medical procedures and diagnostic tests. *Am J Public Health, 83,* 948–954.

9. Sullivan, L. W. (1991). From the Secretary of Health and Human Services. *JAMA, 266,* 2674.

10. Weddington, W. H., Gabel, L. L., Peet, G. M., & Stewart, S. O. (1992). Quality of care and black American patients. *J Natl Med Assoc, 84,* 569–575.

11. Whittle, J., Conigliaro, J., Good, C. B., & Joswiak, M. (1997). Do patient preferences contribute to racial differences in cardiovascular procedure use? *J Gen Intern Med, 12,* 267–273.

12. Geiger, H. J. (1996). Race and health care: An American dilemma? *N Engl J Med, 335,* 815–816.

13. Louis Harris and Associates. (1994). *Health care services and minority groups: A comparative survey of whites, African-Americans, Hispanics, and Asian-Americans.* New York: Author.

14. Veit, C. T., & Ware, J. E., Jr. (1983). The structure of psychological distress and well-being in general populations. *J Consult Clin Psychol, 51,* 730–742.

15. Keith, S. N., Bell, R. M., Swanson, A. G., & Williams, A. P. (1985). Effects of affirmative action in medical schools: A study of the class of 1975. *N Engl J Med, 313,* 1519–1525.

16. Moy, E., & Bartman, B. A. (1995). Physician race and care of minority and medically indigent patients. *JAMA, 273,* 1515–1520.

17. Komaromy, M., Grumbach, K., Drake, M., et al. (1996). The role of black and Hispanic physicians in providing health care for underserved populations. *N Engl J Med, 334,* 1305–1310.

18. Xu, G., Fields, S. K., Laine, C., Veloski, J. J., Barzansky, B., & Martini, C. J. (1997). The relationship between the race/ethnicity of generalist physicians and their care for underserved populations. *Am J Public Health, 87,* 817–822.

19. Association of American Medical Colleges. (1994). *Minority students in medical education.* Washington, DC: Author.

20. Cleary, P. D., & McNeil, B. J. (1988). Patient satisfaction as an indicator of quality care. *Inquiry, 25,* 25–36.

21. Ware, J. E., Jr., & Hays, R. D. (1988). Methods for measuring patient satisfaction with specific medical encounters. *Med Care, 26,* 393–402.

22. Ware, J. E., Jr., & Davies, A. R. (1983). Behavioral consequences of consumer dissatisfaction with medical care. *Eval Program Plan, 6,* 291–297.

23. Institute of Medicine. (1993). *Access to health care in America.* Washington, DC: National Academy Press.

24. Aday, L., & Andersen, R. (1975). *Development of indices of access to medical care.* Ann Arbor, MI: Health Administration Press.

25. Gordon, N. P., Hiatt, R. A., & Lampert, D. I. (1993). Concordance of self-reported data and medical record audit for six cancer screening procedures. *J Natl Cancer Inst, 85,* 566–570.

26. Hennekens, C. H., & Buring, J. E. (1987). *Epidemiology in medicine.* Boston: Little, Brown.

27. Ware, J. E., Jr., Davies, A. R., & Rubin, H. R. (1988). Patients' assessments of their care. In Office of Technology Assessment, *The quality of medical care: Information for consumers* (pp. 231–247). Washington, DC: U.S. Government Printing Office.

28. Rubin, H. R., Gandek, B., Rogers, W. H., Kosinski, M., McHorney, C. A., & Ware, J. E., Jr. (1993). Patients' ratings of outpatient visits in different practice settings: Results from the Medical Outcomes Study. *JAMA, 270,* 835–840.

29. Schmittdiel, J., Selby, J. V., Grumbach, K., & Quesenberry, C. P. (1997). Choice of a personal physician and patient satisfaction in a health maintenance organization. *JAMA, 278,* 1596–1599.

30. Gamble, V. N. (1997). Under the shadow of Tuskegee: African Americans and health care. *Am J Public Health, 87,* 1773–1778.

31. Kelsey, J. L., Whittemore, A. S., Evans, A. S., & Thompson, W. D. (1996). *Methods in observational epidemiology* (2nd ed.). New York: Oxford University Press.

32. National Center for Health Statistics. (1995). *Health, United States, 1994.* Hyattsville, MD: U.S. Public Health Service.

33. Bindman, A. B., Grumbach, K., Osmond, D., Vranizan, K., & Stewart, A. L. (1996). Primary care and receipt of preventive services. *J Gen Intern Med, 11,* 269–276.

34. Stewart, A. L., Grumbach, K., Osmond, D. H., Vranizan, K., Komaromy, M., & Bindman, A. B. (1997). Primary care and patient perceptions of access to care. *J Fam Pract, 44,* 177–185.

35. Weissman, J. S., Stern, R., Fielding, S. L., & Epstein, A. M. (1991). Delayed access to health care: Risk factors, reasons, and consequences. *Ann Intern Med, 114,* 325–331.

36. Rask, K. J., Williams, M. V., Parker, R. M., & McNagny, S. E. (1994). Obstacles predicting lack of a regular provider and delays in seeking care for patients at an urban public hospital. *JAMA, 271,* 1931–1933.

37. Kaplan, S. H., & Ware, J. E., Jr. (1989). The patient's role in health care quality assessment. In N. Goldfield & D. B. Nash (Eds.), *Providing quality care: The challenge to clinicians* (pp. 25–69). Philadelphia: American College of Physicians.

38. Lurie, N., Slater, J., McGovern, P., Ekstrum, J., Quam, L., & Margolis, K. (1993). Preventive care for women: Does the sex of the physician matter? *N Engl J Med, 329,* 478–482.

39. Manson, A. (1988). Language concordance as a determinant of patient compliance and emergency room use in patients with asthma. *Med Care, 26,* 1119–1128.

40. Woloshin, S., Schwartz, L. M., Katz, S. J., & Welch, H. G. (1997). Is language a barrier to the use of preventive services? *J Gen Intern Med, 12,* 472–477.

41. Wallace, A. (1997, August 1). UC San Diego Medical School takes no blacks for fall class: With affirmative action ban in effect, there are also no Native Americans and far fewer Latinos. *Los Angeles Times,* p. A3.

42. Srinivisan, K. (1997, November 2). Fewer minorities entering medical schools: Rollback of affirmative action is blamed. *Seattle Times,* p. A13.

CHAPTER THIRTY-SEVEN

Racial Differences in the Use of Cardiac Catheterization After Acute Myocardial Infarction

Jersey Chen
Saif S. Rathore
Martha J. Radford
Yun Wang
Harlan M. Krumholz

Numerous studies have reported that black patients with coronary artery disease are less likely than white patients to undergo cardiac catheterization.[1-9] Many aspects of the physician-patient relationship that may account for treatment decisions have been described.[10] Factors associated with a difference in race between physicians and patients, such as cross-cultural miscommunication,[11,12] lack of rapport or trust,[13,14] and reduced willingness on the part of the patient to undergo an intervention,[15] may lead to the use of fewer procedures among black patients. Alternatively, bias on the part of physicians—due to subconscious perceptions, incorrect assumptions regarding the preferences of patients, or overt discrimination—may contribute to racial differences in the use of cardiac catheterization.[16,17] However, whether racial differences in the use of cardiac catheterization vary according to the race of the physician is unknown.

In previous studies, it has been observed that patients treated by physicians of a race other than their own participated less in decision making[13] and may have been less willing to consider cardiac interventions than patients whose physicians were of the same race as themselves.[15] We sought to examine whether the race of the physician contributes to racial differences in the use of cardiac catheterization. We hypothesized that if racial differences in the use of

This work was supported by a contract (500-96-P549) with the Health Care Financing Administration, U.S. Department of Health and Human Services. We are indebted to Maria Johnson for editorial assistance.

cardiac catheterization were associated with the race of the physician, then differences between black patients and white patients in the rate of cardiac catheterization would vary according to the race of the physician. We analyzed data from patients in the national Cooperative Cardiovascular Project to assess whether differences in the rate of cardiac catheterization and in survival after acute myocardial infarction were related to differences between the race of physicians and the race of patients.

METHODS

Patients

We performed a retrospective analysis of data from the Cooperative Cardiovascular Project, a Health Care Financing Administration quality-improvement initiative for patients with acute myocardial infarction.[18] The Cooperative Cardiovascular Project provided data on 234,769 hospitalizations among Medicare patients on a fee-for-service basis in 1994 or 1995 who had a discharge diagnosis of acute myocardial infarction (code 410 of the *International Classification of Diseases, 9th Revision, Clinical Modification* [*ICD-9-CM*]).[19] Patients with the following characteristics were excluded from our study: age of less than sixty-five years (17,591 patients); absence of a clinically confirmed diagnosis of acute myocardial infarction (defined as documentation in the patient's chart of either a serum creatine kinase MB fraction above 0.05, a serum lactate dehydrogenase level more than 1.5 times the upper limit of normal, with the level of isoenzyme 1 exceeding the level of isoenzyme 2, or at least two of the following three conditions: chest pain, a serum creatine kinase level more than double the upper limit of normal, or evidence of a new acute myocardial infarction on an electrocardiogram) (31,179); previous percutaneous transluminal coronary angioplasty or coronary artery bypass graft surgery (43,143); concurrent terminal illness (4,616); hospitalization after transfer from another acute care hospital (42,277); readmission (25,185); unavailability of Medicare Part A data at time of analysis (34,187); or hospitalization outside the fifty states of the United States (1,760). Patients whose data could not be linked with American Hospital Association data were also excluded (2,363). Some patients met more than one of the exclusion criteria. Of the remaining 118,953 patients, the cohort we considered was limited to the 75,893 patients in hospitals that had admitted at least one black patient with acute myocardial infarction in the Cooperative Cardiovascular Project during the study period.

Data on physicians were successfully matched for 73,846 of these 75,893 patients (97.3 percent), although data on the physician's race were not available for 24,452 of the 75,893 patients (32 percent). Patients with cardiovascular surgeons as attending physicians (1,806 patients) were excluded because many of them were probably undergoing elective coronary artery bypass graft surgery.

The following patients were also excluded: patients whose race could not be confirmed as either white or black (2,324), and patients who were treated by physicians who were neither white nor black (9,106). Some patients met more than one of these exclusion criteria.

Dependent Variables

We evaluated Medicare Part A billing records for the use of cardiac catheterization (procedure codes 37.22, 37.23, and 88.53 through 88.57 of *ICD-9-CM*) within sixty days after admission with acute myocardial infarction. We ascertained death within three years after admission with acute myocardial infarction by supplementing information on vital status in the Cooperative Cardiovascular Project with data from the Death Master File of the Social Security Administration.[20]

Independent Variables

Race of the Patients and Physicians. The race of the patients in the Cooperative Cardiovascular Project was abstracted from medical records. The race of the attending physicians was identified with use of their unique physician identification numbers as recorded in Medicare Part A claims. The attending physician is regarded as "the clinician who is primarily and largely responsible for the care of the patient from the beginning of the hospital episode."[21] We linked the identification numbers of the attending physicians with the Physician Masterfile of the American Medical Association. The Physician Masterfile is a comprehensive, validated database of information on physicians' characteristics,[22] collected from medical school matriculation forms, surveys of physicians, and residency training programs (P. L. Havlicek, personal communication).

Other Independent Variables. Because the severity of disease and the presence of coexisting illnesses influence the decision to use cardiac catheterization, we adjusted for the following predictive variables (drawn from published studies[23-26]) and clinically relevant factors: age; sex; Killip class at the time of admission; left ventricular ejection fraction; systolic blood pressure; heart rate; anatomical site of the acute myocardial infarction; presence or absence of a history of previous acute myocardial infarction or congestive heart failure; current smoking status; presence or absence of hypertension, diabetes mellitus, stroke, peripheral vascular disease, or renal dysfunction (blood urea nitrogen above 40 mg per deciliter [14 mmol per liter] or serum creatinine level above 2 mg per deciliter [177 μmol per liter]); and use or nonuse of thrombolytic therapy. We also adjusted for several nonclinical factors: characteristics of the hospitals, according to the American Hospital Association 1994 survey of hospitals (teaching status, ownership, and availability of on-site facilities for cardiac procedures);[27] characteristics of the physicians, according to the American Medical Association Physician Masterfile (specialty, sex, decade of graduation, country of medical school, employment type, and type of training [osteopathic or allopathic]); and number of the physician's patients enrolled in the Cooperative Cardiovascular Project. Hospital volume (estimated from Medicare Part A data) and patients' income and education level (from 1990 U.S. Census data[28]) were classified into quintiles.

The survival analyses included the presence or absence of the following additional factors: inability to walk, urinary incontinence, dementia, admission from a nursing home, chronic obstructive pulmonary disease, liver disease, infection with the human immunodeficiency virus or other immunologic compromise, trauma within the previous month, a serum albumin level below 3 g per deciliter, a hematocrit below 30 percent, and use of aspirin, beta-blockers, or angiotensin-converting-enzyme inhibitors during hospitalization or prescribed at discharge. Dummy variables indicating missing values were included in the multivariate analyses.

Statistical Analysis

Differences in the characteristics of the patients, the rate of cardiac catheterization, and mortality were assessed by means of chi-square tests for categorical variables and analysis of variance for continuous variables. We examined whether racial differences in the rate of cardiac catheterization or in survival persisted after adjustment for differences in the characteristics of the patients, the physicians, and the hospitals through a series of multivariate logistic regression models. The effect of the race of the physician on differences between black patients and white patients in the use of cardiac catheterization was examined with the use of models incorporating interaction terms. We transformed odds ratios to relative risks by the method of Zhang and Yu.[29] We used Cox proportional-hazards regression models to assess the relative risks of death. All the regression models incorporated Huber-White robust standard errors, adjusted for clustering according to physician.[30] (We used Stata statistical software [Version 6.0; Stata, College Station, TX] to conduct the analyses.)

RESULTS

Patients

Our cohort consisted of 35,676 white and 4,039 black Medicare beneficiaries who were treated for acute myocardial infarction by 17,550 white physicians and 588 black physicians. The mean (±SD) age of the patients was 77 ± 7.6 years (range, 65 to 108). Blacks represented 9 percent of the patients treated by white physicians and 53 percent of the patients treated by black physicians. Black patients were more likely than white patients to have hypertension, diabetes mellitus, renal dysfunction, previous heart failure, stroke, or peripheral vascular disease, regardless of the race of their physicians (Table 37.1). Other

Table 37.1. Characteristics of the Patients

Characteristic	White Physicians		Black Physicians	
	White Patients (n = 35,176)	Black Patients (n = 3476)	White Patients (n = 500)	Black Patients (n = 563)
Age, years	77.3 ± 7.6	75.9 ± 7.6*	76.6 ± 7.3†	76.1 ± 7.5
Female sex (%)	47.5	41.2*	50.2	35.0‡§
Clinical history (%)				
Hypertension	60.4	77.9*	62.2	82.1‡§
Diabetes mellitus	28.7	41.2*	29.4	42.5‡
Previous myocardial infarction	23.8	25.1	21.2	22.7
Previous heart failure	20.8	25.5*	19.6	27.5‡
Current smoker	14.7	18.3*	18.2†	17.9
Previous stroke	13.5	18.5*	11.4	18.5‡
Peripheral vascular disease	10.1	11.6*	10.4	13.3
Characteristics on admission (%)				
Systolic blood pressure <100 mmHg	7.2	7.0	9.2	8.0
Pulse >100 beats/min	26.6	29.3*	27.0	31.3
Renal dysfunction	11.8	20.9*	11.6	18.7‡
Site of infarction				
Anterior	47.9	47.1	46.8	48.1
Inferior	46.9	44.1*	47.6	43.2
Left ventricular ejection fraction				
≥55%	13.1	13.0	15.4	13.5
40–54%	32.5	29.6*	27.0†	30.7
20–39%	19.9	19.6	22.4	21.0
<20%	1.7	2.2*	1.8	2.8
Unknown	32.8	35.7*	33.4	32.0

Medications used during hospitalization or at discharge (%)				
Aspirin	80.9	79.8	77.2†	75.7§
Beta-blockers	47.8	43.8*	47.6	39.4‡
Thrombolytic agents	18.3	13.5*	22.0†	12.8‡
Angiotensin-converting-enzyme inhibitors	38.1	43.1*	35.4	41.9‡
Specialty of attending physician (%)				
Internal medicine	24.2	21.9*	26.6	24.2
Cardiology	27.2	23.9*	30.8	12.3‡§
Other internal medicine subspecialty	11.0	13.5*	7.0†	7.1§
Family practice	15.4	16.3	12.2	14.0
Characteristics of hospital (%)				
Cardiac catheterization available	70.9	66.6*	63.4	68.2‡
Teaching	41.7	46.5*	31.8†	49.2‡
Public	11.0	21.0*	10.2	19.7‡
Private, not-for-profit	79.8	69.0*	80.0	70.7‡
Socioeconomic characteristics				
Annual household income ($)	31,738 ± 11,851	23,697 ± 9,308*	28,571 ± 9,575†	22,953 ± 8,791‡
Population with at least a high school diploma (%)	50.1	41.1*	47.0†	40.5‡

Note: Plus-minus values are means ±SD.

*p < .05 for the comparison between black patients treated by white physicians and white patients treated by white physicians.

†p < .05 for the comparison between white patients treated by black physicians and white patients treated by white physicians.

‡p < .05 for the comparison between black patients treated by black physicians and white patients treated by black physicians.

§p < .05 for the comparison between black patients treated by black physicians and black patients treated by white physicians.

clinical characteristics of the two groups of patients were generally similar, whether they were treated by white or black physicians. Black patients were less likely to have board-certified cardiologists as attending physicians, were more likely to be treated in public or teaching hospitals, and on average lived in neighborhoods with lower levels of income and education than white patients, regardless of the race of their physicians.

Use of Cardiac Catheterization

We found that black patients were significantly less likely than white patients to undergo cardiac catheterization within sixty days after admission, regardless of whether their attending physicians were white or black ($p < .001$ for both comparisons) (Table 37.2). The rate of cardiac catheterization among white patients did not differ significantly according to whether their physicians were white or black (45.7 percent and 49.6 percent, respectively; $p = .08$). Similarly, the rate of cardiac catheterization among black patients did not differ significantly according to whether their physicians were white or black (38.4 percent and 38.2 percent, respectively; $p = .94$).

In analyses that adjusted for the characteristics of the patients, the physicians, and the hospitals, black patients remained less likely to undergo cardiac catheterization than white patients treated by white doctors, regardless of the race of the

Table 37.2. Rate of Use of Cardiac Catheterization Within 60 Days After Acute Myocardial Infarction Among Black Patients and White Patients According to the Race of Their Physicians

	White Physicians		Black Physicians	
	White Patients ($n = 35,176$)	Black Patients ($n = 3476$)	White Patients ($n = 500$)	Black Patients ($n = 563$)
Rate		Percentage (95% CI)		
Unadjusted	45.7	38.4*	49.6	38.2*
Adjusted	45.7§	32.9 (30.1–36.1)†	53.4 (43.4–65.8)	36.5 (29.2–45.2)‡

Note: In the adjusted analyses, adjustments were made for the characteristics of the patients, the physicians, and the hospitals. There were no significant differences in the rates of cardiac catheterization among either the white patients or the black patients according to the race of their physicians. CI = confidence interval.

*$p < .001$ for the comparison between black patients and white patients, regardless of the race of their physician.

†$p < .001$ for the comparison between black patients treated by white physicians and white patients treated by white physicians.

‡$p = .04$ for the comparison between black patients treated by black physicians and white patients treated by black physicians.

§These patients served as the reference group.

black patients' attending physicians (Table 37.2). The difference between white patients and black patients in the adjusted rates of cardiac catheterization was 12.8 percentage points (45.7 percent and 32.9 percent, respectively) among those treated by white doctors and 16.9 percentage points (53.4 percent and 36.5 percent) among those treated by black doctors. In multivariate analyses of the use of cardiac catheterization, we did not find a significant interaction between the patient's race and the physician's race ($p = .73$), indicating that black patients treated by black physicians did not undergo cardiac catheterization at a different rate from black patients treated by white physicians.

Mortality

Unadjusted thirty-day mortality rates were lower among black patients than among white patients, regardless of the race of their attending physicians (Table 37.3). By the end of three years, unadjusted mortality rates were higher among black patients than among white patients, regardless of the race of their physicians. In multivariate analyses, however, thirty-day mortality rates were significantly lower among black patients—both those treated by white physicians and those treated by black physicians—than among white patients treated by white physicians (Table 37.4). Three-year adjusted mortality rates among black patients treated by white physicians were also lower than the rates among white patients treated by white physicians; the same was true of black patients treated by black physicians as compared with white patients treated by white physicians. The results were consistent when analyses were limited either to patients who underwent cardiac catheterization or to those who did not undergo the procedure.

Table 37.3. Unadjusted Mortality Among Black Patients and White Patients According to the Race of Their Physicians

	White Physicians		Black Physicians	
Follow-up	White Patients	Black Patients	White Patients	Black Patients
		Percentage		
30 days	19.4	17.3*	20.4	18.5
1 year	32.8	33.1	31.2	36.8
2 years	40.0	41.1	38.2	44.9†
3 years	46.0	48.5*	43.2	52.4†

Note: There were no significant differences in the mortality rates among either the white patients or the black patients according to the race of their physicians.

*$p < .05$ for the comparison between black patients treated by white physicians and white patients treated by white physicians.

†$p < .05$ for the comparison between black patients treated by black physicians and white patients treated by black physicians.

Table 37.4. Adjusted Mortality Among Black Patients and White Patients
According to the Race of Their Physicians

	White Physicians		Black Physicians	
Follow-up	White Patients	Black Patients	White Patients	Black Patients
	Hazard ratio (95% CI)			
30 days	1.00	0.78 (0.72–0.86)	0.99 (0.79–1.25)	0.74 (0.59–0.92)
1 year	1.00	0.87 (0.81–0.93)	0.91 (0.76–1.08)	0.88 (0.76–1.03)
2 years	1.00	0.87 (0.82–0.93)	0.91 (0.78–1.06)	0.89 (0.77–1.02)
3 years	1.00	0.89 (0.84–0.95)	0.90 (0.79–1.04)	0.91 (0.80–1.03)

Note: Adjustments were made for the characteristics of the patients, the physicians, and the hospitals. CI = confidence interval. White patients treated by white physicians served as the reference group.

DISCUSSION

Our findings are consistent with those of previous studies that reported differences between white and black Medicare beneficiaries[7] and other white and black populations[1-6,8,9] in the rate of cardiac catheterization. In addition, our study found that black patients underwent cardiac catheterization less frequently after acute myocardial infarction than white patients, regardless of the race of their physicians. The absence of an interaction between the race of the patient and the race of the physician suggests that racial discordance between the patient and the physician does not explain differences between black patients and white patients in the use of cardiac catheterization.

What factors could potentially explain the lower rate of use of cardiac catheterization in black patients, regardless of the physician's race? Differences in clinical characteristics among races are one possible explanation. Black patients are less likely than white patients to describe typical chest pains after acute myocardial infarction[12,31] and are more likely to have nondiagnostic electrocardiograms at the time of presentation.[6] These factors might reduce the likelihood that black patients will undergo cardiac catheterization, although they would be expected to be less important once the diagnosis of acute myocardial infarction has been confirmed.

It is possible that black patients may be less willing than white patients to undergo cardiac procedures because of different thresholds for procedure-related risks, different levels of trust in the medical system, or different degrees of familiarity with these treatments.[14,15] In previous studies, black patients were more likely to refuse to undergo cardiac procedures than white patients.[32] Conversely, white patients may be more aggressive in seeking such procedures. Other interactions between patients and physicians that are related to race may also play a part in ways that have not yet been defined.[13]

Unmeasured or unmeasurable differences in socioeconomic factors may also have contributed to the lower rate of cardiac procedures among blacks, regardless of the race of their physicians. Although we adjusted for income and education according to local U.S. Census data, we cannot exclude the possibility of residual confounding due to heterogeneity of these factors within neighborhoods. Furthermore, although Medicare paid the hospital bills of all the patients in our study, there still may have been differences in their ability to pay for care. For example, our study was unable to assess the effects of supplemental "Medigap" insurance, which pays for outpatient visits, medications, and out-of-pocket expenses, including deductibles and co-payments. Because nonwhite Medicare beneficiaries are less likely to have supplemental insurance than white beneficiaries are,[33] the prospect of incurring substantial out-of-pocket costs may have been a strong disincentive to undergoing cardiac catheterization. Important social factors, such as the availability of family support, may also have an important role. For example, it has been reported that patients who are married may be more likely to undergo a cardiac procedure than those who are not married,[1] and according to the same study, blacks are less likely to be married than whites.

Whether differences in the rate of cardiac procedures between black patients and white patients are associated with differences in outcomes is uncertain. Several studies found that black patients have poorer long-term survival after acute myocardial infarction than white patients.[34,35] Other studies showed that although blacks underwent fewer cardiac procedures, their survival after hospitalization for acute myocardial infarction was equivalent to or better than that of whites.[1,4,6,7] We found that thirty-day mortality rates were lower in blacks than in whites, and this trend, though it diminished, persisted up to three years of follow-up.

Differences in the unmeasured clinical characteristics of patients of different races are one potential reason why blacks may have had a lower rate of death after acute myocardial infarction than white patients. Nonwhite race is associated with failure to hospitalize for acute myocardial infarction,[36] and if black patients with more severe infarctions died before admission, the proportion of hospitalized black patients with less severe infarctions would be greater than that of hospitalized white patients.[37] Studies showing that blacks have higher rates of out-of-hospital death from infarction[38] and cardiac arrest[39] are consistent with this hypothesis. Although it is not clear whether the differences in mortality according to race in our study were due to differences in the clinical characteristics or medical treatment of the patients, our findings do not support the hypothesis that the lower rate of use of cardiac catheterization in black patients is associated with worse survival.

Given the design of our study, we were unable to assess whether cardiac procedures were underused, appropriately used, or overused in either black patients or white patients. We were also unable to examine potential interactions between the patients and the specialists consulted by attending physicians who were not cardiologists. However, the decision to initiate consideration for catheterization by requesting consultation with a cardiac specialist or by transferring the patient to an outside hospital with a cardiac catheterization laboratory is typically the responsibility of the attending physician. We were unable to evaluate the decision to refer a patient for catheterization because we examined only the actual use of the procedure. Finally, we cannot rule out the possibility that institutional factors and attitudes common to black and white physicians contribute to lower rates of cardiac catheterization in black patients than in white patients. Despite these limitations, our findings indicate that there is no interaction between the race of the physician and the race of the patient in the use of cardiac catheterization. The observation that racial differences in the use of cardiac catheterization are similar among patients treated by black physicians and white physicians suggests that racial discordance between patients and physicians does not explain racial differences in the use of this procedure.

Notes

1. Ferguson, J. A., Tierney, W. M., Westmoreland, G. R., et al. (1997). Examination of racial differences in management of cardiovascular disease. *J Am Coll Cardiol, 30,* 1707–1713.

2. Giles, W. H., Anda, R. F., Casper, M. L., Escobedo, L. G., & Taylor, H. A. (1995). Race and sex differences in rates of invasive cardiac procedures in U.S. hospitals: Data from the National Hospital Discharge Survey. *Arch Intern Med, 155,* 318–324.

3. Mirvis, D. M., Burns, R., Gaschen, L., Cloar, F. T., & Graney, M. (1994). Variation in utilization of cardiac procedures in the Department of Veterans Affairs Health Care System: Effect of race. *J Am Coll Cardiol, 24,* 1297–1304.

4. Peterson, E. D., Wright, S. M., Daley, J., & Thibault, G. E. (1994). Racial variation in cardiac procedure use and survival following acute myocardial infarction in the Department of Veterans Affairs. *JAMA, 271,* 1175–1180.

5. Stone, P. H., Thompson, B., Anderson, H. V., et al. (1996). Influence of race, sex, and age on management of unstable angina and non-Q-wave myocardial infarction: The TIMI III Registry. *JAMA, 275,* 1104–1112.

6. Taylor, H. A., Canto, J. G., Sanderson, B., Rogers, W. J., & Hilbe, J. (1998). Management and outcomes for black patients with acute myocardial infarction in the reperfusion era. *Am J Cardiol, 82,* 1019–1023.

7. Udvarhelyi, I. S., Gatsonis, C., Epstein, A. M., Pashos, C. L., Newhouse, J. P., & McNeil, B. J. (1992). Acute myocardial infarction in the Medicare population: Process of care and clinical outcomes. *JAMA, 268,* 2530–2536.

8. Wenneker, M. B., & Epstein, A. M. (1989). Racial inequalities in the use of procedures for patients with ischemic heart disease in Massachusetts. *JAMA, 261,* 253–257.

9. Whittle, J., Conigliaro, J., Good, C. B., & Lofgren, R. P. (1993). Racial differences in the use of invasive cardiovascular procedures in the Department of Veterans Affairs Medical System. *N Engl J Med, 329,* 621–627.

10. Eisenberg, J. M. (1979). Sociologic influences on decision-making by clinicians. *Ann Intern Med, 90,* 957–964.

11. Hooper, E. M., Comstock, L. M., Goodwin, J. M., & Goodwin, J. S. (1982). Patient characteristics that influence physician behavior. *Med Care, 20,* 630–638.

12. Summers, R. L., Cooper, G. J., Carlton, F. D., Andres, M. E., & Kolb, J. C. (1999). Prevalence of atypical chest pain descriptions in a population from the southern United States. *Am J Med Sci, 318,* 142–145.

13. Cooper-Patrick, L., Gallo, J. J., Gonzales, J. J., et al. (1999). Race, gender, and partnership in the patient-physician relationship. *JAMA, 282,* 583–589.

14. Doescher, M. P., Saver, B. G., Franks, P., & Fiscella, K. (2000). Racial and ethnic disparities in perceptions of physician style and trust. *Arch Fam Med, 9,* 1156–1163.

15. Whittle, J., Conigliaro, J., Good, C. B., & Joswiak, M. (1997). Do patient preferences contribute to racial differences in cardiovascular procedure use? *J Gen Intern Med, 12,* 267–273.

16. van Ryn, M., & Burke, J. (2000). The effect of patient race and socio-economic status on physicians' perceptions of patients. *Soc Sci Med, 50,* 813–828.

17. Schulman, K. A., Berlin, J. A., Harless, W., et al. (1999). The effect of race and sex on physicians' recommendations for cardiac catheterization. *N Engl J Med, 340,* 618–626.

18. Marciniak, T. A., Ellerbeck, E. F., Radford, M. J., et al. (1998). Improving the quality of care for Medicare patients with acute myocardial infarction: Results from the Cooperative Cardiovascular Project. *JAMA, 279,* 1351–1357.

19. Health Care Financing Administration. (1997). *International classification of diseases, 9th revision, clinical modification: ICD-9-CM* (6th ed.). Washington, DC: U.S. Government Printing Office.

20. U.S. Department of Health and Human Services. (1999). Social Security Administration's death master file (NTS Order No. SUB-525IINQ.). Washington, DC: National Technical Information Service.

21. Iezzoni, L. I. (1994). Data sources and implications: Administrative data bases. In L. I. Iezzoni (Ed.), *Risk adjustment for measuring health care outcomes* (pp. 119–175). Ann Arbor, MI: Health Administration Press.

22. Kenward, K. (1996). The scope of the data available in the AMA's Physician Masterfile. *Am J Public Health, 86,* 1481–1482.

23. Krumholz, H. M., Chen, J., Wang, Y., Radford, M. J., Chen, Y. T., & Marciniak, T. A. (1999). Comparing AMI mortality among hospitals in patients 65 years of age and older: Evaluating methods of risk adjustment. *Circulation, 99,* 2986–2992.

24. Lee, K. L., Woodlief, L. H., Topol, E. J., et al. (1995). Predictors of 30-day mortality in the era of reperfusion for acute myocardial infarction: Results from an international trial of 41,021 patients. *Circulation, 91,* 1659–1668.

25. Mark, D. B., Nelson, C. L., Califf, R. M., et al. (1994). Continuing evolution of therapy for coronary artery disease: Initial results from the era of coronary angioplasty. *Circulation, 89,* 2015–2025.

26. Peterson, E. D., Shaw, L. K., DeLong, E. R., Pryor, D. B., Califf, R. M., & Mark, D. B. (1997). Racial variation in the use of coronary-revascularization procedures. *N Engl J Med, 336,* 480–486.

27. American Hospital Association. (1994). *The annual survey of hospitals database: Documentation for 1994 data.* Chicago: Author.

28. U.S. Bureau of the Census. (1991, August). *State and metropolitan area data book, 1991.* Washington, DC: U.S. Government Printing Office.

29. Zhang, J., & Yu, K. F. (1998). What's the relative risk? A method of correcting the odds ratio in cohort studies of common outcomes. *JAMA, 280,* 1690–1691.

30. White, H. A. (1980). A heteroskedasticity-consistent covariance matrix estimator and a direct test for heteroskedasticity. *Econometrica, 48,* 817–838.

31. Raczynski, J. M., Taylor, H., Cutter, G., Hardin, M., Rappaport, N., & Oberman, A. (1994). Diagnoses, symptoms, and attribution of symptoms among black and white inpatients admitted for coronary heart disease. *Am J Public Health, 84,* 951–956.

32. Sedlis, S. P., Fisher, V. J., Tice, D., Esposito, R., Madmon, L., & Steinberg, E. H. (1997). Racial differences in performance of invasive cardiac procedures in a Department of Veterans Affairs Medical Center. *J Clin Epidemiol, 50,* 899–901.

33. Rice, T., & McCall, N. (1985). The extent of ownership and the characteristics of Medicare supplemental policies. *Inquiry, 22,* 188–200.

34. Castaner, A., Simmons, B. E., Mar, M., & Cooper, R. (1988). Myocardial infarction among black patients: Poor prognosis after hospital discharge. *Ann Intern Med, 109,* 33–35.

35. Tofler, G. H., Stone, P. H., Muller, J. E., et al. (1987). Effects of gender and race on prognosis after myocardial infarction: Adverse prognosis for women, particularly black women. *J Am Coll Cardiol, 9,* 473–482.

36. Pope, J. H., Aufderheide, T. P., Ruthazer, R., et al. (2000). Missed diagnoses of acute cardiac ischemia in the emergency department. *N Engl J Med, 342,* 1163–1170.

37. Roig, E., Castaner, A., Simmons, B., Patel, R., Ford, E., & Cooper, R. (1987). In-hospital mortality rates from acute myocardial infarction by race in U.S. hospitals: Findings from the National Hospital Discharge Survey. *Circulation, 76,* 280–288.

38. Keil, J. E., Saunders, D. E., Lackland, D. T., et al. (1985). Acute myocardial infarction: Period prevalence, case fatality, and comparison of black and white cases in urban and rural areas of South Carolina. *Am Heart J, 109,* 776–784.

39. Becker, L. B., Han, B. H., Meyer, P. M., et al. (1993). Racial differences in the incidence of cardiac arrest and subsequent survival. *N Engl J Med, 329,* 600–606.

NAME INDEX

SUBJECT INDEX

CREDITS

Grateful acknowledgment is made for permission to reprint the following articles.

Krieger N. (1987). Shades of difference: theoretical underpinnings of the medical controversy on black/white differences in the United States, 1830–1870. *International Journal of Health Services.* 17(2):259–78. Used by permission of Baywood Publishing Company, Inc.

Gamble VN. (1997). Under the shadow of Tuskegee: African Americans and health care. *American Journal of Public Health.* 87(11):1773. Used by permission of the American Public Health Association.

Vega WA, Amaro H. (1994). Latino outlook: good health, uncertain prognosis. *Annual Review of Public Health.* 15:39–67. © 1994 Annual Reviews. Used by permission. www.AnnualReviews.org.

LaVeist TA. (1993). Segregation, poverty, and empowerment: health consequences for African Americans. *Milbank Quarterly.* 71(1):41–64. Originally published by the Milbank Memorial Fund. Used by permission.

Cooper R. (1984). A note on the biologic concept of race and its application in epidemiologic research. *American Heart Journal.* 108(3 Part 2):715–22. Used by permission.

Bullard, RD. (1983). Solid waste sites and the black Houston community. *Sociological Inquiry.* 53(2/3):273–288. Used by permission.

LaVeist TA, Wallace JM Jr. (2000). Health risk and inequitable distribution of liquor stores in African American neighborhood. *Social Science and Medicine.* Aug; 51(4):613–7.

Lillie-Blanton M, Anthony JC, Schuster CR. (1993). Probing the meaning of racial/ethnic group comparisons in crack cocaine smoking. *Journal of the American Medical Association.* 1993, Feb 24; 269(8):993–7.

Todd KH, Deaton C, D'Adamo AP, Goe L. (2000). Ethnicity and analgesic practice. *Annals of Emergency Medicine.* Jan; 35(1):11–6. Used by permission.

Schulman KA, Berlin JA, Harless W, Kerner JF, Sistrunk S, Gersh BJ, Dube R, Taleghani CK, Burke JE, Williams S, Eisenberg JM, Escarce JJ. (1999) The effect of race and sex on physicians' recommendations for cardiac catheterization. *New England Journal of Medicine.* Feb 25; 340(8):618–26. Copyright © 1999 Massachusetts Medical Society. All rights reserved.

Sleath B, Svarstad B, Roter D. (1998). Patient race and psychotropic prescribing during medical encounters, *Social Science and Medicine.* 34:227–238. Copyright © 1998 Elsevier Science Ireland Ltd. Reprinted with permission from Elsevier Science.

van Ryn M, Burke J. (2000). The effect of patient race and socio-economic status on physicians' perception of patients. *Social Science and Medicine.* 50:813–828. Copyright © 2000 Elsevier Science Ltd. Reprinted with permission from Elsevier Science.

Whittle J, Conigliaro J, Good CB, Joswiak M. (1997). Do patient preferences contribute to racial differences in cardiovascular procedure use? *Journal of Internal Medicine.* May; 12(5):267–73. Used by permission.

Diala, Chamberlain, Carles Muntaner, Christine Walrath, Kim Nickerson, Thomas LaVeist, Philip Leaf. (2000). Racial differences in attitudes toward professional mental health care and in the use of services. *American Journal of Orthopsychiatry,* Vol. 70, no. 4 (October), pp. 455–464. © 2000 American Orthopsychiatric Association, Inc. Used by permission.